# Musculoskeletal Diseases 2013-2016
*Diagnostic Imaging and Interventional Techniques*

J. Hodler · G.K. von Schulthess · Ch.L. Zollikofer (Eds)

# MUSCULOSKELETAL DISEASES 2013-2016

## DIAGNOSTIC IMAGING AND INTERVENTIONAL TECHNIQUES

**45th International Diagnostic Course
in Davos (IDKD)**
*Davos, April 2-6, 2013*

*including the*
Nuclear Medicine Satellite Course "Diamond"
Davos, April 1-2, 2013

Pediatric Radiology Satellite Course "Kangaroo"
Davos, April 1, 2013

Breast Imaging Satellite Course "Pearl"
Davos, April 1, 2013

and additional IDKD Courses 2013-2016

presented by the Foundation for the
Advancement of Education in Medical Radiology, Zurich

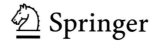 Springer

Editors

J. Hodler
Radiology
University Hospital
Zurich, Switzerland

G. K. von Schulthess
Nuclear Medicine
University Hospital
Zurich, Switzerland

Ch. L. Zollikofer
Kilchberg/Zurich, Switzerland

DOI 10.1007/978-88-470-5292-5

ISBN 978-88-470-5291-8            e-ISBN 978-88-470-5292-5

Springer Milan Dordrecht Heidelberg London New York

Library of Congress Control Number:  2013931950

Cover design: Simona Colombo, Milan, Italy
Typesetting: C & G di Cerri e Galassi, Cremona, Italy
Printing and binding: Grafiche Porpora, Segrate (MI), Italy
*Printed in Italy*

Springer-Verlag Italia S.r.l., Via Decembrio 28, 20137 Milan

Springer is a part of Springer Science+Business Media (www.springer.com)

# Preface

The International Diagnostic Course in Davos (IDKD) is a unique learning experience for imaging specialists in training. The course is also useful for experienced radiologists and clinicians looking for an update on the current state of the art and the latest developments in the fields of imaging.

This course deals with imaging of the musculoskeletal system, including pediatric issues. This field is highly relevant in most practices with regard to numbers of patients. In addition, there are still relevant advances in this subject, driven by clinical as well as technological developments. The authors are internationally renowned experts in their field. They have contributed chapters that are disease-oriented and cover all relevant imaging modalities, including standard radiographs, magnetic resonance imaging, computed tomography, and others.

As a result, this book offers a comprehensive review of the state-of-the art in musculoskeletal imaging. It is particularly relevant for general radiologists, radiology residents, rheumatologists, physiatrists, orthopaedic surgeons, and other clinicians wishing to update their knowledge in this discipline.

The Syllabus is designed to be an "aide-mémoire" for the course participants so that they can fully concentrate on the lectures and participate in the discussions without the need of taking notes.

Additional information can be found on the IDKD website: www.idkd.org

J. Hodler
G.K. von Schulthess
Ch.L. Zollikofer

# Table of Contents

## Nuclear Medicine Satellite Course "Diamond"

## Pediatric Radiology Satellite Course "Kangaroo"

## Breast Imaging Satellite Course "Pearl"

# List of Contributors

# WORKSHOPS

# Shoulder: Instability

William E. Palmer[1], Michael J. Tuite[2]

[1] Department of Radiology, Massachusetts General Hospital, Boston, MA
[2] Department of Radiology, University of Wisconsin, Madison, WI, USA

## Shoulder Stability and Function

The glenohumeral joint is vulnerable to injury and instability due to its extreme mobility and range of motion. The inherent lack of osseous constraint requires dynamic stabilization by the rotator cuff and other muscles. Joint stability also depends heavily on static structures providing passive constraint. The glenoid labrum and glenohumeral ligaments are the most important static restraints and nearly always demonstrate characteristic abnormalities on magnetic resonance (MR) images in unstable shoulders. The clinical spectrum of instability ranges from obvious recurrent dislocations to equivocal, inconclusive symptoms that may mimic other shoulder disorders, such as rotator cuff tear and biceps tendon dislocation. When instability is obvious, imaging studies are useful for lesion characterization and preoperative planning. When clinical symptoms are inconclusive, the emphasis shifts to diagnostic interpretation for choice of treatment options.

Osseous geometry provides minimal functional stability because the glenoid cavity is small and shallow compared with the humeral articular surface. The labrum enhances both the depth and the surface area of the glenoid cavity, thereby improving congruity of the articular surfaces. It partly functions as a "chock block" to resist translational forces during movement, and partly functions as a gasket to boost shoulder stability by creating a suction seal with the joint capsule [1]. Most importantly, the labrum acts as a point of attachment for the superior, middle and inferior glenohumeral ligaments (GHLs) [2]. At the extremes of motion, the glenohumeral ligaments (GHLs) contribute most to stability, especially the inferior labral-ligamentous complex [3].

## Anterior Instability

### Biomechanical Considerations

The functional anatomy of the inferior labral-ligamentous complex enables a biomechanical approach to the diagnosis of anterior shoulder instability. The inferior GHL comprises the anterior band, posterior band and intervening axillary pouch. Compared with the superior and middle GHLs, the anterior band of the inferior GHL provides critical joint stabilization as the primary static restraint to inferior humeral translation. It courses from the humeral metaphysis to the anteroinferior labrum, which anchors the ligament to the glenoid rim, and functions as a unit with the labrum by forming a sleeve of continuous tissue with the glenoid periosteum (Fig. 1).

The inferior GHL becomes taut in abduction-external rotation (ABER), creating a stress point on the labrum. During shoulder dislocation or ABER, tension is transmitted through the inferior GHL to the labral attachment site. Excessive tension can avulse the labrum from the glenoid rim or strip its periosteal sleeve along the glenoid neck. If the inferior GHL is attached to a labrum that is torn from the glenoid rim or stripped medially along the glenoid neck, it loses its labral anchor and becomes incompetent. Thus, the shoulder becomes unstable. Rupture of the inferior GHL is a much less common cause of anterior instability than avulsion of inferior labral-ligamentous complex from the glenoid rim.

## MR Imaging

In the acute setting, arthrographic MR imaging has little or no role because conventional MR images clearly demonstrate periarticular edema or hemorrhage, depict the location and severity of osseous injuries, and elucidate the traumatic mechanism. Effusion, or hemarthrosis, provides an arthrographic effect by distending the joint capsule and outlining intra-articular structures.

Once the acute situation has passed, MR arthrography becomes an option assuming that fluoroscopy or other imaging modality is available to guide needle placement. Some referring physicians are satisfied with conventional MR, whereas others prefer arthrographic MR and the diagnostic confidence provided by intra-

J. Hodler et al. (eds.), *Musculoskeletal Diseases 2013-2016,*
DOI: 10.1007/978-88-470-5292-5_1 © Springer-Verlag Italia 2013

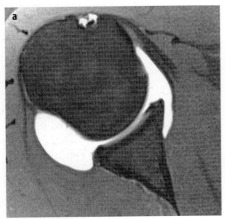 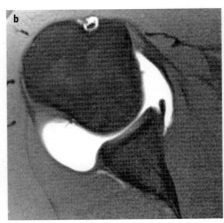 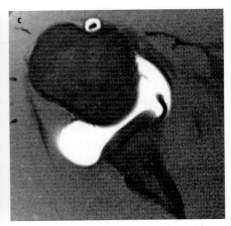

**Fig. 1 a-c.** Normal inferior glenohumeral ligament. Sequential axial, fat-suppressed arthrographic magnetic resonance images show the anterior band of the inferior glenohumeral ligament as it courses towards the humeral head from its labral and periosteal attachment site on the glenoid rim

articular contrast. MR arthrography has its greatest role in the assessment of younger individuals with suspected instability, when subtle labral-ligamentous abnormalities have profound influences on shoulder function, prognosis and management [4]. Another potential advantage of MR arthrography is ABER positioning, which can improve the detection of subtle anteroinferior labral tears [5]. Nondisplaced labral tears may not fill with contrast on arthrographic MR images obtained in the usual adducted position, but may become visible on ABER images because the labrum becomes displaced from the glenoid rim. The ABER position is achieved by flexing the elbow and placing the patient's hand posterior to the contralateral aspect of the head or neck. In the ABER position, MR images of the shoulder are prescribed in an axial oblique plane from a coronal localizer image, parallel to the long axis of the humerus. Computed tomography (CT) is preferable to MR imag-

ing when searching for small fracture fragments of the glenoid rim, or assessing bone stock in patients with recurrent dislocations.

## MR Imaging Findings

In the acute setting, MR images show bone marrow contusions. Over several weeks or months, as healing occurs, bone marrow edema dissipates and, eventually, completely resolves. Compared with the hard, wedge-shaped cortex of the anterior glenoid rim, the flat contour and softer trabecular bone of the humeral head make it susceptible to impaction fracture (Fig. 2). The location, orientation and size of a Hill-Sachs defect depend on the position of the humeral head during dislocation and the magnitude of force. Following first-time anterior dislocation, 25% of shoulders show Hill-Sachs defects at arthroscopy [6]. Prevalence increases to 40-90% in

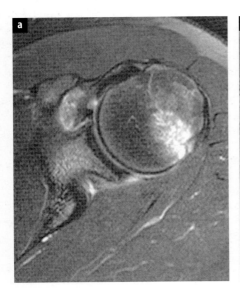 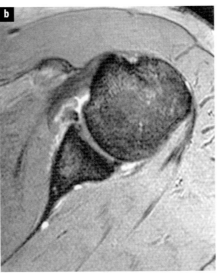

**Fig. 2 a, b.** Hill-Sachs fracture, Bankart lesion. **a** At the level of the upper glenoid, an axial, fat-suppressed T2-weighted image demonstrates a mildly depressed Hill-Sachs fracture with underlying bone marrow edema indicating recent injury. **b** At the level of the lower glenoid, an axial gradient echo image shows a Bankart lesion with anterior labral detachment and displacement from the glenoid rim

**Fig. 3 a, b.** Anterior labral-ligamentous periosteal sleeve avulsion. **a** At the level of the lower glenoid, the anteroinferior labrum is deficient and irregular in contour on an axial, fat-suppressed arthrographic magnetic resonance (MR) image. **b** In a comparable location at the anteroinferior glenoid rim, the labral-ligamentous complex is displaced from the bone with its periosteal sleeve on a fat-suppressed, arthrographic MR abduction-external rotation image

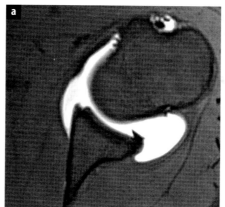 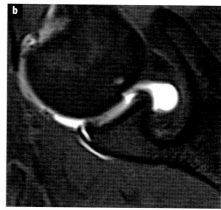

patients with repeated dislocations [7]. Hill-Sachs defects rarely require operative treatment unless they are large enough to cause mechanical symptoms or repeatedly engage the glenoid rim.

The vast majority of unstable shoulders demonstrate abnormalities of the inferior labral-ligamentous complex on MR images. Specific criteria can be used in the differentiation of stable and unstable shoulders because MR images can show the location and length of labral abnormalities relative to the origin of the inferior GHL. If the torn labral segment extends into the attachment site of the inferior GHL, there is a high likelihood of anterior instability. The inferior GHL is best visualized on arthrographic MR images, with or without ABER positioning, and on conventional MR images in the presence of effusion. Because the inferior GHL is a constant anatomical structure, its attachment site to the anteroinferior labrum can be presumed with confidence even though the lack of effusion prevents its visualization. Less commonly, shoulders develop instability due to ligamentous stretching and laxity without labral tear. Both MR imaging and MR arthrography are less valuable in these cases because the entire inferior labral-ligamentous complex appears intact. Currently, no accurate MR imaging criteria are recognized in the diagnosis of capsular laxity.

The classic Bankart lesion refers to complete labral tear at the origin of the inferior GHL, resulting in disruption of the scapular periosteum and detachment of the labrum from the glenoid rim (Fig. 2). Because the scapular periosteum is torn, the inferior labral-ligamentous complex floats away from the glenoid rim at arthroscopy. Partial Bankart lesion refers to incomplete labral detachment. Osseous Bankart lesion indicates an osteochondral fracture of the glenoid rim at the inferior labral-ligamentous attachment site. In contrast to Hill-Sachs defects, anterior glenoid fractures are highly destabilizing. Although larger defects of the glenoid rim invariably lead to recurrent dislocation, even small defects predispose to instability because the inferior labral-ligamentous complex becomes incompetent.

The lexicon of glenohumeral instability has evolved into a complex assortment of eponyms and acronyms that represent either variants of the Bankart lesion, such as Perthes, ALPSA and GLAD, or injuries of the inferior GHL, such as HAGL and BHAGL. These eponyms and acronyms are less important to know than the structural changes that lead to glenohumeral instability. Since many referring physicians, including orthopedists, may not understand these terms or may have different understandings, radiologists should emphasize a descriptive approach in their reports.

In the Perthes lesion, the labrum is torn from the glenoid rim but remains attached to the scapular periosteum, which is stripped medially on the glenoid neck. The torn labral fragment appears normal or nearly normal in location and, therefore, can be difficult to detect by conventional MR imaging. The tear may become synovialized or filled with granulation tissue, preventing the sublabral leak of contrast solution on arthrographic MR images, and leading to the false-negative diagnosis of intact labrum. In the ABER position, traction on the inferior GHL is transmitted to the labrum, displacing the torn labral-ligamentous complex from the glenoid rim.

Anterior labral-ligamentous periosteal sleeve avulsion (ALPSA) is similar to the Perthes lesion, except the inferior labral-ligamentous complex becomes bunched and retracted medially (Fig. 3). The torn labral-ligamentous complex rolls back with the intact periosteum along the glenoid neck, like a sleeve, and scars down to bone. The ALPSA lesion represents a chronic stage of the Perthes lesion. The labrum may re-approximate its normal position in the Perthes lesion, but is permanently displaced from the glenoid rim in the ALPSA lesion. Both conventional and arthrographic MR images can show ALPSA lesions. The healing process can create a smooth, synovialized surface that obscures the ALPSA lesion at arthroscopy.

Glenolabral articular disruption (GLAD) refers to a partial anteroinferior labral tear that is associated with an adjacent articular cartilage defect involving the glenoid fossa (Fig. 4). The GLAD lesion may not always be associated with anterior instability, but may progress to rapid joint degenerative with intra-articular loose bodies. Loose bodies may also result from cartilage defects involving the humeral head.

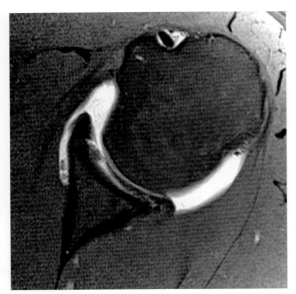

**Fig. 4.** Glenolabral articular disruption. At the level of the lower glenoid, the anterior labrum is partially undercut by contrast material on an axial, fat-suppressed arthrographic magnetic resonance image. Extensive delamination involves articular cartilage. Several small loose bodies are present in the anterior perilabral recess

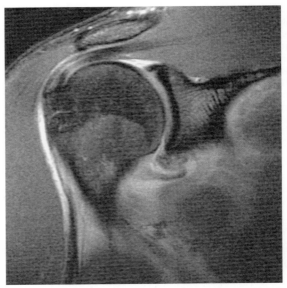

**Fig. 5.** Humeral avulsion of the glenohumeral ligament. Coronal, fat-suppressed T2-weighted image demonstrates laxity of the axillary pouch and high-grade tear of the inferior inferior glenohumeral ligament at its humeral attachment site with adjacent soft tissue edema or hemorrhage

Humeral avulsion of the glenohumeral ligament (HAGL) is a relatively uncommon cause of anterior instability. MR imaging is far more valuable in the days and weeks following traumatic injury because extra-articular edema and hemorrhage localize to the humeral neck and outline the retracted stump of the torn inferior GHL (Fig. 5). In the chronic setting, once the healing process has produced scarring and tissue remodeling, the inferior GHL and capsular contours can appear normal despite mechanical insufficiency. If the inferior GHL does not scar back onto the humerus, the capsular defect enables the development of a pseudo-pouch adjacent to the normal axillary pouch. At MR or CT arthrography, contrast fills this pseudo-pouch and flows distally along the humerus into the quadrilateral space near the axillary nerve, giving the appearance of two axillary pouches. In the months and years following trauma, this pseudo-pouch provides the greatest confidence in the diagnosis of HAGL lesion.

Although arthrographic MR images have demonstrated greater than 90% accuracy in the detection of anteroinferior labral tears, diagnostic confidence may be further increased when the shoulder is imaged in ABER. In the ABER position, the anterior band of the inferior GHL is stretched, transmitting tension to the labrum. Therefore, an anteroinferior labral fragment that is nondisplaced when the shoulder is neutral in position can become displaced from the glenoid rim and more conspicuous when the shoulder is in ABER. In Perthes and ALPSA lesions, ABER images may better demonstrate the degree of medial stripping of the scapular periosteum along the glenoid neck.

## Posterior Instability

Unidirectional posterior instability cannot be predicted based on the mere presence of posterior labral tear. Nondisplaced posterior labral tears may be associated with pain rather than instability. Abnormalities of the glenoid rim (retroversion), articular cartilage, joint capsule or periosteum increase the probability of posterior instability [8]. On MR images, findings that are most specific for posterior instability include labral displacement from the glenoid rim and medial stripping of the joint capsule or periosteum along the glenoid neck (Fig. 6). Nondisplaced posterior labral tear is important to identify in the setting of anterior instability because anterior stabilization procedure may shift the humeral head posteriorly, exacerbating the posterior labral tear and leading to posterior instability.

## Superior Labrum Anterior-Posterior Tears

Superior labrum anterior-posterior (SLAP) tears are tears of the superior labrum that extend in an anterior to posterior direction, as distinct from radial tears of the labrum. SLAP tears are one of the more common tears of the glenoid labrum, with a prevalence at arthroscopy of 5-38% [9, 10]. These tears can result from labral degeneration, acutely after a fall on an outstretched hand, or from either acute or repetitive biceps traction on the superior labrum.

Although SLAP tears have some anterior to posterior involvement of the superior labrum, they can be a variety

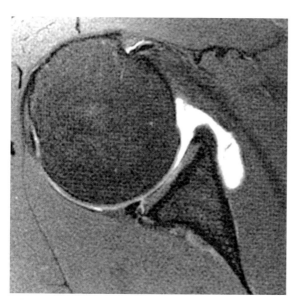

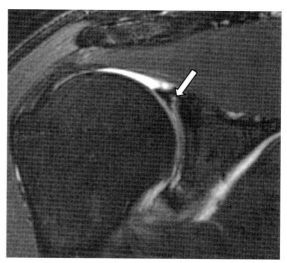

**Fig. 7.** Superior labrum anterior-posterior (SLAP) tear. Oblique coronal fat-suppressed T2-weighted image shows irregular, mainly vertically oriented high signal in the superior labrum (*arrow*)

**Fig. 6.** Posterior labral tear in unstable shoulder. Axial, fat-suppressed arthrographic magnetic resonance image shows posterior labral tear, mild displacement of the labrum from the glenoid rim, periosteal stripping and posterior translocation of the humeral head. These findings are closely associated with posterior glenohumeral instability

of shapes that are identified by subtypes. For example, degenerative fraying of the superior labrum is called a Type 1 tear. The higher "Type" SLAP tears are longitudinal tears of the superior labrum, and these tears may require surgery to alleviate symptoms. Higher type SLAP tears can either be isolated to the superior labrum, or extend into adjacent structures such as the biceps tendon or the anterior labrum.

The original description of SLAP tears included four types, with Type 1 as mentioned above and with the most common higher type SLAP tear being a partial thickness or Type 2 SLAP tear. These tears can either have a stable or unstable biceps anchor depending on their size and specific site of involvement. Distinguishing a stable from an unstable Type 2 SLAP tear can be difficult on MR images, but in general larger tears at the base of the labrum that weaken the biceps anchor are more unstable. The length of the tear can also vary, with some involving the entire anterior to posterior superior labrum, while others involve only the anterior or the posterior portion of the superior labrum. The posterior Type 2 SLAP tears are sometimes seen in overhead throwing athletes and in patients with a spinoglenoid notch paralabral cyst. A Type 3 SLAP tear is a full thickness tear resulting in a bucket handle torn labral segment. Type 3 SLAP tears tend to have a stable biceps anchor. A Type 4 SLAP tear extends into the biceps tendon. There are currently some 12 types of SLAP tears described, and the Type 5 and above tears mainly involve extension to other adjacent structures.

SLAP tears appear on MR images as increased signal either within the superior labrum or at the labral chondral

junction, which extends to the inferior surface of the labrum (Fig. 7). Because some patients have a normal variant superior recess at the labral chondral junction, there are several MR signs that have been proposed to help distinguish a recess from a tear. The findings of a tear include labral detachment, irregular high signal, signal that curves laterally, two high signal lines (a medial recess and a more lateral tear, called the "double oreo" sign), or signal width >2 mm on MR or 3 mm at MR arthrography. High signal at the labral chondral junction posterior to the biceps anchor has been proposed as a possible MR sign of a SLAP tear; however, several studies have found that at MR arthrography a superior recess can have this appearance in up to 90% of individuals.

## Internal Impingement Labral Tears

Internal impingement is a clinical diagnosis that is seen in overhead throwing athletes. These athletes complain of pain in the late cocking phase of the throwing motion, and decreased throwing velocity. There are various theories as to the cause of internal impingement, but there are two main processes that are believed to lead to labral injury. The first is repetitive forceful contact between the greater tuberosity and the posterosuperior glenoid rim during abduction and external rotation, which causes fraying or tears of the posterosuperior labrum. The other is longitudinal twisting with excessive tension on the longhead biceps tendon at full external rotation of the humerus, causing the biceps anchor to also be twisted resulting in a "peel-back" SLAP tear.

The SLAP tears with internal impingement appear similar to other SLAP tears although they tend to involve the posterior portion of the superior labrum [11]. On MR

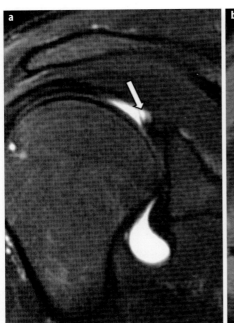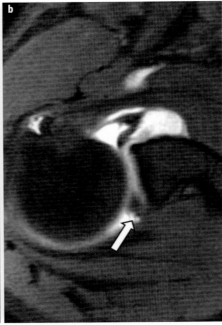

**Fig. 8 a, b.** Internal impingement. Oblique coronal (**a**) and axial (**b**) fat-suppressed T2-weighted images in a young athlete show fraying of the posterosuperior labrum (*arrows*)

images they demonstrate the typical irregular laterally curved high signal. The smaller labral tears of internal impingement may be difficult to identify on conventional MR images, but are usually better seen on MR arthrography with ABER images. ABER images can often show even the fraying of the posterosuperior labrum that occurs early in the injury in these athletes (Fig. 8).

There are several additional findings in the shoulder associated with internal impingement. Patients may have an articular surface partial thickness cuff tear of the posterior supraspinatus or anterior infraspinatus tendon. They may also have prominent posterior humeral head cysts or a "pseudo Hill-Sachs" lesion, or a thickened posterior band inferior GHL/capsule.

## Spinoglenoid Notch Cyst and Labral Tear

Labral tears in the posterosuperior labrum are particularly associated with a paralabral cyst. The labrum in this region is adjacent to the fat plane between the supraspinatus and infraspinatus tendons lateral to the scapular spine, an area called the spinoglenoid notch. Joint fluid can leak through a posterosuperior labral tear into this low-pressure fat plane and form a ganglion cyst. If this cyst is large enough, it can cause compression of the distal portion of the suprascapular nerve. This nerve has both sensory and motor fibers, so the patient will complain of shoulder pain and weakness. The distal motor fibers of the suprascapular nerve innervate the infraspinatus muscle, so the weakness will be with external rotation of the humerus. Very large cysts will typically extend superiorly into the suprascapular notch region and may compress

the suprascapular nerve at or proximal to the take-off of the motor branch to the supraspinatus muscle. These patients will have supraspinatus muscle weakness in addition to pain and external rotation weakness.

On MR, the cyst will appear as a well-defined T2 high-signal mass medial and adjacent to the posterosuperior labrum (Fig. 9) [12]. On MR arthrography, there is variable filling of the cyst with intra-articular contrast. Eighty-five percent of cysts are associated with a labral tear, either isolated to the posterosuperior labrum or from posterior extension of a SLAP tear. Initially the infraspinatus muscle may appear normal, but with time larger cysts in the spinoglenoid notch will usually cause increased T2 signal in the infraspinatus muscle from denervation edema. If the cyst is left untreated, the patient may develop fatty atrophy of the muscle. If a cyst is large and extends up to the suprascapular notch region, there may also be T2 high signal in the supraspinatus muscle. Again, if a large cyst is left untreated the patient may develop fatty atrophy of the supraspinatus as well as the infraspinatus muscle.

## Normal Labral Variants

One of the difficulties with accurately diagnosing labral tears is the presence of normal variants of the labrum. The labral variants take several forms and have different names depending on their location around the glenoid rim, but most involve the labrum being partially or completely unattached from the hyaline cartilage.

Although a small cleft at the labral chondral junction can occur at any point around the glenoid rim, there are

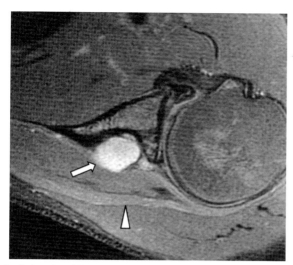

**Fig. 9.** Spinoglenoid notch cyst. Axial fat-suppressed intermediate-weighed image shows the cyst (*arrow*) and mild denervation edema with increased signal in the infraspinatus muscle (*arrowhead*)

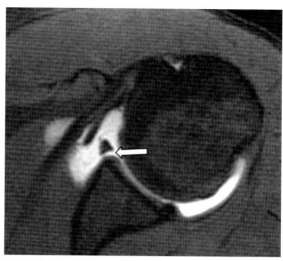

**Fig. 10.** Sublabral foramen. Axial fat-suppressed intermediate-weighted image shows an unattached anterosuperior labrum (*arrow*)

two main sites of normal labral variants: the anterosuperior labrum and the superior labrum. In the anterosuperior (1:00-3:00) labrum there are three subtypes that occur between the origins of the middle and inferior GHLs. One is the sublabral foramen where the labrum is focally unattached to the glenoid rim, and is present in 10-15% of individuals (Fig. 10) [13]. The second is the Buford complex where the anterosuperior portion of the labrum is absent and there is a thick, cord-like middle GHL, and this is seen in 1-2% of individuals [14]. The third is an anterosuperior sublabral recess where the labrum is only attached to the glenoid rim at its periphery, and its prevalence is unknown [15]. In the superior labrum between 11:00 and 1:00, a similar partially unattached labrum results in a superior recess that is seen in up to 73% of individuals. There is an increased association of this superior recess with an anterosuperior labral variant.

On MR images, the anterosuperior labral variants will appear as high signal between the glenoid rim and the labrum (sublabral foramen or recess), or the anterosuperior labrum will be absent with a thick middle GHL lying against the glenoid rim (Buford complex). A superior recess will demonstrate smooth medially curving linear high signal at the labral-chondral junction which does not extend across the entire base of the labrum.

There is controversy whether these variants are in fact a normal variation, or represent an old post-traumatic detachment. There are several studies that suggest that these variants are developmental. For example, De Palma found that the superior recess became more prevalent with age and therefore believed it was an acquired lesion, possibly due to chronic repetitive traction [16, 17]. Tena-Arregui et al. found that a superior recess was not present in still-born fetal specimens [18]. Others, however, have found no correlation between age and the presence of a

labral variant. For example, Lee et al. looked at a population with an average age of 45 years and found that 46% of the labral-chondral clefts in the posterior half of the labrum were in patients <30 years old [19]. Tuite et al. found no association between a 2-3 mm deep recess in the anterior, inferior and posterior regions and increasing age [20]. One of the normal variants, the Buford complex, is an absent anterosuperior labrum associated with a thick cord-like middle GHL, and it is difficult to see how this would be developmental. In any case, multiple arthroscopy articles have stated that a superior recess or an anterosuperior labral variant is an asymptomatic incidental finding at surgery and if "repaired" will only worsen symptoms [15, 21, 22].

## References

1. Veeger HE, van der Helm FC (2007) Shoulder function: the perfect compromise between mobility and stability. J Biomech 40:2119-2129
2. Clark JM, Harryman DT II (1992) Tendons, ligaments, and capsule of the rotator cuff. Gross and microscopic anatomy. J Bone Joint Surg Am 74:713-725
3. O'Connell PW, Nuber GW, Mileski RA, Lautenschlager E (1990) The contribution of the glenohumeral ligaments to anterior stability of the shoulder joint. Am J Sports Med 18:579-584
4. Shankman S, Bencardino J, Beltran J (1999) Glenohumeral instability: evaluation using MR arthrography of the shoulder. Skeletal Radiol 7:365-382
5. Saleem AM, Lee JK, Novak LM (2008) Usefulness of the abduction and external rotation views in shoulder MR arthrography. AJR Am J Roentgenol 191:1024-1030
6. Calandra JJ, Baker CL, Uribe J (1989) The incidence of Hill-Sachs lesions in initial anterior shoulder dislocations. Arthroscopy 5:254-257
7. Hintermann B, Gachter A (1995) Arthroscopic findings after shoulder dislocation. Am J Sports Med 23:545-551

8.  Shah N, Tung GA (2009) Imaging signs of posterior gleno-humeral instability. AJR Am J Roentgenol 192:730-735
9.  Phillips JC, Cook C, Beaty S et al (2012) Validity of noncontrast magnetic resonance imaging in diagnosing superior labrum anterior-posterior tears. J Shoulder Elbow Surg. Epub 2012/09/04
10. Mohana-Borges A, Chung C, Resnick D (2003) Superior labral anteroposterior tear: classification and diagnosis on MRI and MR arthrography. AJR Am J Roentgenol 181:1449-1462
11. Ouellette H, Labis J, Bredella M et al (2008) Spectrum of shoulder injuries in the baseball pitcher. Skeletal Radiol 37:491-498
12. Mellado JM, Salvado E, Camins A et al (2002) Fluid collections and juxta-articular cystic lesions of the shoulder: spectrum of MRI findings. Eur Radiol 12:650-659
13. Tuite MJ, Orwin JF (1996) Anterosuperior labral variants of the shoulder: appearance on gradient-recalled-echo and fast spin-echo MR images. Radiology 199:537-540
14. Tirman PF, Feller JF, Palmer WE et al (1996) The Buford complex—a variation of normal shoulder anatomy: MR arthrographic imaging features. AJR Am J Roentgenol 166:869-873
15. Kanatli U, Ozturk BY, Bolukbasi S (2010) Anatomical variations of the anterosuperior labrum: prevalence and association with type II superior labrum anterior-posterior (SLAP) lesions. J Shoulder Elbow Surg 19:1199-1203
16. DePalma A (1973) Surgery of the shoulder. 2nd ed. JB Lippincott, Philadelphia, pp 206-235
17. DePalma AF, Gallery G, Bennett G (1949) Variational anatomy and degenerative lesions of the shoulder joint. In: Edwards J (Ed) Instructional course lectures: the American Academy of Orthopedic Surgeons. 6. Mosby, St. Louis, pp 225-281
18. Tena-Arregui J, Barrio-Asensio C, Puerta-Fonolla J, Murillo-Gonzalez J (2005) Arthroscopic study of the shoulder joint in fetuses. Arthroscopy 21:1114-1119
19. Lee GY, Choi JA, Oh JH et al (2009) Posteroinferior labral cleft at direct CT arthrography of the shoulder by using multidetector CT: is this a normal variant? Radiology 253:765-770
20. Tuite MJ, Currie JW, Orwin JF et al (2012) Sublabral clefts and recesses in the anterior, inferior, and posterior glenoid labrum at MR arthrography. Skeletal Radiol. Epub 2012/08/16
21. Ilahi OA, Labbe MR, Cosculluela P (2002) Variants of the anterosuperior glenoid labrum and associated pathology. Arthroscopy 18:882-886
22. Rao AG, Kim TK, Chronopoulos E, McFarland EG (2003) Anatomical variants in the anterosuperior aspect of the glenoid labrum: a statistical analysis of seventy-three cases. J Bone Joint Surg Am 85-A:653-659

# Shoulder: Rotator Cuff and Impingement Syndromes

Theodore T. Miller[1], Klaus Woertler[2]

[1] Department of Radiology and Imaging, Hospital for Special Surgery, New York, NY, USA
[2] Department of Diagnostic and Interventional Radiology, Technische Universität München, Munich, Germany

## Impingement Syndromes

Impingement syndromes are a group of abnormalities characterized by shoulder pain with the arm in certain positions, and can be divided into external and internal categories. External impingement is caused by structural changes outside of the joint and is classified as primary, secondary and subcoracoid types. Internal impingement is secondary to rotator cuff and capsular dysfunction, and is subdivided into posterosuperior (classic internal impingement), anterosuperior, anterior and entrapment of the long head of the biceps tendon subtypes. The role of imaging is to demonstrate structural findings that can corroborate a clinical impression of impingement or demonstrate findings that are suggestive of impingement, but the diagnosis of an impingement syndrome is always clinical.

## Primary and Secondary External Impingement Syndromes

Both primary and secondary impingement refer to compression of the subacromial-subdeltoid bursa and supraspinatus tendon due to narrowing of the supraspinatus outlet, a fibro-osseous tunnel in which the subacromial-subdeltoid bursa and supraspinatus tendon are located, and which is bounded by the humeral head inferiorly and the acromion, acromioclavicular joint and the coraco-acromial ligament superiorly (Fig. 1). In primary impingement, the narrowing is caused by anterior acromial morphology and/or degenerative changes of the acromioclavicular joint, whereas secondary impingement is caused by elevation of the humeral head as a result of glenohumeral instability.

Clinically, pain can be elicited during abduction and external rotation of the arm or elevation with internal rotation. To provoke a classic Neer impingement sign on physical examination, the examiner raises the patient's arm forward while simultaneously stabilizing the scapula with another hand, causing the greater tuberosity to impinge against the acromion. If this motion is painful at 90 degrees of forward flexion, it is considered to be positive impingement. The positive result can be confirmed by injection of local anesthetic under the anterior acromion, which will relieve the pain. The Hawkins modification of the Neer maneuver reproduces impingement pain by forced internal rotation at 90 degrees of forward elevation and 30 degrees of forward flexion, which brings the greater tuberosity directly under the coracoacromial ligament, thus simulating the throwing position.

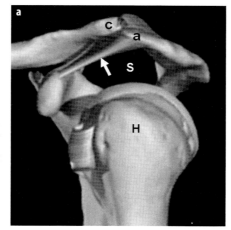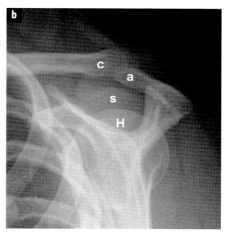

**Fig. 1 a, b.** Supraspinatus outlet. **a** Diagram shows the supraspinatus outlet (*S*) bounded by the humeral head (*H*), the coracoacromial ligament (*arrow*), acromioclavicular joint and the acromion (*a*), and the clavicle (*c*). (Courtesy of Primal Pictures.) **b** Outlet radiograph shows the density of the supraspinatus muscle and tendon (*s*) between the clavicle (*c*), acromion (*a*) and humeral head (*H*)

J. Hodler et al. (eds.), *Musculoskeletal Diseases 2013-2016,*
DOI: 10.1007/978-88-470-5292-5_2 © Springer-Verlag Italia 2013

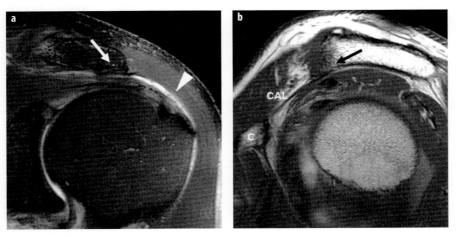

**Fig. 2 a, b.** Subacromial impingement. Coronal intermediate weighted TSE image with fat-suppression (**a**) and sagittal T1-weighted TSE (**b**) images show subacromial spur (*arrows*) at acromial insertion of coracoacromial ligament (*CAL*), subacromial/subdeltoid bursitis, and bursal-sided partial tear of supraspinatus tendon (*arrowhead*). *C*, coracoid process

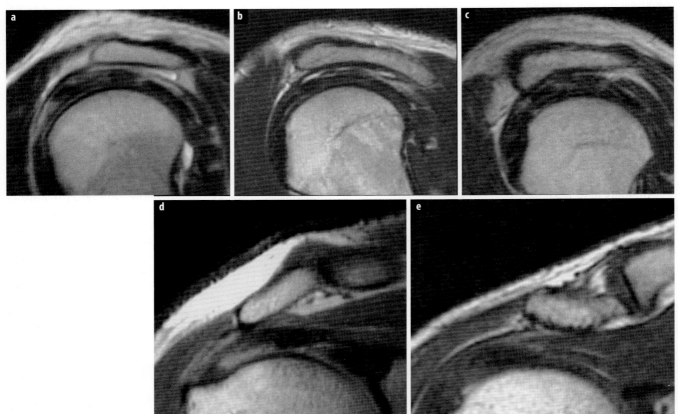

**Fig. 3 a-e.** Acromial morphology. **a** Flat acromion (sagittal T2-weighted TSE image). **b** Curved acromion (sagittal T2-weighted TSE image). **c** Hooked acromion (sagittal T2-weighted TSE image). **d** Laterally downsloping acromion (coronal T1-weighted SE image). **e** Inferior convex acromion (coronal T1-weighted SE image)

Impingement leads to inflammation of the subacromial bursa and mechanical wear of the tendon. Continued activity can then lead to fibrosis of the subacromial bursa and tendinosis of the supraspinatus tendon. Progression of this condition can lead to partial or full thickness tears of the supraspinatus (Fig. 2). The modified Neer classification system is generally used to describe the stages of impingement as:

- Type I: inflammation with no tearing
- Type II: partial tear
- Type III: full thickness tear

Bigliani et al. described three types of acromial morphology (Fig. 3a-c) on outlet radiographs: flat (Type I), curved (Type II) and hooked (Type III), and found the highest incidence of rotator cuff lesions with Type III acromia and the lowest with Type I. However, a hooked morphology as a cause of impingement is controversial since other investigators using both radiographs and magnetic resonance imaging (MRI) have found no association between morphology and cuff tears. Other acromial morphologies that have been described include an inferiorly convex configuration ("Type IV") and a laterally downsloping acromion in the coronal plane (Fig. 3d, e). These shapes are also not agreed upon as causes of impingement. On the other hand, hypertrophic changes at the acromioclavicular joint, whether a result of degeneration or prior trauma, can also narrow the supraspinatus outlet space and cause extrinsic impingement of the supraspinatus tendon.

## Subcoracoid Impingement

Subcoracoid impingement refers to compression of the subscapularis tendon, the subcoracoid bursa, and the anterior joint capsule between the coracoid and the lesser tuberosity due to narrowing of the coracohumeral interval (Fig. 4). The narrowing may be congenital due to an elongated coracoid, post-traumatic as a result of deformity of either the coracoid or the humeral head, or iatrogenic such as from a glenoid osteotomy or coracoplasty. Patients typically present with anteromedial shoulder pain and tenderness of the anterior shoulder over the coracoid process. The coracoid impingement test consists of placing the arm in cross-arm adduction, internal rotation and forward flexion to accentuate the pain.

Attempts have been made to characterize and measure the coracohumeral interval on imaging in order to predict subcoracoid impingement, but there is no consensus. The normal coracohumeral distance has been shown to be 8.4-11 mm, and is on average 1.4-3 mm smaller in

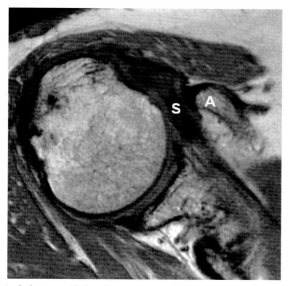

**Fig. 4.** Subcoracoid impingement. Axial proton density image shows the acromion (*A*) indenting a tendinotic subscapularis tendon (*S*)

females than in males. Subcoracoid stenosis is defined as coracohumeral interval of less than 6 mm, but controversy exists regarding the relationship between coracohumeral distance as determined on magnetic resonance (MR) images and the clinical diagnosis of subcoracoid impingement. Friedman et al. used cine MRI and shoulder rotation to measure the coracohumeral interval during 10 degree increments from internal to external rotation. Utilizing this technique, they found that, in asymptomatic patients, the normal coracohumeral distance averaged 11 mm in maximum internal rotation, while in symptomatic patients the distance measured 5.5 mm, and there was compression of the subscapularis tendon and other soft tissue structures between the lesser tuberosity and the coracoid process while the shoulder was maximally internally rotated. On the other hand, Giaroli et al., using axial MR images obtained with the humerus in neutral or external rotation, found that none of nine patients in whom subcoracoid impingement was suggested based on the coracohumeral interval measurement alone (average 5.1 mm) had surgical evidence of subcoracoid impingement, whereas a group of seven patients with clinical suspicion of subcoracoid impingement had a coracohumeral distance of 6.2 mm average. Their data showed a poor positive predictive value of MRI, and concluded that subcoracoid impingement could be only supported or suggested by MRI, and not definitively diagnosed.

The arthroscopic definition of subcoracoid impingement is direct contact of the coracoid against the lesser tuberosity. Lo and Burkhart arthroscopically observed the coracoid indenting the subscapularis tendon in patients with subcoracoid impingement and described the tendon rolling over the indentation during internal and external rotation. Based on this "roller-wringer effect" they postulated that indentation of the subscapularis tendon creates tensile forces on the articular surface of tendon, leading to "tensile undersurface fiber failure" (TUFF) of the subscapularis tendon and eventually articular surface tears.

## Internal Impingement Syndromes

The internal impingement syndromes involve the articular surface fibers rather than the bursal surface fibers of the rotator cuff, and consist of posterosuperior (glenoid) impingement (classic internal impingement), anterosuperior impingement, anterior impingement and entrapment of the long head of the biceps tendon.

Posterosuperior (glenoid) impingement refers to entrapment of the articular surface fibers of the supraspinatus and infraspinatus tendons between the posterosuperior glenoid labrum and the humeral head. This impingement may occur when the shoulder is placed in the abducted and externally rotated (ABER) position, typically encountered during the late cocking-early acceleration phase of throwing but also experienced in other overhead activities such as tennis and swimming. The "posterior

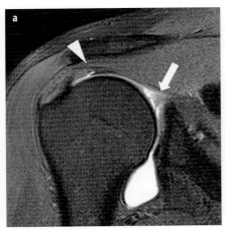 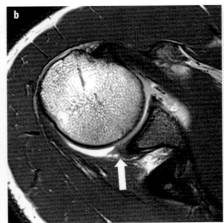 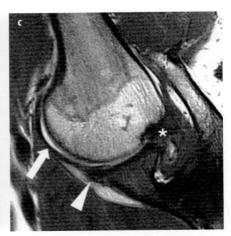

**Fig. 5 a-c.** Posterosuperior impingement (volleyball player). Coronal T1-weighted magnetic resonance (MR) arthrogram with fat suppression (**a**) and transverse T1-weigted MR arthrogram (**b**) show an articular-sided partial tear at the posterior portion of the supraspinatus tendon (*arrowhead*) as well as degeneration and fraying of the posterosuperior glenoid labrum (*arrows*). **c** T1-weighted MR arthrogram obtained in the abduction and external rotation (ABER) position reveals direct contact of the undersurface of the supraspinatus tendon and the posterosuperior labrum (*asterisk*), degenerative changes of the anteroinferior labrum (*arrowhead*) and elongation of the IGHL (*arrow*). [From: Woertler K (2010)]

impingement maneuver" on physical examination is positive when posterior shoulder pain is elicited with supine arm abduction of 90-110 degrees and maximal external rotation.

Possible findings on MRI and MR arthrography include: tearing and degeneration of the articular surface of the posterior aspect of the supraspinatus and/or infraspinatus tendons, tear of the posterosuperior glenoid labrum, impaction of the posterosuperior aspect of the humeral head, anterior capsule laxity, and/or posterior capsule thickening (Fig. 5). In baseball pitchers these findings might be associated with a Bennett's lesion (chronic bone formation at the posterior glenoid rim due to capsular stripping).

Posterior capsular tightening shifts the glenohumeral contact point posterosuperiorly, thus permitting hyperextension in the ABER position and increased external rotation, with resultant glenohumeral internal rotation deficit (GIRD) and the so-called "dead arm" sensation. These altered glenohumeral mechanics increase the sheer forces and torsional load on the posterosuperior rotator cuff and may also cause rotator cuff undersurface tears. Increased sheering at the biceps anchor and posterosuperior labral attachment can cause superior labrum anterior-posterior (SLAP) IIB lesions.

Anterosuperior impingement refers to entrapment of the articular surface of the superior margin of the subscapularis tendon and the humeral insertion of the biceps pulley (the superior glenohumeral and coracohumeral ligaments) between the humeral head and the anterior superior glenoid rim when the arm is horizontally adducted, maximally internally rotated, and anteriorly elevated to varying degrees. Long head of the biceps tendon abnormalities and undersurface tears of the anterior margin of the supraspinatus tendon may also occur.

Anterior impingement, in which an articular surface tear of the supraspinatus tendon compresses against the anterior superior labrum, clinically mimics the symptoms of classic subacromial impingement, but patients with anterior impingement are usually younger. Arthroscopy may demonstrate: partial articular surface tears of the supraspinatus and subscapularis tendons, SLAP IIA lesions, and internal impingement of the fragmented rotator cuff tissue against the superior labrum just anterior to the biceps anchor during intraoperative performance of the Hawkins test.

Repetitive compression of the long head of the biceps tendon between the humeral head and the glenoid may result in marked hypertrophy of the intra-articular portion of the tendon, having an "hourglass" appearance. The caliber of the hypertrophied intra-articular portion of the long head of the biceps tendon may exceed that of the bicipital groove and thus fail to enter the groove when the arm is elevated. The tendon becomes incarcerated in the joint, and the patient experiences pain and restricted range of motion. Clinically, the patient presents with chronic anterior shoulder pain that is accentuated upon forward elevation of the arm above the head. On physical examination, tenderness is elicited in the region overlying the bicipital groove, and there is loss of the final 10-20 degrees of passive elevation. Imaging can demonstrate the hypertrophied tendon, and most cases are associated with rupture of the rotator cuff.

## Rotator Cuff Disease

Rotator cuff disease is by far the most common cause of shoulder pain and dysfunction in adults. The etiology of this disorder is probably multifactorial with age-related degeneration, metabolic disturbances, impingement, chronic overuse and repetitive microtrauma representing potential contributors. The majority of rotator cuff lesions result from degenerative changes in older individuals with subacromial impingement syndrome. "Traumatic" tears are commonly found with pre-existing degeneration or they might be associated with shoulder dislocation. In athletes, repetitive eccentric stress and intrinsic impingement due to microinstability play a major role in development of rotator cuff tendon lesions at young age.

## Tendinopathy

Tendinopathy (tendinosis) represents mucoid tendon degeneration without macroscopic fiber disruption. This process is reflected by increased intrasubstance signal, which is most pronounced on MR images with short echo times. On images with T2 contrast, the signal intensity of the abnormal area is not as high as that of fluid. The affected tendon might become thickened but does not show evidence of fiber discontinuity.

## Partial Tears

Partial (partial-thickness) rotator cuff tears can be classified as articular-sided (undersurface), bursal-sided or intratendinous (intrasubstance or interstitial tear). The undersurface of the tendon represents the most common location. With respect to their depth, partial tears can be further characterized with use of the classification system suggested by Ellman:
- Grade 1: <3 mm or <¼ of tendon thickness
- Grade 2: 3-6 mm or <½ of tendon thickness
- Grade 3: >6 mm or >½ of tendon thickness

On conventional MRI, fluid-like intratendinous signal intensity on images with T2 contrast represents the diagnostic criterion for diagnosis of a rotator cuff tear. In a partial tear, fluid signal traverses a portion but not the entire thickness of the tendon (Fig. 6). The sensitivity of MRI for the detection of partial rotator cuff tears is limited. It can be increased to over 80% with the use of MR arthrography by improving the detection of articular-sided lesions.

In recent years some specific types of partial rotator cuff lesions have been described. A delamination tear is typically an articular-sided partial tear in combination with a horizontal intrasubstance tear (horizontal component), which separates the articular and bursal tendon fibers and might lead to medial retraction of the torn articular fibers. This type of tear most commonly occurs in the supraspinatus tendon and has also been described as the PAINT (Partial Articular-sided tear with INTratedinous extension) lesion. In contrast, noncommunicating intratendinous tears have been termed concealed interstitial delaminations (CID). Due to an intact undersurface of the involved tendon, these partial tears might be invisible at arthroscopy and therefore are important to be depicted at imaging.

The term "rim rent tear" describes an articular-sided partial-thickness tear involving the insertional fibers ("footprint") of the tendon. It is virtually synonymous with the PASTA (partial articular-sided supraspinatus tendon avulsion) lesion. Footprint lesions can also evolve on the bursal surface ("reverse" PASTA lesion) or from the midsubstance of the tendon and appear to represent the most common form of rotator cuff injury in patients younger than 40 years of age.

## Complete Tears

Complete (full-thickness) tears are transtendinous in at least one portion of the involved tendon and lead to communication between the glenohumeral joint and the subacromial/subdeltoid bursa. According to their size, full-thickness tears can be classified as small (<1 cm), intermediate (1-3 cm), large (3-5 cm), or massive (>5 cm).

On T2-weighted MR images, fluid-like signal traversing the entire thickness of the tendon and complete

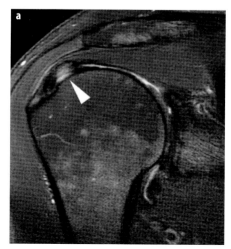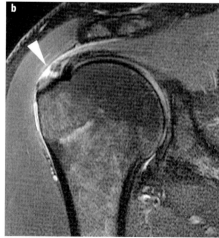

**Fig. 6 a, b.** Partial-thickness rotator cuff tears. Coronal intermediate-weighted TSE images with fat-suppression show articular-sided (**a**) and bursal-sided (**b**) partial tears (*arrowheads*) of supraspinatus tendon. Note articular cartilage defect of humeral head in **b**

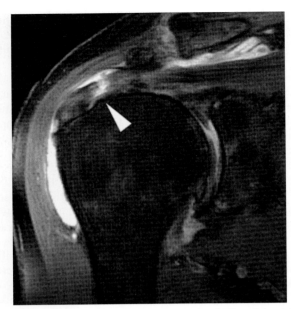

**Fig. 7.** Full-thickness rotator cuff tear. Coronal T2-weighted TSE image with fat-suppression reveals full-thickness tear (*arrowhead*) of supraspinatus tendon and large bursal effusion in a patient with advanced degenerative changes of the glenohumeral joint

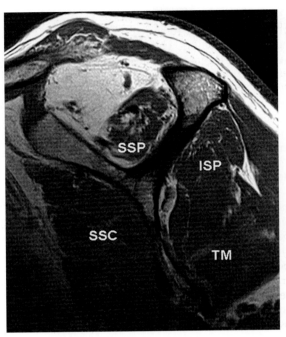

**Fig. 8.** Muscle degeneration consecutive to supraspinatus tendon tear. Sagittal T1-weighted SE image shows marked atrophy and fatty degeneration of supraspinatus muscle (grade 2-3) with otherwise normal appearance of muscle bellies. *ISP* infraspinatus, *SSC* subscapularis, *SSP* supraspinatus, *TM* teres minor

discontinuity of tendon fibers are seen at least on one section (Fig. 7). MR arthrography demonstrates trans-tendinous leakage of contrast media into the subacromial/subdeltoid bursa. High sensitivity and specificity for the diagnosis of complete rotator cuff tears is provided by both conventional MRI and MR arthrography. Conventional MRI, therefore, is usually sufficient to image the rotator cuff in older patients with degenerative changes and subacromial impingement, where partial tears are less relevant, whereas MR arthrography is indicated in young patients and particularly in athletes. The information provided by MRI that is essential to treatment planning and which therefore should be described in the radiologist's report includes: involved tendon(s), size of the tear, presence of tendon retraction, quality of muscles, presence of associated lesions. The size of the tear should be measured in two dimensions on images with T2 contrast or MR arthrograms. According to Patte and coworkers, tendon retraction in full-thickness tears can be quantified as follows:

- Grade 1: tendon retracted but lateral to humeral equator
- Grade 2: tendon medial to humeral equator but lateral to glenoid
- Grade 3: tendon medial to glenoid

Rotator cuff tears induce muscle atrophy and with time irreversible fatty degeneration of the muscle bellies. Since the extent of muscle degeneration correlates with the clinical outcome of surgical repair procedures, muscular quality should routinely be evaluated on MR images. Semiquantitative assessment of fatty degeneration

can be performed with use of the grading system proposed by Goutallier and coworkers on the most lateral sagittal oblique section of a T1- or T2-weighted sequence that shows the scapular spine and coracoid process in continuity with the scapular body (Fig. 8):

- Grade 0: normal muscle, no fat
- Grade 1: muscle contains some streaks of fat
- Grade 2: significant fatty infiltration, but still less fat than muscle
- Grade 3: fatty infiltration with equal amounts of fat and muscle
- Grade 4: fatty infiltration with more fat than muscle

Advanced muscular degeneration (>grade 2) is regarded as an exclusion criterion for anatomic rotator cuff repair in most cases.

### Supraspinatus Tendon Tears

The supraspinatus tendon represents the most commonly torn portion of the rotator cuff. Degenerative tears typically develop at the most anterior aspect of the supraspinatus tendon from where they propagate in a posterior direction and might extend into the infraspinatus tendon. Larger supraspinatus tendon tears can also involve the rotator interval and the superior portion of the subscapularis tendon. In athletes, supraspinatus tendon lesions tend to be located more posteriorly, in particular if caused by posterosuperior glenoid impingement.

**Fig. 9 a, b.** Non-displaced greater tuberosity fracture. Coronal T1-weighted SE image (**a**) and intermediate-weighted TSE image with fat-suppression (**b**) show fracture line and associated bone marrow edema at the greater tuberosity. The fracture was invisible on plain radiographs (not shown)

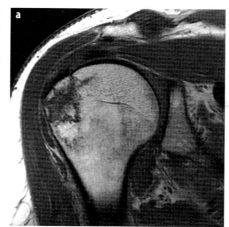
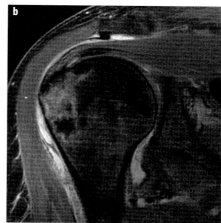

Supraspinatus tendon tears might lead to reactive bone marrow changes and cyst formation at the greater tuberosity of the humeral head.

### Subscapularis Tendon Tears

Subscapularis tendon tears more often occur in combination with supraspinatus tendon tears than in isolation. Isolated subscapularis tears are commonly traumatic and might develop during anterior shoulder dislocation in association with lesions of the inferior glenohumeral ligament. Contributing to the fact that tears of the subscapularis tendon typically progress in a craniocaudad direction, a specific classification system has been proposed by Fox and Romeo:
• Grade 1: partial tear
• Grade 2: complete tear of upper 25% of subscapularis tendon
• Grade 3: complete tear of upper 50% of subscapularis tendon
• Grade 4: complete rupture (100%) of subscapularis tendon

### Intramuscular "Cysts"

Intramuscular fluid collections can develop from leakage of fluid through a rotator cuff defect. These so-called "cysts" are most often observed in the supraspinatus muscle in association with a delaminating tear. Intramuscular ganglia have a similar appearance on MRI, but can occur in the absence of a tendon tear. They typically originate from the region of the myotendinous junction of the affected muscle.

### Differential Diagnosis

The clinical symptoms of a rotator cuff tendon tear can be mimicked by several other conditions that might affect the shoulder.

Fractures of the greater tuberosity of the humeral head can occur with direct or indirect trauma or as a sequel of shoulder dislocation. If nondisplaced, these injuries are often radiographically occult. Greater tuberosity fractures are most common in individuals younger than 40 years of age and are typically not associated with a rotator cuff tear. MRI shows an area of edema-like signal intensity at the greater tuberosity and a vertically oriented fracture line (Fig. 9).

Muscle strains of the rotator cuff are usually seen in younger adults after indirect trauma. As in other locations, the myotendinous junction represents the typical site of injury. The supraspinatus and infraspinatus muscles are most commonly involved.

Suprascapular nerve palsy can develop as a result of traumatic injury, neural compression or inflammation. The nerve can be compromised by acute (scapular fracture) or chronic traumatization (overhead sports) or during shoulder surgery (rotator cuff repair, tumor surgery). Ganglia originating from the glenoid labrum ("paralabral cysts") and extending into the spinoglenoid notch represent the most common cause of suprascapular nerve entrapment. Involvement of the brachial plexus by inflammatory conditions is not uncommon. The Parsonage-Turner syndrome (neuralgic shoulder amyotrophy) is a postviral form of neuritis that typically affects the suprascapular nerve, but also might involve the axillary and, rarely, the subscapular nerve. Regardless of the cause, neural damage can be diagnosed on MRI if denervation edema, atrophy or fatty degeneration of the dependent muscles is seen. Compromise of the suprascapular nerve typically results in denervation of the infraspinatus alone or the infra- and supraspinatus in combination.

The shoulder is by far the most common site of calcific tendonitis/bursitis as a manifestation of calcium hydroxyapatite crystal deposition disease (CHADD), and the supraspinatus tendon is the most frequently affected structure. Since crystal deposits might otherwise be misdiagnosed, MR images should not be interpreted without corresponding radiographs. Bone involvement with cortical erosion and marrow extension at the greater tuberosity of the humeral head might also be observed.

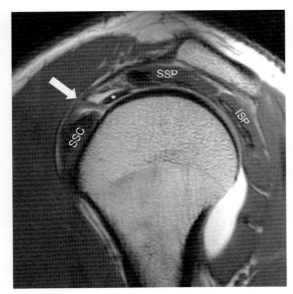

**Fig. 10.** Rotator interval. Sagittal T1-weighted magnetic resonance arthrogram of the shoulder demonstrates normal anatomy of the rotator interval. *SSC* subscapularis tendon, *SSP* supraspinatus, *ISP* infraspinatus, *arrow* pulley sling, *asterisk* long head of biceps tendon

## Rotator Interval Lesions

The rotator interval is a triangular-shaped space that is exclusively covered by capsular structures and is bordered by the anterior free edge of the supraspinatus tendon superiorly, the superior free edge of the subscapularis tendon inferiorly, and the coracoid process medially (Fig. 10). The intertubercular sulcus and transverse ligament represent the apex of this triangle, the coracoid process its base. As the long head of biceps tendons (LHBT) passes through the rotator interval and changes its course

from a horizontal to a vertical orientation, it is stabilized by two structures that form a ligamentous sling termed the "reflection pulley" of the biceps tendon: the coraco-humeral ligament (CHL) and the superior glenohumeral ligament (SGHL).

The term "rotator interval lesion" is an umbrella term for different injuries that can occur at this anatomic site. Horizontally oriented capsular tears at the rotator interval are typically seen following anterior shoulder dislocation. Injuries of the SGHL (pulley lesions) can occur in isolation or in association with rotator cuff tears, and are clinically more important because they result in inferior and medial instability of the LHBT. The Habermeyer classification describes four different types of pulley lesions:

- Type 1: isolated SGHL tear
- Type 2: SGHL and supraspinatus tendon tear
- Type 3: SGHL and subscapularis tendon tear
- Type 4: SGHL and subscapularis and supraspinatus tendon tear

Rotator interval lesions are difficult to detect on conventional MRI. MR arthrography has a sensitivity and specificity of >80 % for the diagnosis of pulley lesions, with caudal displacement of the LHBT, discontinuity of the SGHL and tendinopathy of the LHBT on oblique sagittal images representing the most accurate criteria. Medial displacement of the LHBT on transverse images is usually only seen if the lesion of the reflection pulley is associated with a subscapularis tendon tear (Fig. 11).

Three different types of medial dislocation of the LHBT can be distinguished: intratendinous, intraarticular and extracapsular. In intratendinous dislocation, the biceps tendon cuts in between the CHL and torn fibers of the subscapularis tendon. This lesion may progress to complete detachment of the subscapularis tendon, thus allowing the biceps tendon to dislocate intra-articularly. Extracapsular dislocation with displacement of the biceps tendon superficial to the CHL and subscapularis tendon is uncommon.

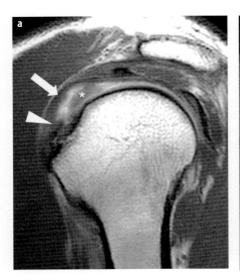

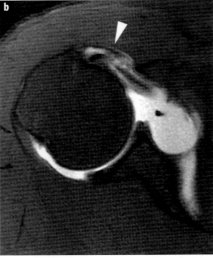

**Fig. 11 a, b.** Pulley lesion and subscapularis tendon tear (type 3 pulley lesion). **a** Sagittal T1-weighted magnetic resonance (MR) arthrogram shows discontinuity of superior glenohumeral ligament (*arrow*), partial tear of superior portion of subscapularis tendon (*arrowhead*) and increased signal intensity and thickening of inferiorly displaced biceps tendon (*asterisk*). **b** Transverse fat-suppressed T1-weighted MR arthrogram demonstrates subscapularis tendon tear and slight medial subluxation of biceps tendon (*arrowhead*)

## Biceps Tendinopathy and Tear

Tendinopathy of the LHBT can result from chronic overuse or tendon instability. However, the majority of degenerative lesions are associated with impingement and rotator cuff pathology. Degenerative changes most commonly affect the horizontal portion of the biceps tendon, and therefore are usually best depicted on sagittal MR images. MR findings associated with tendinosis include increased caliber, irregular contour and increased signal intensity of the tendon on short TE images (Fig. 11a). Although these signs have a high sensitivity, their specificity is relatively low.

Complete tears of the LHBT represent the end stage of chronic degeneration that follows tendinosis and partial tearing. Spontaneous rupture therefore usually occurs with minor trauma or even during a normal movement. The "Popeye sign" is a pathognomonic clinical presentation that results from distal retraction of the muscle belly following complete rupture of the LHBT. Nonetheless, the deformity is not produced by all tears, because dislocation of the distal portion of the tendon can be prevented or limited by fibrous tissue that was formed adjacent to the tendon during the degenerative process prior to the tear, fibrous adherence to the subscapularis tendon, or mechanical fixation of the thickened tendon within the bicipital groove ("autotenodesis"). Partial tears can present with thickening and increased T1- and T2-weighted signal intensity as well as thinning of the tendon. MR findings with complete tears range from discontinuity of the horizontal portion of the tendon to complete absence of visualization.

## Suggested Reading

Ahrens PM, Boileau P (2007) The long head of biceps and associated tendinopathy. J Bone Joint Surg 89-B:1001-1009
Boileau P, Ahrens PM, Hatzidakis AM (2004) Entrapment of the long head of the biceps tendon: the hourglass biceps—a cause of pain and locking of the shoulder. J Shoulder Elbow 13:249-257
Balich SM, Sheley RC, Brown TR et al (1997) MR imaging of the rotator cuff: intraobserver agreement and analysis of interpretative errors. Radiology 204:191-194
Beltran LS, Nikac V, Beltran J (2012) Internal impingement syndromes. Magn Reson Imaging Clin N Am 20:201-211
Bigliani LU, Morrison DS, April EW (1986) The morphology of the acromion and its relationship to rotator cuff tears. Orthop Trans 10:228
Bright AS, Torpey B, Magid D et al (1997) Reliability of radiographic evaluation for acromial morphology. Skeletal Radiol 26:718-721
Burkhart SS (2006) Internal impingement of the shoulder. Instr Course Lect 55:29-34.
Chang EY, Moses DA, Babb JS, Schweitzer ME (2006) Shoulder impingement: objective 3D shape analysis of acromial morphologic features. Radiology 239:497-505
Dines DM, Warren RF, Inglis AE et al (1990) The coracoid impingement syndrome. J Bone Joint Surg 72B:314-316.
Ellman H (1990) Diagnosis and treatment of partial-thickness rotator cuff tears Clin Orthop Relat Res 254:64-74
Farley TE, Neumann CH, Steinbach LS, Petersen SA (1994) The coracoacromial arch: MR evaluation and correlation with rotator cuff pathology. Skeletal Radiol 23:641-645

Friedman RJ, Bonutti PM, Genez B (1998) Cine magnetic resonance imaging of the subcoracoid region. Orthopedics 21:545-548
Gaskin CM, Helms CA (2006) Parsonage-Turner syndrome: MR imaging findings and clinical information of 27 patients. Radiology 240:501-507
Gerber C, Sebesta A (2000) Impingement of the deep surface of the subscapularis tendon and the reflection pulley on the anterosuperior glenoid rim: a preliminary report. J Shoulder Elbow Surg 9:483-490
Giaroli EL, Major NM, Lemley DE, Lee J (2006) Coracohumeral interval imaging in subcoracoid impingement syndrome on MRI. AJR Am J Roentgenol 186:242-246
Giaroli EL, Major NM, Higgins LD (2005) MRI of internal impingement of the shoulder. AJR Am J Roentgenol 185:925-929
Goutallier D, Postel JM, Bernageau J et al (1994) Fatty muscle degeneration in cuff ruptures. Clin Orthop Rel Res 304:78-83
Habermeyer P, Magosch P, Pritsch M et al (2004) Anterosuperior impingement of the shoulder as a result of pulley lesions: a prospective arthroscopic study. J Shoulder Elbow Surg 13:5-12
Jobe CM (1995) Posterior superior glenoid impingement: expanded spectrum. Arthroscopy 11:530-536
Kaplan LD, McMahon PJ, Towers J (2004) Internal impingement: findings on magnetic resonance imaging and arthroscopic evaluation. Arthroscopy 20:701-704
Kassarjian A, Bencardino JT, Palmer WE (2004) MR imaging of the rotator cuff. Magn Reson Imaging Clin N Am 12:39-60
Kassarjian A, Torriani M, Ouelette H, Palmer WE (2005) Intramuscular rotator cuff cysts: association with tendon tears on MRI and arthroscopy. AJR Am J Roentgenol 180:160-165
Lo IK, Burkhart SS (2003) The etiology and assessment of subscapularis tendon tears: a case of subcoracoid impingement, the roller-wringer effect and TUFF lesions of the subscapularis. Arthroscopy 19:1142-1150
Morag Y, Jacobson JA, Shields G et al (2005) MR arthrography of rotator interval, long head of the biceps brachiii, and biceps pulley of the shoulder. Radiology 235:21-30
Neer CS 2nd (1983) Impingement lesions. Clin Orthop 173:70-77
Palmer WE, Brown JH, Rosenthal DI (1993) Rotator cuff evaluation with fat-suppressed MR arthrography. AJR Am J Roentgenol 188:683-687
Peh WC, Farmer TH, Totty WG (1995) Acromial arch shape: assessment with MR imaging. Radiology 195:501-505
Richards DP, Burkhart SS, Campbell SE (2005) Relationship between narrowed coracohumeral distance and subscapularis tears. Arthroscopy 21:1223-1228.
Schaeffeler C, Mueller D, Kirchhoff C et al (2011) Tears at the rotator cuff footprint: prevalence and imaging characteristics in 305 MR arthrograms of the shoulder. Eur Radiol 21:1477-1484
Schaeffeler C, Waldt S, Holzapfel K et al (2012) Lesions of the biceps pulley: Diagnostic accuracy of MR arthrography of the shoulder and evaluation of established and new diagnostic criteria. Radiology 264:504-513
Tirman PFJ, Bost FW, Gravin GJ et al (1994) Posterosuperior glenoid impingement of the shoulder: findings at MR imaging and MR arthrography with arthroscopic correlation. Radiology 193:431-436
Tuite MJ, Petersen BD, Wise SM et al (2007) Shoulder MR arthrography of the posterior labrocapsular complex in overhead throwers with pathologic internal impingement and internal rotation deficit. Skeletal Radiol 36:495-502
Walch G, Boileau P, Noel E, Donell ST (1992) Impingement of the deep surface of the supraspinatus tendon on the posterior superior glenoid rim: an arthroscopic study. J Shoulder Elbow Surg 1:238-245
Waldt S, Bruegel M, Mueller D et al (2006) Rotator cuff tears: assessment with MR arthrography in 275 cases with arthroscopic correlation. Eur Radiol 17:491-498

Walz DM, Miller TT, Chen S, Hofman J (2007) MR imaging of delamination tears of the rotator cuff. Skeletal Radiol 36:411-416

Weishaupt D, Zanetti M, Tanner A et al (1999) Lesions of the reflection pulley of the long biceps tendon: MR arthrographic findings. Invest Radiol 34:463-469

Woertler K (2010) Shoulder injuries in overhead sports. Radiologe 50:453-459

Zanetti M, Weishaupt D, Gerber C, Hodler J (1998) Tendinopathy and rupture of the tendon of the long head of the biceps brachii muscle: evaluation with MR arthography. AJR Am J Roentgenol 170:1557-1561

# Elbow Imaging with an Emphasis on Magnetic Resonance Imaging

Mark W. Anderson[1], Lynne S. Steinbach[2]

[1] Department of Radiology, University of Virginia, Charlottesville, VA, USA
[2] Department of Radiology, University of California San Francisco, San Francisco, CA, USA

## Introduction

The elbow is a complex joint made up of three separate articulations within a common capsule. The proximal ulna articulates with the trochlea and functions as a hinge joint, while the proximal radioulnar joint provides for rotational movement of the forearm. The radiocapitellar joint allows for both hinge and rotational movement. Together, these allow for flexion and extension of the arm and, in conjunction with the distal radioulnar joint at the wrist, pronation and supination.

The elbow is subjected to the same types of articular pathology as other joints, but also demonstrates unique injuries related to the complex forces that occur during throwing and other overhead activities. This article will discuss the normal anatomy of the elbow and the most common types of elbow pathology as well as their appearance on various imaging studies, with an emphasis on magnetic resonance (MR) imaging.

## Bones and Cartilage

### Bones and Cartilage: Normal Anatomy

The humerus, ulna and radius all contribute to the elbow joint [1] (Fig. 1). Two epicondyles project from the distal humerus. The larger medial epicondyle is the site of attachment of the common flexor/pronator tendon along its anteromedial aspect as well as the ulnar collateral ligament along its undersurface. The lateral epicondyle gives rise to the common extensor/supinator tendon from its superolateral surface, while the extensor carpi ulnaris tendon originates on its posterior-inferior aspect [2]. The radial collateral and lateral ulnar collateral ligaments also arise from the lateral epicondyle. The distal articular surface of the humerus is divided into the trough-like trochlea that articulates with the proximal ulna and the rounded capitellum that articulates with the radial head. Dorsally, the deep, triangular olecranon fossa of the

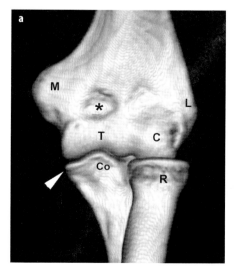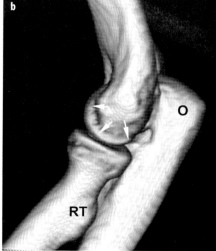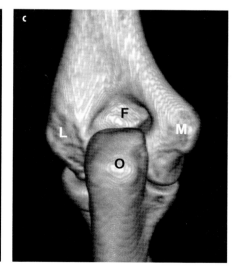

**Fig. 1 a-c.** Normal bones (three-dimensional computed tomography reconstructions). Anterior (**a**), lateral (**b**) and posterior (**c**) views demonstrate the normal osseous features of the elbow; *C* capitellum, *Co* coronoid process, *F* olecranon fossa, *L* lateral epicondyle, *M* medial epicondyle, *O* olecranon, *R* radial head, *RT* radial tuberosity, *T* trochlea. **a** The *arrowhead* points to the sublime tubercle, and the *asterisk* indicates the coronoid fossa. **b** *Arrows* indicate the articular surface of capitellum

J. Hodler et al. (eds.), *Musculoskeletal Diseases 2013-2016*,
DOI: 10.1007/978-88-470-5292-5_3 © Springer-Verlag Italia 2013

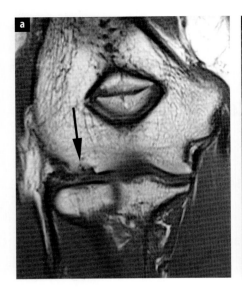 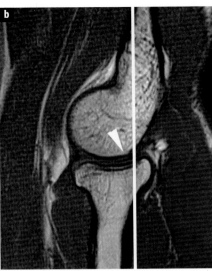

**Fig. 2 a, b.** Pseudodefect of the capitellum. **a** Coronal T1-weighted image shows cortical irregularity along the surface of the capitellum (*arrow*) suggesting an osteochondral lesion. **b** Sagittal T1-weighted image reveals that the slice level of the coronal image (*white line*) is just posterior to the articular surface (*arrowhead*)

humerus accepts the tip of the olecranon when the elbow is extended, while a smaller coronoid fossa along the ventral-medial aspect of the humerus receives the coronoid process when the elbow is flexed. Prominent extrasynovial fat pads are present within both fossae.

In the proximal ulna, the deep, concave trochlear notch lies between the coronoid and olecranon processes and forms a hinge joint with the trochlea. A second concave articular surface, the radial notch, lies along the lateral aspect of the coronoid process and articulates with the radial head to form the proximal radioulnar joint. The slightly concave fovea of the radial head articulates with the capitellum and the small radial tuberosity along the medial aspect of the proximal radius provides the attachment site for the tendons of the short and long heads of the biceps muscle.

The articular cartilage of the elbow is so thin that it is often difficult to evaluate with MR imaging. It is also important to recognize that the articular cartilage of the capitellum is found along its anterior convexity only, and not along its irregular, posterior nonarticular aspect. Also, the cartilage along the margins of the radial head at the proximal radioulnar joint covers approximately 60 degrees of the circumference of the radius where it articulates with the ulna at the proximal radioulnar joint.

## Bones and Cartilage: MR Imaging

Most bone pathology is best identified on fat-saturated T2-weighted or STIR images [3]. T1-weighted images are useful for anatomic definition and to further evaluate abnormalities seen on T2-weighted images. For example, a fracture line is often easier to see on a T1-weighted image if the surrounding edema obscures it on a fat-saturated T2-weighted image. Articular cartilage should be evaluated in all three planes using as high a resolution technique as possible.

## Bones and Cartilage: Potential Pitfalls

With the elbow extended, the border between the articular cartilage of the capitellum and its irregular nonarticular posterior surface may mimic an osteochondral lesion on coronal MR images [4]. This pitfall can be easily avoided by cross-referencing the level of the coronal scan with a sagittal image (Fig. 2). Other osseous variants that may mimic pathology involve the trochlear notch of the ulna [5]. A transverse bony ridge in the mid-trochlear notch is common and may mimic a loose body or osteophyte on sagittal images. Similarly, small cortical notches along the margins of the mid-trochlear groove may mimic osteochondral defects, again when viewed on sagittal images.

## Bones: Pathology

### Acute Trauma

In a patient presenting with elbow pain after an acute injury, often the only radiographic finding is that of an effusion (elevation of the posterior and/or anterior fat pads). Several studies have demonstrated a high incidence of associated osseous contusions or fractures in these patients that are well demonstrated with MR imaging [6-9]. A bone contusion is most easily identified by its edema-like signal intensity on fat-saturated T2-weighted images. In the case of a fracture, a linear component may be seen within the edema on T2-weighted images (Fig. 3), or may be better demonstrated as a low signal intensity line on a T1-weighted image. In the setting of a radiographically apparent fracture, MR imaging is also able to assess any associated ligament or cartilage abnormalities [10-12]. Contusions or fractures involving the radial head and posterior capitellum are commonly

**Fig. 3 a, b.** Radiographically occult fracture. **a** Oblique radiograph of the elbow shows no evidence of fracture. **b** Coronal fat-saturated T2-weighted image reveals a nondisplaced fracture of the radial head (*arrowheads*) with surrounding marrow edema

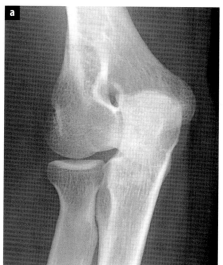
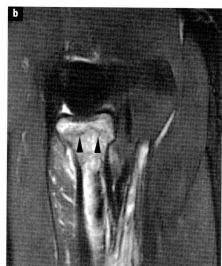

seen after a posterior dislocation, and should prompt close inspection of the collateral ligaments, which are often concurrently disrupted [13].

## Osteochondral Lesions

Osteochondral lesions of the elbow are thought to result from repetitive impaction or shear forces that result in focal damage to the articular cartilage and underlying subchondral bone. Formerly known as osteochondritis dissecans, these injuries occur most often in adolescent throwing athletes or gymnasts [14].

The repetitive valgus forces that occur at the elbow during the late cocking and early acceleration phases of the throwing motion can result in tensile forces across the medial joint that may produce laxity or tearing of the ulnar collateral ligament and/or the common flexor tendon. As these medial stabilizers fail, impaction and shear forces occur across the lateral aspect of the joint resulting in injury to the cartilage and subchondral bone of the capitellum and radial head [15]. This is common in throwing athletes between the ages of 11 and 15 years (often participants of Little League Baseball) [16], and in gymnasts due to axial loading of the joint during activities involving weight-bearing on their hands.

These osteochondral lesions most commonly involve the anterolateral capitellum, but have also been described in the trochlea in young athletes. Lesions involving the medial trochlea most likely result from posteromedial abutment of the olecranon due to ligamentous laxity (see Valgus Overload Syndrome below), whereas lateral trochlear lesions are thought to result from ischemia that arises from a combination of an intrinsically tenuous trochlear blood supply and repetitive hyperextension of the elbow with posterior olecranon abutment leading to vascular compromise [17, 18].

Another mechanism for osteochondral injury of the capitellum is that of posterolateral rotary instability caused by failure of the lateral ulnar collateral ligament (LUCL), a component of the radial collateral ligament complex [19, 20]. This osteochondral lesion has been termed the "Osborne-Cotterill" lesion, named for the authors who first reported the lesion as "an osteochondral fracture in the posterolateral margin of the capitellum with or without a crater or shovel-like defect in the radial head" [21].

On MR images, post-traumatic osteochondral lesions demonstrate irregularity of the chondral surface, disruption or irregularity of the subchondral bone plate, and/or the presence of a fracture line. The primary role of imaging is to provide information regarding the stability of the osteochondral fragment, and both computed tomography (CT) and MR imaging, with and without arthrography, can provide this information to varying degrees. MR imaging, with its excellent soft-tissue contrast, allows direct visualization of the articular cartilage, as well as of the character of the interface of the osteochondral lesion with native bone (Fig. 4). The presence of joint fluid completely encircling the fragment generally indicates an unstable lesion [3, 22]. The direct injection of contrast media into the joint in conjunction with MR imaging can be helpful in two ways: (1) to facilitate the identification of intra-articular bodies, and (2) to establish communication of the bone-fragment interface with the articulation by following the route of contrast, providing even stronger evidence for an unstable fragment [23, 24]. CT arthrography can also be used for this evaluation.

Close inspection of the capitellum on coronal and sagittal MR images is important in order to distinguish a true osteochondral lesion from the normal surface irregularity produced by the pseudodefect of the capitellum described above. Additionally, the pseudodefect does not have bone marrow reactive changes or osteochondral fracture lines.

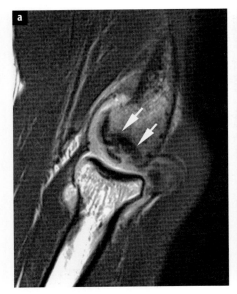
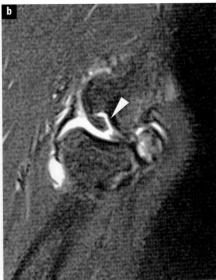

**Fig. 4 a, b.** Osteochondral lesion. **a** Sagittal T1-weighted image (magnetic resonance arthrogram) demonstrates fragmentation of the capitellum in an adolescent baseball pitcher (*arrows*). **b** Fat-saturated T2-weighted image reveals fluid partially undercutting a fragment suggesting instability (*arrowhead*)

## Ligaments

### Ligaments: Normal Anatomy

The primary stabilizing ligaments of the elbow are found along its medial and lateral aspects (Fig. 5). The medial ulnar collateral ligament (UCL) is made up of three bundles. Its anterior bundle courses from the undersurface of the medial epicondyle to the sublime tubercle along the medial margin of the coronoid process. It is the most important stabilizer of the elbow, especially during throwing and other overhead motions. The posterior bundle of the UCL extends from the medial epicondyle in a fan-like distribution to the medial margin of the trochlear notch and forms the floor of the cubital tunnel that contains the ulnar nerve. The small transverse bundle of the UCL runs from the olecranon to the coronoid

process and does not play a significant role in stabilizing the elbow [1, 3].

On the lateral side, the radial collateral ligament lies just deep to the common extensor tendon and courses from the lateral epicondyle to blend with the annular ligament along the volar aspect of the radiocarpal joint. The LUCL also originates on the lateral epicondyle where it is inseparable from the radial collateral ligament, and extends behind the radial head to attach to the supinator crest along the lateral aspect of the proximal ulna. It provides posterolateral stability for the radiocapitellar joint [23]. The annular ligament runs from the ventral aspect of the radial notch around the radial head to attach along with the LUCL along the supinator crest of the ulna and stabilizes the proximal radioulnar joint [24]. Although these are described as individually, more recent studies suggest that these structures function

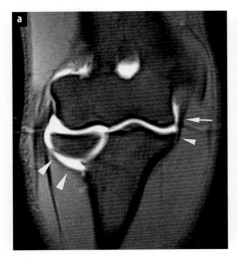
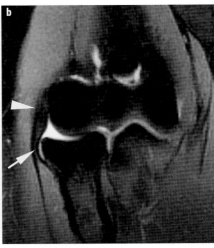

**Fig. 5 a, b.** Normal ligaments. **a** Coronal fat-saturated T1-weighted image (magnetic resonance arthrogram) displays the anterior bundle of the ulnar collateral ligament (*arrow*) and its normal attachment at the sublime tubercle of the ulna (*small arrowhead*). Note also the lateral ulnar collateral ligament coursing posterior to the radial head to its attachment along the supinator crest of the ulna (*arrowheads*). **b** A more ventral coronal fat-saturated T1-weighted image from a magnetic resonance arthrogram shows the radial collateral ligament (*arrow*) just deep to the common extensor tendon (*arrowhead*)

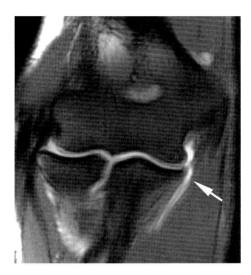

**Fig. 6.** Ulnar collateral ligament (UCL) tear. Coronal T2-weighted image (magnetic resonance arthrogram) demonstrates a tear of the UCL at its distal insertion (*arrow*) with extravasation of fluid into the adjacent soft tissues

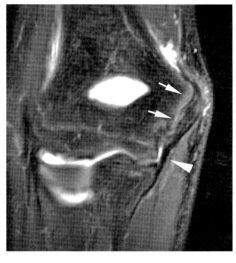

**Fig. 7.** Medial epicondylar epiphysiolysis ("Little Leaguer's elbow"). Coronal fat-saturated T2-weighted image (magnetic resonance arthrogram) displays marrow edema along the medial epicondylar apophysis (*arrows*) in a young baseball player. Note also the normal ulnar collateral ligament (*arrowhead*)

together as a continuous sheet, rather than as individual entities [23, 25].

## Ligaments: MR Imaging Technique

The collateral ligaments of the elbow are best evaluated on coronal and axial images and should appear as low signal intensity structures on all sequences. However, given their collagen structure, ligaments will be susceptible to magic angle artifacts on "short TE" images (T1, proton density, gradient echo).

## Ligaments: Potential Pitfalls

Some degree of increased signal intensity is often present within the proximal portion of the anterior bundle of the UCL on fluid-sensitive MR imaging sequences and can mimic true pathology in this region. The anterior bundle normally may also demonstrate a striated appearance on MR imaging. The same holds true for the LUCL, and it should be noted that this ligament might not be seen in some patients on MR images (up to 15% in one study).

## Ligaments: Pathology

### Valgus Instability

The UCL, and in particular its anterior band, is the most important medial stabilizer of the elbow from 30 to 120 degrees of flexion. The most common mechanisms of ulnar collateral ligament insufficiency are chronic attenuation, as seen in throwers or other athletes using an over-

head motion, and an acute post-traumatic disruption, usually after a fall on an outstretched arm [26]. During the throwing motion, high valgus stresses are placed on the elbow with resulting tensile forces along its medial aspect. The maximum stress on the ulnar collateral ligament occurs during the late cocking and acceleration phases of throwing [27]. Repetitive insults to the ligament produce microscopic tears that progress to significant attenuation or frank tearing within its substance. Complete, full thickness tears are often well demonstrated on conventional MR imaging studies, but partial tears can be subtle and are best seen with MR arthrography (Fig. 6) [28, 29]. While MR imaging facilitates direct visualization of the ligament complex, in chronic cases the development of heterotopic ossification along the course of the ligament has been described [30].

In the skeletally immature patient, the apophysis is the weakest link in the muscle-tendon-bone complex and an acute injury may result in avulsion of the epicondyle into the joint where it may simulate an intra-articular osseous body. Ultrasound [31], CT and MR imaging can show these avulsions. Nonunion can lead to repeated valgus instability.

More commonly, chronic valgus stress may result in a condition known as "Little Leaguer's elbow" in which stress across the physeal plate results in its apparent widening on radiographs (also known as "epiphysiolysis") or displacement or fragmentation of the medial epicondylar apophysis [32]. MR imaging demonstrates extension of physeal cartilage into the metaphysis and/or marrow edema within the apophysis, and also allows for assessment of the UCL, which is usually normal in these patients [33] (Fig. 7).

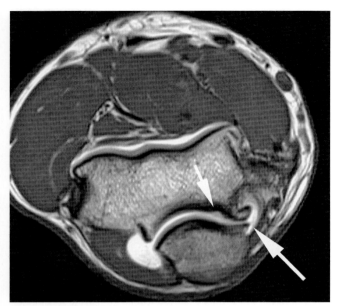

**Fig. 8.** Valgus overload syndrome. Axial T1-weighted image (magnetic resonance arthrogram) demonstrates prominent osteophytes along the posteromedial joint (*large arrow*) as well as a small focus of cartilage loss along the posterior trochlea (*small arrow*)

## Valgus Overload Syndrome

Throwing athletes and others involved in overhead sports often develop a constellation of injuries known as the valgus overload syndrome [34-36]. This is related to the strong valgus forces that occur primarily during the late cocking and early acceleration phases of the throwing motion, which may lead to tensile failure of the UCL, an

osteochondral lesion in the capitellum (related to lateral impaction forces) and subchondral edema, cartilage loss and/or osteophyte formation along the posteromedial trochlea secondary to increased shear forces in that region [37] (Fig. 8). Therefore, a careful inspection of these three areas should be carried out when viewing an MR imaging study in an overhead throwing athlete presenting with elbow pain, but it should be noted that imaging abnormalities at these sites are also common in asymptomatic athletes [38].

## Varus Instability

Lateral elbow instability related to isolated abnormalities of the lateral collateral ligament complex is related to a stress or force applied to the medial side of the articulation, resulting in compression on that side, and tensile forces across the lateral joint producing insufficiency of the radial collateral ligament complex. This most often occurs during an acute injury, but may rarely result from repetitive stress. Other causes of varus instability include dislocation, subluxation and overly aggressive surgical technique during release of the common extensor tendon or resection of the radial head.

## Posterolateral Rotary Instability and Elbow Dislocation

Posterolateral rotary instability (PLRI) is the most common pattern of recurrent elbow instability (Fig. 9). PLRI represents a spectrum of pathology consisting of three stages, according to the degree of soft-tissue disruption. In stage 1, there is posterolateral subluxation of the ulna on the humerus that results in insufficiency or tearing of the LUCL [39-41]. In stage 2, the elbow dislocates incompletely so that the coronoid is perched under the

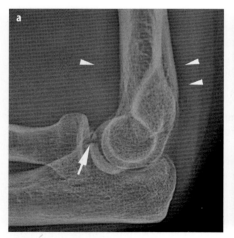
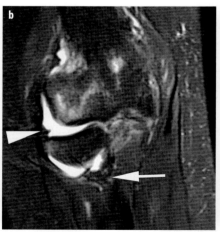
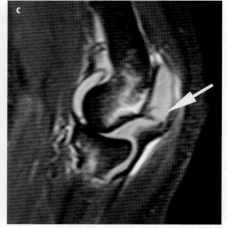

**Fig. 9 a-c.** Elbow dislocation. **a** Lateral radiograph obtained after a fall on an outstretched arm reveals elevation of the anterior and posterior fat pads (*arrowheads*) as well as a nondisplaced fracture of the coronoid process (*arrow*). **b** Coronal fat-saturated T2-weighted image demonstrates lateral subluxation of the radial head, proximal disruption of the lateral ulnar collateral ligament from its humeral attachment (*arrowhead*), and partial tearing of the ligament at its ulnar attachment (*arrow*). **c** Sagittal STIR image reveals bone marrow contusions in the proximal radius and in the posterior capitellum, which is also slightly impacted. The posterior capsule is also disrupted (*arrow*)

trochlea. In this stage, the radial collateral ligament and anterior and posterior portions of the capsule are disrupted, in addition to the LUCL. Finally, in stage 3, the elbow dislocates fully so that the coronoid rests behind the humerus. Stage 3 is subclassified into three further categories. In stage 3A, the anterior bundle of the medial collateral ligament is intact and the elbow is stable to valgus stress after reduction. In stage 3B, the anterior bundle of the medial collateral ligament is disrupted so that the elbow is unstable with valgus stress. In stage 3C, the entire distal humerus is stripped of soft tissues, rendering the elbow grossly unstable even when a splint or cast is applied with the elbow in a semiflexed position. This classification system is helpful, as each stage has specific clinical, radiographic and pathologic features that are predictable and have implications for treatment [40].

Subluxation or dislocation of the elbow can be associated with fractures. Fracture-dislocations most commonly involve the coronoid process and radial head, a constellation of findings referred to as the "terrible triad" of the elbow, since this injury complex is difficult to treat and prone to unsatisfactory results [40].

A shear fracture of the coronoid process of the ulna is commonly seen following elbow dislocations. This fracture is pathognomonic of an episode of elbow subluxation or dislocation, and the larger the coronoid fracture fragment, the higher the degree of posterolateral instability [42]. A fracture of the radial head does not cause clinical instability. Injuries of the articular surfaces may occur during elbow subluxation, as described in the section on osteochondral lesions.

Another consideration with respect to elbow dislocation is that, as the ring of soft tissues is disrupted from its posterolateral to medial aspects, tearing of the capsule allows joint fluid to escape into the periarticular tissues and, as a result, radiographic signs of an effusion, indirect evidence of elbow trauma, might not be present.

## Plicae

### Plicae: Normal Anatomy and Pathology

Synovial plicae represent embryologic remnants that are commonly found within asymptomatic elbows. The most common of these synovial folds is the posterolateral plica [43] (also known as the radiohumeral plica, radiocapitellar plica or "synovial fringe"); anterior and posterior plica are less common (Fig. 10).

The posterolateral plica is present in 86% of cadavers and up to 98% of asymptomatic patients on MR imaging [43, 44]. Even so, it has been implicated as a cause of lateral elbow pain known as the "synovial fringe syndrome" [45]. This is thought to result from dynamic entrapment of the plica between the radial head and capitellum and often produces snapping, popping or even locking of the elbow [46-49]. Histologically, the plica becomes thickened and fibrotic and this

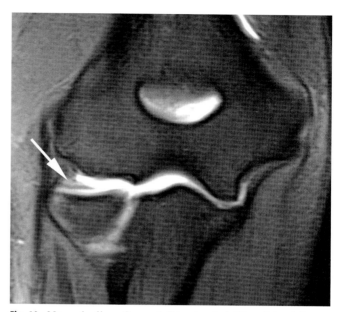

**Fig. 10.** Normal plica. Coronal fat-saturated T1-weighted image (magnetic resonance arthrogram) demonstrates a lateral radiocapitellar plica (*arrow*)

may result in focal cartilage loss along the lateral aspect of the radial head. The MR imaging findings of a plica measuring greater than 3 mm in thickness or covering more than one-third of the articular surface of the radial head should raise suspicion for the diagnosis, but must be correlated with clinical findings since there is an overlap in the MR imaging appearance of the posterolateral plica in symptomatic and asymptomatic patients.

## Tendons and Muscles

### Tendons and Muscles: Normal Anatomy

The biceps tendon courses across the elbow anteriorly to insert on the radial tuberosity and is best seen in the axial plane (Fig. 11). The bicipital aponeurosis (lacertus fibrosus) is a fascial extension from the short head of the biceps that extends over the biceps tendon and provides some tendon stability in this region. The long and short heads of the tendon can usually be distinguished on cross-sectional imaging and should not be mistaken for a longitudinal tear near its insertion [50]. Immediately deep to the biceps lies the brachialis muscle and its very short tendon that attaches to the ventral aspect of the coronoid process of the ulna.

Posteriorly, the triceps tendon attaches along the dorsal aspect of the olecranon, distal to its tip. The small anconeus muscle lies along the posterolateral aspect of the elbow, arising from the posterior aspect of the lateral epicondyle and inserting along the proximal ulna.

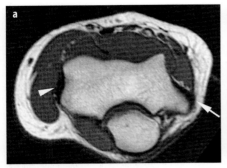
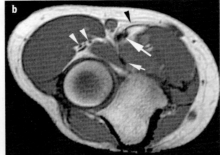
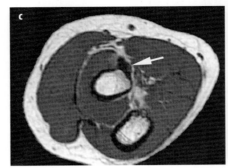
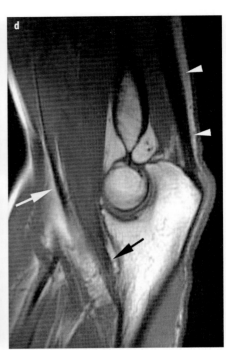

**Fig. 11 a-d.** Normal tendons. Axial T1-weighted images show: **a** the common flexor/ pronator (*arrow*) and common extensor (*arrowhead*) tendons, **b** the biceps tendon (*large arrow*), lacertus fibrosis/bicipital aponeurosis (*black arrowhead*), brachialis tendon (*small arrow*) and branches of the radial nerve within the radial tunnel (*white arrowheads*), **c** the distal biceps tendon at its insertion on the radial tuberosity (*arrow*). **d** Sagittal T1-weighted image again demonstrates the biceps tendon (*white arrow*), brachialis tendon (*black arrow*) and triceps tendon (*arrowheads*)

The flexor/pronator muscles of the forearm originate via a common tendon from the medial epicondyle, while the common extensor/supinator tendon originates on the lateral epicondyle. The supinator muscle arises from the lateral epicondyle, the radial collateral and annular ligaments and the proximal-lateral aspect of the ulna. It then encircles the proximal radius and inserts along its proximal aspect.

## Tendons and Muscles: MR Imaging Technique

Axial images are excellent for evaluating the biceps and brachialis tendons while the common flexor and extensor tendons are well evaluated in both the axial and the coronal planes. The triceps tendon is best assessed on sagittal images. Tendons should be of low signal intensity on all MR imaging sequences but, like ligaments, may demonstrate magic angle artifacts on "short TE" images (T1, proton density, gradient echo). Acute muscle pathology will be most conspicuous on fat-saturated T2-weighted images. Chronic muscle atrophy is best identified on T1-weighted non-fat-saturated images.

## Tendons and Muscles: Potential Pitfalls

The anconeus epitrochlearis is an anomalous muscle, seen in approximately 10% of individuals, that lies along the medial aspect of the olecranon. While this is usually an asymptomatic normal variant, it may produce symptoms of ulnar neuropathy due to compression of the nerve within the adjacent cubital tunnel (Fig. 12) [51].

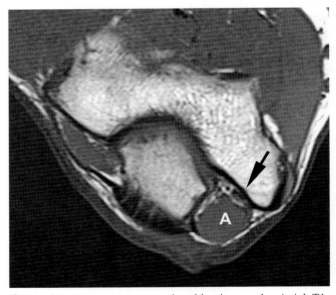

**Fig. 12.** Accessory anconeus epitrochlearis muscle. Axial T1-weighted image reveals the presence of an accessory anconeus epitrochlearis muscle (*A*) at the level of the cubital tunnel where it compresses the ulnar nerve (*arrow*)

## Tendons and Muscles: Pathology

The vast majority of pathology encountered in the flexor and extensor groups will be isolated to the common flexor and common extensor tendons. The classification of tendon injuries about the elbow can be organized by

**Fig. 13 a, b.** Lateral epicondylitis. **a** Axial fat-saturated T2-weighted image displays partial tearing of the proximal common extensor tendon at its humeral origin (*arrowhead*). **b** Coronal fat-saturated T2-weighted image again demonstrates the tendon pathology (*arrowhead*) as well as partial tearing of the underlying radial collateral ligament (*arrow*)

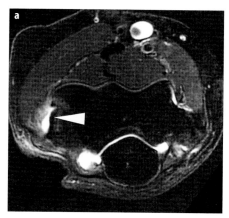
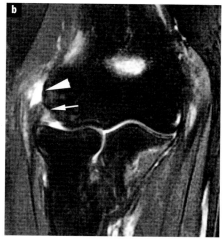

location, acuity and degree of injury. Tendon injury related to a single isolated event is uncommon, although exceptions to this rule do occur. More commonly, tendon pathology in the elbow relates to chronic repetitive microtrauma. MR imaging and ultrasound are particularly well suited to diagnose tendon pathology.

As elsewhere in the body, the tendons about the elbow should be smooth, linear structures of low signal intensity on MR imaging [52]. Abnormal morphology (attenuation or thickening) can be seen in tendinosis (also termed tendinopathy) or tear. If signal intensity becomes increased within the substance of a tendon on fluid-sensitive sequences, a tear is present. Tears can be further characterized as partial or complete. A complete tear is characterized by complete discontinuity.

## Epicondylitis and Overuse Syndromes

Chronic stresses applied to the common flexor and extensor tendons result in medial and lateral "epicondylitis," though this is a misnomer since the underlying pathology relates to chronic degeneration and partial tendon tearing rather than an acute inflammatory reaction. The injury is believed to result from repetitive tensile overload of the tendon that produces microscopic tears that do not heal appropriately.

The imaging findings reflect chronic changes in the tendon, with intermediate intrasubstance signal intensity indicating tendinosis and areas of higher T2-weighted signal intensity in partial or complete tendon tears. Ultrasound is useful for evaluating epicondylitis, but, in those patients with a normal ultrasound, MR imaging is able to better demonstrate other pathology in a symptomatic elbow [53].

## Lateral Epicondylitis

Lateral epicondylitis is associated with excessive, repetitive use of the wrist extensors and is the most common athletic injury in the elbow. It has been termed "tennis el-

bow," but this is somewhat misleading since 95% of cases of lateral epicondylitis occur in non-tennis players [54]. Moreover, it has been estimated that 50% of people involved in any sport with overhead arm motion will develop this process [55].

The pathology most commonly affects the extensor carpi radialis brevis at the origin of the common extensor tendon [56].

The underlying pathology has been well described and includes necrosis, round-cell infiltration, focal calcification and scar formation [57]. In addition, invasion of blood vessels, fibroblastic proliferation and lymphatic infiltration are seen (the combination of which are referred to as angiofibroblastic hyperplasia), and over time these changes ultimately lead to mucoid degeneration [58]. The absence of a significant inflammatory response has been emphasized repeatedly, and may explain the inadequacy of the healing process.

The imaging findings of epicondylitis may include those of tendinosis, thickening or attenuation with intrasubstance intermediate signal intensity, and/or partial- or full-thickness tears (Fig. 13). T2 signal hyperintensity in the adjacent marrow and peritendinous soft tissues may also be seen. Close scrutiny of the underlying ligamentous complex is necessary to exclude concomitant injury. In particular, thickening and tears of the LUCL have been encountered with lateral epicondylitis [59]. Ultrasound has demonstrated high sensitivity but low specificity in the detection of symptomatic lateral epicondylitis [60, 61].

## Medial Epicondylitis

Medial epicondylitis involves similar pathology of the common flexor tendon and is associated primarily with the sports of golfing, pitching and tennis. It has also been reported with javelin throwers, racquetball and squash players, swimmers and bowlers. The pronator teres and flexor carpi radialis tendons are involved most frequently, resulting in pain and tenderness to palpation over the anterior aspect of the medial epicondyle of the humerus and origin of the common flexor tendon. The mechanism of injury includes repetitive valgus strain with pain resulting from resisting pronation of the forearm or flexion of the wrist. The imaging findings in this process are exactly those seen with lateral epicondylitis. As on the lateral side, when assessing the tendon, it is necessary to closely scrutinize the underlying collateral ligament complex to ensure its integrity.

## Biceps Tendon

Rupture of the tendon of the biceps brachii muscle at the elbow is rare and constitutes less than 5% of all biceps tendon injuries [62]. It usually occurs in the dominant arm of males. Injuries to the musculotendinous junction have been reported, but the most common injury is complete avulsion of the tendon from the radial tuberosity. Although the injury often occurs acutely after a single traumatic event, the failure is thought to be due to pre-existing changes in the distal biceps tendon, intrinsic tendon degeneration, enthesopathy at the radial tuberosity, or radiobicipital bursal inflammation. The typical mechanism of injury relates to forced hyperextension applied to a flexed and supinated forearm. Athletes involved in strength sports, such as competitive weightlifting, football and rugby, often sustain this injury. Clinically the patient describes a history of feeling a "pop" or sudden, sharp pain in the antecubital fossa. The classic presentation of a complete distal biceps rupture is that of a mass in the distal upper arm due to proximal migration of the biceps tendon and muscle belly. Accurate diagnosis is more difficult in a partial tear of the tendon, or in the case of a complete tear of the tendon without retraction which can occur with an intact bicipital aponeurosis, which tethers the ruptured tendon to the pronator flexor muscle group (Fig. 14). A

flexed abducted supinated or FABS (flexed elbow with the shoulder abducted and the forearm in supination view) positioning of the elbow for MR imaging can aid in evaluation of subtle tears of the distal biceps [63].

Imaging of distal biceps tendon pathology becomes important in patients who do not present with the classic history or mass in the antecubital fossa, or for evaluation of the integrity of the lacertus fibrosus [64]. MR imaging diagnosis of tendon pathology, as previously mentioned, is largely dependent on morphology, signal intensity and the identification of areas of tendon discontinuity. An important indirect sign of biceps tendon pathology is the presence of radiobicipital bursitis (see below).

## Triceps Tendon

Rupture of the triceps tendon is quite rare [65]. The mechanism of injury has been reported to result from a direct blow to the triceps insertion, or a deceleration force applied to the extended arm with contraction of the triceps, as in a fall. Tears may be partial or complete and usually occur at its insertion site on the olecranon, although musculotendinous junction and muscle belly injuries have been reported. Associated findings may include olecranon bursitis, subluxation of the ulnar nerve, or fracture of the radial head. Accurate clinical diagnosis relies on the presence of local pain, swelling, ecchymosis, a palpable defect, and partial or complete loss of the ability to extend the elbow.

For MR imaging diagnosis of triceps tendon pathology, it is imperative to be aware that the triceps tendon appearance is largely dependent on arm position. The tendon will appear lax and redundant when imaged in full extension, whereas it is taut in flexion. The MR imaging features of a tear are similar to those associated with any other tendon [52].

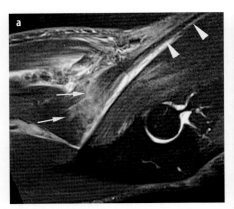 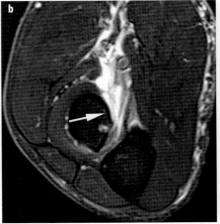 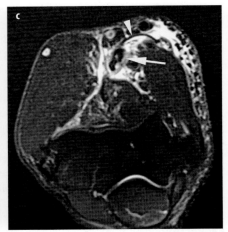

**Fig. 14 a-c.** Biceps tendon tear. **a** Sagittal fat-saturated T2-weighted image shows abnormal signal intensity and ill-definition of the distal biceps tendon (*arrows*), with a taut, normal appearance of the proximal portion of the tendon (*arrowheads*) suggesting this may represent a partial tear. **b** Axial fat-saturated T2-weighted image at the level of the radial tuberosity (*arrow*) reveals absence of the tendon compatible with a complete tear. **c** Axial fat-saturated T2-weighted image at a slightly more proximal level demonstrates the biceps tendon (*arrow*) with an intact bicipital aponeurosis (*arrowhead*) that limited the degree of retraction of the tendon

**Fig. 15 a, b.** Olecranon bursitis. **a** Sagittal fat-saturated T2-weighted image reveals marked distention of the olecranon bursa with fluid. **b** Sagittal fat-saturated T1-weighted image after intravenous administration of gadolinium contrast shows striking enhancement of the thickened synovium

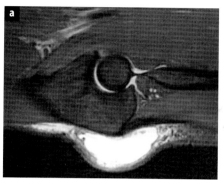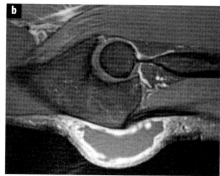

## Bursae

### Bursae: Normal Anatomy and Pathology

The large olecranon bursa lies in the subcutaneous tissues overlying the dorsal aspect of the proximal ulna. Two other bursae are related to the distal biceps tendon near its insertion on the radial tuberosity [66]. The radiobicipital bursa lies between the distal tendon and adjacent radius, allowing for gliding of the tendon with pronation and supination of the arm. The interosseous bursa lies on the medial side of the tendon, between it and the ulna, and may communicate with the radiobicipital bursa. It is important to note that there is no tendon sheath at the level of the distal biceps tendon, so peritendinous fluid in this region indicates distention of one or both of these bursae.

Bursal inflammation may result from infection, trauma or an inflammatory or crystalline arthropathy such as rheumatoid arthritis or gout. MR imaging findings include bursal distention with high signal intensity fluid or, in the case of infection or hemorrhage, more heterogeneous material on T2-weighted images, and pronounced synovial enhancement on T1-weighted images after the intravenous administration of gadolinium contrast [67] (Fig. 15).

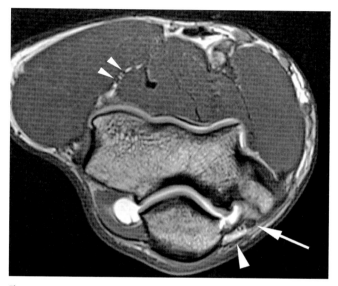

**Fig. 16.** Normal nerves. Axial T1-weighted image (magnetic resonance arthrogram) demonstrates the ulnar nerve within the cubital tunnel (*arrow*) and overlying cubital tunnel retinaculum (*large arrowhead*), as well as the superficial and deep branches of the radial nerve (*small arrowheads*) within the radial tunnel

## Nerves

### Nerves: Normal Anatomy

The ulnar nerve courses along the periphery of the medial head of the triceps muscle in the upper arm and into the cubital tunnel along the posteromedial elbow where it lies superficial to the posterior bundle of the UCL and deep to the cubital tunnel retinaculum (Fig. 16).

After spiraling around the midhumeral shaft, the radial nerve courses through the radial tunnel, a space along the volar-lateral aspect of the elbow between the brachioradialis and brachialis muscles, where it divides into its deep and superficial branches. The deep branch then passes under the arcade of Froshe, pierces the supinator muscle and continues as the posterior interosseous nerve.

The median nerve travels along the medial upper arm with the brachial vessels and then courses between the two heads of the pronator teres muscle and gives off the anterior interosseous nerve more distally.

### Nerves: MR Imaging Technique

The median, ulnar and radial nerves are best evaluated on axial images. T1-weighted images are best for demonstrating anatomic detail while fat-saturated T2-weighted images are most sensitive for detecting nerve pathology and form the basis for most MR neurography protocols.

### Nerves: Potential Pitfalls

The position of the ulnar nerve may be somewhat variable as it courses through the cubital tunnel, with medial subluxation of the nerve seen in 10-16% of asymptomatic patients on MR imaging studies [68]. While increased signal intensity within the ulnar nerve is seen on fluid-sensitive sequences in patients with ulnar neuropathy [69], it is also a common finding in asymptomatic patients and thus must be viewed in conjunction with other findings (nerve enlargement, heterogeneous fascicle size, etc.) when considering the diagnosis of ulnar neuritis [70, 71].

If the ulnar nerve is not seen within the cubital tunnel, it has likely been previously surgically transposed to the volar aspect of the elbow either deep or superficial to the proximal flexor muscles. To locate the nerve after transposition, it is easiest to locate it on T1-weighted images between the medial muscles in the proximal forearm where it is surrounded by bright fat, and then trace its course proximally from there.

## Nerves: Pathology

Pathology involving the nerves of the upper extremity may result from nerve compression/entrapment or a "non-entrapment" etiology such as infection, polyneuropathy, acute trauma or iatrogenic injury during arthroscopy [72, 73]. Most types of nerve pathology will result in changes within the muscles they innervate: high signal intensity "edema" on T2-weighted images with an acute process and high signal intensity on T1-weighted images, indicating fatty atrophy, with more chronic processes. These muscle findings are often more conspicuous on MR images than are abnormalities of the nerve itself.

## Entrapment Neuropathies

### Ulnar Nerve

The ulnar, median and radial nerves may become compressed at the elbow, leading to symptoms of an entrapment neuropathy. Abnormal nerves may demonstrate increased signal intensity on T2-weighted images, focal changes in size, or deviation in their course resulting from subluxation or displacement by an adjacent mass [74].

Ulnar nerve entrapment most commonly occurs in the cubital tunnel. Nerve compression may be caused by a medial trochlear osteophyte, an anomalous anconeus epitrochlearis muscle, or an adjacent soft tissue mass such as a ganglion [75]. Ulnar neuropathy may also arise from repetitive subluxation of the nerve due to absence of the cubital tunnel retinaculum, which occurs with flexion of the elbow in about 10% of patients. If this is suspected, axial imaging with the elbow in flexion should be considered. Other causes of ulnar neuritis include thickening of the overlying ulnar collateral ligament, medial epicondylitis, adhesions, muscle hypertrophy, direct trauma, and callus from a fracture of the medial epicondyle. A snapping medial head of the triceps muscle may also

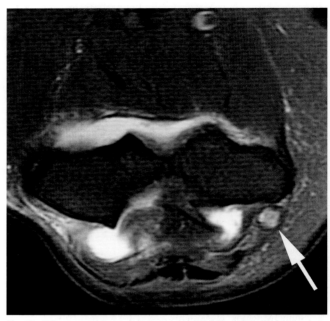

**Fig. 17.** Ulnar neuritis. Axial fat-saturated T2-weighted image in a patient with symptoms of ulnar neuropathy demonstrates increased intrinsic signal intensity and enlargement of the ulnar nerve in the cubital tunnel (*arrow*)

produce displacement and compression of the ulnar nerve, again shown best with elbow flexion [76]. On MR imaging, ulnar neuritis should be considered when the nerve is enlarged and demonstrates increased signal intensity on T2-weighted images, although this latter sign can be seen in asymptomatic patients and therefore must be correlated with other imaging and clinical information. A cross-sectional area threshold of greater the 0.08 cm$^2$ is also useful as a baseline to consider the nerve to be pathologically enlarged [71] (Fig. 17).

If conservative treatment fails, the nerve can be transposed anteriorly, deep to the flexor muscle group, or more superficially, in the subcutaneous tissue. One can follow these patients with MR imaging postoperatively if they become symptomatic, to determine whether symptoms are secondary to scarring or infection around the area of nerve transposition.

### Median Nerve

Compression of the median nerve may occur at several sites and may result from anatomic variants, soft-tissue masses or dynamic forces. In patients with a supracondylar process emanating from the anterior cortex of the distal humerus, the nerve may become compressed by an associated ligament of Struthers (supracondylar process syndrome). The nerve may also become entrapped as it passes between the two heads of the pronator teres and under the fibrous arch of the flexor digitorum profundus (pronator syndrome). More distally, the anterior interosseous nerve may be injured or may be compressed by an adjacent mass (anterior interosseous nerve syndrome) [77].

### Radial Nerve

The radial nerve may be injured from direct trauma, or may be compressed at various sites, the most common being where it penetrates the supinator muscle (the arcade of Frohse), a fibrous band found at that level in 30-50% of patients [72]. The nerve may also be compressed by an adjacent space-occupying mass, an overlying cast, or from dynamic compression as a result of repeated pronation, forearm extension and wrist flexion, as is seen in violinists and swimmers. Motor neuropathy of the hand extensors is a dominant feature when the posterior interosseous nerve is entrapped [78].

## References

1. Stein JM, Cook TS, Simonson S, Kim W (2011) Normal and variant anatomy of the elbow on magnetic resonance imaging. Magn Reson Imaging Clin N Am 19:609-619
2. Zoner CS, Buck FM, Cardoso FN et al (2010) Detailed MRI-anatomic study of the lateral epicondyle of the elbow and its tendinous and ligamentous attachments in cadavers. AJR Am J Roentgenol 195:629-636
3. Kijowski R, Tuite M, Sanford (2004) Magnetic resonance imaging of the elbow, Part I: Normal anatomy, imaging technique, and osseous abnormalities. Skeletal Radiol 33:685-697
4. Rosenberg ZS, Beltran J, Cheung YY (1994) Pseudodefect of the capitellum: potential MR imaging pitfall. Radiology 191:821-823
5. Rosenberg ZS, Beltran J, Cheung Y, Broker M (1995) MR imaging of the elbow: normal variant and potential diagnostic pitfalls of the trochlear groove and cubital tunnel. AJR Am J Roentgenol 164:415-418
6. Al-Aubaidi Z, Torfing T (2012) The role of fat sign in diagnosing occult elbow fractures in the pediatric patient: a prospective magnetic resonance imaging study. J Pediatr Orthop B 21:515-519
7. O'Dwyer H, Sullivan PO, Fitzgerald D et al (2004) The fat pad sign following elbow trauma in adults. J Comput Assist Tomogr 28:562-565
8. Major NM, Crawford ST (2002) Elbow effusions in trauma in adults and children: is there an occult fracture? AJR Am J Roentgenol 178:413-418
9. Griffith JF, Roebuck DJ, Cheng JCY et al (2001) Acute elbow trauma in children: spectrum of injury revealed by MR imaging not apparent on radiographs. AJR Am J Roentgenol 176:53-60
10. Kass L, Turkenburg J, van Riet RP et al (2010) Magnetic resonance imaging findings in 46 elbows with a radial head fracture. Acta Orthopaedica 81:373-376
11. Nalbantoglu U, Gereli A, Kocaoglu B et al (2008) Capitellar cartilage injuries concomitant with radial head fractures. J Hand Surg 33A:1602-1607
12. Itamura J, Roidis N, Mirzayan R et al (2005) Radial head fractures: MRI evaluation of associated injuries. Shoulder Elbow Surg 14:421-424
13. Rosenberg ZS, Blutreich SI, Schweitzer ME et al (2008) MRI features of posterior capitellar impaction injuries. AJR Am J Roentgenol 190:435-441
14. van den Ende KIM, McIntosh AL, Adams JE, Steinmann SP (2011) Osteochondritis dissecans of the capitellum: a review

of the literature and a distal ulnar portal. Arthroscopy: The Journal of Arthroscopic and Related Surgery 27:122-128
15. Ruchelsman DE, Hall MP, Youm T (2010) Osteochondritis dissecans of the capitellum: current concepts. J Am Acad Orthop Surg 18:557-567
16. Bradley JP, Petrie RS (2001) Osteochondritis dissecans of the humeral capitellum. Diagnosis and treatment. Clin Sports Med 20:565-590
17. Patel N, Weiner SD (2002) Osteochondritis dissecans involving the trochlea: report of two patients (three elbows) and review of the literature. J Pediatr Orthop 22:48-51
18. Marshall KW, Marshall DL, Busch MT, Williams JP (2009) Osteochondral lesions of the humeral trochlea in the young athlete. Skeletal Radiol 38:479-491
19. Jeon IH, Micic ID, Yamamoto N, Morrey BF (2008) Osborne-Cotterill lesion: an osseous defect of the capitellum associated with instability of the elbow. AJR Am J Roentgenol 191:727-729
20. Rosenberg ZS, Blutreich SI, Schweitzer ME et al (2008) MRI features of posterior capitellar impaction injuries. AJR Am J Roentgenol 190:435-441
21. Osborne G, Cotterill P (1966) Recurrent dislocation of the elbow. J Bone Joint Surg Br 48:340-346
22. Jans LBO, Ditchfield M, Anna G et al (2012) MR imaging findings and MR criteria for instability in osteochondritis dissecans of the elbow in children. European Journal of Radiology 81:1306-1310
23. Charalambous CP, Stanley JK (2008) Posterolateral rotatory instability of the elbow. J Bone Joint Surg (BR) 90:272-279
24. Sanal HT, Chen L, Haghighi P et al (2009) Annular ligament of the elbow: MR arthrography appearance with anatomic and histologic correlation. AJR Am J Roentgenol 193:W122-W126
25. Seki A, Olsen BS, Jensen SL et al (2002) Functional anatomy of the lateral collateral ligament complex of the elbow: configuration of the Y and its role. J Shoulder Elbow Surg 11:53-59
26. Richard MJ, Aldridge JM III, Wiesler ER, Ruch DS (2008) Traumatic valgus instability of the elbow: pathoanatomy and results of direct repair. J Bone Joint Surg Am 90:2416-2422
27. Phillips CS, Segalman KA (2002) Diagnosis and treatment of post-traumatic medial and lateral elbow ligament incompetence. Hand Clin 18:149-159
28. Schwartz ML, Al-Zahrani S, Morwessel RM et al (1995) Ulnar collateral ligament injury in the throwing athlete: evaluation with saline-enhanced MR arthrography. Radiology 197:297
29. Steinbach LS, Schwartz M (1998) Elbow arthrography. Rad Clin NA 36:635-649
30. Mulligan SA, Schwartz ML, Broussard MF, Andrews JR (2000) Heterotopic calcification and tears of the ulnar collateral ligament: radiographic and MR imaging findings. AJR Am J Roentgenol 175:1099-1102
31. May DA, Disler DG, Jones EA, Pearce DA (2000) Using sonography to diagnose an unossified medial epicondyle avulsion in a child. AJR Am J Roentgenol 174:1115-1117
32. Iyer RS, Thapa MM, Khanna PC, Chew FS (2012) Pediatric bone imaging: imaging elbow trauma in children – a review of acute and chronic injuries. AJR Am J Roentgenol 198:1053-1068
33. Wei AS, Khana S, Limpisvasti O et al (2010) Clinical and magnetic resonance imaging findings associated with little league elbow. J Pediatr Orthop 30:715-719
34. Ouellette H, Bredella M, Labis J et al (2008) MR imaging of the elbow in baseball pitchers. Skeletal Radiol 37:115-121
35. Anderson MW, Alford BA (2010) Overhead throwing injuries of the shoulder and elbow. Radiol Clin North Am 48:1137-1154
36. Limpisvasti O, ElAttrache NS, Jobe FW (2007) Understanding shoulder and elbow injuries in baseball 15:139-147

37. Cohen SB, Valko C, Zoga A et al (2011) Posteromedial elbow impingement: magnetic resonance imaging findings in over head throwing athletes and results of arthroscopic treatment. Arthroscopy: The Journal of Arthroscopic and Related Surgery 27:1364-1370

38. Hurd WJ, Eby S, Kaufman, Murthy NS (2011) Magnetic resonance imaging of the throwing elbow in the uninjured high school-aged baseball pitcher. The American Journal of Sports Medicine 39:722-728

39. Dunning CE, Zarzour ZD, Patterson SD et al (2001) Ligamentous stabilizers against posterolateral rotatory instability of the elbow. J Bone Joint Surg Am 83-A:1823-1828

40. Potter HG, Weiland AJ, Schatz JA et al (1997) Posterolateral rotatory instability of the elbow: usefulness of MR imaging in diagnosis. Radiology 204:185-189

41. O'Driscoll SW, Bell DF, Morrey BF (1991) Posterolateral rotatory instability of the elbow. J Bone Joint Surg 173-A:440-446

42. Pollock JW, Brownhill J, Ferreira L et al ( 2009) The effect of anteromedial facet fractures of the coronoid and lateral collateral ligament injury on elbow stability and kinematics. J Bone Joint Surg Am 91:1448-1458

43. Husarik DB, Saupe N, Pfirrmann CWA et al (2010) Ligaments and plicae of the elbow: normal MR imaging variability in 60 asymptomatic subjects. Radiology 257:185-194

44. Duparc F, Putz R, Michot C et al (2002) The synovial fold of the humeroradial joint: anatomical and histological features, and clinical relevance in lateral epicondylalgia of the elbow. Surg Radiol Anat 24:302-307

45. Ruiz de Luzuriage BC, Helms CA, Kosinski AS, Vinson EN (2012) Elbow MR imaging findings in patients with synovial fringe syndrome. Skeletal Radiol DOI 10.11007/s00256-1523-1

46. Meyers AB, Kim HK, Emery KH (2012) Elbow plica syndrome: presenting with elbow locking in a pediatric patient. Pediatr Radiol 42:1263-1266

47. Kang TT, Kim TH (2010) Lateral sided snapping elbow caused by meniscus: two case reports and literature review. Knee Surg Sports Traumatol Arthrosc 18:840-844

48. Steinert AF, Goebel S, Rucker A, Barthel T (2010) Snapping elbow caused by hypertropic synovial plica in the radiohumeral joint: a report of three cases and review of literature. Arch Orthop Trauma Surg 130:347-351

49. Awaya H, Schweitzer ME, Feng SA et al (2001) Elbow synovial fold syndrome: MR imaging findings. AJR Am J Roentgenol 177:1377-1381

50. Dirim B, Brouha SS, Pretterklieber ML et al (2008) Terminal bifurcation of the biceps brachii muscle and tendon: anatomic considerations and clinical implications. AJR Am J Roentgenol 191:W248-255

51. Li X, Dines JS, Gorman M et al (2012) Anconeus epitrochlearis as a source of medial elbow pain in baseball pitchers. Orthopedics 35:e1129-1132

52. Chung CB, Chew FS, Steinbach L (2004) MR imaging of tendon abnormalities of the elbow. Magn Reson Imaging Clin N Am 12:233-245, vi

53. Miller TT, Shapiro MA, Schultz E, Kalish PE (2002) Comparison of sonography and MRI for diagnosing epicondylitis. J Clin Ultrasound 30:193-202

54. Frostick SP, Mohammad M, Ritchie DA (1999) Sport injuries of the elbow. Br J Sports Med 33:301-311.

55. Field LD, Savoie FH (1998) Common elbow injuries in sport. Sports Med 26:193-205

56. Hayter CL, Alder RS (2012) Injuries of the elbow and the current treatment of tendon disease. AJR Am J Roentgenol 199:546-557

57. Nirschl RP, Pettrone FA (1979) Tennis elbow. The surgical treatment of lateral epicondylitis. J Bone Joint Surg Am 161:832-839

58. Regan W, Wold LE, Coonrad R, Morrey BF (1992) Microscopic histopathology of chronic refractory lateral epicondylitis. Am J Sports Med 20:746-749

59. Bredella MA, Tirman PFJ, Fritz RC (1999) MR imaging findings of lateral ulnar collateral ligament abnormalities in patients with lateral epicondylitis. AJR Am J Roentgenol 173:1379-1382

60. Levin D, Nazarian LN, Miller TT et al (2005) Lateral epicondylitis of the elbow: US findings. Radiology 237:230-234

61. Struijs PA, Spruyt M, Assendelft WJ, van Dijk CN (2005) The predictive value of diagnostic sonography for the effectiveness of conservative treatment of tennis elbow. AJR Am J Roentgenol 185:1113-1118

62. Quach T, Jazayeri R, Sherman OH, Rosen JE (2012) Distal biceps tendon injuries current treatment options. Bulletin of the NYU Hospital for Joint Diseases 68:103-111

63. Giuffre BM, Moss MJ (2004) Optimal positioning for MRI of the distal biceps brachii tendon: flexed abducted supinated view. AJR Am J Roentgenol 182:944-946

64. Williams BD, Schweitzer ME, Weishaupt D et al (2001) Partial tears of the distal biceps tendon: MR appearance and associated clinical findings. Skeletal Radiol 30:560-564

65. Koplas MC, Schneider E, Sundaram M (2011) Prevalence of triceps tendon tears on MRI of the elbow and clinical correlation. Skeletal Radiol 40:587-594

66. Skaf AY, Boutin RD, Dantas RWM et al (1999) Bicipitoradial bursitis: MR imaging findings in eight patients and anatomic data from contrast material opacification of bursae followed by routine radiography and MR imaging in cadavers. Radiology 212:111-116

67. Floemer F, Morrison WB, Bongartz G, Ledermann HP (2004) MRI characteristics of olecranon bursitis. AJR Am J Roentgenol 183:29-34

68. Bozentka DJ (1998) Cubital tunnel syndrome pathophysiology. Clin Orthop Rel Res 351:90-94

69. Baumer P, Dombert T, Staub F et al (2011) Ulnar neuropathy at the elbow: MR neurography – nerve T2 signal increase and caliber. Radiology 260:199-206

70. Husarik DB, Saupe N, Pfirrmann CW et al (2009) Elbow nerves: MR findings in 60 asymptomatic subjects – normal anatomy, variants, and pitfalls. Radiology 252:148-156

71. Keen NN, Chin CT, Engstrom JW et al (2012) Diagnosing ulnar neuropathy at the elbow using magnetic resonance neurography. Skeletal Radiol 41:401-407

72. Andreisek G, Crook DW, Burg D et al (2006) Peripheral neuropathies of the median, radial, and ulnar nerves: MR imaging features. Radio Graphics 26:1267-1287

73. Maak TG, Osei D, Delos D et al (2012) Peripheral nerve injuries in sports-related surgery: presentation, evaluation, and management. J Bone Joint Surg Am 94:e121 (1-10)

74. Bencardino JT, Rosenberg ZS (2006) Entrapment neuropathies of the shoulder and elbow in the athlete. Clin Sports Med 25:465-487, vi-vii

75. Kim YS, Yeh LR, Trudell D, Resnick D (1998) MR imaging of the major nerves about the elbow: cadaveric study examining the effect of flexion and extension of the elbow and pronation and supination of the forearm. Skeletal Radiol 27:419-426

76. Spinner RJ, Goldner RD (1998) Snapping of the medial head of the triceps and recurrent dislocation of the ulnar nerve. J Bone Joint Surg 80A:239-247

77. Dunn AJ, Salonen DC, Anastakis DJ (2007) MR imaging findings of anterior interosseous nerve lesions. Skeletal Radiol 36:1155-1162

78. Yanagisawa H, Okada K, Sashi R (2001) Posterior interosseous nerve palsy caused by synovial chondromatosis of the elbow joint. Clin Radiol 56:510-514

# Wrist and Hand

Louis A. Gilula

Mallinckrodt Institute of Radiology, Barnes Jewish Hospital, Washington University, MO, USA

## Introduction

This course will emphasize the general principles for approaching a variety of lesions of the hand and wrist. An approach to analysis of wrist and hand bones will be provided, followed by applications of these principles with respect to trauma, infection, neoplasia, arthritis and metabolic bone disease. Obviously it is impossible to cover all of musculoskeletal imaging and pathology in a short course such as this; however, some major points will be emphasized in each of these different areas, with most emphasis placed on complex carpal trauma.

## Overview of Analysis

As described by Debbie Forrester [1], looking at any part of the musculoskeletal system can be divided into the A, B, C, D'S, starting with S. "S" stands for soft tissues, "A" is for alignment, "B" is bone mineralization, "C" is cortex, cartilage and joint space abnormalities, and "D" is distribution of abnormalities. Utilizing these principles will help keep one from missing major observations. Starting with "S" for soft tissues will keep one from forgetting to evaluate soft tissues. Recognizing soft tissue abnormalities will point to an area of abnormality and should alert one to look a second or third time at the center of the area of soft tissue swelling to see if there is an underlying abnormality. The soft tissues dorsally over the carpal bones are normally concave. When the soft tissues over the dorsum of the wrist are straight or convex, swelling is suspected. The pronator fat line lying volar to the distal radius suggests deep swelling. When this fat line is convex outward, when normally it should be straight or concave [2], deep swelling should be suspected. Soft tissue swelling along the radial and ulnar styloid processes may be seen with synovitis or trauma. Swelling along the radial or ulnar side of a finger joint can be suspect for collateral ligament injury. Exceptions to this exist along the radial side of the index finger and

the ulnar side of the small finger. Focal swelling circumferentially around one interphalangeal or metacarpophalangeal joint is highly suspect for capsular or joint swelling. Tenosynovitis can be another cause of diffuse swelling along one side of the wrist or finger.

"A" stands for alignment. Evaluation of alignment is utilized to recognize deviations from normal. Angular deformities are commonly seen with arthritis. Dislocations and carpal instabilities can be recognized with abnormalities in alignment. "B" stands for bone mineralization. One can see different types of bone mineralization. Acute bone demineralization can be recognized with subcortical bone loss in the metaphyseal areas and ends of bones, in areas of increased vascularity of bones. This is typified by the young person who has an injured part of the body placed in a cast, with development of rapid demineralization. Diffuse, even demineralization is that which commonly develops over longer periods of time and may be seen in older people with diffuse osteopenia of age and also from prolonged disuse. Focal osteopenia, especially associated with cortical loss, raises the question of infection or a more acute inflammatory process in that area of local bone demineralization. Representing cartilage space and cortex, "C" reminds us to look at all of the joint spaces and also the margins of these joints and bones for cartilage space narrowing, erosions and other cortical abnormalities. "D" refers to distribution of abnormalities. This is most vividly exemplified by the distribution of erosions, as classically might be seen distally in psoriasis and more proximally in rheumatoid arthritis.

Three major concepts in the wrist relate to alignment and can be especially applied to the carpal bones. These three concepts are "parallelism", "overlapping articular surfaces" and "three carpal arcs" [3-5]. The first two concepts are applicable through the entire body. The concept of parallelism is valuable throughout the body, and refers to the fact that any anatomic structure that normally articulates with an adjacent anatomic structure should show parallelism between the articular cortices

J. Hodler et al. (eds.), *Musculoskeletal Diseases 2013-2016*,
DOI: 10.1007/978-88-470-5292-5_4 © Springer-Verlag Italia 2013

of those adjacent bones. This relates to exactly how jig-saw puzzles work. If there is a piece of a jigsaw puzzle out of place, you could see that piece losing its "parallelism" to adjacent pieces. In that situation there would be "overlapping articular surfaces". Therefore the concept of parallelism and overlapping articular surfaces are related. If there is overlapping of normally articulating surfaces, there should be dislocation or subluxation at the site of those overlapping surfaces. This does not apply if one bone is foreshortened or bent, as with overlapping phalanges on a posteroanterior view of a flexed finger. In that situation, one phalanx would overlap the adjacent phalanx, but in that flexed posteroanterior position one would not normally see parallel articular surfaces at that joint.

The last concept is that of three normal carpal arcs. Three carpal arcs can be drawn in any normal wrist where the wrist and hand are in neutral position. Neutral position is the situation when the third metacarpal and the radius are coaxial. Arc I is a smooth curve along the proximal convex surfaces of the scaphoid, lunate and triquetrum. Arc II is a smooth arc drawn along the distal concave surfaces of these same three carpal bones. Arc III is a smooth arc that is drawn along the proximal convex surfaces of the capitate and hamate [3, 6]. When one of these arcs is broken at a joint or at a bone surface, this indicates that there should be something wrong with that joint, such as disruption of ligaments, or when at a bone, a fracture. Two normal exceptions to the descriptions of these arcs exist. In arc I, the proximal-distal dimension of the triquetrum along its radial surface may be shorter than the opposing portion of the lunate. A broken arc I at the lunotriquetral joint is a congenital variation when this situation arises. Another congenital variation exists where there is a prominent articular surface of the lunate that articulates with the hamate, a type II lunate. (A type I lunate is the lunate with one distal smooth concave surface. A type II lunate has one concave articular surface that articulates with the capitate and a second concavity, the hamate facet of the lunate, which articulates with the proximal pole of the hamate.) When there is a type II lunate, arc II may be broken at the distal surface of the lunate where there is a normal concavity at the lunate hamate joint. Similarly, there can be a slight jog of arc III at the joint between the capitate and hamate in the type of wrist with a type II lunate; however, the overall outer curvatures of the capitate and hamate are still smooth. At the proximal margins of the scapholunate and lunotriquetral joints, these joints may be wider as a result of curvature of these bones. Observe the outer curvature of these carpal bones when analyzing the carpal arcs. Also, for analysis of the scapholunate joint space width, look at the middle of the joint between parallel surfaces of the scaphoid and lunate to see if there is any scapholunate space widening when compared with a normal capitolunate joint width in that same wrist.

Analysis of the hand and wrist can be performed very promptly after first surveying the soft tissues, by looking at the overall alignment, bone mineralization and cortical detail simultaneously, as one looks at the radiocarpal joints, the intercarpal joints of the proximal carpal row, midcarpal joint, intercarpal joints of the distal carpal row, carpometacarpal joints and interphalangeal joints. Analyzing these surfaces and bones on all views leads to a diagnosis. It is preferable to carefully analyze the posteroanterior view of the wrist first, as this view will provide most carpal information, and then the lateral and oblique views are merely used for confirmation and clarification of what is actually present on the posteroanterior view. An exception to this comment is the need to closely evaluate the soft tissues on the lateral, as well as the posteroanterior, view. The following sections will describe application of these principles to more specific abnormalities.

## Trauma

Traumatic conditions of the wrist can be classified basically as fractures, fracture-dislocations and soft tissue abnormalities, which include ligament instabilities. Analysis of the carpal arcs, overlapping articular surfaces and parallelism will help determine what exact traumatic abnormality is present. Recognizing which bones are normally parallel to each other also identifies which bones have moved together as a unit away from a bone that has overlapping adjacent surfaces. A majority of the fractures and dislocations about the wrist are of the perilunate type, where there is a dislocation, with or without adjacent fractures, taking place around the lunate. The additional bones that may be fractured are named first with the type of dislocation mentioned last. For the perilunate type of dislocations, whatever bone (the capitate or lunate) is centered over the radius is considered to be "in place". Therefore, if the lunate is centered over the radius, with other bones dislocated from the lunate, this would be a perilunate type of dislocation. If the capitate is centered over the radius and the lunate is not, this would be a lunate dislocation. Therefore, if there were fractures of the scaphoid and capitate, dorsal displacement of the carpus with respect to the lunate, and the lunate was still articulating or centered over the radius, this would be called a transscaphoid transcapitate dorsal perilunate dislocation. Another group of fracture-dislocations that occur in the wrist are the axial fracture-dislocations, where a severe crush injury might split the wrist along an axis around a carpal bone other than the lunate, as perihamate or peritrapezial axial dislocation, usually with fractures [7, 8].

## Ligamentous Instability

There are many types of ligament instabilities, including very subtle types; however, there are five major types of ligament instabilities that can be recognized readily based on plain radiographs. These refer to the lunate as being an "intercalated segment" between the distal carpal row and the radius, similar to the middle or intercalated segment between two links in a three-link chain. Normally there can be a small amount of angulation between the capitate, lunate and the radius on the lateral view. However, with increasing lunate angulation, especially as seen on the lateral view, an instability pattern can be present. If the lunate tilts too much dorsally, it would be called a dorsal intercalated segmental condition. If the lunate tilts too much volarly, it would be called a volar or palmar intercalated segmental condition. Therefore, if the lunate is tilted too much dorsally (where the capitolunate angle is more than 30 degrees and/or a scapholunate (SL) angle is more than 60-80 - degrees), this would be called a dorsal intercalated segmental instability (DISI) pattern. If the lunate is tilted too much volarly or palmarly (a capitolunate angle of more than 30 degrees or scapholunate angle of less than 30 degrees), this would be a volar intercalated segmental instability (VISI) or palmar intercalated segmental instability (PISI) pattern. When there is a "pattern" of instability, a true instability can be further evaluated with a dynamic wrist instability series performed under fluoroscopic control [9, 10]. When there is abnormal intercarpal motion in addition to abnormal alignment, this supports the radiographic diagnosis of carpal instability. Using the opposite wrist for comparison, the wrist in question can be evaluated for instability with lateral flexion, extension and neutral views, posteroanterior and anteroposterior views with radial, neutral and ulnar deviation views. Fist compression views in the supine position, especially with ulnar deviation, can help widen the SL joint in some patients. Ulnar carpal translation is a third type of carpal instability [9]. If the entire carpus moves too much ulnarly, as recognized by more than one-half of the lunate positioned ulnar to the radius when the wrist and hand are in neutral position, this would be an ulnar carpal translation type I. If the scaphoid is in normal position related to the radial styloid, but there is scapholunate dissociation and the remainder of the carpus moves too much ulnarly, as mentioned for ulnar carpal translation type I, this is called ulnar carpal translation type II. The fourth and fifth types of carpal instabilities relate to the carpus displacing dorsally and volarly off the radius. If the carpus, as identified by the lunate, has lost its normal articulation with the radius in the lateral view and is displaced dorsally off the radius, this is called dorsal radiocarpal instability, or dorsal carpal subluxation. This occurs most commonly following a severe dorsally impacted distal radius fracture. If the carpal bones are normally related to the lunate, and the lunate is displaced palmarly with respect to the radius, this would be called a palmar carpal subluxation. Other types of carpal instability patterns that are detected more by physical examination, and are not usually demonstrated by radiography or other imaging, are termed dynamic wrist instabilities and will not be covered in this presentation.

## Infection

Infection should be suspected when there is an area of cortical destruction with pronounced osteopenia. It is not uncommon to have patients present with pain and swelling, and infection might not be a suspected clinical diagnosis when this condition is chronic, as with an indolent type of infection, such as tuberculosis. Soft tissue swelling is a key point for this diagnosis, as for other abnormalities of the wrist, as mentioned above. Therefore, the diagnosis of infection should be most suspected when there is swelling, associated osteopenia and cortical destruction, or even when there is early focal joint space loss without cortical destruction.

## Neoplasia

When there is an area of abnormality, it is helpful to first determine the gross area of involvement, and then look at the center of the abnormality. If the center of abnormality is in bone, then probably the lesion originated within the bone. When the center of abnormality is in the soft tissues, a soft tissue origin for the lesion is suspected. When there is a focal area of bone loss or destruction or even a focal area of soft tissue swelling with or without osteopenia, neoplasia [11] is a major consideration. Whenever neoplasia is a concern on an imaging study, infection should also be considered. To analyze a lesion within a bone, look at the margins of the lesion to see if it is well-defined and if it has a thin to thick sclerotic rim. Evaluate the endosteal surface of the bone to see if there is scalloping or concavities along the surface. Endosteal concavities representing endosteal scalloping are characteristic of cartilage tissue. Such concavities would be typical for the most common intraosseous bone lesion of hand tubular bones, and that is an enchondroma. The matrix of the lesion should also be evaluated to see if there are spots of calcium that can be seen in cartilage, or if there is a more diffuse type of bone formation, as can be seen in an osseous type of tumor, such as from osteosarcoma. As elsewhere in the body, if a lesion is very well-defined and if there is bone enlargement, these are findings for an indolent or a less aggressive type of lesion. The presence of cortical destruction is supportive for the presence of an aggressive lesion, such as malignancy or infection. To determine the extent of a lesion, magnetic resonance imaging (MRI) is the preferred method of imaging. Bone scintigraphy can be very valuable to survey for osseous lesions throughout the body, as many neoplastic conditions spread to other bones or even the lung. Lung computed tomography is important to evaluate extent of disease with osseous neoplasia, as metastases from osseous neoplasia often go to lungs as well as to other bones.

With a soft tissue mass lesion of the hand, especially with pressure effect on an adjacent bone, there is suspicion of a giant cell tumor of the tendon sheath. The ganglion is another cause for a focal swelling in the hand, but usually occurs without underlying bone deformity. Glomus tumor is another less common, but painful, soft tissue lesion that may be detected with ultrasound or MRI. Occasionally a glomus tumor might cause pressure effect on bone, especially on the distal phalanx under the nail bed.

## Arthritis

As for arthritis [12], using the above scheme of analyzing the hand, the wrist and the musculoskeletal system, swelling can indicate capsular involvement and also synovitis. Overall evaluation of alignment shows deviation of fingers at the interphalangeal and metacarpophalangeal joints. Such evaluation also shows subluxation or dislocation at the interphalangeal, metacarpophalangeal, or intercarpal or radiocarpal joints. Joint space loss, the site of erosions, and sites of bone production are important to recognize. Identifying the abnormalities, being certain to look carefully at the metacarpophalangeal joint capsules, especially of the index, long and small fingers to see if they are convex for capsular swelling, can help determine if a case is primarily a synovial arthritis. In some cases, a synovial arthritis exists in combination with osteoarthritis. Synovial arthritis is suspected when there are findings of bony destruction from erosive disease. The most common entities to consider for synovial-based arthritis would be rheumatoid arthritis, then psoriasis. With osteophyte production, osteoarthritis is the most common consideration. However, osteoarthritis associated with erosive disease, especially in the distal interphalangeal joints, is supportive of erosive osteoarthritis. Punched-out or well-defined lucent lesions of bone, especially about the carpometacarpal joints in well-mineralized bones, must also be considered for the robust type of rheumatoid arthritis. For the deposition types of disease, gout is a classic example. Gout is usually associated with normal bone mineralization and "punched-out" lesions of bone. The gouty destruction is related to where the gouty tophi are deposited, whether they are intraosseous, subperiosteal, adjacent to and outside of the periosteum, or intra-articular. Well-defined lytic lesions centered about the carpometacarpal joints are characteristic for robust rheumatoid arthritis or gout.

## Metabolic Bone Disease

A classic condition of metabolic bone disease in the hands is that seen with renal osteodystrophy. Metabolic bone disease is considered when there are multiple sites of bone abnormality throughout the body with or without diffuse osteopenia. However, some manifestations of metabolic bone disease may start first or be more manifest in the hands, feet or elsewhere in the body. One should be very suspicious of renal osteodystrophy when there is subperiosteal resorption, typically along the radial aspect of the bases of the proximal or middle phalanges, but there might also be cortical loss along the tufts of the distal phalanges. Bone resorption can also take place intracortically and endosteally. Again, analysis of the bones involved and associated abnormalities present can help lead to the most likely diagnosis.

## Conclusion

Utilization of the above principles of the A, B, C, D'S, parallelism, abnormal overlapping articular surfaces and carpal arcs can help analyze abnormalities encountered in the hand and wrist that can help make a most reasonable diagnosis for further evaluation of the patient.

## References

1. Forrester DM, Nesson JW (1973) The ABC'S of Arthritis (Introduction) In: Forrester DM, Nesson JW (Eds) The radiology of joint disease. WB Saunders, Philadelphia, PA, p 3
2. Curtis DJ, Downey EF, Jr (1992) Soft tissue evaluation in trauma. In: Gilula LA (Ed) The traumatized hand and wrist. Radiographic and anatomy correlation. WB Saunders, Philadelphia, PA, pp 45-63
3. Gilula LA (1979) Carpal injuries: analytic approach and case exercise. AJR Am J Roentgenol 133:503-517
4. Yin Y, Mann FA, Gilula LA, Hodge JC (1996) Roentgenographic approach to complex bone abnormalities. In: Gilula LA, Yin Y (Eds) Imaging of the wrist and hand. WB Saunders, Philadelphia, PA, pp 293-318
5. Gilula LA, Totty WG (1992) Wrist trauma: roentgenographic analysis. In: Gilula LA (Ed) The traumatized hand and wrist. Radiographic and anatomy correlation. WB Saunders, Philadelphia, PA, pp 221-239
6. Peh WCG, Gilula LA (1996) Normal disruption of carpal arcs. J Hand Surg (Am) 21:561-566
7. Garcia-Elias M, Dobyns JH, Cooney WP, Linscheid RL (1989) Traumatic axial dislocations of the carpus. J Hand Surg 14A:446-457
8. Reinsmith LE, Garcia-Elias M, Gilula LA (in press) Traumatic axial dislocation injuries of the wrist. Radiology
9. Gilula LA, Weeks PM (1978) Post-traumatic ligamentous instabilities of the wrist. Radiology 129:641-651
10. Truong NP, Mann FA, Gilula LA, Kang SW (1994) Wrist instability series: Increased yield with clinical-radiologic screening criteria. Radiology 192:481-484
11. Peh WCG, Gilula LA (1995) Plain film approach to tumors and tumor-like conditions of bone. Br J Hosp Med 54:549-557
12. Forrester DM, Nesson JW (1973) The radiology of joint disease. WB Saunders, Philadelphia PA

# Imaging of the Hand and Wrist

Monique Reijnierse

Department of Radiology, Leiden University Medical Center, Leiden, The Netherlands

## Introduction

This article addresses the imaging modalities that are commonly used in the hand and wrist, and describes their roles in the evaluation of particular wrist and hand pathology. The focus will be on specific bone and soft tissue pathology, evaluated with state-of-the-art techniques, based on recent literature.

## Imaging Modalities

Conventional radiography is usually the first imaging technique performed to identify any bone abnormality. A standardized protocol is the basis, including posteroanterior (PA), lateral and semipronated oblique views. On indication, additional views are available to evaluate fractures, dislocations or malalignment [1]. A PA view of the wrist is taken with the palm flat on the table, elbow abducted to shoulder height and flexed to 90 degrees, with the forearm and wrist in neutral rotation. Arthrography is used to evaluate intra-articular structures such as the triangular fibrocartilage complex (TFCC) and intrinsic and capsular ligaments. Although ultrasound-guided injection is also performed, fluoroscopy has the advantage of direct visualization of the diluted contrast and dynamic examination of the wrist. Single-, double- and triple-compartment injections are used and arthrography is followed by magnetic resonance imaging (MRI). However, multidetector computed tomography (MDCT) can also be used [2].

Computed tomography (CT) provides high resolution of the bony structures with multiplanar and three-dimensional reconstructed images, and thus allows evaluation of fracture healing, alignment and postoperative complications. The role of isotope bone scanning has been superseded by other techniques for most osseous and soft tissue abnormalities, because of its low specificity.

MRI provides high anatomic detail of all anatomic structures. With the use of a short screening protocol in-

cluding T1-weighted and short tau inversion recovery (STIR) sequences, a fracture can be easily excluded or diagnosed. Extremity 1.5T magnetic resonance (MR) is particularly well suited for imaging of the wrist.

MR arthrography after direct contrast injection in the joint, resulting in joint distension, is preferred over indirect contrast administration to evaluate intra-articular pathology [1]. However, intravenous contrast administration has additional value in infection and osteomyelitis to rule out an abscess and in (teno)synovitis to differentiate fluid from enhancing synovial tissue.

Ultrasound (US) is a good alternative for the evaluation of soft tissues of the wrist and hand [3, 4]. The newest US machines have a high spatial resolution, and direct patient contact allows the examiner to focus on the site of complaints. In general, if there is a focal symptom, evaluation with US will be useful. However, in patients with more diffuse symptoms, MRI is preferred. In other words, the "pointers" are well assessed with US, whereas the "waivers" will profit from MRI. A specific advantage of US is the ability to perform dynamic imaging and, if necessary, to perform US-guided injection in the same outpatient visit. The fibrillar structure of the tendons can be well assessed, and movement in the synovial sheath can be observed. US of the tendons can provide detailed anatomic pathology, which is increased by using dynamic imaging. With the use of power Doppler, hypervascularization is visualized and, for instance, the difference between chronic and active synovitis of a joint can be made [5]. In addition, it is easy to confirm the presence of a (occult) ganglion cyst.

## Specific Disorders

Hand and wrist pain is a common clinical problem with a wide differential diagnosis. Several examples of bone and soft tissue pathology, requiring dedicated imaging modalities, will be addressed.

J. Hodler et al. (eds.), *Musculoskeletal Diseases 2013-2016,*
DOI: 10.1007/978-88-470-5292-5_5 © Springer-Verlag Italia 2013

## Bones

### Post-traumatic Wrist: Scaphoid Fracture

Conventional radiographs are the basis for evaluation of patients with post-traumatic hand and wrist pain. Routinely, PA and lateral views are obtained. Supplementary scaphoid views, showing the full length, may be helpful to diagnose a fracture of this carpal bone. Before searching for a nondisplaced scaphoid fracture, a distal radius fracture needs to be excluded, since these are ten times more common than carpal fractures [6]. Follow-up radiographs 10-14 days after the initial trauma are usually performed to rule out an occult scaphoid fracture. 10-15% of scaphoid fractures are initially occult. However, other imaging modalities are available to diagnose this earlier. A recent meta-analysis of 30 clinical studies on the diagnosis of suspected scaphoid fractures, showed that MRI is the most accurate test; follow-up radiographs and CT may be less sensitive, and bone scintigraphy less specific [7]. The availability of high-quality extremity (1.5T) MRI machines aids in early diagnosis. A short protocol including coronal T1-weighted and STIR sequences may be sufficient to rule out a fracture (Fig. 1). A major concern is not to miss a scaphoid fracture, with subsequent complications such as nonunion with displacement and instability. However, avascular necrosis and scaphoid nonunion advanced collapse (SNAC) wrist are major complications. Delaying the diagnosis may lead to poor functional outcome. In order to assess the viability of the proximal pole of the scaphoid in patients with nonunion, MRI with intravenous contrast is recommended [8]. Nondisplaced

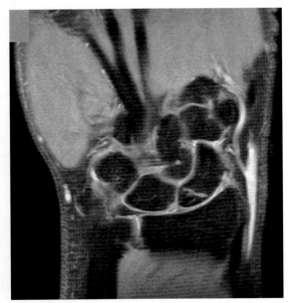

**Fig. 1.** Coronal short tau inversion recovery (STIR) image of the left wrist on a 1.5T extremity magnetic resonance scan. A nondisplaced fracture is visualized in the proximal pole of the scaphoid. No edema is present, consistent with an older fracture

scaphoid fractures are treated with immobilization. Displaced fractures of more than 1 mm require percutaneous fixation with a compression screw. Open reduction and internal fixation (ORIF) with or without a vascularized bone graft may be performed, and salvage procedures include excision and/or arthrodesis of carpals. It should also be mentioned that correlation between symptoms and disease is poor, since only symptomatic patients present for treatment [2, 6, 9].

### Ulnar Impaction Syndrome

Ulnar impaction syndrome is a common cause of ulnar-sided wrist pain. This is often exacerbated by activity and relieved by rest. Impaction between the ulnar carpal bone and the ulnar head may be secondary to positive ulnar variance and leads to degeneration of the ulnar side of the wrist. This can be seen in cases of excessive load-bearing across the ulnar carpus, TFCC and ulnar head [10, 11]. Ulnar variance is the length between the distal end of the ulna and radius measured on PA radiographs. Note that this varies with wrist and forearm pronation and supination, and should only be measured on a standardized PA view [12]. An underlying cause for positive ulnar variance may be shortening of the radius, secondary to a distal radius fracture or a previous surgical procedure. Early changes, such as bone marrow edema and cartilage loss, might be subtle and can be assessed on MRI. Chronic impaction is radiographically evident, showing subchondral cyst formation and sclerosis of the lunate, triquetrum and ulnar head, and joint space narrowing of the ulnocarpal and distal radioulnar joints. However, MR arthrography is the modality of choice to evaluate a degenerative tear of the TFCC and lunotriquetral ligament tear [11]. The treatment most frequently used is ulnar shortening osteotomy (USO). In a retrospective review of 30 patients with ulnocarpal abutment syndrome after a minimum follow-up of 5 years, arthroscopic evaluation of the TFCC at the time of both USO and plate removal was performed. Most TFCC disc tears identified at the initial surgery had healed at long-term arthroscopic follow-up [13].

### Distal Radial Ulnar Joint Instability

Another cause of ulnar-sided pain after trauma is damage to the distal radial ulnar (DRU) joint with instability. It can be the result of an isolated injury of the ligament or be part of a complex lesion such as a Colles or Galleazzi fracture. Diagnosis is a challenge, since standard lateral wrist radiographs can only confirm DRU joint instability if a true lateral neutral view is acquired, which may be difficult. In addition, DRU joint subluxation may not be obvious in the neutral position. Cross-sectional imaging with CT can overcome these limitations. In cases of suspected unilateral distal DRU joint subluxation, bilateral wrist CT might be a good imaging modality. Imaging is performed with a straight elbow in extreme supination and extreme pronation. CT criteria for diagnosing dorsovolar subluxation have been examined by Nakamura et al. [14]. In general, the convex articular surface of lateral distal ulna should be congruent with the sigmoid notch regardless of wrist position. However, there is a large variation in DRU joint translation because of differences in laxity of ligaments and other stabilizing soft tissues. The modified radioulnar line method [14] is commonly used because it is simple, has few false-positive results, and good interobserver agreement. To compare both wrists can be of additional value. Dorsal displacement of the ulna with respect to the distal radius is most commonly found, and this increases by pronation. Volar displacement is rare; however, it can be present after a hypersupination injury. The treatment of chronic volar or dorsal DRU joint instability is surgical. Specific surgical procedures such as distal ulna resection-stabilization are used, with good clinical results [15].

## Soft Tissues

### Ligaments

Scapholunate (SL) and lunotriquetral (LT) ligaments connect the bones in the proximal carpal row and are important stabilizers of the wrist. There is a connection at the dorsal and volar margins of the bones, as well as a central (proximal) membranous component. Imaging modalities used to diagnose ligament tears include radiography in ulnar and radial deviation, arthrography, and CT and MR with and without arthrography [16, 17]. US provides good visualization of the dorsal aspect of the SL ligament, and dynamic imaging (radial and ulnar deviation) may help to diagnose a tear. However, US is not a good method to observe TL tears [18]. With advancing age, the presence of degenerate tear increases [19]. The differentiation between a traumatic and degenerate tear can be made based on the location: a traumatic tear is in the periphery, whereas a degenerate tear is located centrally. A dorsal SL tear is clinically significant and might lead to SL dissociation with wrist instability. Scapholunate advanced collapse, a SLAC wrist, might be the end result [2].

## Triangular Fibrocartilage Complex

Direct MR arthrography is the preferred modality to evaluate TFCC as well as wrist ligaments; however, MDCT arthrography can also be used [20, 21]. There is no role for US in the diagnosis of TFCC tears [16]. Single-, double- and triple-compartment injections are used. On MRI, the normal cartilage disc has a low signal intensity on all sequences. However, the radial and ulnar attachments may show an intermediate to high signal intensity on T1- or T2-weighted images, and this should not be interpreted as pathology [19]. In addition, a central, radial-sided communicating defect of the TFCC is often asymptomatic and bilateral. With increasing age defects and central communication within the TFCC increase in frequency [22].

Note that the presence of fluid in the DRU joint on T2-weighted images can be secondary to synovitis or DRU instability.

Without intra-articular contrast, the identification of clinically meaningful ulnar-sided peripheral tears is difficult to diagnose (Figs. 2, 3).

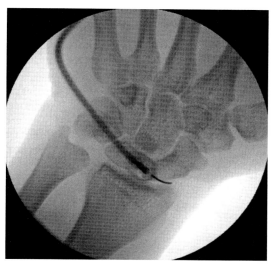

**Fig. 2.** Fluoroscopic image: needle position for radiocarpal joint injection, located radial from the scapholunate ligament

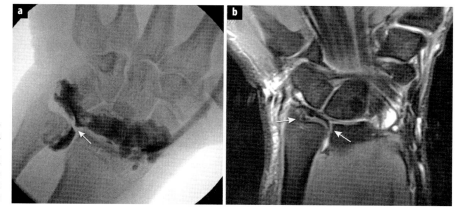

**Fig. 3 a, b. a** Fluoroscopic image of an arthrogram at the radiocarpal joint. Contrast has leaked in the distal radial ulnar joint (*arrow*). **b** Coronal T1-weighted fat-suppressed magnetic resonance arthrogram shows the radial-sided defect of TFCC. Contrast leaks in the soft tissues on the ulnar side (*arrows*)

## Tendons

Tendon pathology is a frequent cause of wrist pain. On MRI, the tendons are described based on changes in morphology, signal intensities and associated findings. Surmenage is an underlying cause of wrist tendon pathology, and acute and chronic changes can coexist. Fluid is the hallmark of acute disease, whereas tendon thickening and synovial hypertrophy are predominantly seen in chronic disease. Tendinosis shows an increase in thickness and focal increase of tendon signal intensity on T1-weighted or proton density images, whereas high signal on T2-weighted images in the tendon correlates with intrasubstance degeneration or a partial tear. However, the signal intensity in some wrist tendons is complicated by the magic angle phenomenon, which can simulate pathology. Classically this phenomenon occurs in ligaments and other ordered structures when they are oriented approximately 55 degrees to the main magnetic field (B0) [23]. The tendons of the extensor pollicis longus (third compartment) and flexor pollicis longus, especially on T1-weighted images, are prone to this phenomenon because of their oblique course [19]. On US, the fibrillar structure of the tendons can be well assessed. Changes in echogenicity and volume of the tendons are well visualized. Using the heel-toe procedure, rocking the transducer, differentiates a normal tendon from a pathologic tendon (Fig. 4). In the axial plane, a normal tendon changes from hyper- to hypoechoic, called anisotropy, whereas a pathologic tendon will keep its hypoechogenicity. In addition, the movement of the tendon in the tendon sheath, passively or actively, can be shown, thus diagnosing triggering or a partial or full thickness tear. With color Doppler, the presence of hypervascularization is seen. If necessary, US-guided injection can be performed.

The wrist tendons can be divided in extensor and flexor tendons. Based on anatomic landmarks, the extensor tendons are subdivided in six dorsal compartments, numbered from radial to ulnar. The deep and superficial flexor tendons for the fingers pass the carpal tunnel together with the flexor pollicis longus and the median nerve.

### Wrist Tendon Pathology

At the level of the wrist, the tendons are surrounded by a synovial sheath. Tenosynovitis, inflammation of the synovial lining, is commonly found. Rheumatoid arthritis (RA) is the number one cause, and tenosynovitis may be one of the first signs of RA (Fig. 5) [24].

US and MRI show fluid in the tendon sheath and/or synovial proliferation. On US, hypervascularization can be present; on MRI, synovial enhancement can be present after intravenous gadolinium administration.

De Quervain's tenosynovitis is typically located in the first extensor compartment, and the diagnosis is made clinically. The abductor pollicis longus and extensor pollicis brevis share this compartment, and are sometimes divided by a septum. The abductor pollicis longus is frequently composed of different bundles. On MRI, this should not be misinterpreted as a longitudinal tear or tendinopathy [19].

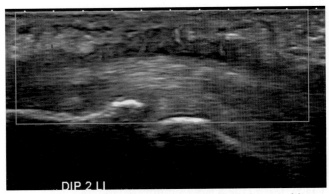

**Fig. 5.** Flexor tendon tenosynovitis. Longitudinal ultrasound image of the index finger at the level of the distal interphalangeal joint. Synovial thickening with hypervascularization is apparent (for color reproduction see p 301)

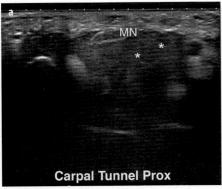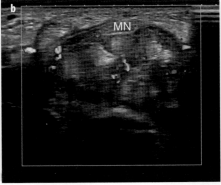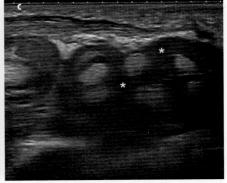

**Fig. 4 a-c.** Axial ultrasound images of the volar wrist at the level of the carpal tunnel (**a**, **b**) and palm of the hand (**c**) demonstrate a diffuse soft tissue mass (*asterisks*, **a**) around the superficial and deep flexor tendons extending distally in the palm of the hand (**c**). Part of the hypoechogenicity is based on anisotrophy (**b**); however, a definite soft tissue mass is present, with hyperemia secondary to an infection. Clinically, carpal tunnel syndrome was evident. *MN* median nerve (for color reproduction see p 301)

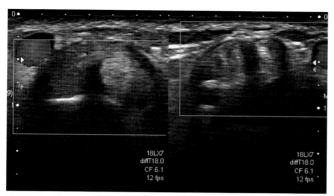

**Fig. 6.** De Quervain's tenosynovitis. Axial ultrasound images of the wrists demonstrate the first extensor compartments, with a normal image (*right*) for comparison. The radial artery is visualized with color Doppler, adjacent to the abductor pollicis longus and extensor pollicis brevis tendons. The image on the *left* demonstrates tendon thickening surrounded by hypoechoic synovium with subtle hypervascularization (for color reproduction see p 301)

In de Quervain's tenosynovitis, there is a specific advantage of US over MRI, notably identification of the thickened retinaculum, which is an early feature (Fig. 6). With knowledge of the anatomy, the exact tendon and division of a compartment can be identified, and corticosteroids can be administered by US-guided injection.

Chronic tendinitis causes tendon thickening and a hypoechoic region; in the presence of active disease, hypervascularity can be seen. However, focal tendon thickening can also be based on rheumatoid nodules, preferably the flexor tendons. The nodules are well defined and hypoechoic [25]. However, the sonographic appearance is nonspecific and a tendon fibroma can show the same characteristics. Incidentally, nodular tenosynovitis is based on a giant cell tumor of the tendon sheath (GCTTS). This is histologically identical to pigmented villonodular synovitis. GCTTS is the most common soft tissue tumor of the hand and wrist and is usually seen on the volar aspect of the distal fingers. It arises from the tendon sheath, is hypoechoic and hypervascular, and can erode the bone [26].

A ganglion cyst can arise from a joint or from the tendon sheath, and a connection with the sheath can be shown with US.

Complication of chronic tendon disease is a tendon tear. The tendons at the dorsal side of the wrist are vulnerable because of their superficial location at the dorsum of the hand and wrist. Tear of an extensor tendon can be caused by a perforating trauma or RA. The extensor pollicis longus can show a tear secondary to a trauma with a bony fragment of, for example, the scaphoid or orthopedic hardware rubbing the tendon, or repetitive stress, which may be work or sports related [27]. US can provide preoperative information on the position of the two tendon stumps.

The role of imaging in the diagnosis of carpal tunnel syndrome is limited. This is considered a clinical diagno-

sis. However, in cases of external compression of the median nerve, US and MRI are important (Fig. 4). Knowledge of synovial sheath anatomy aids in understanding the spread of a bacterial or fungal infection. The common flexor sheath, the ulnar bursa, is in connection with the flexor tendon sheath of the fifth finger. It is important to realize the presence of a gap between the ulnar bursa and the flexor tendons of the second, third and fourth fingers. The radial bursa envelops the tendon of the flexor pollicis longus [28].

The flexor pulleys keep the flexor tendons to the bone. In cases of tendinitis, a typical image is seen of fluid surrounding the tendon with indentations caused by the annular pulleys. Pulley lesions, typical in rock climbers, are increasingly found in regions without mountains, as a result of an increase in the popularity of climbing walls. A typical grip in climbing, with enormous weight on the fingers, can cause the pulleys to tear. A2 and A4 pulley tears are most frequently seen. US plays an important role in diagnosis. In professionals, these tears will be repaired [29].

Abnormalities of movement include tendon clicks and snaps, and no other imaging technique (apart from US) is capable of directly demonstrating these. A trigger finger is often idiopathic; however, repetitive movement may lead to chronic stenosing tenosynovitis, with secondary thickening of the A1 pulley. An additional advantage of US is the possibility of US-guided treatment either by injecting corticosteroids in the tendon sheath or cleavage of the thickened pulley [30, 31].

Flexor tendon tears are less common than extensor tears. Surgeons may require preoperative imaging to differentiate superficial from deep flexor tendon tears and to identify the distance between the two stumps. A retracted tendon may be found in the mid-palm. Both MRI and US are used for this purpose.

## Summary and Conclusion

Wrist and hand pain is a common complaint and has a large differential diagnosis. History and examination of the patient are essential in order to decide which imaging modality will be first choice. Conventional radiographs are used as a screening examination in posttraumatic cases. Knowledge of the advantage and limitations of different imaging modalities is essential. In general, patients with focal pain might benefit from an initial US, and patients with diffuse pain might benefit from MR.

## References

1. Gupta P, Gilula LA (2008) The normal wrist. In: Imaging of the musculoskeletal system. Saunders, Philadelphia, pp 272-308
2. Crema MD, Zentner J, Guermazi A et al (2012) Scapholunate advanced collapse and scaphoid nonunion advanced collapse: MDCT arthrography features. AJR Am J Roentgenol 199: W202-207

3. Bianchi S, Martinoli C (2007) Wrist. In: Ultrasound of the musculoskeletal system. Springer, Berlin Heidelberg New York, pp 425-494

4. Bianchi S, Martinoli C (2007) Hand. In: Ultrasound of the musculoskeletal system. Springer, Berlin Heidelberg New York, pp 495-548

5. McNally EG (2008) Ultrasound of the small joints of the hands and feet: current status. Skelet Radiol 37:99-113

6. Rao N, Hrehorovich P, Mathew M (2008) Acute osseous injury to the wrist. In: Imaging of the musculoskeletal system. Saunders, Philadelphia pp 309-321

7. Yin ZG, Zhang JB, Kan SL, Wang XG (2012) Diagnostic accuracy of imaging modalities for suspected scaphoid fractures: meta-analysis combined with latent class analysis. J Bone Joint Surg Br 94:1077-1085

8. Schmitt R, Christopoulos G, Wagner M et al (2011) Avascular necrosis (AVN) of the proximal fragment in scaphoid nonunion: is intravenous contrast agent necessary in MRI? Eur J Radiol 77:222-227

9. Buijze GA, Ochtman L, Ring D (2012) Management of scaphoid nonunion. J Hand Surg Am 37:1095-1100

10. Watanabe A, Peter S, Vezeridis PS et al (2010) Ulnar-sided wrist pain. II. Clinical imaging and treatment. Skeletal Radiol 39:837-857

11. Cerezal L, del Piñal F, Abascal F et al (2002) Imaging findings in ulnar-sided wrist impaction syndromes. Radiographics 22:105-121

12. Fedlinsky A, Kauer JM, Jonsson K (1995) Evaluation of the true neutral position of the wrist: the groove for extensor carpi ulnaris as a landmark. J Hand Surg (Am) 20:511-512

13. Tatebe M, Shinohara T, Okui N (2012) Clinical, radiographic, and arthroscopic outcomes after ulnar shortening osteotomy: a long-term follow-up study. J Hand Surg Am 37:2468-2474

14. Nakamura R, Horii E, Imaeda T, Nakao E (1996) Criteria for diagnosing distal radioulnar joint subluxation by computed tomography. Skeletal Radiol 25:649-53

15. Mansat P, Ayel JE, Bonnevialle N (2010) Long-term outcome of distal ulna resection-stabilisation procedures in post-traumatic radio-ulnar joint disorders. Orthop Traumatol Surg Res 96:216-221

16. Finlay K, Lee R, Friedman L (2004) Ultrasound of intrinsic wrist ligament and triangular fibrocartilage injuries. Skeletal Radiol 33:85-90

17. Schweitzer ME, Brahme SK, Hodler J et al (1992) Chronic wrist pain: spin-echo and short tau inversion recovery MR imaging and conventional and MR arthrography. Radiology 182:205-211

18. Timins ME, Jahnke JP, Krah SF et al (1995) MR imaging of the major carpal stabilizing ligaments: normal anatomy and clinical examples. Radiographics 15:575-587

19. Pfirrman CWA, Zanetti M (2005) Variants, pitfalls and asymptomatic findings in wrist and hand imaging. Eur J of Radiol 56:286-295

20. Zanetti M, Saupe N, Nagy L (2007) Role of MR imaging in chronic wrist pain. Eur Radiol 17:927-938

21. Moser T, Khoury V, Harris PG et al (2009) MDCT arthrography or MR arthrography for imaging the wrist joint? Semin Musculoskelet Radiol 13:39-54

22. Zanetti M, Linkous MD, Gilula LA, Hodler J (2000) Characteristics of triangular fibrocartilage defects in symptomatic and contralateral asymptomatic wrists. Radiology 216:840-845

23. Erickson SJ, Cox IH, Hyde JS et al (1991) Effect of tendon orientation on MR imaging signal intensity: a manifestation of the "magic angle" phenomenon. Radiology 181:389-92

24. Navalho M, Resende C, Rodrigues AM et al (2012) Bilateral MR imaging of the hand and wrist in early and very early inflammatory arthritis: tenosynovitis is associated with progression to rheumatoid arthritis. Radiology 264:823-33

25. Kotob H, Kamel M (1999) Identification and prevalence of rheumatoid nodules in the finger tendons using high frequency ultrasonography. J Rheumatol 26:1264-1268

26. Murphey MD, Rhee JH, Lewis RB et al (2008) Pigmented villonodular synovitis: radiologic-pathologic correlation. Radiographics 28:1493-1518

27. Santiago FR, Plaza PG, Fernandez JMT (2008) Sonography findings in tears of the extensor pollicis tendon and correlation with CT, MRI and surgical findings. Eur J Radiol 66:112-116

28. Netter FH, Woodburne RT, Crelin ES et al (1987) Upper limb: hand and wrist. In: Musculoskeletal System Part 1. Anatomy, physiology and metabolic disorders. Ciba-Geigy Corporation, Summit, New Jersey, pp 61-64

29. Klauser A, Frauscher F, Bodner G et al (2002) Finger pulley injuries in extreme rock climbers: depiction with dynamic US. Radiology 222:755-761

30. Peters-Veluthamaningal C, van der Windt DA, Winters JC, Meyboom-de Jong B (2009) Corticosteroid injection for trigger finger in adults. Cochrane Database Syst Rev 1

31. Rajeswaran G, Lee JC, Eckersley R et al (2009) Eur Radiol 19:2232-2237

# Hip

Apostolos H. Karantanas[1], Christian W.A. Pfirrmann[2]

[1] Medical Imaging, University Hospital, Stavrakia, Heraklion, Greece
[2] Radiology, University Hospital Balgrist, University of Zurich, Zurich, Switzerland

## Introduction

The painful hip is often a difficult clinical problem because the clinical tests may be nonspecific in many disorders that share the same symptoms and clinical findings. In addition, hip pain may be difficult to attribute to a single underlying cause by using imaging techniques. Plain radiographs remain the first imaging method for hip joint evaluation. Advanced imaging, including computed tomography (CT), magnetic resonance (MR) imaging and combination of both with arthrography [CT arthrography (CTa), magnetic resonance arthrography (MRa)], is often required for further evaluation. MR imaging provides direct imaging of the bone marrow because of its ability to discriminate fat from other tissues. In addition, it provides detailed anatomic overview of the articular, mainly by applying MRa, and peri-articular soft tissue structures. CTa is useful in the postoperative painful hip, when metallic implants exist in the field of view. This chapter will focus on common clinical problems such as benign bone marrow disorders, osteoarthritis and clinical syndromes associated with abnormal contact between the femur and the acetabulum.

## Avascular Necrosis

Femoral head avascular necrosis (FHAVN), or osteonecrosis or ischemic necrosis, is a common disease entity. FHAVN affects mainly young men at their late 30s and early 40s, is characterized by nonspecific symptoms and is initially unilateral with progression to bilateral femoral head involvement in up to 72% of patients. If left untreated, the disease will progress to secondary osteoarthritis in 80% of cases and eventually require total hip arthroplasty [1]. The choice of treatment remains one of the more complex problems for orthopedic surgeons. Two main categories of FHAVN treatment exist: (1) joint-preserving procedures, and (2) joint-replacing procedures. In order to optimize treatment, it is important to use an accurate method of classification and staging based on a reliable and accurate imaging diagnosis. The

most critical point of all classification systems is the loss of the spherical surface of the femoral head. Other significant features of FHAVN are the size and the location of the lesion. The above are important factors that are related to the prognosis and the possibility of collapse [2-4]. MR imaging has been shown to be more sensitive than CT or scintigraphy for early detection of FHAVN in patients with normal radiographs (stage I). The presence of a circumscribed subchondral "band like" lesion with low signal intensity (SI) on T1-weighted sequences is considered pathognomonic of FHAVN (Fig. 1a) [5]. The "double line" sign seen on non-fat suppressed T2-weighted spin-echo (SE) and turbo/fast SE images, despite its artifactual origin, is virtually diagnostic of osteonecrosis (Fig. 1b) [4, 5]. Subchondral fractures in osteonecrosis typically occur as low SI lines on T1-weighted MR images. When fluid is present, the fractures exhibit high SI on T2-weighted images, fat-suppressed proton density (PD) weighted images and short TI inversion recovery (STIR) MR images. They can be differentiated from subchondral insufficiency fractures seen in elderly and in osteoporotic women based on the shape of the lesion (Fig. 1c) [6]. Joint effusion, probably secondary to FHAVN-related synovitis, is seen in 58% to 72% of patients regardless of the presence of articular collapse and is usually found in association with bone marrow edema (BME) (92%) in advanced disease (Fig. 1d). It has been shown that plain radiographs can miss important information in stages II and III, as they overestimate stage II, underestimate stage III lesions, and are inaccurate in estimating the collapse size, which is an important parameter in therapeutic decisions [7]. The wider use of MR imaging in any classification system could improve the accuracy and prognostic value by means of discriminating between early and advanced stages. In advanced disease, there is no need for additional imaging beyond plain radiographs.

The lesion size and extent of femoral head involvement are important parameters in predicting outcome and determining treatment in FHAVN [8]. The size of lesions on plain radiographs may be difficult to assess and might not correlate with the size on MR imaging. The lesion

J. Hodler et al. (eds.), *Musculoskeletal Diseases 2013-2016*,
DOI: 10.1007/978-88-470-5292-5_6 © Springer-Verlag Italia 2013

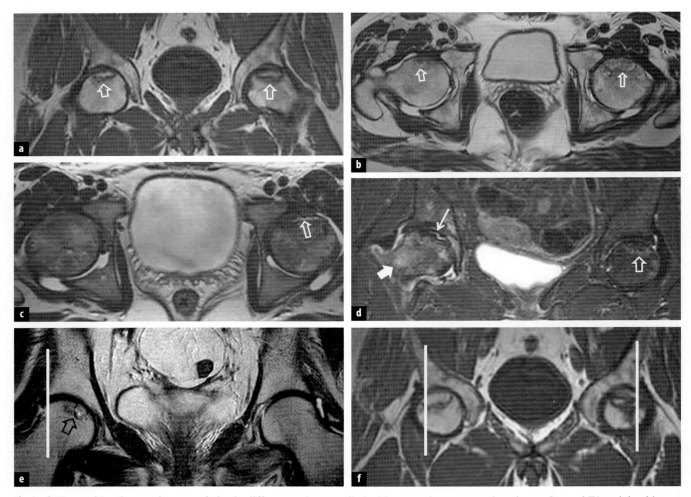

**Fig. 1 a-f.** Femoral head avascular necrosis in six different patients studied with magnetic resonance imaging. **a** Coronal T1-weighted image shows the typical "band-like" sign (*arrows*). **b** Axial T2-weighted image shows the "double-line" sign (*arrows*). **c** Axial T2-weighted image shows the subchondral fracture ("crescent" sign), in keeping with advanced disease (*arrow*). **d** Coronal STIR image in a 50-year-old woman, with known asymptomatic bilateral osteonecrosis and recent pain in the right hip, shows the subchondral fracture (*thin arrow*), bone marrow edema (*thick arrow*) and joint effusion. The osteonecrotic lesion on the left side (*open arrow*) is not associated with bone marrow edema. **e** On coronal T2-weighted image, the lesion (*arrow*) is well contained within the acetabulum. **f** Coronal T1-weighted image in a 45-year-old man shows a noncontained lesion of the noncollapsed right femoral head, extending slightly outside the lip of the acetabulum. The left hip shows a noncontained lesion

location is also an important parameter in predicting femoral head collapse. It has been shown that a hip with an intact articular surface, combined with a well contained from the acetabulum necrotic lesion, has the best functional outcome following joint preserving surgery (Fig. 1e,f) [8]. The presence of BME in patients with known FHAVN seems to correlate with pain and progression of the disease in terms of articular collapse. Following surgery with free vascularized fibular grafting, persistent or increased marrow edema and low SI within the upper part of the graft suggest failure [9].

## Transient Osteoporosis/Regional Migration Osteoporosis

Transient osteoporosis of the hip (TOH), or transient BME syndrome, usually involves healthy middle-aged men; it rarely affects women, almost exclusively during the third trimester of pregnancy or the immediate postpartum period [10]. The syndrome is characterized by acute disabling pain in the hip and functional disability without a history of previous trauma. It has been considered by many authors as an initial and reversible form of FHAVN or alternatively as a variety of algodystrophy syndromes. Currently, it is believed to represent a distinct clinical entity without any sequelae following conservative treatment. With few exceptions, in patients with TOH, the clinical course is relatively short and may last up to 6-8 months, with rapid aggravation of pain and functional restriction of the hip during the first month after the onset [10, 11]. Osteopenia of the proximal femur may be present on plain radiographs at 3-6 weeks after the onset of the symptoms. Spontaneous clinical and radiological recovery is the rule. A characteristic BME

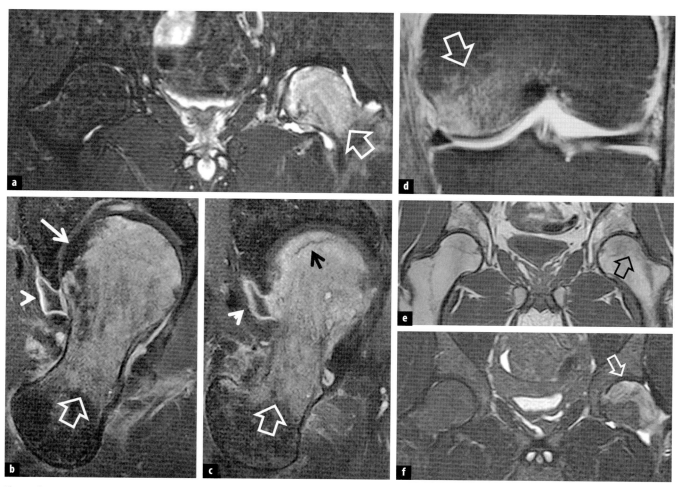

**Fig. 2 a-f.** A 40-year-old man with 2-month left hip pain and complete resolution of pain 8 months after onset of symptoms. **a** Coronal STIR magnetic resonance (MR) image shows the high signal intensity bone marrow edema-like area (*arrow*). **b, c** Oblique axial contrast-enhanced fat-suppressed T1-weighted MR images show homogeneous enhancement of the edematous marrow lesion (*open arrows*), sparing of subchondral area medially (*thin arrow*), a microtrabecular subchondral fracture (*black arrow*) and mild synovitis (*arrowheads*). A 35-year-old man with regional migrating osteoporosis. **d** Originally, the bone marrow edema lesion was located in the medial femoral condyle, as shown in the coronal fat-suppressed proton density weighted MR image (*arrow*). Coronal T1-weighted (**e**) and STIR (**f**) MR images 18 months after **d** show bone marrow edema-like lesion in the left femoral head, in keeping with recent hip joint pain (*arrows*). The DEXA of the spine 16 months after the onset of symptoms showed marked osteoporosis (*Z*-score, -3.3)

signal on T1-weighted and fat-suppressed PD or STIR MR images has been demonstrated in patients with TOH (Fig. 2a-c) [11]. Sparing of the subchondral bone marrow, particularly on the medial aspect of the femoral head, is a well-recognized finding in TOH [11]. Joint effusion and mild synovitis, combined with periarticular soft tissue edema, are constant findings. The BME area is enhancing following contrast administration. In about 5% of patients, linear subchondral changes may appear and probably represent reversible microtrabecurar fractures.

Regional migratory osteoporosis (RMO) is defined as sequential polyarticular arthralgia of the weight-bearing joints, limited to the lower appendicular skeleton [12, 13]. The pattern of shifting symptoms is typically proximal to distal, with a mean migration interval of 4-9 months. In patients with TOH, migration occurs in 5% to 41% [11]. Usually, the joint nearest the diseased one is the next to be involved, i.e., contralateral hip, or either ipsilateral knee or ankle. Rarely, the disorder migrates from the peripheral joints to the more proximal ones (Fig. 2d-f). As the MR imaging findings are identical to those of TOH, with a similar duration of symptoms, the diagnosis of RMO mainly depends on its clinical behavior [12, 13]. There are reports suggesting that systemic osteopenia or osteoporosis may coexist with RMO. Densitometric evaluation, preferably by means of spinal DEXA, may significantly contribute to treatment planning.

## Stress Injuries

Osseous stress injuries represent a spectrum of disorders ranging from a stress reaction to a frank fracture. Stress fractures are classified as fatigue (abnormal forces applied

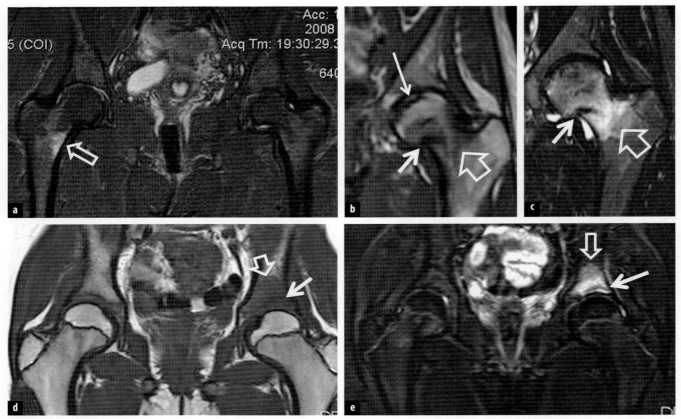

**Fig. 3 a-e. a** A 30-year-old obese woman who started playing tennis in an attempt to lose weight is referred with right hip pain after practicing for 6 weeks. The coronal STIR magnetic resonance (MR) image shows bone marrow edema in the medial femoral metaphysis in keeping with stress reaction (*arrow*). **b, c** A 22-year-old long-distance female runner presents with pain in the left hip joint. The coronal T1-weighted (**b**) and STIR (**c**) MR images show a fatigue fracture (*thick arrows*) surrounded by bone marrow edema (*open arrows*) and an old subchondral fatigue fracture (**b**) with no associated bone marrow edema (*thin arrow*). Coronal T1 (**d**) and STIR (**e**) MR images of a 9-year-old female elite dancer show a fatigue fracture in the acetabulum (*arrows*) surrounded by bone marrow edema (*open arrows*)

on normal bone) and insufficiency (normal forces applied on weakened bone) [13]. The former are overuse injuries primarily afflicting competitive and recreational athletes and military recruits, and they account for more than 10% of all sports-related injuries. The latter occur in the elderly, mainly postmenopausal osteoporotic women, and are located most commonly in the pelvic girdle followed by the proximal femur and the spine. A combined fatigue and insufficiency fracture may occur in (a) young female anorexic gymnasts or long distance runners, and (b) osteoporotic middle-aged avid runners.

Early diagnosis and intervention are essential for prompt and effective rehabilitation, often preventing progression to a complete fracture. MR imaging has become the modality of choice in the evaluation of patients with a high index of suspicion for a stress injury. The application of fluid-sensitive sequences is mandatory for early diagnosis. In addition, MR imaging allows accurate grading of these injuries and provides useful information regarding prognosis and clinical management as it is able to detect different causes of associated symptoms. Sites of stress injuries with pain referred to the hip include the

inferomedial femoral neck, superior and inferior pubic rami, acetabular roof, subcortical femoral head and very rarely the sacrum.

Stress response or stress reaction is a pre-fracture condition characterized by low signal on T1-weighted and high signal on T2-weighted and STIR sequences, and is caused by repetitive trauma to the bone marrow, without any fracture line (Fig. 3a) [14, 15]. Stress reactions are distinguished from (a) fatigue fractures, by the absence of a distinct fracture line, and (b) bone contusion only with history, by means of one single traumatic effect occurring in the latter. Bone bruise is rare in the hip, both in the growing skeleton and in adults.

Fatigue fractures are shown as low SI linear structures on all pulse sequences, extending up to the cortex. The fractures are surrounded by hypointense areas on T1-weighted images and hyperintense areas on fat-supressed PD/T2-weighted or STIR images because of the BME and hemorrhage (Fig. 3b-e) [14, 15]. MR imaging has been shown to be 100% accurate in differentiating stress fractures from other causes of sports-related disorders in the hip. MR imaging can be quite useful for the follow-

**Fig. 4 a, b.** A 19-year-old elite soccer player suffering from a cam-type femoroacetabular impingement. Anteroposterior radiograph (**a**) of the left hip shows a laterally increasing radius of the femoral head (*black arrowheads*) consistent with a pistol grip deformity. The lateral cross table view (**b**) shows a marked waist deficiency of the femoral neck (*white arrowheads*)

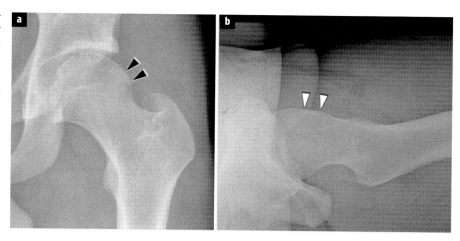

up of elite athletes because, by using fat-suppressed sequences, it allows the depiction of return of the bone marrow signal to normal in about 3 months. The majority of stress fractures have a good prognosis and are healed in a few weeks with conservative treatment. Surgical operation is required for displacement of a stress fracture, usually in cases of delayed diagnosis or when it develops on the outer aspect of the femoral neck, where tensile forces predominate and it might become unstable. Insufficiency fractures exhibit imaging findings that are identical to those of fatigue fractures.

## Femoroacetabular Impingement and Osteoarthritis

Femoroacetabular impingement (FAI) is caused by a conflict between the acetabulum and the femur [16]. This may be due to an abnormal shape of the femur, overcoverage of the acetabulum or supraphysiologic range of motion [17]. Extra-articular factors, such as abnormal torsional alignment of the femur, can also cause FAI. Commonly, several of these factors are combined. FAI results in premature osteoarthritis of the hip.

### Femoral Cause: Cam Femoroacetabular Impingement

The typical femoral cause for FAI is an eccentric femoral head with a laterally increasing radius, often aggravated by a deficiency of the femoral waist and an osseous bump at the femoral neck (Fig. 4). The deformity is termed "Cam deformity". The typical location for the cam deformity is anterosuperior [18]. The cam deformity is usually diagnosed on plain radiographs; for example, on a cross-table lateral view with internal rotation of the leg. On cross-sectional imaging the cam deformity might not be visible on standard planes, because of its anterosuperior location. Therefore radial imaging around the axis of the femoral neck is often recommended. The alpha angle is a measurement to quantify the cam deformity. The alpha angle is typically calculated on axial oblique image,

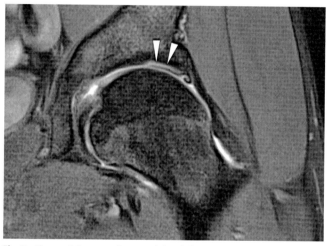

**Fig. 5.** Coronal intermediate-weighted fat-saturated magnetic resonance arthrography image of the left hip in a patient with cam femoroacetabular impingement demonstrates fluid (*arrowheads*) underneath the acetabular cartilage layer consistent with cartilage delamination

between a line representing the axis of the femoral neck and a line connecting the center of the femoral head and the point where a circle, placed on the femoral head, leaves the anterior outline of the femoral head. Again, the best location to assess the alpha angle is anterosuperior [19], and therefore these measurements are often performed on radial images. The optimal threshold for the alpha angle is 60 degrees [19]. The cam deformity leads to an outside-in abrasion of the cartilage. Cartilage damage occurs typically on the acetabular side and is typically located at the anterosuperior aspect. Sagittal MR images are well suited to recognize these damages. The sheer forces on the acetabular cartilage lead to carpet-like delamination of the acetabular cartilage. These cartilage delaminations may be invisible on MR or MRa. Fluid underneath the cartilage layer is a specific but rare finding (Fig. 5). Signal changes within the acetabular cartilage

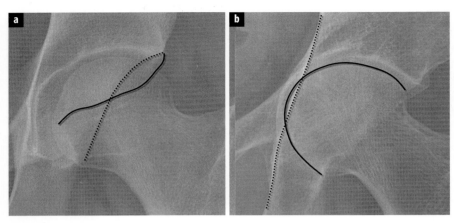

**Fig. 6 a,b.** Femoroacetabular impingement of the pincer type. **a** Acetabular retroversion: anteroposterior radiograph of the hip shows an acetabular retroversion with a "crossing" sign. In the superior aspect of the hip, the anterior rim of the acetabulum (*continuous line*) is lateral to the posterior rim of the acetabulum (*dotted line*). **b** Protrusio acetabuli: the outline of the femoral head (*dotted line*) lies medial to the ilio-ischial line (*continuous line*)

layer (not at the interface between the two cartilage layers), especially hypointensities of the acetabular cartilage on PD or T1-weighted MR images, should raise the suspicion for a cartilage delamination [20]. The typical patient with cam impingement is a young athletic male.

## Acetabular Cause: Pincer Femoroacetabular Impingement

The reason for an acetabular cause for the FAI is an overcoverage of the femoral head [16]. The overcoverage may be general, for example in hips with a deep acetabulum or even a protrusio acetabuli. The overcoverage may also be focal, as in hips with an acetabular retroversion (Fig. 6). The overcoverage is generally well diagnosed on plain radiographs; however on cross-sectional imaging, the findings might not be very obvious [18]. The typical patient for a pincer FAI is a middle-aged woman. The pattern of damage to the joint differs from that of cam FAI. In pincer FAI, the labral damage tends to occur more frequently and earlier than in cam FAI. However, the cartilage damage is often much less pronounced than in cam FAI. The cartilage damage in pincer FAI is usually limited to the acetabular rim region. There may be a characteristic cartilage damage to the posteroinferior region of the acetabulum, the so called "contre-coup lesion". The sagittal imaging plane may be the most relevant to see this contre-coup cartilage lesion.

## Torsional Malalignment

Torsional malalignment may be an important cofactor for FAI, or even the only factor to explain the impaired internal rotation of the hip joint. A retrotorsion of the femoral neck impairs internal rotation to a significant degree [21]. A retrotorsion of the femoral neck may be diagnosed on CT or MR using transverse sections through the proximal and the distal femur.

## Role of Imaging in Femoroacetabular Impingement

Usually, FAI may be sufficiently characterized by clinical examination and plain radiographs. The main role for MR

or MRa is to stage the extent of joint damage before surgery and to give additional three-dimensional information about the deformity. In cases with advanced cartilage damage, especially with involvement of the femoral cartilage, joint preserving surgery often has unfavorable outcome.

## Developmental Dysplasia of the Hip

Developmental dysplasia of the hip (DDH) is characterized by an insufficient lateral or anterior coverage of the femoral head by the acetabulum, leading to premature osteoarthritis. DDH can be well diagnosed and quantified on plain radiographs. The Tönnis angle or acetabular index is formed with a horizontal line (connecting bases of the teardrops) and a line at the acetabular sourcil (the sclerotic weight-bearing portion of the acetabulum). Normal values for the acetabular index are between 0 degrees and 10 degrees. Increased angles are linked to structural instability, as in DDH. Decreased angles are seen with pincer-type FAI. The Wiberg angle or lateral center-edge angle (CE-angle) is measured between a vertical line through the center of the femoral head and a line extending through the center of the femoral head to the lateral sourcil. The normal CE-angle is between 25 degrees and 45 degrees. A CE-angle of less than 20 degrees is diagnostic of DDH. Lequesne's angle is the anterior CE-angle [22]. The anterior CE-angle measures the anterior dysplasia on a false profile view. The anterior CE-angle is formed by a vertical line through the center of the femoral head and a line extending through the center of the femoral head to the anterior end of the sourcil. Normal values are between 25 degrees and 50 degrees. An anterior CE-angle of less than 20 degrees is diagnostic of DDH. At MR imaging, DDH is characterized by a hypertrophic labrum. Often perilabral ganglion cysts and labral tears are seen [23]. The cartilage in the acetabular rim region shows premature damage. There is often an increased centrum collum diaphyseal angle, a high riding fovea and tears of the ligamentum teres at the femoral attachment.

# Trochanteric Pain: Greater Trochanter

The greater trochanter is the attachment site for the abductor tendons. Pain around the greater trochanter is very common and often patients refer to this as "hip pain". The greater trochanter has four distinct bony facets [24]. At the anterior facet the gluteus minimus tendon is attaching. At the lateral facet the lateral portion of the gluteus medius tendon is attaching. The main tendon of the gluteus medius attaches to the posterosuperior facet. The posterior facet of the greater trochanter is only covered by the trochanteric bursa and does not have a tendinous attachment. Tendon lesions most commonly occur at the anterolateral location involving the gluteus minimus and the lateral part of the gluteus medius. Typically these lesions are found in elderly women. Trochanteric bursitis is easily diagnosed by ultrasound or MR imaging demonstrating increased fluid in the trochanteric bursa. Whenever a trochanteric bursitis is seen, the reason for the bursitis should be investigated. In many cases a tear of the abductor tendons may be seen.

# References

1. Mont MA, Hungerford DS (1995) Non-traumatic avascular necrosis of the femoral head. J Bone Joint Surg Am 77:459-474
2. ARCO (1992) ARCO (Association Research Circulation Osseous): Committee on Terminology and classification. ARCO news 4:41-46
3. Steinberg ME, Steinberg DR (2004) Classification systems for osteonecrosis: an overview. Orthop Clin North Am 35:273-283
4. Malizos KN, Karantanas AH, Varitimidis SE et al (2007) Osteonecrosis of the femoral head: etiology, imaging and treatment. Eur J Radiol 63:16-28
5. Mitchell DG, Rao VM, Dalinka MK et al (1987) Femoral head avascular necrosis: correlation of MR imaging, radiographic staging, radionuclide imaging, and clinical findings. Radiology 162:709-715
6. Ikemura S, Yamamoto T, Motomura G et al (2010) MRI evaluation of collapsed femoral heads in patients 60 years old or older: Differentiation of subchondral insufficiency fracture from osteonecrosis of the femoral head. AJR Am J Roentgenol 195:W63-68
7. Zibis AH, Karantanas AH, Roidis NT et al (2007) The role of MR imaging in staging femoral head osteonecrosis. Eur J Radiol 63:3-9
8. Bassounas AE, Karantanas AH, Fotiadis DI, Malizos KN (2007) Femoral head osteonecrosis: volumetric MRI assessment and outcome. Eur J Radiol 63:10-15
9. Karantanas AH, Drakonaki EE (2012) The role of MR imaging in avascular necrosis of the femoral head. Semin Musculoskelet Radiol 15:281-300
10. Korompilias AV, Karantanas AH, Lykissas MG, Beris AE (2008) Transient osteoporosis. J Am Acad Orthop Surg 16:480-489
11. Malizos KN, Zibis AH, Dailiana Z et al (2004) MR imaging findings in transient osteoporosis of the hip. Eur J Radiol 50:238-244
12. Karantanas AH (2007) Acute bone marrow edema of the hip: role of MR imaging. Eur J Radiol 17:2225-2236
13. Lakhanpal S, Ginsburg WW, Luthra HS, Hunder GG (1987) Transient regional osteoporosis. A study of 56 cases and review of the literature. Ann Intern Med 106:444-450
13. Berger FH, de Jonge MC, Maas M (2007) Stress fractures in the lower extremity. The importance of increasing awareness amongst radiologists. Eur J Radiol 62:16-26
14. Navas A, Kassarjian A (2011) Bone marrow changes in stress injuries. Semin Musculoskelet Radiol 15:183-97
15. Krestan CR, Nemec U, Nemec S (2011) Imaging of insufficiency fractures. Semin Musculoskelet Radiol 15:198-207
16. Ganz R, Parvizi J, Beck M et al (2003) Femoroacetabular impingement: a cause for osteoarthritis of the hip. Clin Orthop Relat Res 417:112-120
17. Kolo FC, Charbonnier C, Pfirrmann CW et al (2012) Extreme hip motion in professional ballet dancers: dynamic and morphological evaluation based on magnetic resonance imaging. Skeletal Radiol DOI 10.1007/s00256-012-1544-9
18. Pfirrmann CW, Mengiardi B, Dora C et al (2006) Cam and pincer femoroacetabular impingement: characteristic MR arthrographic findings in 50 patients. Radiology 240:778-785
19. Sutter R, Dietrich TJ, Zingg PO, Pfirrmann CW (2012) How useful is the alpha angle for discriminating between symptomatic patients with cam-type femoroacetabular impingement and asymptomatic volunteers? Radiology 264:514-521
20. Pfirrmann CW, Duc SR, Zanetti M et al (2008) MR arthrography of acetabular cartilage delamination in femoroacetabular cam impingement. Radiology 249:236-241
21. Sutter R, Dietrich TJ, Zingg PO, Pfirrmann CW (2012) Femoral antetorsion: comparing asymptomatic volunteers and patients with femoroacetabular impingement. Radiology 263:475-483
22. Zingg PO, Werner CM, Sukthankar A et al (2009) The anterior center edge angle in Lequesne's false profile view: interrater correlation, dependence on pelvic tilt and correlation to anterior acetabular coverage in the sagital plane. A cadaver study. Arch Orthop Trauma Surg 129:787-791
23. James S, Miocevic M, Malara F et al (2006) MR imaging findings of acetabular dysplasia in adults. Skeletal Radiol 35:378-384
24. Pfirrmann CW, Chung CB, Theumann NH et al (2001) Greater trochanter of the hip: attachment of the abductor mechanism and a complex of three bursae-MR imaging and MR bursography in cadavers and MR imaging in asymptomatic volunteers. Radiology 221:469-477

# Pelvis and Groin

William B. Morrison[1], Suzanne E. Anderson[2]

[1] Department of Radiology, Thomas Jefferson University Hospital, Philadelphia, PA, USA
[2] Medical Imaging, The University of Notre Dame Australia, Sydney School of Medicine, Sydney, NSW; Clinical School of Medicine, Melbourne, VIC, Australia

## Introduction

Pain in the hip, groin and buttock region can be related to a variety of conditions; it may be difficult to clinically differentiate pain originating from the hip from referred pain related to pathology outside of the joint. This chapter will discuss a variety of conditions of the groin and the pelvis external to the hip joint, and will discuss imaging modalities and findings associated with each condition.

## Stress Injury

Stress injury is seen in young and old patients alike. Young athletic patients are prone to fatigue fractures. These injuries occur during the training phase; the bone requires breakdown and remodeling before it strengthens, resulting in transient weakening of its structure as a repetitive stress is applied (Wolff's law). Muscle training results in a consistent strengthening over the short term, without a prolonged breakdown period. This disparity results in a period where the bone is weaker and the muscle is stronger. During this period the elastic limit of bone is more easily overcome, the repetitive recurrence of which causes stress fracture (Fig. 1). Older patients with osteoporosis or radiation therapy are susceptible, especially to fractures at the sacral alae or supra-acetabular region [1, 2]. Patients treated with bisphosphonates are more likely to acquire insufficiency fractures of the lateral aspect of the proximal femoral shaft, which can progress to complete fracture (Fig. 2) [3].

On radiographs, bony stress injuries initially may be invisible, although if the injury occurs in an area with periosteal covering, a faint periosteal reaction may be visible. In the early stage, magnetic resonance imaging (MRI) will show a curvilinear subcortical rim of edema. As the injury becomes more established, radiographs or

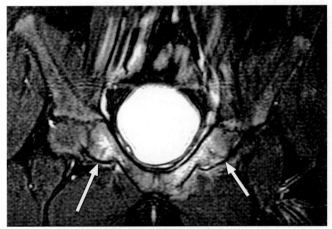

**Fig. 1.** Stress fractures of the superior pubic rami (*arrows*) on coronal STIR image of the pelvis in a 15-year-old gymnast

computed tomography (CT) show a sclerotic line extending from the cortex into the medullary bone, perpendicular to the major trabecular lines of stress. MRI shows a low signal line corresponding to the sclerotic line (representing trabecular reparative callus) surrounded by marrow edema [1-6].

Common locations for stress fracture in young adults include the pubic rami and femoral neck. Stress fractures can also develop in the proximal femoral shaft related to adductor insertion avulsive stress, also known as "thigh splints" (Fig. 3) [4].

Stress fractures occasionally occur in the subchondral bone of the femoral head [5, 6]. The associated hyperemia results in calcium resorption and can result in appearance of osteopenia on radiographs and CT. Because of the radiographic appearance this entity was formerly referred to as "transient osteoporosis of the hip". It is seen on MRI as intense bone marrow edema within the femoral head extending into the intertrochanteric region. A subchondral crescent of low signal is seen which represents the fracture

J. Hodler et al. (eds.), *Musculoskeletal Diseases 2013-2016*,
DOI: 10.1007/978-88-470-5292-5_7 © Springer-Verlag Italia 2013

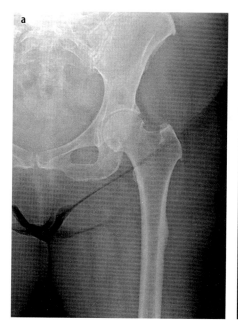
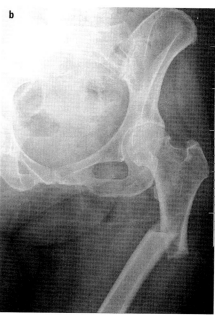
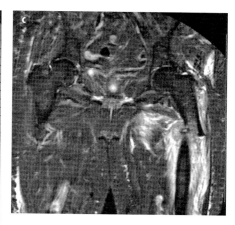

**Fig. 2 a-c.** Insufficiency fracture of the proximal femur in an 80-year-old woman on bisphosphonate therapy. **a** Initial radiograph shows thickening of the lateral cortex. **b** Radiograph 1 week later showing a displaced fracture. **c** Coronal STIR image showing fracture with hemorrhage

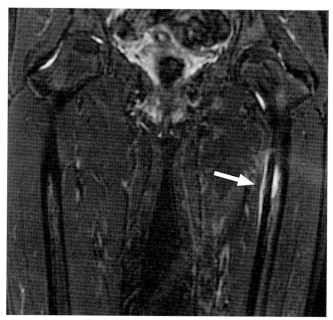

**Fig. 3.** Thigh splints. Coronal STIR image of the femur showing periostitis and subcortical bone marrow edema (*arrow*)

line (Fig. 4). The MRI appearance is similar to that of avascular necrosis, but the latter entity generally shows increased bone density on radiographs and CT.

## Muscle Strain/Tendon Avulsion

Muscle strain is extremely common in athletes. A variety of muscles can be injured, the pattern depending on the specific movement or mechanism involved. Most muscle strains are diagnosed clinically and treated with physical therapy. For more significant injuries or those that do not improve with rest and time, MRI may be obtained. Ultrasound can be used for a targeted exam whereas MRI provides a global assessment of the injury pattern [7]. Strains are graded by MRI on a scale from 1 to 3. Grade 1 strain is a minor injury, exhibiting mild edema without disruption of fibers. Grade 2 strain is synonymous with a partial muscle tear, where more soft tissue edema is observed along with discontinuity of some fibers; there may be fascial edema as well, and the disrupted fibers may retract along the central tendon complex arising from the myotendinous junction, resulting in a low signal center with surrounding edema at the injury site that is characteristic of a muscle injury. Grade 3 strain is the same as a complete muscle tear with complete discontinuity. With this injury there is extensive soft tissue edema and often hematoma [7-12].

Direct muscle injury (e.g., from traumatic impact) generally occurs in large muscle groups and is centered at the muscle belly; the mid thigh is a common location (Fig. 5). Muscle damage related to indirect injury (e.g., eccentric contraction where the muscle is contracting as it is forced to stretch) is far more prevalent and most commonly occurs at the myotendinous junction [13-15].

Avulsion fractures occur around the pelvis after acute trauma, but in adolescents stress-related apophyseal injuries can occur (Fig. 6) [16-18]. These are common at the sartorius muscle origin at the anterior-superior iliac spine, at the rectus femoris origin at the anterior-inferior iliac spine and at the hamstring origin at the ischial spine. Older patients are prone to avulsions at the greater trochanter (insertion site of the gluteus medius/minimus and obturator externus). These injuries can be diagnosed on radiographs. If confirmation is necessary, MRI will show edema at the junction indicating underlying pathology.

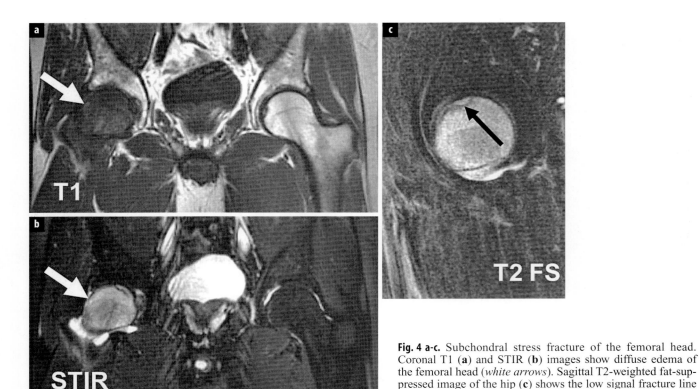

**Fig. 4 a-c.** Subchondral stress fracture of the femoral head. Coronal T1 (**a**) and STIR (**b**) images show diffuse edema of the femoral head (*white arrows*). Sagittal T2-weighted fat-suppressed image of the hip (**c**) shows the low signal fracture line (*black arrow*)

**Fig. 5 a, b.** Muscle direct injury: quadriceps tear in an 18-year-old man presenting with a painful lump at the anterior thigh after a football game. **a** Axial T2-weighted fat-suppressed magnetic resonance image shows edema at the muscle belly of the rectus femoris (*arrows*) representing a partial tear from direct injury. **b** Sagittal STIR image of the thigh shows extensive edema along the muscle (*arrows*)

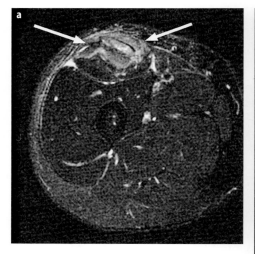
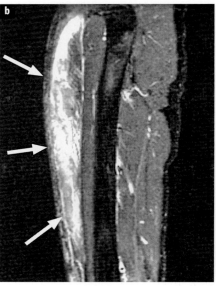

## Groin Pain and Athletic Pubalgia (Previously Known as "Sports Hernia")

A key part of the anterior pelvic anatomy that forms the fulcrum for many of the forces is the pubic symphysis (Fig. 7). The muscles that attach to the fulcrum play a major role in stability. One can think in terms of there being four sets of forces and their counterforces that interact with the symphysis fulcrum. For convenience, we think of these forces as residing in three different compartments. The anterior compartment consists mainly of the abdominal muscles with some complex interdigitations composed of fibers from the thighs and medial and posterior pelvis. The posterior compartment primarily encompasses the hamstrings, a portion of the adductor magnus, and several key nerves and an artery. The medial

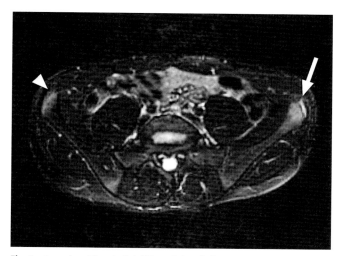

**Fig. 6.** Apophysitis. Axial T2-weighted fat-suppressed magnetic resonance image shows edema at the anterior superior iliac spine (ASIS) growth center, at the origin of the sartorius muscle bilaterally (more pronounced on the left, *arrow*, compared with the right, *arrowhead*) in this 16-year-old male athlete with chronic pain at the ASIS during activity

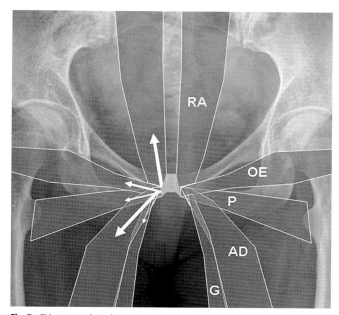

**Fig. 7.** Diagram showing anatomy of the muscle groups attaching to the pubis. *RA* rectus abdominis, *OE* obturator externus, *P* pectineus, *AD* adductors, *G* gracilis. *Arrows* show force vectors upon the pubis resulting from muscle action (for color reproduction see p 302)

compartment is composed of the most important thigh components, which include the gracilis, the three adductors and the obturator externus.

## Clinical Presentation

Most commonly individuals who present with athletic pubalgia are males (approximately 10:1 males to females),

and typically young and athletic, ranging from high-performance to recreational sports. The injuries occur in the most athletically stressed, hence the fittest of athletes.

Participants of sports involving pivoting and/or contact are especially susceptible (i.e., hockey, American football, baseball, rugby and soccer). Patients present with pain anywhere from the pubic symphysis to the hip, and it may not be clear regarding anatomic origin of the symptoms. Pain and tenderness is often referred to the external inguinal ring, leading to previous misconception that the pathology was related to a hernia in this location, which may at times still be the case.

## Imaging findings

Radiographs are generally noncontributory. MRI and ultrasound are the primary modalities used for diagnosis.

The pubic symphysis is marginated by a thick capsule and supporting ligaments, which are normally black on all sequences. The normal symphyseal joint contains a fibrocartilage disc extending in sagittal orientation through the joint which then attaches to the capsule. The rectus abdominis extends down the midline of the abdomen and over the anterior capsule of the pubic symphysis, where it inserts into to the common adductor origin, thereby creating a rectus-adductor aponeurosis. This aponeurosis appears black on all sequences and is tightly attached to the anterior pubis; no fluid should extend from the symphysis into the capsule or aponeurosis ("cleft" sign). Nor should fluid extend between the aponeurosis and pubis (aponeurotic separation). The common adductor origin (composed of the pectineus and adductor longus, magnus and brevis) is incorporated into the aponeurosis inferiorly [19-22]. In order to diagnose injuries to the aponeurosis a small field-of-view specialized MRI protocol (available at www.bone.tju.edu) of the pubic symphysis is recommended. Injury patterns involving the pubic symphysis include acute osteitis pubis (seen as diffuse bone marrow edema around the joint), subchondral stress fracture (with a low signal line in the marrow adjacent to the symphysis with surrounding edema) or osteoarthritis (spurs, sclerosis). This injury pattern may be initiated by disruption of the joint capsule and resultant instability of the articulation. With injury to the rectus-adductor aponeurosis, this common attachment can "peel off" the capsule of the pubic symphysis and cause severe pain and tenderness over the inguinal ring with limited leg adduction (this is why the incorrect term of "sports hernia" was originally applied). Alternatively the common adductor tendon can tear or avulse and retract. With these lesions MRI provides optimal global evaluation, with fluid seen under or within the aponeurosis (Fig. 8) [20-22]. There is a variable degree of associated adductor muscle strain (usually involving the adductor longus). Ultrasound can also be used, showing focal hypoechogenicity at the adductor origin (Fig. 9).

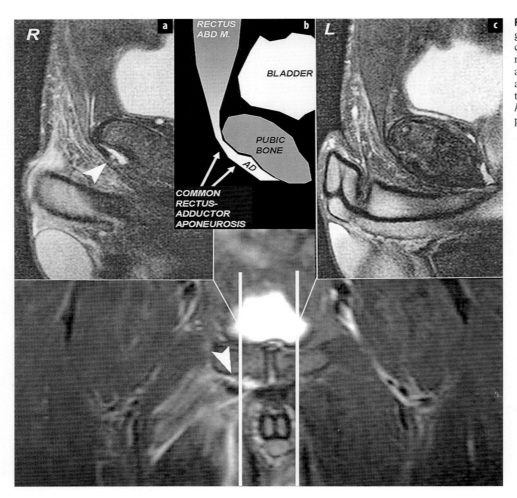

**Fig. 8 a-c.** Athletic pubalgia. Diagram (**b**) shows formation of a common aponeurosis at the attachment of the rectus abdominis and adductors. Magnetic resonance images (**a**, **c**) show a tear of the attachment on the right (**a**, *arrowheads*) in a professional baseball player with groin pain

## Bursitis

Bursitis is usually a clinical diagnosis, and MRI is only obtained after failure of conservative management to rule out other pathology. Bursitis is common at the hip and pelvis, and may be a sign of additional underlying pathology. Most tendon origins and insertions about the pelvis are associated with an anatomic bursa, and the bursa can be thought of as a window to tendon pathology. For example, when greater trochanteric bursal fluid is seen on an MRI or ultrasound, one should direct their attention to the adjacent gluteus medius tendon, which may be torn (Fig. 10) [23]. Alternatively, if the patient has a snapping hip this could be a manifestation of a tight iliotibial band resulting in snapping over the greater trochanter. Similarly, iliopsoas bursitis can be related to snapping of the tendon over a ridge at the anterior acetabulum [24, 25]. Hamstring bursitis is another common entity, and is usually related to tendinosis or tear of the tendon origin.

Bursitis may be classified by the location of involvement, or the etiology (i.e., mechanical/infectious/noninfectious inflammatory/crystalline). Additionally, osseous prominence can result in abnormal osseous apposition and acquired bursitis related to friction of the sur-

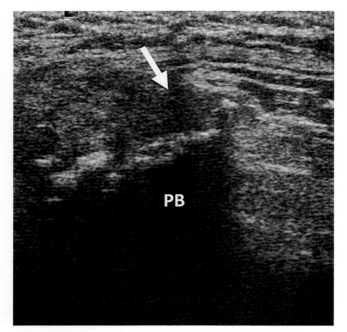

**Fig. 9.** Athletic pubalgia on ultrasound. Transverse image through the right pubis shows focal tear of the adductor origin (*arrow*). *PB* pubic bone

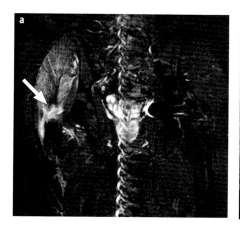

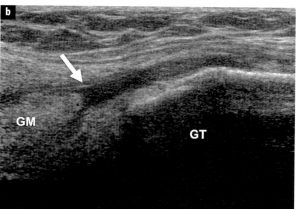

**Fig. 10 a, b.** Gluteus medius and minimus tear at the greater trochanter in a 69-year-old man with sudden onset of right lateral hip pain and inability to bear weight on the right leg. **a** Coronal STIR image of the pelvis; note: retraction of fibers (*arrow*) and associated fluid in the greater trochanteric bursa. **b** Longitudinal ultrasound image showing a tear of the gluteus minimus attachment (*arrow*). *GT* greater trochanter, *GM* gluteus minimus

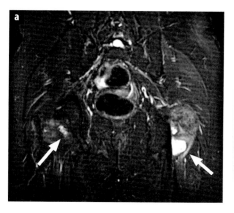

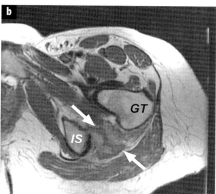

**Fig. 11 a, b.** Ischiofemoral impingement. Friction from the trochanters against the ischium can result in a painful bursitis at the interval between the structures, and this can cause pain and a palpable lump. Coronal STIR (**a**) and axial proton density (**b**) images show complex fluid in this region (*arrows*). *GT* greater trochanter, *IS* ischium

faces. For example, a prominent lesser trochanter can abut the ischium and result in posterior pain and bursitis (ischiofemoral impingement, Fig. 11) [26].

## Summary

There are numerous causes of hip, groin and buttock pain originating outside of the hip joint. Consideration should be given to these entities when evaluating patients with lower extremity pain.

## References

1. Kiuru MJ, Pihlajamaki HK, Ahovuo JA (2003) Fatigue stress injuries of the pelvic bones and proximal femur: evaluation with MR imaging. Eur Radiol 13:605-611
2. Hodnett PA, Shelly MJ, MacMahon PJ et al (2009) MR imaging of overuse injuries of the hip. Magn Reson Imaging Clin N Am 17:667-679, vi
3. La Rocca Vieira R, Rosenberg ZS et al (2012) Frequency of incomplete atypical femoral fractures in asymptomatic patients on long-term bisphosphonate therapy. AJR Am J Roentgenol 198:1144-1151
4. Anderson MW, Kaplan PA, Dussault RG (2001) Adductor insertion avulsion syndrome (thigh splints): spectrum of MR imaging features. AJR Am J Roentgenol 177:673-675
5. Buttaro M, Della Valle AG, Morandi A et al (2003) Insufficiency subchondral fracture of the femoral head: report of 4 cases and review of the literature. J Arthroplasty 18:377-382
6. Vande Berg BC, Lecouvet FE, Koutaissoff S (2008) Bone marrow edema of the femoral head and transient osteoporosis of the hip. Eur J Radiol 67:68-77
7. Rybak LD, Torriani M (2003) Magnetic resonance imaging of sports-related muscle injuries. Top Magn Reson Imaging 14:209-219
8. Steinbach LS, Fleckenstein JL, Mink JH (1994) Magnetic resonance imaging of muscle injuries. Orthopedics 17:991-999
9. Shelly MJ, Hodnett PA, MacMahon PJ et al (2009) MR imaging of muscle injury. Magn Reson Imaging Clin N Am 17:757-773, vii
10. Palmer WE, Kuong SJ, Elmadbouh HM (1999) MR imaging of myotendinous strain. AJR Am J Roentgenol 173:703-709
11. Brandser EA, el-Khoury GY, Kathol MH et al (1995) Hamstring injuries: Radiographic, conventional tomographic, CT, and MR imaging characteristics. Radiology 197:257-262
12. Hancock CR, Sanders TG, Zlatkin MB (2009) Flexor femoris muscle complex: grading systems used to describe the complete spectrum of injury. Clinical Imaging 33:130-135
13. Nikolaou PK, Macdonald BL, Glisson RR (1987) Biomechanical and histochemical evaluation of muscle after controlled strain injury. Am J Sports Med 15:9-14
14. Taylor DC, Dalton JD Jr, Seaber AV, Garrett WE Jr (1993) Experimental muscle strain injury. Early functional and structural deficits and the increased risk for reinjury. Am J Sports Med 21:190-194

15. Garrett WE Jr, Nikolaou PK, Ribbeck BM et al (1988) The effect of muscle architecture on the biomechanical failure properties of skeletal muscle under passive extension. Am J Sports Med 16:7-12

16. Hébert KJ, Laor T, Divine JG et al (2008) MRI appearance of chronic stress injury of the iliac crest apophysis in adolescent athletes. AJR Am J Roentgenol 190:1487-1491

17. Sanders TG, Zlatkin MB (2008) Avulsion injuries of the pelvis. Semin Musculoskelet Radiol 12:42-53.

18. Stevens MA, El-Khoury GY, Kathol MH et al (1999) Imaging features of avulsion injuries. Radiographics 19:655-672

19. Meyers WC, McKechnie A, Philippon MJ et al (2008) Experience with "sports hernia" spanning two decades. Ann Surg 248:656-665

20. Shortt CP, Zoga AC, Kavanagh EC, Meyers WC (2008) Anatomy, pathology, and MRI findings in the sports hernia. Semin Musculoskelet Radiol 12:54-61

21. Omar IM, Zoga AC, Kavanagh EC (2008) Athletic pubalgia and "sports hernia": optimal MR imaging technique and findings. RadioGraphics 28:1415-1438

22. Zajick DC, Zoga AC, Omar IM, Meyers WC (2008) Spectrum of MRI findings in clinical athletic pubalgia. Semin Musculoskelet Radiol 12:3-12

23. Blankenbaker DG, Ullrick SR, Davis KW (2008) Correlation of MRI findings with clinical findings of trochanteric pain syndrome. Skeletal Radiol 37:903-909

24. Blankenbaker DG, Tuite MJ (2008) Iliopsoas musculotendinous unit. Semin Musculoskelet Radiol 12:13-27

25. Janzen DL, Partridge E, Logan PM (1996) The snapping hip: clinical and imaging findings in transient subluxation of the iliopsoas tendon. Can Assoc Radiol J 47:202-208

26. Torriani M, Souto SC, Thomas BJ et al (2009) Ischiofemoral impingement syndrome: an entity with hip pain and abnormalities of the quadratus femoris muscle. AJR Am J Roentgenol 193:186-190

# Imaging of the Knee

David A. Rubin[1], Mario Maas[2]

[1] Mallinckrodt Institute of Radiology, Washington University School of Medicine, St Louis, MO, USA
[2] Musculoskeletal Section, Department of Radiology, Academic Medical Center, University of Amsterdam, Amsterdam, The Netherlands

## Imaging Modalities

Conventional radiographs are the initial imaging study in most suspected knee disorders. A minimum radiographic examination consists of an anteroposterior (AP) and lateral projection. For the early detection of articular cartilage loss, a posteroanterior (PA) radiograph of both knees with the patient standing and knees mildly flexed (the Rosenberg projection) is a useful adjunct: a joint space difference of 2 mm side-to-side correlates with grade III and higher chondrosis [1]. In patients with anterior knee symptoms, an axial projection of the patellofemoral joint, such as a Merchant view, can evaluate the patellofemoral joint space and alignment [2].

Sonography is largely limited to evaluation of the extra-articular soft tissues of the knee, but, with careful technique, at least partial visualization of the synovium and ligaments is also possible [3]. Ultrasound is most commonly used to evaluate the patellar tendon, popliteal (Baker's) cysts and other fluid-containing structures [4, 5].

Computed tomography (CT) is useful for evaluation of intra-articular fractures about the knee, for planning complex orthopedic procedures, and for postoperative evaluation. Typically, images are reformatted into orthogonal planes and/or three-dimensional (3D) surface projections [6]. An advantage of CT over magnetic resonance imaging (MRI) is the ability to acquire images of both knees simultaneously, to compare symmetry and use the normal knee as a control. To facilitate multiplanar reconstructions, CT is best done with multidetector-row helical acquisitions and thin collimation (submillimeter, if possible) [7]. Combining helical CT with arthrography makes it a viable examination for the detection of internal derangements, including meniscal and articular cartilage abnormalities, typically when there is a contraindication to MRI [8-10].

MRI is the most sensitive, noninvasive test for bone and soft tissue disorders in and around the knee. MRI provides information that can be used to grade pathology, guide therapy, prognosticate conditions, and evaluate treatment for a wide variety of orthopedic conditions in the knee. Multiple studies have found that MRI can be cost effective when used as a triage tool in the evaluation of patients with selected acute and nonacute presentations, and in patients in whom arthroscopy is planned [11-14]. Magnetic resonance (MR) arthrography following the direct intra-articular injection of gadolinium-based contrast agents can increase accuracy in the postoperative knee, improve staging of chondral and osteochondral infractions, and facilitate discovery of intra-articular loose bodies [15-17].

High-quality knee MRI can be performed with high-field or low-field systems including those with open, closed or dedicated-extremity designs, as long as proper technique is followed [18-20]. A local (extremity) coil encircling only the knee of interest is mandatory to maximize signal-to-noise ratio [21]. Images are acquired in transverse, coronal and sagittal planes, with some studies suggesting that oblique imaging planes may be useful in selected circumstances [22, 23]. A combination of different pulse sequences, which can be spin-echo, fast spin-echo or gradient-recalled echo, provides tissue contrast. T1-weighted images demonstrate hemorrhage, as well as abnormalities of bone marrow, and extra-articular structures that are surrounded by fat [24, 25]. Proton-density-weighted (long TR, short effective-TE) sequences are best for imaging the menisci [26]. T2 or T2*-weighted images are used for the evaluation of abnormalities of the muscles, tendons, ligaments and articular cartilage [27, 28]. Suppressing the signal from fat increases the sensitivity for detecting marrow and soft tissue edema on water-sensitive sequences [29, 30]; some practices also add fat suppression to the proton density weighted sequences, but this practice does not appear to increase the accuracy of the examination for meniscal tears [29]. 3D acquisitions can provide supplemental imaging of articular cartilage [31-34], or provide isotropic images for multiplanar reconstruction of other tissues [35-37]. To visualize the critical structures in the knee, standard MRI should be done with a field-of-view no greater than 16 cm, 3 or

J. Hodler et al. (eds.), *Musculoskeletal Diseases 2013-2016*,
DOI: 10.1007/978-88-470-5292-5_8 © Springer-Verlag Italia 2013

4 mm slice thickness, and imaging matrices of at least 256 × 256. Depending on the MR system and coil design, in order to achieve this spatial resolution with adequate signal-to-noise, optimizing other parameters, such as the number of signals averaged and the receiver bandwidth, is necessary [21].

## Specific Disorders: Bone, Marrow and Articular Cartilage

Bone pathology in the knee encompasses a spectrum of traumatic, reactive, ischemic, infectious and neoplastic conditions. Radiographs, CT, scintigraphy and MRI each have a diagnostic role for these disorders.

### Trauma

Most fractures are visible radiographically. For tibial plateau fractures, the amount of depression and the articular surface congruence determine the treatment and prognosis; CT with multiplanar reconstructions [6] or MRI can be used for this purpose [38]. MR examination can not only show the number and position of fracture planes, but also demonstrates associate soft tissue lesions, such as meniscus and ligament tears, that often affect surgical planning [39, 40]. Fractures of the intercondylar eminence and spines of the tibia often involve the cruciate ligament attachments [41]. Other avulsion fractures may signal serious ligament disruptions. For example, a (Segond) fracture of the lateral tibial is a strong predictor of anterior cruciate ligament disruption [42, 43], while an avulsion of the medial head of the fibula (arcuate fracture) indicates a posterolateral corner injury [43, 44].

Bone scintigraphy, CT and MRI are all sensitive to radiographically occult fractures. A positive bone scan, however, is nonspecific, and when a fracture is present, scintigraphy does not show the number and position of fracture lines, and this impacts treatment. For these reasons, CT and MR have largely replaced bone scanning for occult fractures. MR probably has an advantage over CT because, when there is no fracture present, MR shows more of the soft tissue injuries that may clinically mimic an occult fracture. Additionally, unlike bone scintigraphy and CT, MR does not contribute to the patient's radiation dose. Non-fat-suppressed, T1-weighted images best demonstrate fracture lines, where they appear as very low-signal intensity linear or stellate lines surrounded by marrow edema. On gradient-recalled, proton-density-weighted and non-fat-suppressed T2-weighted images, fractures lines and marrow edema are often not visible. Marrow edema is most conspicuous on fat-suppressed T2-weighted or short tau inversion recovery (STIR) images, but the amount of edema may obscure underlying fracture lines.

In children, injuries to the ends of the long bones are usually osteochondral, while in adults they may be purely chondral. Osteochondral defects are visible radiographically, but MRI is used to stage these lesions [45]. In skeletally mature patients, a thin line of fluid-intensity

signal surrounding the base of the fragment (on T2-weighted images) combined with disruption of the articular surface indicates an unstable lesion [46]. Similarly, cysts in the base of the crater or an empty crater also predict fragment instability [47]. In skeletally immature knees, the same criteria are not as specific. Before the physes close, a diagnosis of fragment instability requires a distinct cleavage plane at the base of a lesion in combination with disruption of the subchondral plate, or the presence of large or multiple bone cysts [48, 49]. For equivocal cases, direct MR arthrography may be useful: injected contrast tracking around the base of the lesion indicates a loose, in situ fragment [10, 50].

Chondral injuries in the knee mimic meniscal tears clinically. Arthroscopy, MRI with or without arthrography, or CT arthrography can show these injuries [51]. Fast spin-echo sequences, with intermediate-to-long TE values, or spoiled gradient-echo sequences are needed to demonstrate contrast between articular cartilage and joint fluid [52]. Arthrographic images show contrast filling a defect in the articular cartilage. A focus of overlying subchondral edema may be a clue to subtle chondral defects [53]. Most traumatic cartilage injuries are full-thickness and have sharp, vertically-oriented walls (unlike degenerative cartilage lesions, which may be partial-thickness or full-thickness with sloped walls). Occasionally, focal delamination will occur without extension to the articular surface [54].

Stress fractures, whether of the fatigue or insufficiency type, are initially radiographically occult, but can be detected with either bone scintigraphy or MRI [55]. Like the case for traumatic fractures, MR images show a low signal intensity fracture line surrounded by a larger region of marrow edema. The proximal tibia is a common location for insufficiency fractures, especially in elderly, osteoporotic patients. Subchondral insufficiency fractures also occur in the femoral condyles, frequently associated with tears of the posterior meniscal roots and/or osteoarthritis [56-58].

The term "bone bruise" or "bone contusion" describes trabecular microfractures due to impaction, which can be due to external blunt force trauma, or more commonly from two bones striking each other after ligament injuries. Bone bruises appear as reticulated, ill-defined regions in the marrow isointense to muscle on T1-weighted images and hyperintense on fat-suppressed T2-weighted or STIR images [30, 59]. Granulation tissue and fibrosis dominate the histologic appearance of this "bone marrow edema pattern" [60]. Bone bruises are an important clue to the mechanism of injury, can contribute to a patient's pain, and may prognosticate eventual cartilage degeneration [61, 62]. However, the radiologist should avoid the temptation to label any area of marrow edema as a "bone bruise," a term reserved for instances where there is good clinical or imaging evidence of trauma. The bone marrow edema pattern is nonspecific, seen in a variety of other ischemic, reactive, neoplastic and infectious conditions, as well as following injuries.

## Ischemia and Infarction

Marrow infarcts result from a variety of insults including endogenous and exogenous steroids, collagen vascular diseases, alcoholism and hemoglobinopathies. An idiopathic form also occurs in the femoral condyles [63, 64], although many cases that were designated as spontaneous osteonecrosis in the past likely represent subchondral insufficiency fractures [56, 57]. True subchondral infarcts (termed osteonecrosis, avascular necrosis or AVN) can lead to formation of a subchondral crescent and articular surface collapse. Established infarcts have a serpiginous, sclerotic margin. On MR images, infarctions initially appear as geographic areas of abnormal marrow signal. As an infarct evolves, a peripheral reactive margin becomes visible, often with a pathognomonic double-line sign on T2-weighted images: a low signal intensity zone surrounded by a parallel high signal intensity line [65, 66].

## Replacement

The most common marrow alteration encountered around the knee is hyperplastic red marrow. This can be seen in physiologic conditions caused by anemia, obesity and cigarette smoking, as well as in athletes and persons living at high altitudes [67, 68]. Unlike the case for pathologic marrow replacement, the signal intensity of expanded hematopoietic marrow is isointense to muscle, foci of residual yellow marrow separate islands of red marrow islands, and the process spares the epiphyses. However, in extreme cases, such as due to hemolytic anemia, the hyperplastic marrow will partially or completely replace the epiphyseal marrow [69].

Other alterations in marrow composition are less common, but relatively characteristic in their MR appearances. Irradiated and aplastic marrow may be entirely yellow marrow [70]. Fibrotic marrow is low in signal intensity on all pulse sequences, and marrow in patients with hemosiderosis shows near complete absence of signal [71].

## Destruction

Tumors and infections destroy the trabecular and/or cortical bone, and infiltrate the bone marrow. In subacute and chronic osteomyelitis, the primary role of cross-sectional imaging is to stage infection. For example, CT is useful for surgical planning to identify a sequestrum or foreign body [72], while MRI can show soft tissue abscesses and assess the viability of the infected bone (with the use of intravenous contrast). On MR images, acute osteomyelitis demonstrates the marrow edema pattern, but a specific diagnosis of osteomyelitis requires demonstrating cortical destruction, or an adjacent soft tissue abscess, sinus tract or ulcer (at least in adults, where direct inoculation is much more common than hematogenous spread of infection) [73, 74].

Both benign and malignant bone neoplasms occur commonly around the knee. Radiographs should be the initial imaging study in these patients, and are essential to identify mineralized matrix and predict the biologic behavior. The intraosseous extent of tumor and the presence and type of matrix are easiest to asses with CT examination. For staging beyond the bone (into the surrounding soft tissues, as skip lesions to other parts of the same bone, and to regional nodes), MR or CT are approximately equally effective [75]. The radiologist should have a high index of suspicion when encountering unexpected bone findings in MR studies that were requested to evaluate athletic injuries or for internal derangements; it is not unusual for a bone tumor to occur as an incidental finding or to be misinterpreted as an injury in these patients [76-78].

## Degeneration

Chondrosis (or chondropathy) refers to degeneration of articular cartilage. With progressive cartilage erosion, radiographs show the typical findings of osteoarthritis, namely nonuniform joint space narrowing and osteophyte formation. Earlier diagnosis requires direct visualization of articular cartilage. While CT arthrography using dilute contrast can show areas of degeneration [9, 79], MRI is the most commonly used imaging modality to examine degenerated cartilage.

On standard MR sequences, internal signal intensity changes do not reliably correlate with cartilage degeneration [80, 81]. Seeing joint fluid (or injected contrast) within chondral defects along the joint surface is more accurate [82]. The most commonly used MR sequences are long-TR, fast spin-echo (intermediate-weighted or T2-weighted) sequences with or without fat suppression [28, 32, 83]. Some practices use 3D volume acquisitions using gradient-echo-recalled or fast spin-echo sequences to achieve thinner sections [31, 84, 85]. MR arthrography uses T1-weighted sequences [86]. Reactive marrow edema in the subjacent bone (analogous to the subchondral uptake seen on bone scans) is often associated with deep chondral defects. These subchondral marrow lesions can be a clue alerting the radiologist to the presence of cartilage degeneration, may be associated with clinical symptoms, and have prognostic value in predicting progression of osteoarthritis [87-89]. Newer quantitative MR techniques, including T2-mapping, delayed gadolinium-enhanced MRI of cartilage (dGEMRIC), ultra-short TE, diffusion, sodium and T1-rho imaging, are often used as research tools for the interrogation of the different constituents of articular cartilage [90], but their added value for routine clinical use is not yet certain.

## Specific Disorders: Soft Tissues

MRI is the imaging study of choice for most soft tissue conditions in and around the knee. Ultrasound can also visualize relatively superficial structures.

## Menisci

The fibrocartilagenous menisci distribute the load of the femur on the tibia, and function as shock absorbers. There are two criteria for meniscal tears on MR images. The first is intrameniscal signal on a short-TE (typically proton density weighted) image that unequivocally contacts an articular surface of the meniscus, ideally on two or more images [91]. Intrameniscal signal that only equivocally touches the meniscal surface is no more likely torn than a meniscus containing no internal signal [92, 93]. The second criterion is abnormal meniscal shape [26]. The normal menisci in cross-section are triangular or bow tie shaped, with sharp inner margins. Any variation from the normal shape, other than in discoid menisci or following partial meniscectomy, represents a meniscal tear.

The radiologist should describe the features of each identified meniscal tear that may affect treatment. These properties include the location of the tear (medial or lateral; anterior horn, body, posterior horn or roots; periphery or inner margin), the shape of the tear (longitudinal, horizontal, radial or complex), the approximate length of the tear, the completeness of the tear (whether it extends partly or completely through the meniscus), and the presence of associated meniscal cysts. Special attention to tears of the posterior meniscal roots is important, as these tears greatly affect biomechanics, predisposing the compartment to articular cartilage degeneration, subchondral insufficiency fractures and osteonecrosis. For root tears, the posterior coronal images will show a radial defect in the meniscus, while sagittal images can demonstrate an absent ("ghost") segment of the meniscus [94-96]. Displaced meniscal fragments, which commonly occur in the intercondylar notch or outer gutters, also affect arthroscopic management [97, 98].

Like any study, MRI is not perfect for diagnosing meniscal tears. Sensitivity is lower for lateral meniscal tears, while specificity is lower for medial meniscal tears [99, 100]. Although some incorrect diagnoses are due to observer error or failure to recognize normal variants and anatomy [101], others are unavoidable. Examples include "false-positive" MR diagnoses of peripheral longitudinal medial meniscal tears that heal spontaneously by the time of arthroscopy, and false-negative diagnoses of stable posterior horn lateral meniscus tears in knees with torn anterior cruciate ligaments [102, 103].

A meniscal tear that heals spontaneously or following surgical repair will frequently still show intrameniscal signal on short-TE images contacting the meniscal surface. When there is a displaced meniscal fragment or when this finding occurs in a new location, the radiologist can confidently diagnose a recurrent meniscal tear [104]. MR or CT examination performed after direct intra-articular contrast injection is useful in uncertain cases. Visualizing injected contrast within the substance of a repaired meniscus is diagnostic of a recurrent or residual tear [17, 105]. Diagnosis is more difficult after partial meniscectomy, where both the meniscal shape and internal signal are un-

reliable signs. Again, MR arthrography is the most useful noninvasive test for diagnosing recurrent meniscal tears following partial meniscectomy [16, 106].

## Ligaments

T2-weighted images demonstrate ruptures of the cruciate and collateral ligaments, and the patellofemoral retinacula [107]. Both long-axis and cross-sectional images are important to examine. The direct sign of a ligament tear is partial or complete disruption of the ligament fibers [108]. While edema typically surrounds acutely torn ligaments, edema enveloping an intact ligament is nonspecific, present in bursitis and other soft tissue conditions [109]. Chronic ligament tears have a more varied appearance. Nonvisualization of any ligament fibers or abnormal orientation of the scarred ligament fibers may be the only MR signs [110]. Secondary findings of ligament tears, such as bone contusions and joint subluxation, are useful when present, but do not supplant the primary findings, and do not reliably distinguish acute from chronic injuries [111].

Mucoid ligament degeneration sometimes occurs with aging. The anterior cruciate ligament is most often affected. MR images show high-signal intensity amorphous material between the intact ligament fibers on T2-weighted images [112]. The ligament may appear enlarged in cross-section, and often there is associated intraosseous cyst formation near the ligament attachment points [113]. Degenerated ligaments are stable and do not require surgical intervention [114], and so should be distinguished from torn ligaments.

## Muscles and Tendons

The muscles around the knee are susceptible to strains due to eccentric (stretching) injuries. On MRI, a strain demonstrates edema centered at the myotendinous junction, with partial or complete disruption of the tendon from the muscle in more severe cases [115]. Strains commonly involve the distal quadriceps, proximal gastrocnemius, soleus and popliteus muscles.

Chronic overuse results in degeneration or "tendonopathy." While tendonopathy can be painful or asymptomatic, it weakens tendons, placing them at risk of rupture. The condition affects the patellar, quadriceps and distal semimembranosus tendons around the knee. Sonographically, a degenerated tendon appears enlarged, with loss of the normal parallel fiber architecture, focal hypoechoic or hyperechoic regions, or regions of increased Doppler flow. However, hypoechoic and hypervascular zones by themselves do not correlate with symptoms, and if seen in asymptomatic athletes, do not prognosticate later disease [116, 117]. A gap between the tendon fibers indicates that the process has progressed to partial or complete tear [118]. Similarly, on MR images focal or diffuse enlargement of a tendon with loss of its sharp margins, with or without foci of high signal intensity on T2-weighted images indicates tendonopathy [4, 119]. Partial or complete fiber disruption represents a tendon tear on MRI [120]. When macroscopic tearing is present, the radiologist should also examine the corresponding muscle belly for fatty atrophy (which indicates chronicity) or edema (suggesting a more acute rupture). If a tear is complete, the retracted stump should be located on the images as well. These last two tasks may require repositioning of the MR coil.

## Synovium

Fluid distention of a synovial structure has water attenuation on CT images, signal isointense to fluid on MR images, and is hypoechoic or anechoic with enhanced through transmission on ultrasound images. All imaging modalities easily show popliteal or Baker's cysts, which represent distention of the posteromedial semimembranosus-gastrocnemius recess of the knee [5, 121]. At least 11 other named bursae occur around the knee. The most commonly diseased ones are probably the prepatellar, superficial infrapatellar, pes anserinus and semimembranosus-tibial collateral ligament bursae [122-124].

Synovitis due to infection, trauma, inflammatory arthritis or crystal disease is readily identifiable in the knee on both ultrasound and MR images. Power Doppler ultrasound or the use of ultrasound contrast agents may increase sensitivity for active synovitis [125]. On MR examination, thickening of the usually imperceptibly thin synovial membrane or enhancement of the synovium following intravenous contrast administration indicates active synovitis [126-128].

In juvenile idiopathic arthritis, synovitis represents the principle pathological process, which can be most sensitively evaluated with MRI [129]. The inflamed synovial membrane is thickened, irregular and can have wavy outlines. The signal intensity of this hypertrophic synovial membrane is low to intermediate on T1-weighted images and high on T2-weighted images, similar to joint effusion [130]. To provide an optimal discrimination between synovium and joint effusion, obtaining MR images following intravenous administration of a gadolinium-based contrast is essential [131].

Synovial metaplasia and neoplasia are uncommon. In the knee, primary synovial osteochondromatosis appears as multiple cartilaginous bodies within the joint on MR images, or on radiographs or CT when the bodies are calcified [132]. Diffuse pigmented villonodular synovitis and focal nodular synovitis demonstrate proliferative synovium, which enhances following contrast administration [133, 134]. Hemosiderin deposition in the synovium, which demonstrates very low signal on all MR pulse sequences with blooming on gradient-echo images, is an important, though inconstant, clue to these diagnoses [135].

## References

1. Rosenberg TD, Paulos LE, Parker RD et al (1988) The forty-five-degree posteroanterior flexion weight-bearing radiograph of the knee. The Journal of Bone and Joint Surgery American Volume 70:1479-1483
2. Jones AC, Ledingham J, McAlindon T et al (1993) Radiographic assessment of patellofemoral osteoarthritis. Annals of the Rheumatic Diseases 52:655-658
3. Bouffard JA, Dhanju J (1998) Ultrasonography of the knee. Seminars in Musculoskeletal Radiology 2:245-270
4. Khan KM, Bonar F, Desmond PM et al (1996) Patellar tendinosis (jumper's knee): findings at histopathologic examination, US, and MR imaging. Victorian Institute of Sport Tendon Study Group. Radiology 200:821-827
5. Ward EE, Jacobson JA, Fessell DP et al (2001) Sonographic detection of Baker's cysts: comparison with MR imaging. AJR Am J Roentgenol 176:373-380
6. Wicky S, Blaser PF, Blanc CH et al (2000) Comparison between standard radiography and spiral CT with 3D reconstruction in the evaluation, classification and management of tibial plateau fractures. European Radiology 10:1227-1232
7. Buckwalter KA, Farber JM (2004) Application of multidetector CT in skeletal trauma. Seminars in Musculoskeletal Radiology 8:147-156
8. Mutschler C, Vande Berg BC, Lecouvet FE et al (2003) Postoperative meniscus: assessment at dual-detector row spiral CT arthrography of the knee. Radiology 228:635-641
9. Vande Berg BC, Lecouvet FE, Poilvache P et al (2002) Assessment of knee cartilage in cadavers with dual-detector spiral CT arthrography and MR imaging. Radiology 222:430-436
10. Kalke RJ, Di Primio GA, Schweitzer ME (2012) MR and CT arthrography of the knee. Seminars in Musculoskeletal Radiology 16:57-68
11. Bui-Mansfield LT, Youngberg RA, Warme W et al (1997) Potential cost savings of MR imaging obtained before arthroscopy of the knee: evaluation of 50 consecutive patients. AJR Am J Roentgenol 168:913-918
12. Vincken PW, ter Braak BP, van Erkell AR et al (2002) Effectiveness of MR imaging in selection of patients for arthroscopy of the knee. Radiology 223:739-746
13. Vincken PW, ter Braak AP, van Erkel AR et al (2007) MR imaging: effectiveness and costs at triage of patients with nonacute knee symptoms. Radiology 242:85-93
14. Oei EH, Nikken JJ, Ginai AZ et al (2009) Costs and effectiveness of a brief MRI examination of patients with acute knee injury. European Radiology 19:409-418
15. Chung CB, Isaza IL, Angulo M et al (2005) MR arthrography of the knee: how, why, when. Radiologic Clinics of North America 43:733-746, viii-ix
16. Ciliz D, Ciliz A, Elverici E et al (2008) Evaluation of postoperative menisci with MR arthrography and routine conventional MRI. Clinical Imaging 32:212-219
17. Cardello P, Gigli C, Ricci A et al (2009) Retears of postoperative knee meniscus: findings on magnetic resonance imaging (MRI) and magnetic resonance arthrography (MRA) by using low and high field magnets. Skeletal Radiology 38:149-156
18. Barnett MJ (1993) MR diagnosis of internal derangements of the knee: effect of field strength on efficacy. AJR Am J Roentgenol 161:115-118
19. Kinnunen J, Bondestam S, Kivioja A et al (1994) Diagnostic performance of low field MRI in acute knee injuries. Magnetic Resonance Imaging 12:1155-1160
20. Magee T (2007) Three-Tesla MR imaging of the knee. Radiologic Clinics of North America 45:1055-1062, vii
21. Rubin DA, Kneeland JB (1994) MR imaging of the musculoskeletal system: technical considerations for enhancing image quality and diagnostic yield. AJR Am J Roentgenol 163:1155-1163
22. Buckwalter KA, Pennes DR (1990) Anterior cruciate ligament: oblique sagittal MR imaging. Radiology 175:276-277
23. Yu JS, Salonen DC, Hodler J et al (1996) Posterolateral aspect of the knee: improved MR imaging with a coronal oblique technique. Radiology 198:199-204

24. Vande Berg BC, Malghem J, Lecouvet FE, Maldague B (1998) Classification and detection of bone marrow lesions with magnetic resonance imaging. Skeletal Radiology 27:529-545

25. Bush CH (2000) The magnetic resonance imaging of musculoskeletal hemorrhage. Skeletal Radiology 29:1-9

26. Rubin DA, Paletta GA, Jr (2000) Current concepts and controversies in meniscal imaging. Magnetic Resonance Imaging Clinics of North America 8:243-270

27. Ha TP, Li KC, Beaulieu CF et al (1998) Anterior cruciate ligament injury: fast spin-echo MR imaging with arthroscopic correlation in 217 examinations. AJR Am J Roentgenol 170:1215-1219

28. Sonin AH, Pensy RA, Mulligan ME, Hatem S (2002) Grading articular cartilage of the knee using fast spin-echo proton density-weighted MR imaging without fat suppression. AJR Am J Roentgenol 179:1159-1166

29. Lee SY, Jee WH, Kim SK, Kim JM (2011) Proton density-weighted MR imaging of the knee: fat suppression versus without fat suppression. Skeletal Radiology 40:189-195

30. Kapelov SR, Teresi LM, Bradley WG et al (1993) Bone contusions of the knee: increased lesion detection with fast spin-echo MR imaging with spectroscopic fat saturation. Radiology 189:901-904

31. Kijowski R, Blankenbaker DG, Woods M et al (2011) Clinical usefulness of adding 3D cartilage imaging sequences to a routine knee MR protocol. AJR Am J Roentgenol 196:159-167

32. Lee SY, Jee WH, Kim SK et al (2010) Differentiation between grade 3 and grade 4 articular cartilage defects of the knee: fat-suppressed proton density-weighted versus fat-suppressed three-dimensional gradient-echo MRI. Acta Radiol 51:455-461

33. Friedrich KM, Reiter G, Kaiser B et al (2011) High-resolution cartilage imaging of the knee at 3T: basic evaluation of modern isotropic 3D MR-sequences. European Journal of Radiology 78:398-405

34. Ai T, Zhang W, Priddy NK, Li X (2012) Diagnostic performance of CUBE MRI sequences of the knee compared with conventional MRI. Clinical Radiology 67:e58-63

35. Jung JY, Jee WH, Park MY et al (2012) Meniscal tear configurations: categorization with 3D isotropic turbo spin-echo MRI compared with conventional MRI at 3 T. AJR Am J Roentgenol 198:W173-180

36. Ren AH, Zheng ZZ, Shang Y, Tian CY (2012). An anatomical study of normal meniscal roots with isotropic 3D MRI at 3T. European Journal of Radiology 81:e783-788

37. Subhas N, Kao A, Freire M et al (2011) MRI of the knee ligaments and menisci: comparison of isotropic-resolution 3D and conventional 2D fast spin-echo sequences at 3 T. AJR Am J Roentgenol 197:442-450

38. Yacoubian SV, Nevins RT, Sallis JG et al (2002) Impact of MRI on treatment plan and fracture classification of tibial plateau fractures. Journal of Orthopaedic Trauma 16:632-637

39. Mustonen AO, Koivikko MP, Lindahl J, Koskinen SK (2008) MRI of acute meniscal injury associated with tibial plateau fractures: prevalence, type, and location. AJR Am J Roentgenol 191:1002-1009

40. Mui LW, Engelsohn E, Umans H (2007) Comparison of CT and MRI in patients with tibial plateau fracture: can CT findings predict ligament tear or meniscal injury? Skeletal Radiology 36:145-151

41. Prince JS, Laor T, Bean JA (2005) MRI of anterior cruciate ligament injuries and associated findings in the pediatric knee: changes with skeletal maturation. AJR Am J Roentgenol 185:756-762

42. Campos JC, Chung CB, Lektrakul N et al (2001) Pathogenesis of the Segond fracture: anatomic and MR imaging evidence of an iliotibial tract or anterior oblique band avulsion. Radiology 219:381-386

43. Huang GS, Yu JS, Munshi M et al (2003) Avulsion fracture of the head of the fibula (the "arcuate" sign): MR imaging findings predictive of injuries to the posterolateral ligaments and posterior cruciate ligament. AJR Am J Roentgenol 180:381-387

44. Lee J, Papakonstantinou O, Brookenthal KR et al (2003) Arcuate sign of posterolateral knee injuries: anatomic, radiographic, and MR imaging data related to patterns of injury. Skeletal Radiology 32:619-627

45. Quatman CE, Quatman-Yates CC, Schmitt LC, Paterno MV (2012) The clinical utility and diagnostic performance of MRI for identification and classification of knee osteochondritis dissecans. The Journal of Bone and Joint Surgery American 94:1036-1044

46. O'Connor MA, Palaniappan M, Khan N, Bruce CE (2002) Osteochondritis dissecans of the knee in children. A comparison of MRI and arthroscopic findings. The Journal of Bone and Joint Surgery British 84:258-262

47. De Smet AA, Ilahi OA, Graf BK (1996) Reassessment of the MR criteria for stability of osteochondritis dissecans in the knee and ankle. Skeletal Radiology 25:159-163

48. Kijowski R, Blankenbaker DG, Shinki K et al (2008) Juvenile versus adult osteochondritis dissecans of the knee: appropriate MR imaging criteria for instability. Radiology 248:571-578

49. Wall EJ, Vourazeris J, Myer GD et al (2008) The healing potential of stable juvenile osteochondritis dissecans knee lesions. The Journal of Bone and Joint Surgery American 90:2655-2664

50. Kramer J, Stiglbauer R, Engel A et al (1992) MR contrast arthrography (MRA) in osteochondrosis dissecans. Journal of Computer Assisted Tomography 16:254-260

51. Hughes RJ, Houlihan-Burne DG (2011) Clinical and MRI considerations in sports-related knee joint cartilage injury and cartilage repair. Seminars in Musculoskeletal Radiology 15:69-88

52. Kim CW, Jaramillo D, Hresko MT (1997) MRI demonstration of occult purely chondral fractures of the tibia: a potential mimic of meniscal tears. Pediatric Radiology 27:765-766

53. Rubin DA, Harner CD, Costello JM (2000) Treatable chondral injuries in the knee: frequency of associated focal subchondral edema. AJR Am J Roentgenol 174:1099-1106

54. Kendell SD, Helms CA, Rampton JW et al (2005) MRI appearance of chondral delamination injuries of the knee. AJR Am J Roentgenol 184:1486-1489

55. Spitz DJ, Newberg AH (2002) Imaging of stress fractures in the athlete. Radiologic Clinics of North America 40:313-331

56. Ramnath RR, Kattapuram SV (2004) MR appearance of SONK-like subchondral abnormalities in the adult knee: SONK redefined. Skeletal Radiology 33:575-581

57. Yao L, Stanczak J, Boutin RD (2004) Presumptive subarticular stress reactions of the knee: MRI detection and association with meniscal tear patterns. Skeletal Radiology 33:260-264

58. Karantanas AH, Drakonaki E, Karachalios T et al (2008) Acute non-traumatic marrow edema syndrome in the knee: MRI findings at presentation, correlation with spinal DEXA and outcome. European Journal of Radiology 67:22-33

59. Arndt WF 3rd, Truax AL, Barnett FM et al (1996) MR diagnosis of bone contusions of the knee: comparison of coronal T2-weighted fast spin-echo with fat saturation and fast spin-echo STIR images with conventional STIR images. AJR Am J Roentgenol 166:119-124

60. Zanetti M, Bruder E, Romero J, Hodler J (2000) Bone marrow edema pattern in osteoarthritic knees: correlation between MR imaging and histologic findings. Radiology 215:835-840

61. Sanders TG, Medynski MA, Feller JF, Lawhorn KW (2000) Bone contusion patterns of the knee at MR imaging: footprint of the mechanism of injury. Radiographics 20:S135-151

62. Boks SS, Vroegindeweij D, Koes BW et al (2007) MRI follow-up of posttraumatic bone bruises of the knee in general practice. AJR Am J Roentgenol 189:556-562

63. Marti CB, Rodriguez M, Zanetti M, Romero J (2000) Spontaneous osteonecrosis of the medial compartment of the knee: a MRI follow-up after conservative and operative treatment, pre-

liminary results. Knee Surgery, Sports Traumatology, Arthroscopy 8:83-88

64. Yates PJ, Calder JD, Stranks GJ et al (2007) Early MRI diagnosis and non-surgical management of spontaneous osteonecrosis of the knee. The Knee 14:112-116

65. Mitchell DG, Rao VM, Dalinka MK et al (1987) Femoral head avascular necrosis: correlation of MR imaging, radiographic staging, radionuclide imaging, and clinical findings. Radiology 162:709-715

66. Karimova EJ, Rai SN, Ingle D et al (2006) MRI of knee osteonecrosis in children with leukemia and lymphoma: Part 2, clinical and imaging patterns. AJR Am J Roentgenol 186:477-482

67. Deutsch AL, Mink JH, Rosenfelt FP, Waxman AD (1989) Incidental detection of hematopoietic hyperplasia on routine knee MR imaging. AJR Am J Roentgenol 152:333-336

68. Shellock FG, Morris E, Deutsch AL et al (1992) Hematopoietic bone marrow hyperplasia: high prevalence on MR images of the knee in asymptomatic marathon runners. AJR Am J Roentgenol 158:335-338

69. Rao VM, Mitchell DG, Rifkin MD et al (1989) Marrow infarction in sickle cell anemia: correlation with marrow type and distribution by MRI. Magnetic Resonance Imaging 7:39-44

70. Remedios PA, Colletti PM, Raval JK et al (1988) Magnetic resonance imaging of bone after radiation. Magnetic Resonance Imaging 6:301-304

71. Lanir A, Aghai E, Simon JS et al (1986) MR imaging in myelofibrosis. Journal of Computer Assisted Tomography 10:634-636

72. Hernandez RJ (1985) Visualization of small sequestra by computerized tomography. Report of 6 cases. Pediatric Radiology 15:238-241

73. Erdman WA, Tamburro F, Jayson HT et al (1991) Osteomyelitis: characteristics and pitfalls of diagnosis with MR imaging. Radiology 180:533-539

74. Bancroft LW (2007) MR imaging of infectious processes of the knee. Radiologic Clinics of North America 45:931-941, v

75. Panicek DM, Gatsonis C, Rosenthal DI et al (1997) CT and MR imaging in the local staging of primary malignant musculoskeletal neoplasms: Report of the Radiology Diagnostic Oncology Group. Radiology 202:237-246

76. Stacy GS, Heck RK, Peabody TD, Dixon LB (2002) Neoplastic and tumorlike lesions detected on MR imaging of the knee in patients with suspected internal derangement: Part I, intraosseous entities. AJR Am J Roentgenol 178:589-594

77. Kransdorf MJ, Peterson JJ, Bancroft LW (2007) MR imaging of the knee: incidental osseous lesions. Radiologic Clinics of North America 45:943-954, v

78. Muscolo DL, Ayerza MA, Makino A et al (2003) Tumors about the knee misdiagnosed as athletic injuries. The Journal of Bone and Joint Surgery American 85-A:1209-1214

79. Li J, Zheng ZZ, Li X, Yu JK (2009) Three dimensional assessments of knee cartilage in cadavers with high resolution MR-arthrography and MSCT-arthrography. Academic Radiology 16:1049-1055

80. Brown TR, Quinn SF (1993) Evaluation of chondromalacia of the patellofemoral compartment with axial magnetic resonance imaging. Skeletal Radiology 22:325-328

81. Disler DG, McCauley TR, Wirth CR, Fuchs MD (1995) Detection of knee hyaline cartilage defects using fat-suppressed three-dimensional spoiled gradient-echo MR imaging: comparison with standard MR imaging and correlation with arthroscopy. AJR Am J Roentgenol 165:377-382

82. Gagliardi JA, Chung EM, Chandnani VP et al (1994) Detection and staging of chondromalacia patellae: relative efficacies of conventional MR imaging, MR arthrography, and CT arthrography. AJR Am J Roentgenol 163:629-636

83. Kijowski R, Blankenbaker DG, Davis KW et al (2009) Comparison of 1.5- and 3.0-T MR imaging for evaluating the articular cartilage of the knee joint. Radiology 250:839-848

84. Gold GE, Hargreaves BA, Vasanawala SS et al (2006) Articular cartilage of the knee: evaluation with fluctuating equilibrium MR imaging—initial experience in healthy volunteers. Radiology 238:712-718

85. Kijowski R, Davis KW, Woods MA et al (2009) Knee joint: comprehensive assessment with 3D isotropic resolution fast spin-echo MR imaging—diagnostic performance compared with that of conventional MR imaging at 3.0 T. Radiology 252:486-495

86. Mathieu L, Bouchard A, Marchaland JP et al (2009) Knee MR-arthrography in assessment of meniscal and chondral lesions. Orthopaedics & Traumatology, Surgery & Research 95:40-47

87. Roemer FW, Guermazi A, Javaid MK et al (2009) Change in MRI-detected subchondral bone marrow lesions is associated with cartilage loss: the MOST Study. A longitudinal multicentre study of knee osteoarthritis. Annals of the Rheumatic Diseases 68:1461-1465

88. Dore D, Quinn S, Ding C et al (2010) Natural history and clinical significance of MRI-detected bone marrow lesions at the knee: a prospective study in community dwelling older adults. Arthritis Research & Therapy 12:R223

89. Yusuf E, Kortekaas MC, Watt I et al (2011) Do knee abnormalities visualised on MRI explain knee pain in knee osteoarthritis? A systematic review. Annals of the Rheumatic Diseases 70:60-67

90. Crema MD, Roemer FW, Marra MD et al (2011) Articular cartilage in the knee: current MR imaging techniques and applications in clinical practice and research. Radiographics 31:37-61

91. De Smet AA, Tuite MJ (2006) Use of the "two-slice-touch" rule for the MRI diagnosis of meniscal tears. AJR Am J Roentgenol 187:911-914

92. De Smet AA, Norris MA, Yandow DR et al (1993) MR diagnosis of meniscal tears of the knee: importance of high signal in the meniscus that extends to the surface. AJR Am J Roentgenol 161:101-107

93. Kaplan PA, Nelson NL, Garvin KL, Brown DE (1991) MR of the knee: the significance of high signal in the meniscus that does not clearly extend to the surface. AJR Am J Roentgenol 156:333-336

94. Lee SY, Jee WH, Kim JM (2008) Radial tear of the medial meniscal root: reliability and accuracy of MRI for diagnosis. AJR Am J Roentgenol 191:81-85

95. De Smet AA, Blankenbaker DG, Kijowski R et al (2009) MR diagnosis of posterior root tears of the lateral meniscus using arthroscopy as the reference standard. AJR Am J Roentgenol 192:480-486

96. Choi SH, Bae S, Ji SK, Chang MJ (2012) The MRI findings of meniscal root tear of the medial meniscus: emphasis on coronal, sagittal and axial images. Knee Surgery, Sports Traumatology, Arthroscopy 20:2098-2103

97. Vande Berg BC, Malghem J, Poilvache P et al (2005) Meniscal tears with fragments displaced in notch and recesses of knee: MR imaging with arthroscopic comparison. Radiology 234:842-850

98. Ververidis AN, Verettas DA, Kazakos KJ et al (2006) Meniscal bucket handle tears: a retrospective study of arthroscopy and the relation to MRI. Knee Surgery, Sports Traumatology, Arthroscopy 14:343-349

99. Oei EH, Nikken JJ, Verstijnen AC et al (2003) MR imaging of the menisci and cruciate ligaments: a systematic review. Radiology 226:837-848

100. De Smet AA, Mukherjee R (2008) Clinical, MRI, and arthroscopic findings associated with failure to diagnose a lateral meniscal tear on knee MRI. AJR Am J Roentgenol 190:22-26

101. De Smet AA (2012) How I diagnose meniscal tears on knee MRI. AJR Am J Roentgenol 199:481-499

102. De Smet AA, Nathan DH, Graf BK et al (2008) Clinical and MRI findings associated with false-positive knee MR diagnoses of medial meniscal tears. AJR Am J Roentgenol 191:93-99

103. Van Dyck P, Gielen J, D'Anvers J et al (2007) MR diagnosis of meniscal tears of the knee: analysis of error patterns. Archives of Orthopaedic and Trauma Surgery 127:849-854

104. Lim PS, Schweitzer ME, Bhatia M et al (1999) Repeat tear of postoperative meniscus: potential MR imaging signs. Radiology 210:183-188

105. Sciulli RL, Boutin RD, Brown RR et al (1999) Evaluation of the postoperative meniscus of the knee: a study comparing conventional arthrography, conventional MR imaging, MR arthrography with iodinated contrast material, and MR arthrography with gadolinium-based contrast material. Skeletal Radiology 28:508-514

106. Applegate GR, Flannigan BD, Tolin BS et al (1993) MR diagnosis of recurrent tears in the knee: value of intraarticular contrast material. AJR Am J Roentgenol 161:821-825

107. Rubin DA, Kettering JM, Towers JD, Britton CA (1998) MR imaging of knees having isolated and combined ligament injuries. AJR Am J Roentgenol 170:1207-1213

108. Tung GA, Davis LM, Wiggins ME, Fadale PD (1993) Tears of the anterior cruciate ligament: primary and secondary signs at MR imaging. Radiology 188:661-667

109. Schweitzer ME, Tran D, Deely DM, Hume EL (1995) Medial collateral ligament injuries: evaluation of multiple signs, prevalence and location of associated bone bruises, and assessment with MR imaging. Radiology 194:825-829

110. Vahey TN, Broome DR, Kayes KJ, Shelbourne KD (1991) Acute and chronic tears of the anterior cruciate ligament: differential features at MR imaging. Radiology 181:251-253

111. Brandser EA, Riley MA, Berbaum KS et al (1996) MR imaging of anterior cruciate ligament injury: independent value of primary and secondary signs. AJR Am J Roentgenol 167:121-126

112. McIntyre J, Moelleken S, Tirman P (2001) Mucoid degeneration of the anterior cruciate ligament mistaken for ligamentous tears. Skeletal Radiology 30:312-315

113. Makino A, Pascual-Garrido C, Rolon A et al (2011) Mucoid degeneration of the anterior cruciate ligament: MRI, clinical, intraoperative, and histological findings. Knee Surgery, Sports Traumatology, Arthroscopy 19:408-411

114. Bergin D, Morrison WB, Carrino JA et al (2004) Anterior cruciate ligament ganglia and mucoid degeneration: coexistence and clinical correlation. AJR Am J Roentgenol 182:1283-1287

115. Nguyen B, Brandser E, Rubin DA (2000) Pains, strains, and fasciculations: lower extremity muscle disorders. Magnetic Resonance Imaging Clinics of North America 8:391-408

116. Cook JL, Khan KM, Kiss ZS et al (2001) Asymptomatic hypoechoic regions on patellar tendon ultrasound: A 4-year clinical and ultrasound followup of 46 tendons. Scandinavian Journal of Medicine & Science in Sports 11:321-327

117. Terslev L, Qvistgaard E, Torp-Pedersen S et al (2001) Ultrasound and Power Doppler findings in jumper's knee - preliminary observations. European Journal of Ultrasound 13:183-189

118. La S, Fessell DP, Femino JE et al (2003) Sonography of partial-thickness quadriceps tendon tears with surgical correlation. Journal of Ultrasound in Medicine 22:1323-1329

119. Shalaby M, Almekinders LC (1999) Patellar tendinitis: the significance of magnetic resonance imaging findings. The American Journal of Sports Medicine 27:345-349

120. Zeiss J, Saddemi SR, Ebraheim NA (1992) MR imaging of the quadriceps tendon: normal layered configuration and its importance in cases of tendon rupture. AJR Am J Roentgenol 159:1031-1034

121. Marti-Bonmati L, Molla E, Dosda R et al (2000) MR imaging of Baker cysts —prevalence and relation to internal derangements of the knee. MAGMA 10:205-210

122. Viegas FC, Aguiar RO, Gasparetto E et al (2007) Deep and superficial infrapatellar bursae: cadaveric investigation of regional anatomy using magnetic resonance after ultrasound-guided bursography. Skeletal Radiology 36:41-46

123. McCarthy CL, McNally EG (2004) The MRI appearance of cystic lesions around the knee. Skeletal Radiology 33:187-209

124. Tschirch FT, Schmid MR, Pfirrmann CW et al (2003) Prevalence and size of meniscal cysts, ganglionic cysts, synovial cysts of the popliteal space, fluid-filled bursae, and other fluid collections in asymptomatic knees on MR imaging. AJR Am J Roentgenol 180:1431-1436

125. Carotti M, Salaffi F, Manganelli P et al (2002) Power Doppler sonography in the assessment of synovial tissue of the knee joint in rheumatoid arthritis: a preliminary experience. Annals of the Rheumatic Diseases 61:877-882

126. Adam G, Dammer M, Bohndorf K et al (1991) Rheumatoid arthritis of the knee: value of gadopentetate dimeglumine-enhanced MR imaging. AJR Am J Roentgenol 156:125-129

127. Bredella MA, Tirman PF, Wischer TK et al (2000) Reactive synovitis of the knee joint: MR imaging appearance with arthroscopic correlation. Skeletal Radiology 29:577-582

128. Singson RD, Zalduondo FM (1992) Value of unenhanced spin-echo MR imaging in distinguishing between synovitis and effusion of the knee. AJR Am J Roentgenol 159:569-571

129. Miller E, Uleryk E, Doria AS (2009) Evidence-based outcomes of studies addressing diagnostic accuracy of MRI of juvenile idiopathic arthritis. AJR Am J Roentgenol 192:1209-1218

130. Hemke R, van Veenendaal M, Kuijpers TW et al (2012) Increasing feasibility and patient comfort of MRI in children with juvenile idiopathic arthritis. Pediatric Radiology 42:440-448

131. Hemke R, van Rossum MA, van Veenendaal M et al (2012) Reliability and responsiveness of the Juvenile Arthritis MRI Scoring (JAMRIS) system for the knee. European Radiology [Epub ahead of print]

132. Crotty JM, Monu JU, Pope TL, Jr (1996) Synovial osteochondromatosis. Radiologic Clinics of North America 34:327-342, xi

133. Bessette PR, Cooley PA, Johnson RP, Czarnecki DJ (1992) Gadolinium-enhanced MRI of pigmented villonodular synovitis of the knee. Journal of Computer Assisted Tomography 16:992-994

134. Huang GS, Lee CH, Chan WP et al (2003) Localized nodular synovitis of the knee: MR imaging appearance and clinical correlates in 21 patients. AJR Am J Roentgenol 181:539-543

135. Lin J, Jacobson JA, Jamadar DA, Ellis JH (1999) Pigmented villonodular synovitis and related lesions: the spectrum of imaging findings. AJR Am J Roentgenol 172:191-197

# Magnetic Resonance of Foot and Ankle

Mark E. Schweitzer[1], Eva Llopis[2]

[1] Department of Diagnostic Imaging, The Ottawa Hospital, Ottawa, ON, Canada
[2] Department of Radiology, Hospital de la Ribera, Alzira, Valencia, Spain

## Tendons

Most tendon disorders of the ankle occur in females, with the exception being Achilles disorders.

Nearly all tendons that tear have underlying degeneration. There are four histologic types of degenerations seen, the most common of which is fibrinoid. Fibrinoid degeneration leads to enlarged tendons without an internal signal. In the foot and ankle this is most common in the Achilles tendon and posterior tibial tendon [1-3].

The next most common type of degeneration is mucoid. In mucoid degeneration, a high signal is seen in the tendon on T2-weighted images. These deposits often have an interrupted pattern, similar to Morse code. This is relatively common in the Achilles tendon, and less so in the peroneals and posterior tibial tendon (PTT) (Fig. 1). When these interstitial deposits coalesce, it is termed interstitial tearing. In this situation, a longitudinal split is seen within the tendon. This is seen in the Achilles tendon. It is also seen in peroneal split syndrome (Figs. 2, 3). The next most common type of tendon degeneration is calcific. The only common location in the ankle where calcific degeneration occurs is in the Achilles tendon. In fact in this location the degeneration is typically ossific rather than calcific and occurs 2-3 cm from the insertion. Ossified and calcified tendons tear infrequently. Lipoid degeneration is age related and shows fat deposits between normal tenocytes, and is not associated with tendon rupture.

Tendon tearing can be thought of as predominantly a chronic process, with the "tear" being a culmination of

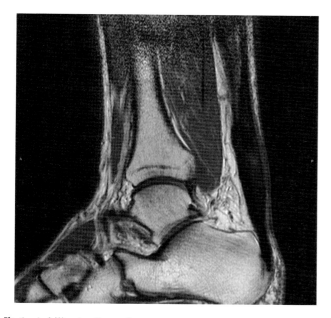

**Fig. 1.** Achilles tendinopathy

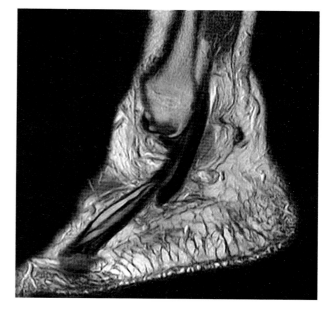

**Fig. 2.** Longitudinal tear of the peroneus tendon

J. Hodler et al. (eds.), *Musculoskeletal Diseases 2013-2016,*
DOI: 10.1007/978-88-470-5292-5_9 © Springer-Verlag Italia 2013

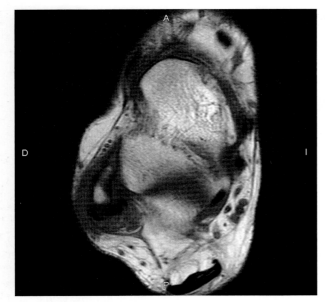

**Fig. 3.** Peronal splint syndrome

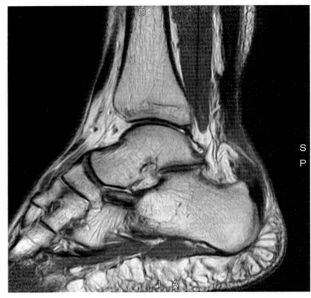

**Fig. 4.** Complete tear of the Achilles tendon

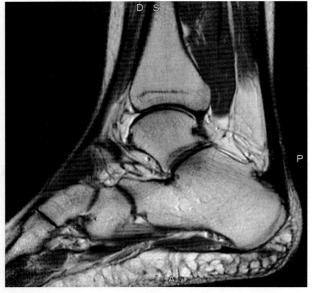

**Fig. 5.** Hadlund syndrome with partial tear of the Achilles tendon

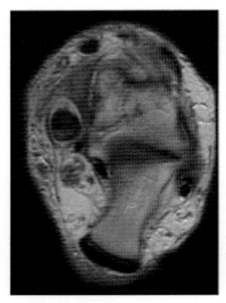

**Fig. 6.** Posterior tibialis tendinopathy

long-standing disease. The degeneration may be silent but is nearly always present. Silent tendonopathy is more commonly fibrinoid (Fig. 4).

## Achilles

Achilles disorders occur usually 2-3 cm from the insertion, and they often have visible, underlying degeneration, and they can be partial, interstitial or complete.

Older patients may have tears that are more proximal, and this is termed a myotendinous tear of the gastrocnemious.

Insertional tears may be seen in runners, or associated with rheumatoid or reactive arthritis. Haglund's syndrome is seen distally, with a congenitally enlarge posterior tubercle, retrocalcaneal bursitis and insertional tendonosis (Fig. 5).

## Posterior Tibial

The posterior tibial tendon has two types of disorder. One type is seen around the malleolus; it is seen in older patients and is more common. Early stages of PTT disorder have associated synovitis, which is more often distal (Fig. 6).

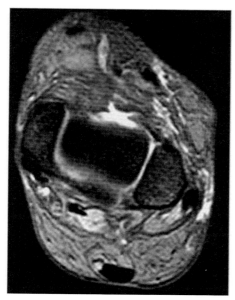

**Fig. 7.** Peroneal tendons subluxation

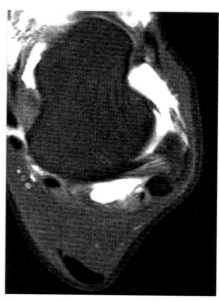

**Fig. 8.** Complete tear of the anterior talofibular ligament

The second type of disorder is seen in young or active patients with seronegative or seropositive spondyloarthropathies. PTT disorders are manifest by a focally enlarged tendon, or less frequently a focal thinned tendon. Internal signal is less common.

Secondary signs of PTT tears include plantar flexion of the talus, talonavicular unroofing, heal valgus with possible impaction, and marrow edema under the course of the tendon [4, 5].

### Peroneus

Peroneal disorders include peroneal splits, which are interstitial tears often secondary to chronic subluxation long tears (Fig. 7). Relatively unique to the peroneal tendons, and also affecting the PTT, is tendon subluxation. This occurs because of a combination of biomechanical factors and anatomic factors such as a shallow groove. The splits that occur are often related to chronic instability of the brevis tendon. This can be related to ankle instability, or complex calcaneal fracture.

Peroneal disorders have a variable association with fluid in the common tendon sheath. Splits and more focal tears occur epicentered at the calcaneocuboid joint [6, 7].

### Anterior Tibial Tendon

Anterior tibial tendons can be clinically silent and can also be associated with arthropathies. These arthropathies include rheumatoid arthritis and gout. These tears are more often seen in the elderly, and very frequently are clinically silent [8].

### Ligament Disorders

The most common ligament tear in the ankle is the anterior talofibular ligament (Fig. 8). It typically tears at its insertion onto the talus. The second most common is the calcaneofibular ligament, which also tends to tear distally, at its insertion onto the calcaneus. When acute, most of these tears demonstrate fluid violating the margins. On coronal images, the fluid dissects upwards in an anterior talofibular ligament injury and downwards in a calcaneofibular ligament injury The posterior talofibular ligament is rarely injured [9-11].

Of somewhat more biomechanical importance are the syndesmotic ligaments. These are often associated with ankle joint instability. Asymmetry of the fibular within the sigmoid sulcus is a useful secondary sign, as is edema in the flexor hallucis muscle belly. Axial imaging for anterior syndesmotic ligament tears is difficult to interpret [12, 13].

### Other Soft Tissues

The plantar fascia will degenerate in a similar way to tendon degeneration, as described above. When it tears, it tears approximately 5 mm from its insertion and demonstrates focal disruption. Tears may also be associated with muscle tearing, usually involving the flexor brevis or occasionally the quadratus plantae. Chronic disorders lead to a thickened fascia, with internal signal. Reactive marrow edema can also be seen in the calcaneus (Fig. 9). Reactive arthritis and rheumatoid arthritis can also lead to disruption of the plantar fascia [14, 15].

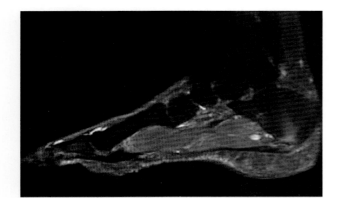

**Fig. 9.** Plantar fasciitis

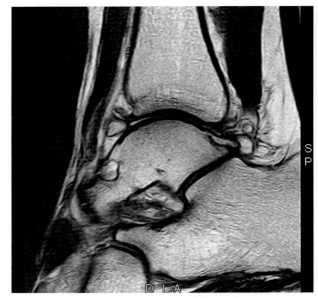

**Fig. 11.** Anterior and posterior bone impingement

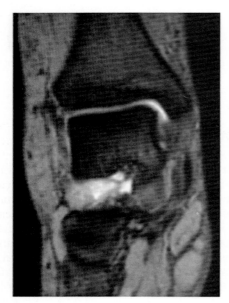

**Fig. 10.** Sinus tarsi syndrome

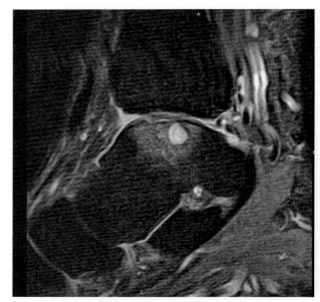

**Fig. 12.** Talus osteochondral instable lesion

Sinus tarsi syndrome is associated with ankle sprains and anthropathies of the subtalar joint. More useful than obliteration of the fat in the sinus is focal edema and disruption of the sinus tarsi ligaments; this should be clearly visible on most imaging protocols. Ganglia often extend laterally from the sinus tarsi, and marrow edema can be seen about the insertions of the ligament (Fig. 10).

Tarsal tunnel syndrome is an infrequent indication for magnetic resonance (MR) imaging. Masses are disproportionately seen in tarsal tunnel syndrome, but still relatively uncommon. These masses include ganglia, varices, synovial cysts and ganglions [16].

Impingement syndromes of the ankle are chronic painful conditions secondary to repetitive friction between bones and soft tissue structures. They can be divided, following anatomic distribution, into: anterior, anterolateral, anteromedial and posterior impingement syn-

dromes (Fig. 11). Anteromedial and anterolateral impingement syndromes are caused by hypertrophic synovial tissue and fibrosis, and MR arthrography might be helpful for accurate diagnosis [17].

## Bone Injuries

Marrow edema in the ankle has many causes, including osteochondral defects (Fig. 12), acute fractures, stress injuries

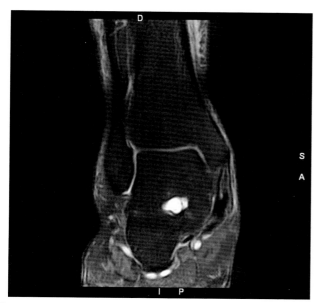

**Fig. 13.** Talocalcaneal coalition

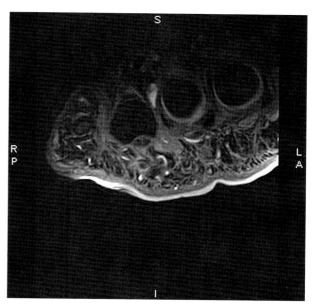

**Fig. 14.** Morton neuroma

and bone bruises; the latter are usually seen in association with ankle sprain, avascular necrosis and very rarely primary tumors, and rarely metastatic tumors [18-21].

Not infrequently, osteomyelitis is seen as a cause of marrow edema. Almost invariably these patients are diabetic and have ulceration, which leads to an exposed bone [22].

Tarsal coalition is an abnormal bridging across two or more tarsal bones. It is a well-recognized cause of decrease range of motion and pain in children and adolescents; however, it is often diagnosed in adults when complications occur. The most frequent coalitions are calcaneo-navicular and talocalcaneal. They can be osseous, cartilaginous or fibrous. Both computed tomography and MR are very at good detecting tarsal coalitions (Fig. 13) [23, 24.]

## Foot

The foot is a focused examination. There may be disorders of the distal tendons, sesamoids, Morton neuroma, fibromatosis or other soft tissue masses (Fig. 14) [25-27].

Fractures of the foot are usually stress fractures, most commonly seen in the metatarsals and occasionally in the mid-foot. When mid-foot fractures are seen, careful attention should be paid to the Lisfranc ligament.

Morton neuromas are most commonly seen in the third interspace as tear-drop-shaped areas of low signal, best seen on short TE imaging. These neuromas are really fibromas and are epicentered somewhat plantarly. Long TE images distinguish these from the similarly positioned intermetatarsal bursitis, which demonstrates uniformly high signal on T2-weighted images [28].

There is some debate as to what is the cause of sesamoid disorders. Certainly abnormal mechanics is one cause, often associated with diffuse, predominantly plantarly positioned low signal within the sesamoids, involving both relatively symmetrically. Also to be considered is articular disease, which is not uncommon in sesamoids but will show "kissing changes" in the metatarsal head. Less commonly, abnormal marrow signal within a single sesamoid is seen. This has sometimes been considered to be inflammatory, sometimes avascular necrosis, sometimes a stress fracture and is most likely a stress fracture, leading to some degree of bone necrosis. Sagittal imaging should be utilized to best visualize the fracture line. If the two fracture fragments are too large to fit together, consider diastases of the synchondrosis between a bipartite sesamoid [29, 30].

Soft tissue masses are common indications for MR of the foot and, to a lesser degree, the ankle; the vast majority of these are benign and represent ganglia, neuromas, foreign body reactions or plantar fibromatosis. The latter is characterized by low T1 and T2, with variable but usually intense enhancement. It also notable that it has a much smaller size on MR than is noticeable clinically.

## References

1. Rosenberg ZS, Beltran J, Bencardino JT (2000) MR imaging of the ankle and foot. Radiographics 20(Spec No):S153-179
2. Schweitzer ME, Karasick D (2000) MR imaging of disorders of the Achilles tendon. AJR Am J Roentgenol 175:613-625
3. Schweitzer ME, Karasick D (2000) MR imaging of disorders of the posterior tibialis tendon. AJR Am J Roentgenol 175:627-635

4. Balen PF, Helms CA (2001) Association of posterior tibial tendon injury with spring ligament injury, sinus tarsi abnormality, and plantar fasciitis on MR imaging. AJR Am J Roentgenol 176:1137-1143

5. Beals TC, Pomeroy GC, Manoli A (1999) Posterior tibial tendon insufficiency: diagnosis and treatment. J Am Acad Orthop Surg 7:112-118

6. Bencardino JT, Rosenberg ZS, Serrano LF (2001) MR imaging features of diseases of the peroneal tendons. Magn Reson Imaging Clin N Am 9:493-505

7. Rademaker J, Rosenberg ZS, Delfaut EM et al (2000) Tear of the peroneus longus tendon: MR imaging features in nine patients.Radiology 214:700-704

8. Khoury NJ, el-Khoury GY, Saltzman CL, Brandser EA (1996) Rupture of the anterior tibial tendon: diagnosis by MR imaging. AJR Am J Roentgenol 67:351-354

9. Cheung Y, Rosenberg ZS (2001) MR imaging of ligamentous abnormalities of the ankle and foot. Magn Reson Imaging Clin N Am 9:507-531

10. Perrich KD, Goodwin DW, Hecht PJ, Cheung Y (2009) Ankle ligaments on MRI: appearance of normal and injured ligaments. AJR Am J Roentgenol 193:687-695

11. Campbell SE, Warner M (2008) MR imaging of ankle inversion injuries. Magn Reson Imaging Clin N Am 16:1-18

12. Uys HD, Rijke AM (2002) Clinical association of acute lateral ankle sprain with syndesmotic involvement: a stress radiography and magnetic resonance imaging study. Am J Sports Med 30:816-822

13. Boonthathip M, Chen L, Trudell DJ, Resnick DL (2010) Tibiofibular syndesmotic ligaments: MR arthrography in cadavers with anatomic correlation. Radiology 254:827-836

14. Narváez JA, Narváez J, Ortega R et al (2000) Painful heel: MR imaging findings. Radiographics 20:333-352

15. Theodorou DJ, Theodorou SJ, Kakitsubata Y (2000) Plantar fasciitis and fascial rupture: MR imaging findings in 26 patients supplemented with anatomic data in cadavers. Radiographics 20(Spec No):S181-197

16. Erickson SJ, Quinn SF, Kneeland JB (1990) MR imaging of the tarsal tunnel and related spaces: normal and abnormal findings with anatomic correlation AJR Am J Roentgenol 155:323-328

17. Cerezal L, Abascal F, Canga A (2003) MR imaging of ankle impingement syndromes. AJR Am J Roentgenol 181:551-559

18. Fernandez-Canton G, Casado O, Capelastegui A (2003) Bone marrow edema syndrome of the foot: one year follow-up with MR imaging. Skeletal Radiol 32:273-278

19. Bencardino JT, Rosenberg ZS (2001) MR imaging and CT in the assessment of osseous abnormalities of the ankle and foot. Magn Reson Imaging Clin N Am 9:567-578

20. Stroud CC, Marks RM (2000) Imaging of osteochondral lesions of the talus. Foot Ankle Clin 5:119-133

21. Pearce DH, Mongiardi CN, Fornasier VL, Daniels TR (2005) Avascular necrosis of the talus: a pictorial essay. Radiographics 25:399-410

22. Moore TE, Yuh WT, Kathol MH (1991) Abnormalities of the foot in patients with diabetes mellitus: findings on MR imaging. AJR Am J Roentgenol 157:813-816

23. Emery KH, Bisset GS 3rd, Johnson ND, Nunan PJ (1998) Tarsal coalition: a blinded comparison of MRI and CT. Pediatr Radiol 28:612-616

24. Newman JS, Newberg AH (2000) Congenital tarsal coalition: multimodality evaluation with emphasis on CT and MR imaging. Radiographics 20:321-332

25. Espinosa N, Brodsky JW, Maceira E (2010) Metatarsalgia. J Am Acad Orthop Surg 18:474-485

26. Espinosa N, Maceira E, Myerson MS (2008) Current concept review: metatarsalgia. Foot Ankle Int 29:871-879

27. Ashman CJ, Klecker RJ, Yu JS (2001) Forefoot pain involving the metatarsal region: differential diagnosis with MR imaging. Radiographics 21:1425-1440

28. Zanetti M, Strehle JK, Kundert HP (1999) Morton neuroma: effect of MR imaging findings on diagnostic thinking and therapeutic decisions. Radiology 213:583-588

29. Taylor JA, Sartoris DJ, Huang GS, Resnick DL (1993) Painful conditions affecting the first metatarsal sesamoid bones. Radiographics 13:817-830

30. Mohana-Borges AV, Theumann NH, Pfirrmann CW (2003) Lesser metatarsophalangeal joints: standard MR imaging, MR arthrography, and MR bursography—initial results in 48 cadaveric joints. Radiology 227:175-182

# Postoperative Imaging of the Knee and Shoulder

Lawrence M. White[1], Laura W. Bancroft[2]

[1] Joint Department of Medical Imaging, University of Toronto, Toronto, ON, Canada
[2] Department of Diagnostic Radiology, Florida Hospital, Orlando, FL, USA

Postoperative imaging poses unique challenges in sports medicine imaging. The interpreting radiologist must first be cognisant of the fact that the patient has had previous surgery, as this may not be communicated in the provided clinical history. Interpretation of imaging studies following surgery requires knowledge of the commonly used surgical techniques and the potential complications of such procedures. Surgery also results in morphological changes to normal structures, and these may simulate pathological processes and may be misinterpreted as a recurrent lesion if conventional diagnostic criteria are employed. Bulk orthopedic hardware can also result in substantial imaging-related artifacts obscuring and distorting the area of interest. Even in the absence of bulk orthopedic hardware, extensive microscopic metallic debris may be shed from surgical instruments, such as high-speed drills and shavers, and this may result in extensive artifact with magnetic resonance imaging (MRI). This may necessitate modification of imaging protocols in the postoperative setting.

Surgical intervention is most commonly performed in the knee and shoulder and these will form the basis of this chapter. Depending on the procedure performed and the nature of the postoperative symptoms, the full range of imaging studies including conventional radiography, ultrasound (US), computer tomography (CT) and magnetic resonance imaging (MRI) may be utilized and provide complementary information. In our experience, MRI with its excellent soft tissue evaluation and multiplanar capability forms the cornerstone of the advanced imaging evaluation of the postoperative patient by allowing a global assessment of soft tissue and osseous structures.

## Imaging Techniques in the Postoperative Patient

Postoperative imaging can be challenging for numerous reasons including, but not limited to, postsurgical changes in articular structural morphology, signal intensity changes related to tissue healing and reconstruction

materials, as well as postoperative artifacts at imaging, which may obscure adjacent anatomy or mimic pathological changes. Such artifacts are important to recognize as modification of user defined imaging parameters and can be of value in diagnostic assessment of the postoperative knee and shoulder.

Postsurgical artifacts at MRI may originate secondary to implanted surgical devices, as well as microscopic metallic debris related to arthroscopic instruments used at the time of joint surgery. Such artifacts resulting secondary to local magnetic field inhomogeneities induced by ferromagnetic materials are generally most marked in the setting of metallic fixation devices or bulk reconstruction hardware. The pattern and degree of such postsurgical metal related artifact at MRI are typically reflective of the type of surgery previously performed, the size and composition of surgically implanted devices, and the pulse sequence parameters utilized for image acquisition.

The choice of pulse sequences and imaging parameters can be crucial to minimizing image distortion and artifacts at postsurgical MRI evaluation. Gradient echo acquisitions, which lack a 180-degree refocusing pulse, are inherently prone to intravoxel dephasing and loss of signal, and in general should be avoided in postoperative imaging. Gradient echo images can be useful, however, to identify microscopic metallic debris if there is doubt as to whether the patient has had prior surgery, and the anatomic pattern of postoperative artifacts may be suggestive of the particular type of operative intervention previously performed. Fast-spin echo sequences, using multiple 180-degree refocusing pulses, minimize the signal loss caused by inhomogeneities in the local magnetic field induced by metal hardware or debris. Such reductions in metal-induced artifacts may be further maximized by reducing/minimizing the interecho spacing on traditional fast or turbo spin echo imaging sequences. Additional important user-defined MRI parameters that can influence the appearance of artifacts at postoperative imaging are the selection of frequency-encoding gradient

J. Hodler et al. (eds.), *Musculoskeletal Diseases 2013-2016,*
DOI: 10.1007/978-88-470-5292-5_10 © Springer-Verlag Italia 2013

readout strength, and the frequency-encoding direction at imaging. Traditional 2-dimensional (2D) MRI acquisitions suffer from misregistration artifacts in the presence of ferromagnetic materials that are inversely proportional to the frequency-encoding gradient strength utilized at imaging. Importantly, such misregistration artifacts are only manifested in the frequency-encoding direction. Using a higher frequency-encoding gradient readout strength, corresponding to use of a widened/higher imaging receiver bandwidth, at imaging might help to reduce magnetic resonance (MR) metal-related artifacts [1]. Similarly, as misregistration artifacts are only manifest in the frequency-encoding direction, selective orientation of the frequency-encoding direction might help orient misregistration artifacts away from areas of anatomic interest. Reducing slice thickness and increasing matrix size might also help to reduce the degree of image distortion at MRI in the vicinity of metal [1].

Spectral fat-saturation techniques are dependent on a homogeneous local magnetic field and, in the presence of metal, inhomogeneous fat suppression results. Short-tau inversion recovery (STIR) sequences are less susceptible to field inhomogeneities and are better suited to imaging around bulk metal hardware, as are water-fat separation strategies such as Dixon imaging techniques [2].

Several new pulse sequences have recently been commercially developed for clinical use to address imaging artifacts in the vicinity of surgical metallic hardware. These acquisition sequences, which have a variety of commercial names, employ intrinsic acquisition artifact reduction strategies including in-plane and through-plane view-angle-tilting techniques, which can result in dramatic improvements in MRI quality in the setting of metal-related magnetic field distortions.

## Postoperative Imaging in Meniscal Surgery

The meniscus has important functions with regards to distributing loads across the knee, maintaining joint congruity and contributing to joint stability. Meniscal tearing is among the most common pathology of the knee joint, with the pathogenesis of meniscal tearing broadly categorized as degenerative or traumatic in etiology. Clinically, meniscal tearing, whether degenerative or traumatic in origin, can manifest with joint pain, joint locking and can significantly alter joint function and biomechanics, and predispose articular cartilage to degenerative changes and osteoarthritis. As a result, a large amount of interest has been directed toward the surgical treatment of meniscal tears.

The natural history of total meniscectomy is well documented as a primary risk factor towards premature chondral loss and degenerative change. As a result, the fundamental principle of modern meniscal surgery is to preserve as much meniscal tissue as possible while addressing the tear and restoring meniscal morphology, function and stability. Modern surgical treatment options in the setting of

a meniscal tear include meniscal repair, meniscectomy and, in some centers, meniscal transplantation in cases of meniscal deficiency [3]. Meniscal tear pattern and presence or absence of vascularity to the tear segment are critical factors for determining the optimal treatment of a meniscal tear. Tears amenable to meniscal repair include linear oblique or longitudinal vertical tears through the peripheral vascular or "red zone" of the meniscus, typically within 3 mm of the meniscocapsular junction. Tears through the "red-white zone", typically between 3 and 5 mm from the meniscocapsular junction, have variable vascularity, whereas those through the central "white zone" of the meniscus demonstrate poor healing unless vascularity is demonstrated at surgery [3]. Similarly, complex or chronic degenerative tears are less likely to heal following meniscal repair. Meniscal repair can be attempted using sutures, tacks, arrows or anchors. Unrepairable complex or degenerative meniscal tears and tears remote from a viable vascular supply are generally treated with partial meniscectomy. Goals of successful meniscectomy are the removal of any unstable or potentially unstable meniscal tissue, with the preservation of as much stable smoothly contoured residual meniscal tissue as possible.

Young patients with subtotal meniscectomy or extensive meniscal tears not amenable to meniscus preserving surgery, and without complications of secondary cartilage loss, may be candidates at some centers for meniscal allograft transplantation. This can be performed as a combined arthroscopic and mini-open procedure. The meniscus is transplanted with either anterior and posterior root bone plugs, which are inserted into the proximal tibia and maintained in position with traction sutures, or a bone bridge attached to the anterior and posterior roots, with the periphery of the meniscus sutured to the adjacent joint capsule [4].

Clinically worrisome symptoms following partial meniscectomy or meniscal repair can be the result of a residual or recurrent tear at the site of prior surgery, a meniscal tear at a new location, or due to other pathology such as chondral or ligamentous injury. If the history of prior meniscal surgery has not been provided on the requisition form, there may be clues on MR images, which may help in establishing whether there has been previous surgery. In the presence of arthroscopy, a linear low signal intensity scar might be seen within Hoffa's fat pad of the anterior knee joint. This can be of variable thickness and prominence and is secondary to arthroscopic portal tract scarring/healing postoperatively. A further clue that might be apparent in some cases is focal thickening of the edge of the patellar tendon through its mid third. Typically there is little or no artifact in the region of the meniscus to alert the reader to presence of prior meniscal surgery, unless meniscal repair has been attempted with a fixation device.

The utility and diagnostic criteria of MRI in the identification of meniscal tears in virgin menisci are well established and extensively validated with an accuracy of over 90% [5]. Diagnostic criteria include intrameniscal

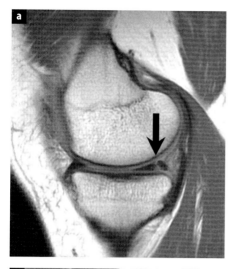

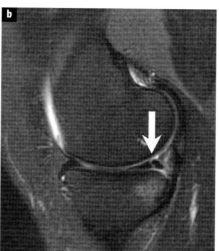

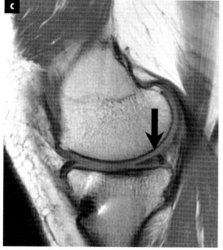

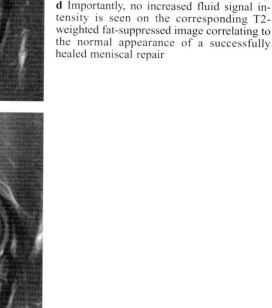

**Fig. 1 a-d.** Normal magnetic resonance (MR) appearance following meniscal repair. Sagittal fast spin echo intermediate weighted (**a**) and T2-weighted fat-suppressed (**b**) images through the medial meniscus illustrate a clearly defined vertical tear (*arrow*, **a**, **b**) extending through the posterior horn of the medial meniscus. **c** Corresponding position matched MR imaging performed 5 years following meniscal repair shows persistent increased intrasubstance signal changes related to the healed meniscal tear site (*arrow*). **d** Importantly, no increased fluid signal intensity is seen on the corresponding T2-weighted fat-suppressed image correlating to the normal appearance of a successfully healed meniscal repair

signal extending to an articular surface (grade III signal) seen on at least two slices on a short TE sequence, alteration of meniscal morphology, loss of meniscal volume or demonstration of a displaced meniscal fragment [6]. Applying these criteria after meniscal surgery yields modest results for detection of residual or recurrent meniscal tears. There are several reasons to account for the overall poor diagnostic value of primary diagnostic criteria of virgin meniscal tear, in evaluation of the postoperative meniscus. First, a healing tear, either following conservative treatment or meniscal repair, will show increased signal intensity on short TE sequences corresponding to fibrovascular tissue during the healing phase [7]. These tears might be stable at arthroscopy but signal changes might be evident even years post surgery (Fig. 1) [7]. Even the presence of a full thickness signal abnormality on short TE sequences does not correlate with a recurrent tear after meniscal repair [8]. Second, following partial meniscectomy, areas of intrasubstance signal change, classified as grade I or grade II on preoperative MRI, may indeed extend to the neoarticular surface and simulate grade III signal following resection of subjacent

unstable meniscal tissue. This phenomenon of "signal conversion" can result in a false-positive diagnosis of a meniscal tear using preoperative criteria of meniscal pathology. Finally, the anatomic morphologic appearances of menisci postoperatively can be highly variable following surgery. Meniscal morphology is dependent on the location and type of previous tear and the technique used to treat them. Surgery can result in distortion, truncation or blunting of the meniscus as a normal postoperative finding. Therefore, the diagnosis of a recurrent or residual tear cannot be based on alteration of normal virgin meniscal morphology, unless a displaced meniscal fragment is concomitantly identified.

The accuracy of MRI in diagnosing meniscal tears following meniscal surgery appears to be related to the amount of meniscal tissue that has been resected. In menisci where there has been resection of <25% of the meniscus, MRI demonstrates accuracy rates of 89-100% utilizing the traditional criteria of grade III signal on short TE sequences [9]. In menisci where >25% of the meniscus has been resected, the presence of grade III signal on short TE sequences is of limited diagnostic utility.

Accuracy rates of 50-65% have been recorded for conventional MRI depending on the degree/extent of prior meniscal resection, the lower figure representing the accuracy in those with >75% of the meniscus resected [9]. Similarly, contour abnormality is of limited accuracy in the diagnosis of a meniscal tear in patients with extensive partial meniscectomy. In one study, all patients who demonstrated marked contour irregularity after resection of more than a third of the meniscus had a negative repeat arthroscopy, while in another study using alteration of meniscal morphology beyond what would be expected following meniscal surgery as the only criteria for a recurrent tear, an accuracy rate of only 67-68% was achieved [10]. Traditional diagnostic criteria of a meniscal tear can still be applied for diagnosis of tears in portions of the meniscus where surgery has not been performed, but this is dependent on access to prior surgical reports and preoperative imaging.

Therefore, it is clear that diagnostic criteria for accurate assessment of meniscal tearing need to be modified following meniscal surgery. The suggested modified criteria for diagnosis of a meniscal tear in a postoperative meniscus include an area of fluid signal intensity extending into the substance of the meniscus on T2-weighted images, and identification of a displaced meniscal fragment or meniscal fragmentation [7]. As identification of fluid signal intensity is critical to diagnosing a recurrent tear, it is worthwhile to obtain T2-weighted images in both the sagittal and the coronal planes. The addition of fat saturation increases the conspicuity of the fluid signal and can be helpful. Indeed, in the group of patients with resection of >75% of the meniscus, the meniscal remnant may be hard to visualize on proton density images and is best seen on T2-weighted images, particularly in the presence of adjacent fluid. Radial tears in particular appear to be more common in the postoperative setting in comparison with virgin menisci, and this is likely related to altered biomechanical properties of a partially resected meniscus [11]. Another potentially useful sign of recurrent or residual meniscal tearing following meniscal repair is widening of the tear repair cleft on serial examinations [8]. In patients with prior meniscal repair, identification of surfacing high T2 signal within a meniscus has a specificity of 88-92% and a sensitivity of 41-69% [7, 9]. However, in applying these diagnostic criteria in the diagnosis of a recurrent or residual meniscal tear, it must be remembered that fluid signal may be seen within a healing cleft without signifying a residual tear within the first 12 weeks following meniscal repair [7].

Identification of fluid signal within a tear is likely to be related to imbibition of joint fluid into a tear gap. In an attempt to utilize this mechanism, direct MR arthrography has been used for evaluation of recurrent or residual meniscal tears. Direct MR arthrography has potential advantages in imaging of a postoperative meniscus through bathing the meniscus completely in a diluted gadolinium mixture and increasing intra-articular pressure by distending the joint, and then the tear cleft is theoretically more likely to be outlined. In addition, T1-weighted imaging, which is typically performed at MR arthrography, has a higher signal-to-noise ratio than T2-weighted acquisitions and may be advantageous for detection of tear clefts. Direct MR arthrography is most commonly performed under fluoroscopic guidance whereby intra-articular position of the needle is confirmed by injection of a small quantity of iodinated contrast, followed by injection of a 20-30 mL gadolinium mixture with a 1:100 to 1:250 dilution. Gentle exercise following the injection can further assist in imbibition of the gadolinium mixture into a potential tear.

Meniscal tears at MR arthrography are diagnosed on the basis of a cleft of similar signal intensity as intra-articular gadolinium. Several studies directly comparing conventional MRI and MR arthrography in each patient have demonstrated a higher accuracy rate with MR arthrography in patients with previous meniscal surgery [9, 12, 13]. Applegate et al. demonstrated an overall accuracy of 66% for conventional MRI and 88% for MR arthrography [9]. Sciulli et al. obtained similar results, with accuracy rates of 77% and 92%, respectively, for conventional MRI and MR arthrography [12]. MR arthrography does not appear to have an advantage over conventional MRI for detection of recurrent tears in the subset of patients where <25% of the meniscus has been resected, with an accuracy of 89% for both techniques [9, 13]. In another study, whereby patients were randomized to either conventional MRI or MR arthrography, there were no statistically significant differences between the two techniques, with conventional MRI demonstrating a sensitivity of 86% and a specificity of 67%, and MR arthrography 89% and 78%, respectively, in the diagnosis of a recurrent or residual meniscal tear [14]. Diagnostic difficulties with direct MR arthrography can still be encountered because of residual increased intrasubstance signal changes seen within a healing or healed meniscal tear on short TE acquisitions, such as T1-weighted sequences traditionally employed at MR arthrography. Volume averaging of signal can occur across residual tear clefts utilizing traditional 2D MR acquisitions with image slice thicknesses of 3-4 mm. Such acquisitions may average voxel signal related to intrameniscal contrast or fluid with adjacent meniscal tissues, resulting in intermediate signal characteristics and diagnostic difficulties at evaluation.

CT arthrography has been utilized for detection of meniscal tears in virgin menisci with a reported sensitivity and specificity of over 90% [15]. CT arthrography has a sensitivity of 100% but a specificity of only 78% in detection of recurrent or residual meniscal tears [15]. The lower specificity is likely to be related to the high spatial resolution of CT arthrography identifying small foci of intrameniscal contrast that may represent stable partial-thickness meniscal tears. Using the criteria of contrast extending throughout the height or depth of the meniscus for a full thickness tear or at least a third of the height or depth of the meniscus for diagnosis of an unstable partial-thickness tear, the specificity of CT arthrography improves to 89%, but with a lower sensitivity of 93% [16].

In the setting of a young patient without pre-existent cartilage loss and an irrepairable extensive meniscal tear resulting in meniscal deficiency post meniscal resection, meniscal transplantation may be performed. MRI plays an important role in the preoperative assessment of potential transplant candidates, providing important information regarding the status of articular cartilage and ligamentous integrity of the joint, and serving as an accurate measure of meniscal transplant size matching requirements [17]. MRI can be used for evaluation of possible complications following meniscal transplantation. Few long-term follow-up MR imaging studies of meniscal transplants have been performed to date. The presence of meniscal transplant tears, healing of meniscal bone plugs, status of the meniscocapsular junction, and extrusion of the meniscus and chondral changes can be evaluated, but there appears to be poor correlation between MRI findings and clinical symptoms [17]. A degree of peripheral displacement of the body of a meniscal transplant can be seen in up to 46-72% of patients post meniscal transplantation [17]. However, frank meniscal transplant extrusion is less commonly seen and is more likely to be associated with symptoms. Additional MRI findings described suggestive of transplant failure include meniscal fragmentation, and progressive adjacent articular cartilage loss [17].

## Imaging of Postoperative Ligaments

### Anterior Cruciate Ligament

The anterior cruciate ligament (ACL) is by far the most frequently completely torn ligament of the knee. Treatment and reconstruction techniques of ligamentous injuries of the knee have improved significantly over the past two decades. Treatment of ACL injury is typically tailored to the patient's lifestyle and age, and the presence or absence of other associated injuries of the joint. In older patients, conservative treatment may be an option, with physiotherapy and muscle training used in attempts to minimize the degree of joint instability and thus avoid or sufficiently delay the early onset of arthritis. In people used to sporting activities or in professional athletes, operative treatment is advocated in order to prevent ongoing joint instability and complications of ACL deficiency, including further ligamentous damage, cartilage loss and meniscal tearing. Primary healing capacity of the ACL after tearing is limited, and primary repair of complete ACL tears without using augmentation grafts has generally been unsuccessful to date. Therefore, primary ACL reconstruction utilizing autologous graft material, allowing for early restoration of joint function, has become the most widely employed method of surgical management of the ACL deficient knee.

Several techniques of ACL reconstruction have been described. Currently, the mainstay of modern surgical re-construction is a single bundle reconstruction to recapitulate the anatomy and function of the anteromedial band of the native ACL. Recommended graft choices for such ACL reconstruction consist of either biologic autograft or allograft material [18]. Reconstruction of the ACL with prosthetic material has met with only limited degrees of success. The patellar tendon autograft is the method used in most orthopedic centers. The hamstring tendon graft has increased in popularity over the past several years, primarily as a result of improved fixation techniques [18]. No significant difference in long-term success between these two different methods of graft reconstruction has been found. However, advantages of hamstring graft ACL reconstruction include a small incision at the harvest site, as well as a decreased incidence of anterior knee symptoms following surgery. Bone-patellar tendon-bone grafts are commonly utilized in young active athletes because high-quality fixation of the graft allows for the earliest possible return to activity [18]. With this method, the middle third of the patellar tendon with bone plugs from the inferior pole of the patella and the tibial tuberosity are harvested. The major disadvantage of bone-patellar tendon-bone graft ACL reconstruction is a comparatively high incidence of symptoms at the harvest site, including anterior knee pain, postoperative arthrofibrosis, patellar tendon rupture, and even patellar fracture in rare cases. On MRI, following graft harvest the patellar tendon is initially thickened, generally illustrating intrasubstance increased T1- and intermediate T2- weighted signal. By about 18 months to 2 years after surgery, the gap in the patellar tendon becomes filled with granulation and scar tissue, demonstrating MRI signal almost identical to that of the original patellar tendon.

During the first couple of months after surgery, it has been have shown that the inserted graft is avascular, illustrating low MR signal intensity on all pulse sequences similar to that of the normal patellar tendon [19]. Within the first 3 months after ACL reconstruction, proliferating synovial tissue envelops the graft and provides its vascular supply. At approximately 6 months following surgery, however, the graft undergoes a remodeling process, during which time the graft experiences revascularization and resynovialization. The process of gradual transformation of the patellar or hamstring tendon graft into tissue very similar to the native ACL is referred to as graft "ligamentization". The strength of the graft is decreased during the period of revascularization and this results in its vulnerability to reinjury during this time period. Normally by 12-24 months the resynovialization process is finished [19]. Persistent intrasubstance graft signal following this was previously hypothesized to be reflective of complications such as possible graft impingement or partial tearing. However, more recently published literature has shown that variable degrees of mild increased intrasubstance graft signal is in fact seen in the majority of patients post ACL reconstruction, with stable joints at biomechanical testing, and excellent clinical function up to 7-10 years postoperatively [19].

Hamstring tendon grafts are derived from resection of the distal segments of the semimembranosus and gracilis tendons. The tendons are harvested from the level of their tibial attachment to the level of the musculotendinous junction. The two tendons are sutured together, doubled back onto one another, and then sutured together again, resulting in a graft composed of four separate bundles. MR signal intensities of the hamstring graft are almost identical to the patellar tendon graft. However, because the hamstring graft is composed of four separate bundles sutured together, MR imaging often demonstrates linear areas of intermediate signal interposed between the separate bundles of the graft. Important clinical considerations for achieving optimal results of ACL reconstruction include isometric graft positioning, avoidance of graft impingement, proper tensioning and fixation of the graft, and appropriate postoperative rehabilitation. The position of the femoral tunnel is critical in obtaining graft isometry. Graft tunnel location is chosen to achieve graft isometry by restoring normal anatomic alignment, and thus limit potential stretching or impingement of the graft, as well as overconstraint of the knee. The position of the femoral tunnel is typically placed at the intersection of the posterior femoral cortex and the posterior physeal scar corresponding to the midpoint in the anatomic origin of the anteromedial and posterolateral bands of the native ACL. The position of the tibial tunnel is typically chosen to correspond to the tibial insertion of the anteromedial band of the native ACL, such that the graft is oriented parallel but posterior to the slope of the intercondylar roof (Blumensaat's line), with the knee in a fully extended position, such as is well depicted on sagittal MR images. An anteriorly located femoral bone tunnel will cause elongation of the graft and result in instability of the knee. Posterior positioning of the tibial tunnel results in too steep a course of the ACL reconstruction, and potential residual ACL instability post reconstruction. In contrast, roof impingement occurs when the tibial tunnel is placed too far anteriorly.

Recent modifications in single bundle ACL surgical technique to address possible issues of posterolateral rotational instability following ACL reconstruction have included lower positioning of the femoral graft tunnel, such that the graft is oriented in a less vertical fashion on coronal images. In general, an orientation of a single bundle ACL graft in the coronal plane should be such that the femoral tunnel and origin of the graft is at the approximate 2:30 position of a clock face, with the graft oriented in a plane less than 75 degrees relative to the tibial plateaus. An additional trend in ACL reconstructive surgery, performed in attempts to recapitulate the full biomechanical function of an ACL reconstruction, is the double bundle anatomic ACL reconstruction. With double bundle reconstructions, anatomic surgical reconstruction of the two native ACL functional (anteromedial, and posterolateral) bundles are performed.

Common clinical symptoms of complication following ACL reconstruction include recurrent ACL instability, limited knee joint extension postoperatively, or new symptoms of joint derangement. MRI plays an important role in the assessment of possible ACL repair complications. ACL grafts are most vulnerable to injury during the first several months following reconstruction. The remodeling process weakens the graft temporarily, but by the end of the first year the graft approaches the strength of the native ACL. Recurrent instability following ACL reconstruction may be seen in the setting of graft tearing, dislodgement or failure of graft fixation, or graft stretching in the setting of an intact graft at MRI, but findings or symptoms of instability at clinical examination. MRI is highly accurate for diagnosing complete ACL graft tears. Integrity of the graft fibers can be well evaluated on MRI, with complete discontinuity of graft fibers seen in the setting of complete graft tears (Fig. 2). However, partial-thickness graft tears may also be seen with discontinuity of some, but not all, ACL graft fibers observed. Clinically, ACL graft tearing is classically associated with instability and history of re-injury of the knee. Another imaging feature that might accompany such clinical findings in the setting of intact graft fibers is dislodgement of a reconstruction graft secondary to fixation failure.

Limited knee extension following ACL reconstruction is typically manifest by loss of the terminal 5-10 degrees of knee extension at clinical examination. One important cause of such complication, which is evaluated by MRI, is graft impingement. Graft impingement is typically observed with surgical tibial tunnel positioning partially or completely anterior to the projected slope of the intercondylar notch (Blumensaat's line). In such instances, the distal half of the intercondylar roof mechanically impinges on the anterior surface of the graft during knee extension, leading to loss of terminal extension of the knee and the potential for progressive graft injury, fibrosis and possible rupture [19]. MRI allows direct visualization of the position of the tibial tunnel and its relationship to Blumensaat's line, as well as the course of the ACL graft and its relationship to the intercondylar roof. The impinged graft demonstrates focal increased signal on T1- and T2-weighted images in the distal two-thirds of the graft fibers. Notchplasty (a surgical procedure that consists of resection of a few millimeters of bone from the anterior outlet of the roof and the lateral wall of the intercondylar notch) can be performed to treat cases of mild graft impingement. Signal intensity changes seen on MR images of impinged grafts usually resolve within several weeks following notchplasty.

Another important cause of limited terminal extension of the knee following ACL reconstruction is postoperative arthrofibrosis. The focal localized nodular form of anterior compartment arthrofibrosis is seen in varying degrees in up to 10% of ACL reconstruction patients. It is believed that this form of arthrofibrosis potentially originates from osteocartilaginous debris or ligament residue at surgery, which incites a localized inflammatory response leading to the development of a fibrotic nodule classically situated immediately anterior to the inferior aspect of the ACL graft. Depending on its size, this

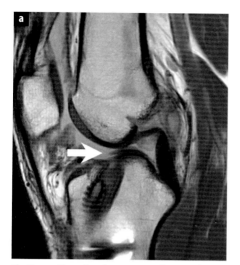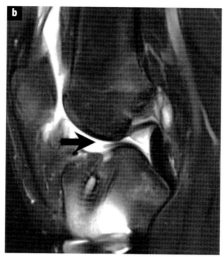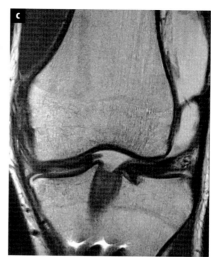

**Fig. 2 a-c.** Completely torn anterior cruciate ligament (ACL) reconstruction graft in a 30-year-old man who sustained an acute injury, 6 years following prior ACL reconstruction. Sagittal fast spin echo intermediate weighted (**a**), T2-weighted fat-suppressed (**b**), and coronal intermediate weighted (**c**) magnetic resonance images show complete discontinuity of ACL graft fibers (*arrows*) immediately adjacent to the tibial tunnel of the patients prior ACL reconstruction. Complete ACL graft tear was confirmed at the time of revision reconstruction surgery

fibrotic nodule may become entrapped between the femur and tibia when the knee is extended and lead to a mechanical block of terminal extension. At arthroscopy, the fibrous lesion has a head-like appearance with focal areas of discoloration that resemble an eye, leading to reference of the lesion as a "cyclops" lesion. Patients with symptomatic extension loss caused by cyclops lesions typically require second arthroscopy to resect the fibrous nodular shaped tissue. On T1-weighted MR images, a cyclops lesion appears as a focal nodular lesion of low signal intensity that is anterior to the graft in the intercondylar notch. Differentiation from adjacent joint fluid may be difficult on T1-weighted images alone. On T2-weighted images, the nodule is heterogeneous but predominantly of low signal intensity, and is well differentiated from high-signal-intensity joint fluid.

Cystic degeneration, or so-called ganglion of the graft, is a late complication of ACL repair that is also commonly accompanied by enlargement of the bone tunnel. Ganglion cysts most commonly arise within the tibial tunnel of the graft construct and may propagate and protrude into the joint proximally or into the subcutaneous soft tissues through the distal opening of the tibial tunnel. Hamstring autografts and fixation of the graft with endobuttons are reported to predispose to cystic degeneration. It has been shown that fluid collections occur normally within the tibial and femoral tunnels during the first year following use of hamstring grafts. Small amounts of fluid may also accumulate between the four separate bundles of the hamstring graft without a relationship to subsequent graft ganglion cyst formation.

Tibial and femoral tunnel enlargement has often been observed after ACL reconstruction with absorbable interference or metallic screws. Possible etiologies for this enlargement include an immune response with resorption and stress shielding proximal to the interference screw that results in resorption or an inflammatory response by the synovium within the tunnel. Other proposed etiologies of tunnel enlargement include bone resorption due to the micromotion of the graft relative to the tunnel wall, or mechanical osseous compression and secondary bony remodeling, or stress shielding caused by graft fixation hardware.

## Posterior Cruciate Ligament

Injury to the posterior cruciate ligament (PCL) is 10-20 times less common than ACL injuries. Unlike ACL injuries, the majority of PCL injuries are partial-thickness tears, which are adequately treated conservatively. Nonoperative treatment is also the common means of managing patients with asymptomatic isolated PCL injuries. However, importantly, PCL injuries are isolated in only 30% of cases, and in patients with multiligamentous knee injury, or those with chronic symptomatic PCL laxity, PCL reconstruction is an important and increasingly popular surgical treatment option for re-establishing stability of the joint. The same graft options that are available for ACL reconstruction are also used for PCL reconstruction. The normal PCL graft should have uniform low signal on all MRI pulse sequences, although it appears to undergo a similar synovialization process to the ACL, illustrating inhomogeneity and mild signal change during the first year. On long-term follow-up the graft demonstrates low signal intensity on all pulse sequences. The contour of the normal PCL graft can range from mildly curved to straight. As with ACL reconstruction, graft rupture is manifested by discontinuity of fibers and extension of fluid into the tear gap. Small amounts of fluid signal intensity may be seen extending longitudinally in between the bundles of a hamstring graft without signifying pathology. PCL graft reconstruction can also lead to arthrofibrosis anterior to the graft construct, and this can be visualized on postoperative MRI studies.

## Collateral Ligaments

As with PCL injuries, collateral ligament injuries are rarely surgically treated as they are often partial injuries that respond well to nonoperative treatment. Even grade III injuries can be treated conservatively. With medial collateral ligament injuries, surgical treatment is reserved for athletes, and patients with complete tears causing instability or chronic tears that have failed to respond to conservative treatment. In such instances where surgery is required, the ligament is typically repaired with sutures and staples rather than reconstructed.

With posterolateral corner injuries, early treatment of complete tears is recommended. Within the first 2-3 weeks, primary repair may be undertaken but thereafter reconstructive techniques are typically required in those with grade III injuries. Treatment of posterolateral corner injury is especially important in those with ACL or PCL reconstruction, as failure to address posterolateral instability has been recognized as an important cause of ACL and PCL reconstruction failure. Primary repair techniques address proximal avulsions of the popliteus and fibular collateral ligament with transosseous tunnels through the lateral femoral condyle. Complete myotendinous injuries of the popliteus can be treated by directly suturing the popliteus onto the posterior tibia. Distal fibular collateral ligament avulsions are treated with drill holes in the fibular styloid or by screw fixation. These repairs may need to be augmented using the iliotibial band or the biceps femoris. Reconstructive techniques in delayed cases can be anatomic or nonanatomic, with the former being preferred. Anatomic techniques use semitendinosus autograft or allograft or an Achilles allograft combined with capsular repair or posterolateral capsular shift to reconstruct the popliteus, the fibular collateral and popliteofibular ligaments.

MRI evaluation of posterolateral corner and medial collateral ligament repairs and reconstructions has not been extensively studied. The use of screws and staples can result in artifact obscuring the reconstructed ligaments. With ligamentous repairs, the ligaments may initially demonstrate abnormal signal intensity and diffuse thickening. Such thickening invariably persists, although the signal intensity tends to diminish with time.

## Rotator Cuff Repair: Normal Postoperative Findings

The postoperative MRI appearance of the rotator cuff will depend upon the extent of the original tear and the surgical procedure that was performed. In the case of partial-thickness rotator cuff tendon tears, the tendon may be debrided, repaired with a transtendon technique or repaired after tear completion by the orthopedic surgeon [20, 21].

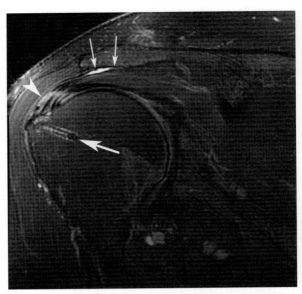

**Fig. 3.** Intact supraspinatus tendon tear after repair with bioabsorbable anchor. Coronal oblique fast spin echo T2-weighted fat-suppressed image demonstrates intermediate signal intensity in the distal supraspinatus tendon (*arrowhead*) without fluid signal to suggest re-tear. Note the intact bioabsorbable anchor (*large arrow*) and acromioplasty (*small arrows*). Of note, only 10% of repaired rotator cuff tendons will demonstrate normal signal intensity

When tears are debrided, they classically have a defect that is "longer than deep" relative to the long axis of the tendon on MRI. However, if the postoperative MRI demonstrates a deep defect extending from the articular to the bursal surface of the cuff, then re-tear should be strongly suspected. Repaired rotator cuff tendons will have a variable appearance with respect to signal intensity on MRI, with an expected temporal evolution on serial imaging [22]. Within 3 months after surgery, rotator cuff tendons typically display intermediate signal intensity and appear most disorganized compared with native tendons, reflecting development of granulation tissue [22-24]. With time, the fibrosis within the tendons leads to lower signal intensity on all sequences, but only 10% of repaired tendons will ever demonstrate normal signal intensity on MRI (Fig. 3) [24].

Rotator cuff tendon tears involving the myotendinous junction or critical zone can be treated with direct suture repair; however, the majority of small full-thickness rotator cuff repairs are performed using the tendon-to-bone repair technique with surgical tacks and suture. Assessment of the repaired rotator cuff tendon must address both the status of the suture anchors and the repaired tendon. Tendon re-tears will demonstrate fluid or intra-articular contrast (if injected) within the recurrent defect; however, radiologists should be aware that even asymptomatic patients may have signal changes suggestive of tendinopathy and have clinically "silent" partial and complete rotator cuff tears [24]. In studies of clinically asymptomatic postoperative patients, individuals can have marked improve-

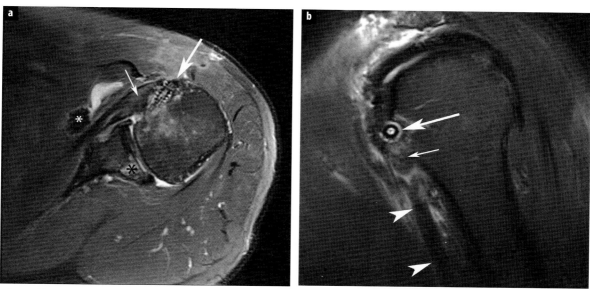

**Fig. 4 a, b.** Intact biceps tenodesis. **a** Axial fast spin echo (FSE) T2-weighted fat-suppressed (FS) image shows bioabsorbable anchor (*large arrow*) extending through the bicipital groove at site of biceps tenodesis. Note the thickened, intermediate signal intensity within the subscapularis tendon (*small arrow*) due to marked tendinopathy and remote tear. *White asterisk* indicates loose bodies in the subscapularis recess; *black asterisk* indicates degenerative edema in the posterior glenoid deep to full-thickness cartilage defects. **b** Sagittal FSE T2-weighted FS image demonstrates tenodesis anchor (*large arrow*) and reattached long head of the biceps tendon (*arrowheads*), with marked tendinopathy of the adjacent subscapularis tendon (*small arrow*)

ment in symptoms without a watertight seal. "Suspension bridge" repair of massive rotator cuff tears can be an effective technique, and complete coverage is not essential to convert debilitating tears into functional cuff tears.

Double row suture anchor repair is done in conjunction with creation of an implantation trough at the junction of the humeral head and greater tuberosity, allowing optimal apposition of tendon to bone [23, 24]. Irreparable massive rotator cuff tears can be repaired using arthroscopic rotator cuff reconstruction with a variety of patch grafts, including artificial synthetic grafts, allogenic freeze-dried tissues, porcine small intestine submucosa or autografts (i.e., long head of the biceps tendon) [23, 24]. Osteolysis around bioabsorbable suture anchors is an expected reaction caused by mechanical forces from drilling or focal necrosis, but these defects should eventually stabilize and become replaced with bone at 2 years [23]. In addition, mild bone marrow edema-like signal changes should be recognized as an expected finding on MRI, and may occur up to 5 years after surgery in asymptomatic patients [24]. However, T1 marrow signal should remain normal. If erosions develop or T1 marrow signal intensity starts to approximate muscle signal intensity, then infection should be strongly suspected.

Tenotomy or tenodesis of the long head of the biceps is performed if there are irreversible structural changes in the tendon, significant atrophy or hypertrophy, partial tearing greater than 25% of the width of the tendon, subluxation of the tendon from its groove, or if certain disorders of the biceps origin exist [25]. Tenodesis remains the preferred treatment for younger patients with biceps dysfunction, and intact repairs will often demonstrate in-

termediate signal intensity within the reattached portion of the tendon (Fig. 4).

## Labral Tear Repair: Normal Postoperative Findings

Direct anatomic repair of labral tears is usually performed by suturing the anterior labrum and joint capsule, and the anterior band of the inferior band of the inferior glenohumeral ligament to the glenoid rim. With MRI or MR arthrography, there should be no separation between the labrocapsular complex and the glenoid margin in intact labral repairs (Fig. 5). If there is a susceptibility artifact from metallic fixation, MRI metal reduction techniques should be implemented as discussed above in the section "Imaging Techniques in the Postoperative Patient". Capsular thickening with an irregular nodular contour is an expected postoperative MRI finding. Comparison with prior MRI studies is of utmost importance to evaluate for re-tear. The overall accuracy of MR arthrography for detecting labral tears after prior instability repair varies in the literature, but is generally greater than 90% [26]. A known pitfall resulting in false-negative MRI interpretation is the presence of intermediate signal intensity granulation tissue within a repaired labral tear, which may prevent joint fluid or injected contrast from outlining a persistent defect.

Paralabral cysts develop through the accumulation of joint fluid extending through labral tears, and may propagate along the spinoglenoid or suprascapular notches. These are known as spinoglenoid notch or suprascapular notch ganglia. Improvements in external rotation strength have been shown in patients who are treated with cyst

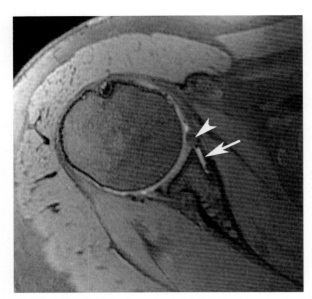

**Fig. 5.** Intact anterior labral repair. Axial double echo steady state image delineates the anterior glenoid bioabsorbable anchor (*arrow*) and reattached anterior labrum (*arrowhead*). Although the reattached labrum is heterogeneous, there is no fluid signal intensity within or subjacent to the labrum to suggest re-tear

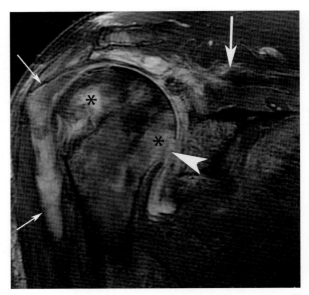

**Fig. 6.** Septic arthritis and osteomyelitis after failed rotator cuff repair. Coronal oblique fast spin echo T2-weighted fat-suppressed image shows extensive abnormal signal intensity throughout the humeral head (*asterisks*) with focal destruction of the medial humeral neck cortex (*arrowhead*), consistent with osteomyelitis. Complex fluid (*small arrows*) within and around the shoulder joint communicated with draining sinus tract (not shown). Notice the retracted, torn supraspinatus tendon (*large arrow*)

decompression and superior labrum anterior and posterior (SLAP) repair, as opposed to SLAP repair alone [27].

Recurrent anterior shoulder dislocation typically results in combined Bankart and Hill-Sachs lesions, although concomitant SLAP lesions can also be present. Arthroscopic Bankart repair after recurrent anterior shoulder dislocation can be performed along with the remplissage technique for treatment of instability with engaging Hill-Sachs lesions [28]. This technique transfers the posterior capsule and infraspinatus tendon into the Hill-Sachs defect to prevent re-engagement of the lesion on the glenoid rim. MRI will show corresponding findings of reattachment of the posterior structures into the defect, along with the metallic or bioabsorbable anchor embedded in the trough [28].

## Postoperative Imaging of Complications of the Shoulder

Complications in the postoperative shoulder may include failure of the repair, hematoma or seroma, adhesive capsulitis, septic arthritis and osteomyelitis (Fig. 6), muscle atrophy, deltoid dehiscence and heterotopic ossification, and regional complex pain syndrome, among others [29, 30]. Of note, the majority of recurrent tendon tears occur in the first 3 months after surgical repair (Figs. 7, 8) [29]. Rotator cuff failure has a myriad of causes, including suture-bone or suture-anchor pullout, suture breakage, knot slippage, tendon pullout, poor quality tendon or bone, muscle atrophy, inadequate initial repair, and improper/overly aggressive physical therapy [29, 30]. The bioabsorbable anchors may fragment before they are re-

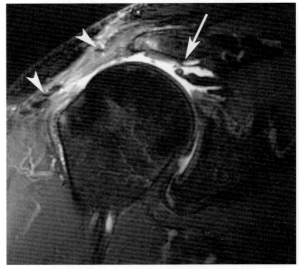

**Fig. 7.** Supraspinatus tendon re-tear and deltoid dehiscence. Coronal oblique fast spin echo T2-weighted fat-suppressed image shows full-thickness rupture of the supraspinatus tendon, with retraction of the tendinous remnant (*arrow*) to the level of the medial humeral head. Also notice focal deltoid dehiscence, with suture susceptibility artifact (*arrowheads*) at the retracted margins after mini-open rotator cuff repair

sorbed, become intra-articular loose bodies and induce synovitis. The likelihood of recurrent rotator cuff tear is much greater if the repaired tendons have associated muscle fatty degeneration and atrophy, so this imaging feature should be noted in all MRI dictations. Of interest, patients

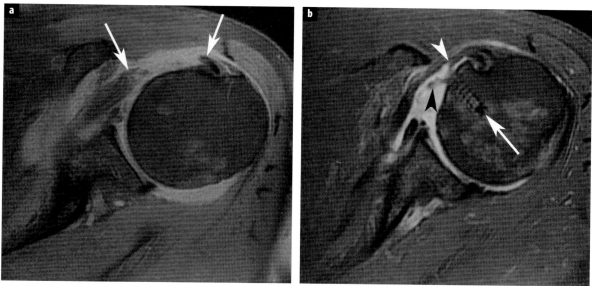

**Fig. 8 a, b.** Partial thickness re-tear of subscapularis tendon. **a** Axial fast spin echo (FSE) T2-weighted fat-suppressed (FS) image shows full-thickness rupture of the subscapularis tendon, with distraction of the tendinous remnants (*arrows*). **b** Postoperative axial FSE T2-weighted FS image shows partial thickness re-tear of the deep fibers of the reattached subscapularis tendon (*arrowheads*) and intact bioabsorbable screw (*arrow*) in the lesser tuberosity of the humerus

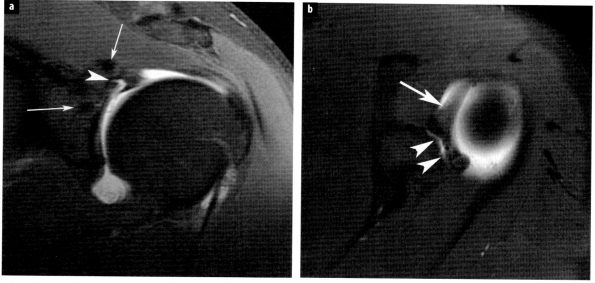

**Fig. 9 a, b.** Superior labral re-tear. Coronal (**a**) and axial (**b**) images from a magnetic resonance arthrogram demonstrate injected contrast (*arrowheads*) extending beneath the detached superior labrum. Two superior glenoid suture anchors (*small arrows*, **a**) are not dislodged. The *large arrow* (**b**) indicates the long head of the biceps tendon

with structural failure or re-rupture may still have significant improvement in pain and function, however, re-tears are usually smaller than the original tears. Occasionally, a retracted full-thickness rotator cuff tear may adhere to the subacromial soft tissues via scar tissue, giving a somewhat confusing MRI appearance. Therefore, direct visualization of a continuous tendon onto the humeral head is required to prevent this misinterpretation.

Finally, complications of labral repair are similar to those of rotator cuff repair in regard to hardware fail-ure points. MRI is particularly useful for identifying labral re-tear, migration of the bioabsorbable tacks or suture anchors, loosened or protruding anchors, which can abut the articular cartilage and result in early cartilage degeneration, and synovitis induced by bioabsorbable tacks [30]. Labral re-tears will be evident on MRI by either abnormal extension of fluid signal or injected contrast into either the substance of the labrum or between the detached labrum and the glenoid (Fig. 9).

## Conclusion

In conclusion, MRI is an excellent technique to address complications after knee and shoulder surgery, and allows for evaluation for meniscal re-tear, integrity of the postoperative cruciate and collateral ligaments, rotator cuff and labral re-tears, hardware integrity, infection, synovitis, soft tissue dehiscence and heterotopic ossification. Review of the preoperative MRI of each patient's knee and shoulder injury and knowledge of the applied surgical procedure is essential to optimize the radiologist's interpretation of the postoperative patient. Radiologists must also be familiar with the expected postoperative appearance of bioabsorbable suture anchors and recognize a variety of complications related to them. Overall, MRI continues to be a highly accurate imaging modality in the work-up of the complicated postoperative patient.

## References

1. Viano AM, Gronemeyer SA, Haliloglu M, Hoffer FA (2000) Improved MR imaging for patients with metallic implants. Magn Reson Imaging 18:287-295
2. Sofka CM, Potter HG (2002) MR imaging of joint arthroplasty. Semin Musculoskelet Radiol 6:79-85
3. Barber FA, McGarry JE (2007) Meniscal repair techniques. Sports Med Arthrosc 15:199-207
4. Toms AP, White LM, Marshall TJ, Donell ST (2005) Imaging the post-operative meniscus. Eur J Radiol 54:189-198
5. De Smet AA, Tuite MJ, Norris MA, Swan JS (1994) MR diagnosis of meniscal tears: analysis of causes of errors. AJR Am J Roentgenol 163:1419-1423
6. De Smet AA, Norris MA, Yandow DR et al (1993) MR diagnosis of meniscal tears of the knee: importance of high signal in the meniscus that extends to the surface. AJR Am J Roentgenol 161:101-107
7. Farley TE, Howell SM, Love KF et al (1991) Meniscal tears: MR and arthrographic findings after arthroscopic repair. Radiology 180:517-522
8. Mariani PP, Santori N, Adriani E, Mastantuono M (1996) Accelerated rehabilitation after arthroscopic meniscal repair: a clinical and magnetic resonance imaging evaluation. Arthroscopy 12:680-686
9. Applegate GR, Flannigan BD, Tolin BS et al (1993) MR diagnosis of recurrent tears in the knee: value of intraarticular contrast material. AJR Am J Roentgenol 161:821-825
10. Smith DK, Totty WG (1990) The knee after partial meniscectomy: MR imaging features. Radiology 176:141-144
11. Magee T, Shapiro M, Williams D (2004) Prevalence of meniscal radial tears of the knee revealed by MRI after surgery. AJR Am J Roentgenol 182:931-936
12. Sciulli RL, Boutin RD, Brown RR et al (1999) Evaluation of the postoperative meniscus of the knee: a study comparing conventional arthrography, conventional MR imaging, MR arthrography with iodinated contrast material, and MR arthrography with gadolinium-based contrast material. Skeletal Radiol 28:508-514
13. Magee T, Shapiro M, Rodriguez J, Williams D (2003) MR arthrography of postoperative knee: for which patients is it useful? Radiology 229:159-163
14. White LM, Schweitzer ME, Weishaupt D et al (2002) Diagnosis of recurrent meniscal tears: prospective evaluation of conventional MR imaging, indirect MR arthrography, and direct MR arthrography. Radiology 222:421-429
15. Vande Berg BC, Lecouvet FE, Poilvache P et al (2002) Anterior cruciate ligament tears and associated meniscal lesions: assessment at dual-detector spiral CT arthrography. Radiology 223:403-409
16. Mutschler C, Vande Berg BC, Lecouvet FE et al (2003) Postoperative meniscus: assessment at dual-detector row spiral CT arthrography of the knee. Radiology 228:635-641
17. Verstraete KL, Verdonk R, Lootens T et al (1997) Current status and imaging of allograft meniscal transplantation. Eur J Radiol 26:16-22
18. Brand J, Weiler A, Caborn DN et al (2000) Graft fixation in cruciate ligament reconstruction. Am J Sports Med 28:761-774
19. Saupe N, White LM, Chiavaras MM et al (2008) Anterior cruciate ligament reconstruction grafts: MR imaging features at long-term follow-up – correlation with functional and clinical evaluation. Radiology 249:581-590
20. Jacobson JA, Miller B, Bedi A, Morag Y (2011) Imaging of the postoperative shoulder. Semin Musculoskelet Radiol 15:320-339
21. Shin SJ (2011) A comparison of 2 repair techniques for partial-thickness articular sided rotator cuff tears. Arthroscopy. Epub ahead of print.
22. Crim J, Burks R, Manaster BJ et al (2010) Temporal evolution of MRI findings after arthroscopic rotator cuff repair. AJR Am J Roentgenol 195:1361-1366
23. Glueck D, Wilson TC, Johnson DL (2005) Extensive osteolysis after rotator cuff repair with a bioabsorbable suture anchor: a case report. Am J Sports Med 33:742-744
24. Spielmann AL, Forster BB, Kokan P et al (1999) Shoulder after rotator cuff repair: MR imaging findings in asymptomatic individuals—initial experience. Radiology 213:705-708
25. Ball C, Galatz LM, Yamaguchi K (2001) Tenodesis or tenotomy of the biceps tendon: why and when to do it. Techn Shoulder Elbow Surg 2:140-152
26. Probyn LJ, White LM, Salonen DC et al (2007) Recurrent symptoms after shoulder instability repair: Direct MR arthrographic assessment – correlation with second-look surgical evaluation. Radiology 245:814-823
27. Pillai G, Baynes JR, Gladstone J, Flatow EL (2011) Greater strength increase with cyst decompression and SLAP repair than SLAP repair alone. Clin Orthop Relat Res 469:1050-1060
28. Zhu YM, Lu Y, Zhang J et al (2011) Arthroscopic Bankart repair combined with remplissage technique for the treatment of anterior shoulder instability with engaging Hill-Sachs lesion: a report of 49 cases with a minimum of 2-year follow-up. Am J Sports Med 39:1640-1647
29. Kluger R, Bock P, Mittlbock M et al (2011) Long-term survivorship of rotator cuff repairs using ultrasound and magnetic resonance imaging analysis. Am J Sports Med 39:3071-3081
30. Mohana-Borges AV, Chung CB, Resnick D (2004) MR imaging and MR arthrography of the postoperative shoulder: spectrum of normal and abnormal findings. RadioGraphics 24:69-85

# Imaging and Staging of Bone and Soft Tissue Tumors: Fundamental Concepts

Mark J. Kransdorf[1], Mark D. Murphey[2]

[1] Department of Radiology, Mayo Clinic, Phoenix, AZ, USA
[2] American Institute for Radiologic Pathology, Silver Spring, MD, USA

## Introduction

The radiologic evaluation of musculoskeletal tumors has undergone dramatic evolution with the advent of computer-assisted imaging; specifically, computed tomography (CT) and magnetic resonance (MR) imaging. Despite the use of these sophisticated imaging modalities, the objectives of initial radiologic evaluation remain unchanged: detecting the suspected lesion, establishing a diagnosis, or, when a definitive diagnosis is not possible, formulating an appropriate differential diagnosis, and determining the radiologic staging of the lesion [1]. As a detailed discussion of all bone and soft tissue tumors is well beyond the scope of this review, we will highlight fundamental principles that should serve as a guide to the initial evaluation and staging of primary musculoskeletal neoplasms.

**Box 1.** Differential diagnoses: multiple musculoskeletal lesions

Bone tumors
    Metastases
    Myeloma
    Lymphoma
    Enchondromatosis (including variants)
    Multiple hereditary exostoses
    Langerhans cell histiocytosis
    Multifocal osteomyelitis
    Hyperparathyroidism with brown tumors

Soft tissue tumors
    Neurofibromatosis
    Schwannomatosis
    Myxomas (Mazabraud syndrome)
    Angiomatosis
    Lipomas (including hereditary lipomasosis)
    Desmoid tumors

## Clinical History

The clinical history is an important factor in establishing an accurate diagnosis and should not be overlooked. In many circumstances it provides key information that suggests or allows a specific diagnosis when imaging is nonspecific. Useful information includes a history of the present illness: how and why did the patient come to medical attention. An incidental finding on an examination for an unrelated cause is more likely (although not invariably) benign. Similarly, lesions that have remained stable in size over time are also more likely to be benign, while a history of continued growth is always suspicious for malignancy. Other useful information includes a history of a previous lesion or underlying malignancy, previous surgery, radiation, notable trauma or anticoagulants. The differential diagnostic criteria for bone and soft tissue tumors are markedly reduced if multiple lesions are present (Box 1).

## Initial Tumor Evaluation

The radiograph remains the initial imaging study for evaluating both bone and soft tissue lesions. For osseous lesions, it is almost invariably the most diagnostic. The radiograph accurately predicts the biologic activity of a bone lesion, which is reflected in the appearance of the margin of the lesion, and the type and extent of accompanying periosteal reaction. In addition, the pattern of associated matrix mineralization may be a key to the underlying histology (e.g., cartilage, bone, fibro-osseous) [2-5]. Although other imaging modalities (MR and CT) are superior to radiographs in staging a bone lesion, the radiograph remains the best modality for establishing a diagnosis, for formulating a differential, and for accurately assessing the biologic activity (separating benign from malignant lesions). In many cases, as in patients with fibroxanthoma (nonossifying fibroma), fibrous dysplasia,

J. Hodler et al. (eds.), *Musculoskeletal Diseases 2013-2016*,
DOI: 10.1007/978-88-470-5292-5_11 © Springer-Verlag Italia 2013

osteochondroma or enchondroma, radiographs may be virtually pathognomonic, and no further diagnostic imaging is required. In other cases, despite not having an unequivocal diagnosis, a benign-appearing, asymptomatic lesion may require only continued radiographic follow-up in order to document long-term stability.

Radiographs are typically considered unrewarding in the assessment of soft tissue masses; however, a recent study of 281 patients showed calcification in 27%, bone involvement in 22% and fat in 11% of cases [6]. Such features may be essential in establishing an appropriate imaging diagnosis, establishing a differential, and in assessing malignant potential. Radiographs may also be diagnostic of a palpable lesion caused by an underlying skeletal deformity (such as exuberant callus related to prior trauma) or exostosis, which may masquerade as a soft tissue mass. The soft tissue calcifications and/or ossification identified on radiographs can be suggestive, and at times highly characteristic, of a specific diagnosis. For example, they may reveal the phleboliths within a hemangioma, the juxta-articular osteocartilaginous masses of synovial chondromatosis, the peripherally more mature ossification of myositis ossificans, or the characteristic bone changes of other processes with associated soft tissue involvement. When not characteristic of a specific process, soft tissue calcification can suggest certain diagnoses. For example, nonspecific dystrophic calcifications within a slowly growing lower extremity mass in an adolescent or young adult should suggest a synovial sarcoma as the diagnosis of exclusion.

## Advanced Imaging Techniques

MR imaging is the preferred modality for evaluating soft tissue lesions. It provides superior soft tissue contrast, allows multiplanar image acquisition, obviates the need for iodinated contrast agents or for ionizing radiation, and is devoid of streak artifact commonly encountered with CT imaging [7-10]. When clinical findings are equivocal, MR imaging evaluation can confirm the presence of a soft tissue lesion or reassuringly identify a suspected "bump" or "mass" as normal tissue [11]. Whereas MR imaging has emerged as the preferred advanced imaging modality for the evaluation of soft tissue lesions, CT and MR imaging are often complimentary modalities for the evaluation of primary osseous tumors [10]. In a study by Tehranzadeh et al., the information obtained from CT and MR imaging was additive in 76% of malignant primary bone neoplasms [10]. CT scanning is superior to MR imaging for the detection and characterization (osteoid or chondroid) of matrix mineralization, cortical involvement and periosteal reaction [9, 10]. Although some studies suggest that CT and MR are equivalent for the evaluation of the local extent of tumor [12], most studies note the superiority of MR imaging [9, 10, 13-15].

## Magnetic Resonance Imaging

While there is no single best tumor protocol, we feel MR imaging should be performed in at least two orthogonal planes, typically including both T1- and T2-weighted images in the axial plane, supplemented by sagittal and/or coronal images, depending on the location of the lesion. The long axis imaging should include both T1 and a water-sensitive sequence, such as short tau inversion-recovery (STIR) or fat-suppressed T2-weighted sequence. It has been our experience that spin-echo imaging is often most useful in establishing a specific diagnosis when possible, and is the most reproducible technique, and the one most often referenced in the tumor imaging literature. It is the imaging technique with which we are most familiar for tumor evaluation, and it has established itself as the standard by which other imaging techniques must be judged [16]. The main disadvantage of spin-echo imaging remains the relatively long acquisition times, particularly for double-echo T2-weighted sequences [16]. This is especially problematic in areas susceptible to respiratory motion. Some time savings have been obtained by increasing the number of echoes collected per excitation, in so-called turbo spin-echo or fast spin-echo (TSE/FSE) sequences, which have now generally replaced the traditional spin-echo sequences. Recent advances have made it possible to extend this concept so that an entire T2-weighted image set can now be obtained in a single breath-hold [17-19].

Rapid, fluid-sensitive imaging techniques comprise both spin-echo and gradient-echo design. Both approaches acquire all the echoes necessary for creation of a single image during the course of a single TR (i.e, after a single excitation pulse, or radio frequency). In a sense, then, these resemble CT, in that slices are obtained separately and sequentially, restricting motion artifact to only those slices acquired while motion is occurring. The term single-shot (SS) is commonly used to describe this approach. Of the SS techniques, the spin-echo-based sequences are the most commonly employed. Depending on the vendor, these are variously labeled HASTE, SS-TSE or SS-FSE. Not only are these relatively motion insensitive, and fast enough to allow for breath-hold imaging, but they are exquisitely sensitive to the presence of fluid, improving contrast with soft tissue [20-22]. HASTE is an important part of the technical arsenal for T2-weighted body MR imaging, where it is, for example, the backbone of magnetic resonance cholangiopancreatography (MRCP) imaging [22]. Because of the modifications of the traditional spin-echo sequence required to shorten it to a breath-hold, a significant drawback of the HASTE-type sequence is a low signal-to-noise ratio (SNR). Sensitivity to the SNR issue is important to avoid starving the images of signal by, for example, over-reduction of slice thickness or field-of-view.

Although also easily acquired in a breath-hold, the gradient-echo (GRE) version of SS imaging (trueFISP/FIESTA/balanced FFE), which is based on steady-state principles, provides a different kind of contrast. Immediately noticeable is the high signal intensity of flowing blood, compared with the usual signal void produced by a spin-echo sequence. This characteristic can be nicely exploited for unenhanced vascular imaging. By the same token, however, the concatenation of bright vessels and bright fluid collections can be visually daunting, and can at times obscure structures of interest. In addition, because trueFISP has mixed T1- and T2-weighting, tissue contrast is less than optimal. On the other hand, an important strength of the trueFISP-like sequences is its improved SNR, which can be exploited in the service of spatial resolution [22-25]. Furthermore, for motion studies, as in cardiac or pelvic floor evaluation, these sequences far outperform the spin-echo-based SS techniques [23]. When incorporating trueFISP or its cousins into a protocol, it is important to consider its GRE origin, since the technique does not perform as well in the presence of metal or air, with greater risk for magnetic susceptibility artifact.

GRE imaging techniques may be a useful supplement for demonstrating hemosiderin because of their greater magnetic susceptibility and, in general, susceptibility artifacts related to metallic material, hemorrhage and air are accentuated on GRE images [26]. STIR sequences are very useful in evaluating subtle marrow abnormalities and can be performed more quickly than T2-weighted spin-echo sequences [27], being frequently added to the conventional spin-echo sequences. Some prefer short TE/TR spin-echo and STIR sequences to typical T1- and T2-weighted spin-echo sequences. Although STIR imaging increases lesion conspicuity [27, 28], it typically has lower SNRs than spin-echo imaging and is also more susceptible to degradation by motion [16, 29]. Additionally, STIR and other fat-suppressed imaging techniques reduce the variations in signal intensities identified on conventional spin-echo MR imaging, variations that are most helpful in tissue characterization.

For suspected malignant extremity lesions, such as when osteosarcoma is a differential consideration, it is essential that at least one long axis sequence be performed through the entire involved bone in order to evaluate for the presence of skip metastases. Skip metastases represent a second site of disease in the same bone as the primary tumor but are separated by an area of normal marrow. The identification of skip lesions has clinical implications, and this additional imaging should be performed in appropriate cases.

## Computed Tomography Scanning

As previously noted, CT scanning is superior to MR imaging in the detection and characterization of matrix mineralization (osteoid or chondroid), cortical involvement and periosteal reaction [9, 29]. CT is uniquely suited to assess internal matrix when such matrix is obscured by lesion marginal sclerosis and not adequately evaluated by radiographs [30]. We find CT especially useful in the assessment of both bone and soft tissue lesions in those areas in which the osseous anatomy is complex, such as in the spine or small bones of the hands and feet, or where the radiographic osseous detail is obscured by overlying soft tissue, such as in the pelvis.

Although initial investigations maintained that CT is superior to MR imaging in detecting destruction of cortical bone [9, 10], more recently it has been suggested that these two modalities are comparable in this regard [31]. It has also been our experience that nonmetallic foreign bodies may be difficult to identify on MR imaging. In such cases, imaging may show the changes associated with the foreign body, although the foreign body itself may have no signal and may be difficult to identify when small.

## Contrast Enhancement

Contrast administration may be a useful adjunct in the assessment of both bone and soft tissue lesions; however, its use is usually dictated by the objectives of the examination. For example, in the CT evaluation of osseous lesions, it is typically not required to assess the presence or character of matrix mineralization, periosteal reaction or marginal sclerosis. On MR imaging, many lesions are well assessed without contrast. As a rule, we find it of little value in the assessment of lipoma or the usual atypical lipomatous tumor (atypical lipoma). In some cases, contrast administration can also cause confusion, blurring the distinction of tumor from peritumoral edema and normal from abnormal marrow [14, 32]. Nevertheless, it may provide essential information and we find contrast imaging especially important in the assessment of lesions containing hemorrhage, myxomatous areas, or necrotic or cystic regions. Only vascularized tissue enhances; therefore, contrast enhanced imaging may be quite useful in directing biopsy to the solid, enhancing portions of a lesion, the portion of the lesion that harbors the diagnostic tissue, as opposed to the cystic, necrotic or hemorrhagic nondiagnostic components. Additionally, the pattern of enhancement may also provide clues to the diagnosis, as in the characteristic peripheral and septal enhancement pattern seen with hyaline cartilage neoplasms.

Contrast-enhanced imaging is not without a price. The use of intravenous contrast increases the length and cost of the examination. Although contrast-enhanced MR imaging may provide additional information, it usually does not increase lesion conspicuity nor replace the diagnostic value of T2-weighted imaging [33]. While MR contrast agents are safer than those used with CT, there is a small, but real, incidence of untoward reactions including hypotension, laryngospasm, bronchospasm and anaphylactic shock [34-36]. Most recently, the association of nephrogenic systemic fibrosis (NSF) with the use of gadolinium-based contrast agents has focused greater attention on its routine administration [37-39]. NSF was first reported in 2000 as a scleroderma-like fibrotic skin disorder in patients with renal insufficiency [38-40]. In a large 10-year study of 8,997 patients receiving gadolinium-based contrast, 15 (0.17%) developed NSF, all of whom had renal failure with glomerular filtration rates of less than 30 mL/min [37]. In a study at four US university tertiary care centers involving over 216,000 patients, NSF was found to be more than 15 times more common with gadodiamide (Omniscan™) than gadopentetate dimeglumine (Magnevist®) [38]. The development of NSF has also been associated with high cumulative doses of gadolinium-based contrast, leading to the recommendation that half-strength contrast be given to patients with glomerular filtration rates of less than 60 mL/min [37, 41-43]. Consequently, contrast-enhanced imaging should be reserved for those cases in which the results influence patient management.

## Bone Scintigraphy

Bone scintigrapy with 99mTc phosphate compounds remains the modality of choice for the identification of multifocal osseous disease. Positron emission tomography (PET) has established itself as the gold standard for metabolic imaging, and while it has not replaced skeletal scintigraphy, it has several intrinsic advantages. It has inherently superior spatial resolution and routinely includes tomographic images with multiplanar capability. Additionally, unlike skeletal scintigraphy, which primarily evaluates only the skeletal system, PET detects disease in both the osseous structures as well in the soft tissues, allowing detection of not only the primary tumor, but pulmonary, as well as nodal, metastasis [44]. Moreover, PET detects the presence of tumor directly, by reflecting its metabolic activity, rather than indirectly as with conventional scintigraphy, by demonstrating tumor involvement due to its increased bone mineral turnover [44].

## Staging

The staging of musculoskeletal tumors is one of the primary functions of imaging. Accurate staging is essential for appropriate planning of therapy and establishing of prognosis. Simply stated, the purpose of a staging system is to provide a standard manner in which to readily communicate the state of a malignancy. Accurate staging is essential to (a) incorporate the most significant prognostic factors into a system that describes progressive degrees of risk to which a patient is subject, (b) delineate progressive stages of disease that have specific implications for surgical management, and (c) provide guidelines to the use of adjunctive therapies [45]. The staging systems most commonly used are the Enneking system and the staging system of the American Joint Committee. Staging requires a knowledge of the histologic grade of the lesion, as well as its anatomic extent, and can only be completed following biopsy.

**Table 1.** Enneking surgical staging of musculoskeletal sarcomas

| Stage | Grade | Site |
|-------|-------|------|
| IA | Low ($G_1$) | Intracompartmental ($T_1$) |
| IB | Low ($G_1$) | Extracompartmental ($T_2$) |
| IIA | High ($G_2$) | Intracompartmental ($T_1$) |
| IIB | High ($G_2$) | Extracompartmental ($T_2$) |
| III | Any (G) | Any (T) with metastases |

Data from [45]

## Enneking Staging System

The surgical staging system most commonly used in the evaluation of musculoskeletal tumors is that of Enneking [45]. The Enneking staging system is based on the surgical grade of a tumor (G), its local extent (T), and the presence or absence of regional or distant metastases (M) [45]. The Enneking staging system was designed for the evaluation of musculoskeletal mesenchymal tumors and was not intended for use with lesions derived from marrow or the reticuloendothelial system, because of their different natural history, surgical management and response to treatment.

Lesions are divided into two grades: low ($G_1$) and high ($G_2$), on the basis of histologic appearance. In general, low-grade lesions are well-differentiated and have a low potential for the development of metastatic disease. In contrast, high-grade lesions are in general poorly-differentiated, with a high mitotic rate and aggressive clinical course. Local extent is divided into lesions that are intracompartmental ($T_1$) and extracompartmental ($T_2$). The designation of intracompartmental indicates the lesion remains confined to the compartment of origin. For osseous lesions, each bone is considered to be a distinct compartment. When a lesion is designated as extracompartmental, this indicates it has extended beyond the compartment of origin. For example, an osteosarcoma is extracompartmental when it has extended from the bone into the adjacent soft tissue or joint. The presence ($M_1$) or absence ($M_0$) of regional or distant metastases is the third and final component of staging. On the basis of these considerations, lesions are staged as shown in Table 1.

### American Joint Committee on Cancer Staging System

The Enneking system is well-suited for the evaluation of extremity lesions because of its emphasis on compartmentalization. It does not, however, consider tumor size or distinguish between regional lymph node and distant metastases. In addition, the division of all lesions into either high- or low-grade may not be sufficient to be applicable to the wide range of all sarcomas. An alternative staging system is that of the American Joint Committee on Cancer (AJCC), which is based on the tumor, node and metastasis (TNM) classification [46]. This system is more complex, with four stages and several subclassifications.

The AJCC staging system addresses the surgical grade of a tumor (G), its size and local extent (T), the presence

**Box 2.** American Joint Committee on Cancer (AJCC) staging of bone sarcomas

The AJCC staging system utilizes the TMN system, described below, to assess the anatomic extent of disease:

T  Extent of primary tumor
N  Absence or presence of regional nodal involvement
M  Absence or presence of distant metastasis

Histologic grade (G):
$G_1$  Well-differentiated
$G_2$  Moderately well-differentiated
$G_3$  Poorly differentiated
$G_4$  Undifferentiated

Primary site (T):
$T_1$  Tumor 8 cm or less in greatest dimension
$T_2$  Tumor more than 8 cm in greatest dimension
$T_3$  Discontinuous tumors in the primary bone site

Nodal involvement (N):
$N_0$  No regional lymph nodal metastases
$N_1$  Regional lymph nodal metastases

Distant Metastasis (M)
$M_0$  No distant metastasis
$M_{1a}$  Lung metastasis present
$M_{1b}$  Metastasis other distant sites, including lymph nodes

Data from [46]

**Table 2.** American Joint Committee on Cancer (AJCC) staging of bone sarcomas

| Stage | T | N | M | Histologic grade (G) |
|---|---|---|---|---|
| IA | $T_1$ | $N_0$ | $M_0$ | $G_{1,2}$ Low grade |
| IB | $T_2$ | $N_0$ | $M_0$ | $G_{1,2}$ Low grade |
| IIA | $T_1$ | $N_0$ | $M_0$ | $G_{3,4}$ High grade |
| IIB | $T_2$ | $N_0$ | $M_0$ | $G_{3,4}$ High grade |
| III | $T_3$ | $N_0$ | $M_0$ | Any G |
| IVA | Any T | $N_0$ | $M_{1a}$ | Any G |
| IVB | Any T | $N_1$ | Any M | Any G |
|  | Any T | Any N | $M_{1b}$ | Any G |

Data from [46]

provides the information needed for accurate staging, diagnosis (or differential diagnosis) begins with the radiograph and is based on the morphology of the lesion, the location of the lesion and the age of the patient. Morphology characterizes the presence and character of the lesion's margin and periosteal reaction; features which are a function of the interaction between the lesion and the host, and are a key to biologic behavior. Morphology also includes an analysis of matrix. If present, a mineralized matrix may be a key to the lesion histology.

The location of a lesion is a major consideration in establishing a diagnosis and structuring a differential diagnosis. There are two components to the location of an osseous lesion: the anatomic location (which bone) and the lesion's location within the bone (epiphysis, metaphysis, metadiaphysis or diaphysis). The latter is critical in assessment of long bone lesions and is an essential principle of diagnosis pictorially presented in Fig. 1. Age is also a critical consideration, since specific lesions tend to occur in specific age groups (Tables 3, 4) [47]. For example, Langerhans cell histiocytosis localized

or absence of nodal involvement (N), and the presence or absence of distal metastasis (M) [46]. Box 2 and Table 2 list the classification criteria and subsequent surgical staging.

## Diagnosis: Bone Tumors

As previously noted, the radiograph remains the most diagnostic imaging study. While more advanced imaging

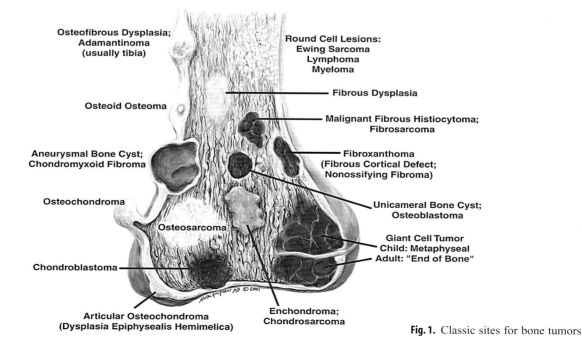

**Fig. 1.** Classic sites for bone tumors

**Table 3.** Age distribution of malignant osseous tumors

| Tumor type | Overall incidence (%) | Incidence by decade (%) | | | | | | | | |
|---|---|---|---|---|---|---|---|---|---|---|
| | | 1 | 2 | 3 | 4 | 5 | 6 | 7 | 8 | 9+ |
| Osteosarcoma | 29.2 | 4.6 | 46.0 | 17.2 | 8.8 | 7.6 | 6.5 | 6.7 | 2.4 | 0.3 |
| Myeloma | 14.4 | | 0.1 | 1.2 | 5.2 | 15.7 | 29.2 | 29.2 | 15.8 | 3.4 |
| Chondrosarcoma | 15.8 | 0.6 | 4.8 | 12.3 | 21.4 | 20.3 | 20.1 | 14.0 | 5.6 | 0.8 |
| Lymphoma | 12.3 | 2.7 | 8.9 | 10.8 | 10.2 | 14.7 | 20.3 | 17.5 | 12.0 | 2.7 |
| Ewing sarcoma | 9.5 | 16.2 | 59.6 | 16.8 | 4.7 | 2.0 | 0.8 | | | |
| Chordoma | 6.3 | 1.1 | 4.2 | 6.2 | 13.5 | 18.5 | 24.4 | 20.5 | 9.3 | 2.2 |
| Fibrosarcoma | 4.5 | 3.1 | 11.4 | 13.3 | 19.2 | 14.5 | 16.7 | 12.9 | 6.3 | 2.4 |
| Chondrosarcoma, dedifferentiated | 2.1 | | 1.7 | 2.5 | 6.7 | 18.3 | 32.5 | 17.5 | 16.7 | 4.2 |
| Malignant fibrous histiocytoma | 1.5 | 1.2 | 15.7 | 10.8 | 13.3 | 19.3 | 9.6 | 21.7 | 6.0 | 2.4 |
| Osteosarcoma, parosteal | 1.2 | | 17.4 | 39.1 | 27.5 | 10.1 | 5.8 | | | |
| Chondrosarcoma, mesenchymal | 0.6 | | 17.6 | 32.4 | 29.4 | 11.8 | 2.9 | | 2.9 | |
| Adamantinoma | 0.6 | 2.9 | 29.4 | 44.1 | 5.9 | 5.9 | 5.9 | | 5.9 | |

Data from [51], based on an analysis of 5,656 malignancies, including 814 cases of myeloma diagnosed on the basis of surgical biopsy. Not included are 2,935 cases of myeloma diagnosed on the basis of bone marrow aspirate, for a total of 8,591 malignancies and an overall incidence of myeloma of 43.6%

**Table 4.** Age distribution of benign osseous tumors

| Tumor type | Overall incidence (%) | Incidence by decade (%) | | | | | | | | |
|---|---|---|---|---|---|---|---|---|---|---|
| | | 1 | 2 | 3 | 4 | 5 | 6 | 7 | 8 | 9+ |
| Osteochondroma | 34.9 | 11.8 | 47.8 | 18.5 | 10.6 | 5.4 | 3.6 | 1.4 | 0.9 | |
| Giant cell tumor | 22.8 | 0.5 | 15.1 | 37.0 | 24.6 | 13.3 | 6.2 | 2.5 | 0.9 | |
| Chondroma (enchondroma) | 13.4 | 10.7 | 21.8 | 17.0 | 17.0 | 17.3 | 8.1 | 6.6 | 1.2 | 0.3 |
| Osteoid osteoma | 13.3 | 13.6 | 51.4 | 21.8 | 9.1 | 1.5 | 0.9 | 1.2 | 0.6 | |
| Chondroblastoma | 4.8 | 2.5 | 58.8 | 14.3 | 10.9 | 4.2 | 8.4 | 0.8 | | |
| Hemangioma | 4.3 | 3.7 | 9.3 | 13.9 | 15.7 | 25.9 | 16.7 | 11.1 | 3.7 | |
| Osteoblastoma | 3.5 | 6.9 | 41.4 | 32.2 | 10.3 | 3.4 | 3.4 | 1.1 | 1.1 | |
| Chondromyxoid fibroma | 1.8 | 11.1 | 24.4 | 31.1 | 13.3 | 8.9 | 8.9 | | 2.2 | |

Data from [51], based on an analysis of 2,496 benign tumors

to bone typically occurs in children and adolescents, while osseous lymphoma is most often encountered in mature adults, usually in the sixth and seventh decades. The final diagnosis, or differential, is then based on the integration of all of the above factors, taken in consideration of the prevalence of tumors within the population.

## Diagnosis: Soft Tissue Tumors

Despite the superiority of MR imaging in delineating soft-tissue tumors, it remains limited in its ability to precisely characterize them, with most lesions demonstrating a nonspecific appearance [48, 49]. There are instances, however, in which a specific diagnosis may be made or strongly suspected on the basis of MR imaging features (Box 3). This is usually done on the basis of lesion signal intensity, pattern of growth, location and associated "signs" and findings. The MR imaging appearance of these lesions has been well reported, and is not reviewed here.

DeSchepper et al. [50] performed a multivariate statistical analysis of ten imaging parameters, individually and in combination. These researchers found that malignancy was predicted with the highest sensitivity when lesions had high signal intensity on T2-weighted images, were larger than 33 mm in diameter, and had heterogeneous signal intensity on T1-weighted images. The signs that had the greatest specificity for malignancy included tumor necrosis, bone or neurovascular involvement, and mean diameter of more than 66 mm. In a recent study of 548 patients by Gielen and colleagues [51], in which imaging and clinical data were available, an accuracy of 85% was reported in differentiating between benign and malignant lesions.

When a specific diagnosis is not possible, it is often useful to formulate a suitably ordered differential diagnosis on the basis of imaging features, suspected biological potential and a knowledge of tumor prevalence based on the patient age and lesion anatomic location. This can be further refined by considering clinical history and radiologic features, such as pattern of growth, signal intensity and localization (subcutaneous, intramuscular, intermuscular, etc.). The most common malignant and benign lesions, by tumor location and patient age, are shown in Tables 5 and 6.

**Box 3.** Specific diagnoses that might be made or suspected on the basis of magnetic resonance imaging

Vascular lesions:
    Aneurysm and pseudoaneurysm
    Arteriovenous hemangioma (AVM)
    Glomus tumor
    Hemangioma
    Hemangiomatosis (angiomatosis)
    Lymphangioma
    Lymphangiomatosis

Bone and cartilage forming lesions:
    Extraskeletal chondroma
    Myositis ossificans
    Panniculitis ossificans
    Synovial chondromatosis

Fibrous lesions:
    Elastofibroma
    Fibroma of tendon sheath
    Fibromatosis coli
    Musculoaponeurotic fibromatosis
    Superficial fibromatosis

Lipomatous lesions:
    Lipoma
    Lipoma arborescens
    Lipoma of tendon sheath
    Lipomatosis
    Lipomatosis of nerve
    Lipoblastoma
    Lipoblastomatosis
    Liposarcoma

    Periosteal lipoma
    Synovial lipoma

Tumor-like lesions:
    Abscess
    Calcific myonecrosis
    Cystic adventitial disease
    Epidermal inclusion cyst
    Fat necrosis
    Ganglion
    Granuloma annulare
    Hematoma
    Hydroxyapatite crystal disease
    Intramuscular myxoma
    Myonecrosis
    Popliteal (synovial) cyst
    Tophus
    Tumoral calcinosis

Peripheral nerve lesions:
    Morton neuroma
    Neurofibroma
    Schwannoma
    Traumatic (stump) neuroma

Synovial lesions:
    Giant cell tumor of tendon sheath
    Nodular synovotis
    Pigmented villonodular synovitis
    Synovial chondromatosis
    Synovial sarcoma

**Table 5.** Distribution of common malignant soft tissue tumors by anatomic location and age

| Age (years) | Hand and wrist | No. (%) | Upper extremity | No. (%) | Axilla and shoulder | No. (%) | Foot and ankle | No. (%) | Lower extremity | No. (%) |
|---|---|---|---|---|---|---|---|---|---|---|
| 0-5 | Fibrosarcoma | 5 (45)[a] | Fibrosarcoma | 9 (29) | Fibrosarcoma | 9 (56) | Fibrosarcoma | 5 (45) | Fibrosarcoma | 24 (45) |
| | Angiosarcoma | 1 (9) | Rhabdomyosarcoma | 7 (23) | Rhabdomyosarcoma | 4 (25) | DFSP | 2 (18) | Rhabdomyosarcoma | 8 (15) |
| | Epithelioid sarcoma | 1 (9) | Angiomatoid MFH | 3 (10) | Angiomatoid MFH | 1 (6) | MPNST | 2 (18) | Giant cell fibroblastoma | 5 (9) |
| | Malignant GCT tendon sheath | 1 (9) | DFSP | 2 (6) | Chondrosarcoma | 1 (6) | Rhabdomyosarcoma | 2 (18) | MPNST | 5 (9) |
| | DFSP | 1 (9) | Giant cell fibroblastoma | 2 (6) | MPNST | 1 (6) | | | Angiomatoid MFH | 3 (6) |
| | MPNST | 1 (9) | MPNST | 2 (6) | | | | | DFSP | 3 (6) |
| | Rhabdomyosarcoma | 1 (9) | MFH | 2 (6) | | | | | Angiosarcoma | 2 (4) |
| | | | Other | 4 (13) | | | | | Other | 3 (6) |
| 6-15 | Epithelioid sarcoma | 9 (21) | Angiomatoid MFH | 30 (33) | Angiomatoid MFH | 8 (21) | Synovial sarcoma | 11 (21) | Synovial sarcoma | 28 (22) |
| | Angiomatoid MFH | 7 (16) | Synovial sarcoma | 14 (15) | MFH | 5 (13) | DFSP | 9 (17) | Angiomatoid MFH | 22 (17) |
| | Synovial sarcoma | 5 (12) | Fibrosarcoma | 8 (9) | Ewing sarcoma | 4 (10) | Rhabdomyosarcoma | 5 (9) | MFH | 13 (10) |
| | MFH | 4 (9) | MPNST | 7 (8) | MPNST | 4 (10) | Angiosarcoma | 4 (8) | Liposarcoma | 11 (9) |
| | Angiosarcoma | 3 (7) | MFH | 7 (8) | Rhabdomyosarcoma | 4 (10) | Clear cell sarcoma | 4 (8) | MPNST | 9 (7) |
| | Rhabdomyosarcoma | 3 (7) | Rhabdomyosarcoma | 7 (8) | Fibrosarcoma | 3 (8) | Fibrosarcoma | 4 (8) | DFSP | 8 (6) |
| | Clear cell sarcoma | 2 (5) | Epithelioid sarcoma | 4 (4) | Synovial sarcoma | 3 (8) | Chondrosarcoma | 3 (6) | Rhabdomyosarcoma | 6 (5) |
| | Other | 10 (23) | Other | 15 (16) | Other | 8 (21) | Other | 13 (25) | Other | 31 (24) |
| 16-25 | Epithelioid sarcoma | 25 (29) | Synovial sarcoma | 32 (23) | Synovial sarcoma | 13 (18) | Synovial sarcoma | 27 (30) | Synovial sarcoma | 76 (22) |
| | MFH | 11 (13) | MFH | 19 (14) | DFSP | 12 (16) | Clear cell sarcoma | 10 (11) | Liposarcoma | 45 (13) |
| | DFSP | 7 (8) | MPNST | 16 (12) | MPNST | 11 (15) | Fibrosarcoma | 7 (8) | MPNST | 44 (13) |
| | Synovial sarcoma | 7 (8) | Fibrosarcoma | 12 (9) | Fibrosarcoma | 8 (11) | DFSP | 7 (8) | MFH | 36 (11) |
| | Rhabdomyosarcoma | 7 (8) | Angiomatoid MFH | 10 (7) | MFH | 8 (11) | MFH | 6 (7) | Fibrosarcoma | 24 (7) |
| | Angiomatoid MFH | 5 (6) | Epithelioid sarcoma | 9 (7) | Rhabdomyosarcoma | 4 (5) | Hemangioendothelioma | 6 (7) | DFSP | 18 (5) |

(continued on the next page)

(→ *cont.*) **Table 5.** Distribution of common malignant soft tissue tumors by anatomic location and age

| Age (years) | Hand and wrist | No. (%) | Upper extremity | No. (%) | Axilla and shoulder | No. (%) | Foot and ankle | No. (%) | Lower extremity | No. |
|---|---|---|---|---|---|---|---|---|---|---|
| | Hemangioendothelioma | 5 (6) | Hemangioendothelioma | 6 (4) | Angiomatoid MFH | 3 (4) | MPNST | 5 (6) | Angiomatoid MFH | 15 (4) |
| | Other | 19 (22) | Other | 34 (25) | Other | 15 (20) | Other | 22 (24) | Other | 80 (24) |
| 26-45 | MFH | 26 (18) | MFH | 65 (28) | DFSP | 55 (33) | Synovial sarcoma | 50 (26) | Liposarcoma | 196 (28) |
| | Epitheliod sarcoma | 24 (16) | MPNST | 29 (12) | MFH | 30 (18) | Clear cell sarcoma | 25 (13) | MFH | 151 (21) |
| | Synovial sarcoma | 21 (14) | Fibrosarcoma | 25 (11) | Liposarcoma | 22 (13) | MFH | 25 (13) | Synovial sarcoma | 78 (11) |
| | Fibrosarcoma | 17 (12) | Synovial sarcoma | 23 (10) | MPNST | 21 (12) | Hemangioendothelioma | 14 (7) | MPNST | 70 (10) |
| | Clear cell sarcoma | 9 (6) | Liposarcoma | 20 (8) | Fibrosarcoma | 10 (6) | DFSP | 13 (7) | DFSP | 47 (7) |
| | Liposarcoma | 9 (6) | DFSP | 18 (8) | Synovial sarcoma | 7 (4) | Liposarcoma | 13 (7) | Leiomyosarcoma | 35 (5) |
| | MPNST | 7 (5) | Epithelioid sarcoma | 13 (6) | Chondrosarcoma | 6 (4) | MPNST | 11 (6) | Fibrosarcoma | 33 (5) |
| | Other | 33 (23) | Other | 43 (18) | Other | 18 ( (11) | Other | 38 (20) | Other | 98 (14) |
| 46-65 | MFH | 16 (19) | MFH | 133 (46) | MFH | 66 (35) | MFH | 39 (25) | MFH | 399 (43) |
| | Synovial sarcoma | 12 (14) | Liposarcoma | 34 (12) | Liposarcoma | 39 (21) | Synovial sarcoma | 27 (17) | Liposarcoma | 232 (25) |
| | Fibrosarcoma | 8 (10) | Leiomyosarcoma | 22 (8) | DFSP | 22 (12) | Leiomyosarcoma | 19 (12) | Leiomyosarcoma | 63 (7) |
| | Epithelioid sarcoma | 7 (8) | Fibrosarcoma | 18 (6) | MPNST | 20 (11) | Kaposi sarcoma | 14 (9) | Synovial sarcoma | 40 (4) |
| | Liposarcoma | 7 (8) | MPNST | 17 (6) | Leiomyosarcoma | 14 (7) | Liposarcoma | 9 (6) | MPNST | 38 (4) |
| | Chondrosarcoma | 7 (8) | Synovial sarcoma | 16 (5) | Fibrosarcoma | 8 (4) | Fibrosarcoma | 8 (5) | Chondrosarcoma | 37 (4) |
| | Clear cell sarcoma | 5 (6) | Hemangioendothelioma | 9 (3) | Synovial sarcoma | 4 (2) | Clear cell sarcoma | 7 (5) | Fibrosarcoma | 24 (3) |
| | Other | 22 (26) | Other | 43 (15) | Other | 15 (8) | Other | 32 (21) | Other | 87 (9) |
| 66+ | MFH | 28 (35) | MFH | 183 (60) | MFH | 67 (50) | Kaposi sarcoma | 49 (37) | MFH | 455 (55) |
| | Leiomyosarcoma | 8 (10) | Liposarcoma | 25 (8) | Liposarcoma | 30 (23) | MFH | 26 (19) | Liposarcoma | 178 (22) |
| | Synovial sarcoma | 6 (8) | Leiomyosarcoma | 23 (8) | MPNST | 12 (9) | Leiomyosarcoma | 20 (15) | Leiomyosarcoma | 86 (10) |
| | Kaposi sarcoma | 5 (6) | MPNST | 20 (7) | DFSP | 6 (5) | Fibrosarcoma | 9 (7) | Fibrosarcoma | 22 (3) |
| | DFSP | 4 (5) | Kaposi sarcoma | 10 (3) | Fibrosarcoma | 4 (3) | Chondrosarcoma | 6 (4) | Chrondrosarcoma | 16 (2) |
| | MPNST | 4 (5) | Fibrosarcoma | 8 (3) | Leiomyosarcoma | 3 (2) | MPNST | 5 (4) | MPNST | 15 (2) |
| | Clear cell sarcoma | 3 (4) | Angiosarcoma | 6 (2) | Chondrosarcoma | 2 (2) | Liposarcoma | 3 (2) | Synovial sarcoma | 11 (1) |
| | Other | 21 (27) | Other | 29 (10) | Other | 9 (7) | Other | 16 (12) | Other | 43 (5) |

| Age (years) | Hip, groin and buttocks | No. (%) | Head and neck | No. (%) | Trunk | No. (%) | Retroperitoneum | No. (%) |
|---|---|---|---|---|---|---|---|---|
| 0-5 | Fibrosarcoma | 7 (32) | Fibrosarcoma | 22 (37) | Fibrosarcoma | 13 (26) | Fibrosarcoma | 4 (20) |
| | Giant cell fibroblastoma | 3 (14) | Rhabdomyosarcoma | 20 (33) | Giant cell fibroblastoma | 8 (16) | Neuroblastoma | 4 (20) |
| | Rhabdomyosarcoma | 3 (14) | Malignant hemangiopericytoma | 3 (5) | Rhabdomyosarcoma | 8 (16) | Rhabdomyosarcoma | 4 (20) |
| | DFSP | 2 (9) | Alveolar soft part sarcoma | 2 (3) | Angiomatoid MFH | 6 (12) | Ganglioneuroblastoma | 3 (15) |
| | MFH | 2 (9) | DFSP | 2 (3) | DFSP | 4 (8) | Angiosarcoma | 2 (10) |
| | Leiomyosarcoma | 1 (5) | MPNST | 2 (3) | Ewing sarcoma | 3 (6) | Leiomyosarcoma | 2 (10) |
| | Synovial sarcoma | 1 (5) | Giant cell fibroblastoma | 2 (3) | Neuroblastoma | 3 (6) | Alveolar soft part sarcoma | 1 (5) |
| | Other | 3 (14) | Other | 7 (12) | Other | 5 (10) | | |
| 6-15 | Angiomatoid MFH | 8 (21) | Rhabdomyosarcoma | 17 (26) | Angiomatoid MFH | 14 (15) | Rhabdomyosarcoma | 9 (31) |
| | Synovial sarcoma | 7 (19) | Fibrosarcoma | 13 (20) | Fibrosarcoma | 13 (14) | MPNST | 5 (17) |
| | Rhabdomyosarcoma | 6 (16) | Synovial sarcoma | 7 (11) | Ewing sarcoma | 12 (13) | Neuroblastoma | 4 (14) |
| | MFH | 4 (11) | MPNST | 6 (9) | DFSP | 12 (13) | Ewing sarcoma | 2 (7) |
| | Epithelioid sarcoma | 2 (5) | MFH | 6 (9) | MPNST | 9 (10) | Fibrosarcoma | 2 (7) |
| | Fibrosarcoma | 2 (5) | Angiomatoid MFH | 4 (6) | Rhabdomyosarcoma | 8 (9) | MFH | 2 (7) |
| | MPNST | 2 (5) | DFSP | 2 (3) | MFH | 3 (3) | Malignant hemangiopericytoma | 2 (7) |
| | Other | 7 (18) | Other | 10 (15) | Other | 20 (22) | Other | 3 (10) |
| 16-25 | Synovial sarcoma | 15 (18) | Fibrosarcoma | 15 (17) | DFSP | 37 (23) | MPNST | 9 (20) |
| | MPNST | 13 (16) | DFSP | 14 (16) | MFH | 21 (13) | Ewing sarcoma | 8 (18) |
| | Liposarcoma | 8 (10) | MPNST | 8 (9) | MPNST | 19 (12) | Leiomyosarcoma | 6 (14) |
| | DFSP | 6 (7) | Synovial sarcoma | 8 (9) | Fibrosarcoma | 15 (9) | Ganglioneuroblastoma | 4 (9) |
| | MFH | 6 (7) | Rhabdomyosarcoma | 8 (9) | Synovial sarcoma | 13 (8) | Neuroblastoma | 4 (9) |
| | Rhabdomyosarcoma | 5 (6) | MFH | 7 (8) | Ewing sarcoma | 12 (7) | Rhabdomyosarcoma | 3 (7) |
| | Leiomyosarcoma | 4 (5) | Angiomatoid MFH | 6 (7) | Angiomatoid MFH | 6 (4) | Malignant khemangiopericytoma | 2 (5) |
| | Other | 26 (31) | Other | 23 (26) | Other | 38 (24) | Other | 8 (18) |
| 26-45 | Liposarcoma | 45 (18) | DFSP | 59 (30) | DFSP | 129 (30) | Leiomyosarcoma | 57 (32) |
| | DFSP | 42 (17) | MPNST | 27 (14) | MFH | 77 (18) | Liposarcoma | 52 (29) |
| | MFH | 38 (16) | Liposarcoma | 18 (9) | MPNST | 45 (10) | MFH | 22 (12) |
| | Leiomyosarcoma | 26 (11) | MFH | 15 (8) | Liposarcoma | 41 (9) | MPNST | 11 (6) |
| | MPNST | 15 (6) | Fibrosarcoma | 14 (7) | Fibrosarcoma | 36 (8) | Fibrosarcoma | 7 (4) |
| | Synovial sarcoma | 13 (5) | Synovial sarcoma | 10 (5) | Synovial sarcoma | 20 (5) | Malignant hemangiopericytoma | 7 (4) |

(*continued on the next page*)

(→ *cont.*) **Table 5.** Distribution of common malignant soft tissue tumors by anatomic location and age

| Age (years) | Hip, groin and buttocks | No. (%) | Head and neck | No. (%) | Trunk | No. (%) | Retroperitoneum | No. (%) |
|---|---|---|---|---|---|---|---|---|
| | Fibrosarcoma | 12 (5) | Angiosarcoma | 9 (4) | Angiosarcoma | 15 (3) | Ewing sarcoma | 3 (2) |
| | Other | 53 (22) | Other | 42 (22) | Other | 70 (16) | Other | 20 (11) |
| 46-66 | Liposarcoma | 67 (24) | MFH | 54 (28) | MFH | 131 (31) | Liposarcoma | 170 (33) |
| | MFH | 66 (23) | DFSP | 28 (15) | Liposarcoma | 80 (19) | Leiomyosarcoma | 154 (30) |
| | Leiomyosarcoma | 40 (14) | MPNST | 23 (12) | DFSP | 60 (14) | MFH | 111 (22) |
| | DFSP | 20 (7) | Liposarcoma | 22 (12) | MPNST | 35 (8) | MPNST | 23 (5) |
| | Fibrosarcoma | 16 (6) | Angiosarcoma | 16 (8) | Leiomyosarcoma | 27 (6) | Malignant mesenchymoma | 10 (2) |
| | Synovial sarcoma | 14 (5) | Atypical fibroxanthoma | 12 (6) | Fibrosarcoma | 24 (6) | Fibrosarcoma | 9 (2) |
| | Chondrosarcoma | 14 (5) | Leiomyosarcoma | 11 (6) | Angiosarcoma | 15 (4) | Malignant hemangiopericytoma | 7 (1) |
| | Other | 46 (16) | Other | 24 (13) | Other | 50 (12) | Other | 27 (5) |
| 66+ | MFH | 111 (46) | MFH | 82 (34) | MFH | 137 (44) | Liposarcoma | 164 (39) |
| | Liposarcoma | 49 (20) | Atypical fibroxanthoma | 41 (17) | Liposarcoma | 56 (18) | Leiomyosarcoma | 118 (28) |
| | Leiomyosarcoma | 24 (10) | Angiosarcoma | 27 (11) | Leiomyosarcoma | 23 (7) | MFH | 93 (22) |
| | Angiosarcoma | 11 (5) | Liposarcoma | 20 (8) | MPNST | 20 (6) | MPNST | 13 (3) |
| | MPNST | 11 (5) | MPNST | 16 (7) | DFSP | 17 (5) | Fibrosarcoma | 8 (2) |
| | Fibrosarcoma | 10 (4) | Leiomyosarcoma | 13 (5) | Fibrosarcoma | 12 (4) | Osteosarcoma | 6 (1) |
| | Chondrosarcoma | 7 (3) | Fibrosarcoma | 10 (4) | Chondrosarcoma | 11 (4) | Malignant mesenchymoma | 5 (1) |
| | Other | 20 (8) | Other | 31 (13) | Other | 35 (11) | Other | 9 (2) |

*DFSP* dermatofibrosarcoma protuberans, *GCT* giant cell tumor, *MFH* malignant fibrous histiocytoma, *MPNST* malignant peripheral nerve sheath tumor

Based on an analysis of 12,370 cases seen in consultation by the Department of Soft Tissue Pathology (Armed Forces Institute of Pathology) over a 10-year period. Modified from [52]

a 5(45) indicates that there were five fibrosarcomas in the hand and wrist of patients 0-5 years, and this represents 45% of all malignant tumors at this location and in this age group

**Table 6.** Distribution of common benign soft tissue tumors by anatomic location and age

| Age (years) | Hand and wrist | No. (%) | Upper extremity | No. (%) | Axilla and shoulder | No. (%) | Foot and ankle | No. (%) | Lower extremity | No. (%) |
|---|---|---|---|---|---|---|---|---|---|---|
| 0-5 | Hemangioma | 15 (15)a | Fibrous hamartoma infancy | 15 (16) | Fibrous hamartoma infancy | 23 (29) | Granuloma annulare | 23 (30) | Granuloma annulare | 42 (23) |
| | Granuloma annulare | 14 (14) | Granuloma annulare | 15 (16) | Hemangioma | 12 (15) | Infantile fibromatosis | 11 (14) | Hemangioma | 26 (14) |
| | Infantile fibromatosis | 13 (13) | Hemangioma | 14 (14) | Lipoblastoma | 11 (14) | Hemangioma | 8 (11) | Myofibromatosis | 16 (9) |
| | Infantile digital fibroma | 8 (8) | Infantile fibromatosis | 12 (13) | Fibrous hamartoma | 7 (9) | Fibromatosis | 8 (11) | Fibrous histiocytoma | 15 (8) |
| | Fibromatosis | 8 (8) | Fibrous histiocytoma | 6 (6) | Myofibromatosis | 6 (8) | Infantile digital fibroma | 7 (9) | Lipoblastoma | 13 (7) |
| | Aponeurotic fibroma | 7 (7) | Juvenile xanthogranuloma | 6 (6) | Lymphangioma | 5 (6) | Lipoblastoma | 6 (8) | Lymphangioma | 10 (6) |
| | Fibrous histiocytoma | 5 (5) | Myofibromatosis | 6 (6) | Nodular fasciitis | 4 (5) | Lipoma | 4 (5) | Juvenile xanthogranuloma | 10 (6) |
| | Other | 27 (28) | Other | 20 (21) | Other | 12 (15) | Other | 9 (12) | Other | 48 (27) |
| 6-15 | Fibrous histiocytoma | 32 (14) | Fibrous histiocytoma | 41 (23) | Fibrous histiocytoma | 25 (34) | Fibromatosis | 35 (22) | Hemangioma | 47 (22) |
| | Hemangioma | 31 (13) | Nodular fasciitis | 39 (21) | Nodular fasciitis | 18 (25) | Granuloma annulare | 21 (13) | Fibrous histiocytoma | 34 (16) |
| | Aponeurotic fibroma | 25 (11) | Hemangioma | 24 (13) | Hemangioma | 7 (10) | Hemangioma | 21 (13) | Nodular fasciitis | 22 (10) |
| | Fibroma tendon sheath | 22 (9) | Granuloma annulare | 12 (7) | Granular cell tumor | 4 (5) | Fibrous histiocytoma | 14 (9) | Granuloma annulare | 20 (9) |
| | GCT tendon sheath | 17 (7) | Fibromatosis | 11 (6) | Neurofibroma | 3 (4) | GCT tendon sheath | 13 (8) | Fibromatosis | 14 (6) |
| | Fibromatosis | 13 (6) | Neurofibroma | 7 (4) | Lymphangioma | 2 (3) | Chondroma | 11 (7) | Lipoma | 13 (6) |
| | Lipoma | 9 (4) | Neurothekeoma | 6 (3) | Myofibromatosis | 2 (3) | Lipoma | 9 (6) | Neurofibroma | 8 (4) |
| | Other | 86 (37) | Other | 42 (23) | Other | 12 (16) | Other | 37 (23) | Other | 58 (27) |
| 16-25 | GCT tendon sheath | 84 (20) | Nodular fasciitis | 130 (35) | Fibrous histiocytoma | 62 (36) | Fibromatosis | 46 (22) | Fibrous histiocytoma | 118 (24) |
| | Fibrous histiocytoma | 57 (14) | Fibrous histiocytoma | 87 (23) | Nodular fasciitis | 35 (20) | GCT tendon sheath | 29 (14) | Nodular fasciitis | 61 (13) |
| | Hemangioma | 40 (10) | Hemangioma | 36 (10) | Fibromatosis | 16 (9) | Granuloma annulare | 25 (12) | Hemangioma | 55 (11) |
| | Fibroma tendon sheath | 40 (10) | Neurofibroma | 24 (6) | Lipoma | 14 (8) | Fibrous histiocytoma | 24 (12) | Neurofibroma | 48 (10) |
| | Nodular fasciitis | 26 (6) | Granuloma annulare | 20 (5) | Neurofibroma | 12 (7) | Hemangioma | 13 (6) | Fibromatosis | 38 (8) |
| | Granuloma annulare | 21 (5) | Granular cell tumor | 17 (5) | Hemangioma | 4 (2) | PVNS | 12 (6) | Lipoma | 22 (5) |
| | Ganglion | 20 (5) | Schwannoma | 11 (3) | Schwannoma | 4 (2) | Neurofibroma | 11 (5) | Schwannoma | 20 (4) |
| | Other | 132 (31) | Other | 51 (14) | Other | 25 (15) | Other | 45 (22) | Other | 122 (25) |
| 26-45 | Fibrous histiocytoma | 167 (18) | Nodular fasciitis | 309 (38) | Lipoma | 105 (28) | Fibromatosis | 99 (21) | Fibrous histiocytoma | 245 (25) |
| | GCT tendon sheath | 148 (16) | Fibrous histiocytoma | 145 (18) | Fibrous histiocytoma | 92 (24) | Fibrous histiocytoma | 74 (16) | Nodular fasciitis | 229 (23) |
| | Fibroma tendon sheath | 106 (11) | Angiolipoma | 48 (6) | Nodular fasciitis | 55 (14) | GCT tendon sheath | 41 (9) | Lipoma | 101 (10) |
| | Hemangioma | 86 (10) | Hemangioma | 43 (5) | Fibromatosis | 29 (8) | Hemangioma | 36 (8) | Neurofibroma | 71 (7) |

(*continued on the next page*)

(→ *cont.*) **Table 6.** Distribution of common benign soft tissue tumors by anatomic location and age

| Age (years) | Hand and wrist | No. (%) | Upper extremity | No. (%) | Axilla and shoulder | No. (%) | Foot and ankle | No. (%) | Lower extremity | No. (%) |
|---|---|---|---|---|---|---|---|---|---|---|
| | Nodular fasciitis | 79 (8) | Schwannoma | 43 (5) | Hemangioma | 17 (4) | Schwannoma | 30 (6) | Schwannoma | 59 (6) |
| | Fibromatosis | 46 (5) | Neurofibroma | 37 (5) | Neurofibroma | 13 (3) | Neurofibroma | 24 (5) | Myxoma | 53 (5) |
| | Chondroma | 42 (4) | Lipoma | 32 (4) | Schwannoma | 12 (3) | Chondroma | 23 (5) | Hemangioma | 52 (5) |
| | Other | 269 (29) | Other | 153 (19) | Other | 57 (15) | Other | 135 (29) | Other | 185 (19) |
| 46-65 | GCT tendon sheath | 143 (23) | Nodular fasciitis | 86 (20) | Lipoma | 189 (58) | Fibromatosis | 83 (25) | Lipoma | 157 (23) |
| | Fibrous histiocytoma | 63 (10) | Lipoma | 80 (19) | Fibrous histiocytoma | 28 (9) | Fibrous histiocytoma | 43 (13) | Myxoma | 109 (16) |
| | Hemangioma | 61 (10) | Fibrous histiocytoma | 44 (10) | Myxoma | 16 (5) | Lipoma | 35 (11) | Fibrous histiocytoma | 93 (14) |
| | Lipoma | 59 (9) | Schwannoma | 30 (7) | Fibromatosis | 14 (4) | Schwannoma | 25 (8) | Nodular fasciitis | 40 (6) |
| | Chondroma | 52 (8) | Neurofibroma | 24 (6) | Nodular fasciitis | 13 (4) | GCT tendon sheath | 21 (6) | Schwannoma | 39 (6) |
| | Fibromatosis | 43 (7) | Myxoma | 24 (6) | Schwannoma | 12 (4) | Chondroma | 21 (6) | Neurofibroma | 31 (5) |
| | Fibroma tendon sheath | 37 (6) | Hemangioma | 19 (4) | Granular cell tumor | 12 (4) | Hemangioma | 16 (5) | Proliferative fasciitis | 28 (4) |
| | Other | 172 (27) | Other | 125 (29) | Other | 44 (13) | Other | 89 (27) | Other | 186 (27) |
| 66+ | GCT tendon sheath | 51 (21) | Lipoma | 39 (22) | Lipoma | 83 (58) | Fibromatosis | 16 (14) | Lipoma | 68 (26) |
| | Hemangioma | 24 (10) | Myxoma | 19 (11) | Myxoma | 14 (10) | Schwannoma | 15 (13) | Myxoma | 44 (17) |
| | Schwannoma | 24 (10) | Nodular fasciitis | 18 (10) | Schwannoma | 6 (4) | Fibrous histiocytoma | 13 (11) | Fibrous histiocytoma | 33 (13) |
| | Chondroma | 24 (10) | Schwannoma | 17 (9) | Fibromatosis | 5 (3) | Chondroma | 11 (9) | Schwannoma | 31 (12) |
| | Neurofibroma | 21 (9) | Glomus tumor | 12 (7) | Fibrous histiocytoma | 5 (3) | Lipoma | 10 (8) | Hemangiopericytoma | 10 (4) |
| | Fibromatosis | 14 (6) | Neurofibroma | 10 (6) | Proliferative fasciitis | 5 (3) | Granuloma annulare | 8 (7) | Neurofibroma | 9 (4) |
| | Lipoma | 13 (5) | Angiolipoma | 10 (6) | Hemangioma | 4 (3) | GCT tendon sheath | 6 (5) | Hemangioma | 8 (3) |
| | Other | 71 (29) | Other | 55 (31) | Other | 22 (15) | Other | 39 (33) | Other | 56 (22) |

| Age (years) | Hip, groin and buttocks | No. (%) | Head and neck | No. (%) | Trunk | No. (%) | Retroperitoneum | No. (%) |
|---|---|---|---|---|---|---|---|---|
| 0-5 | Fibrous hamartoma infancy | 14 (20) | Nodular fasciitis | 47 (20) | Hemangioma | 36 (18) | Lipoblastoma | 7 (37) |
| | Lipoblastoma | 14 (20) | Hemangioma | 43 (18) | Juvenile xanthogranuloma | 24 (12) | Lymphangioma | 5 (26) |
| | Myofibromatosis | 8 (11) | Myofibromatosis | 27 (11) | Myofibromatosis | 24 (12) | Hemangioma | 4 (21) |
| | Lymphangioma | 7 (10) | Fibromatosis | 17 (7) | Nodular fasciitis | 17 (8) | Ganglioneuroma | 2 (11) |
| | Fibrous histiocytoma | 5 (7) | Granuloma annulare | 14 (6) | Lipoblastoma | 17 (8) | Fibrous hamartoma infancy | 1 (5) |
| | Nodular fasciitis | 4 (6) | Fibrous histiocytoma | 13 (5) | Infantile fibromatosis | 15 (7) | | |
| | Infantile fibromatosis | 4 (6) | Infantile fibromatosis | 13 (5) | Fibrous hamartoma infancy | 15 (7) | | |
| | Other | 14 (20) | Other | 63 (27) | Other | 55 (27) | | |
| 6-15 | Nodular fasciitis | 15 (27) | Nodular fasciitis | 75 (33) | Nodular fasciitis | 54 (28) | Lymphangioma | 7 (37) |
| | Fibroma | 7 (13) | Fibrous histiocytoma | 34 (15) | Fibrous histiocytoma | 43 (22) | Ganglioneuroma | 4 (21) |
| | Fibrous histiocytoma | 6 (11) | Neurofibroma | 23 (10) | Hemangioma | 25 (13) | Schwannoma | 2 (11) |
| | Fibromatosis | 5 (9) | Hemangioma | 21 (9) | Lipoma | 9 (5) | Fibromatosis | 2 (11) |
| | Lipoma | 5 (9) | Myofibromatosis | 14 (6) | Neurofibroma | 7 (4) | Paraganglioma | 1 (5) |
| | Lipoblastoma | 3 (5) | Fibromatosis | 12 (5) | Fibromatosis | 6 (3) | Hemangioma | 1 (5) |
| | Neurofibroma | 3 (5) | Lipoma | 6 (3) | Granular cell tumor | 6 (3) | Inflammatory pseudotumor | 1 (5) |
| | Other | 11 (20) | Other | 43 (19) | Other | 45 (23) | Other | 1 (5) |
| 16-25 | Neurofibroma | 20 (16) | Nodular fasciitis | 61 (21) | Nodular fasciitis | 112 (24) | Fibromatosis | 14 (20) |
| | Fibromatosis | 18 (15) | Hemangioma | 48 (17) | Fibromatosis | 72 (16) | Schwannoma | 10 (14) |
| | Fibrous histiocytoma | 18 (15) | Fibrous histiocytoma | 45 (16) | Fibrous histiocytoma | 71 (15) | Neurofibroma | 9 (13) |
| | Nodular fasciitis | 12 (10) | Neurofibroma | 37 (13) | Hemangioma | 52 (11) | Hemangiopericytoma | 8 (11) |
| | Hemangioma | 9 (7) | Schwannoma | 19 (7) | Neurofibroma | 38 (8) | Lymphangioma | 8 (11) |
| | Lipoma | 8 (7) | Fibromatosis | 11 (4) | Lipoma | 21 (5) | Ganglioneuroma | 6 (8) |
| | Hemangiopericytoma | 8 (7) | Lipoma | 10 (4) | Schwannoma | 17 (4) | Hemangioma | 4 (6) |
| | Other | 29 (24) | Other | 56 (19) | Other | 79 (17) | Other | 12 (17) |
| 26-45 | Lipoma | 57 (17) | Lipoma | 168 (22) | Lipoma | 178 (19) | Schwannoma | 38 (23) |
| | Neurofibroma | 38 (12) | Nodular fasciitis | 145 (19) | Nodular fasciitis | 150 (16) | Fibromatosis | 30 (18) |
| | Fibrous histiocytoma | 37 (11) | Fibrous histiocytoma | 137 (18) | Fibromatosis | 148 (16) | Hemangiopericytoma | 25 (15) |
| | Fibromatosis | 36 (11) | Hemangioma | 97 (13) | Fibrous histiocytoma | 98 (10) | Neurofibroma | 13 (8) |
| | Nodular fasciitis | 31 (9) | Neurofibroma | 57 (8) | Hemangioma | 78 (8) | Angiomyolipoma | 10 (6) |
| | Hemangiopericytoma | 24 (7) | Hemangiopericytoma | 37 (5) | Neurofibroma | 65 (7) | Hemangioma | 9 (5) |
| | Myxoma | 22 (7) | Schwannoma | 27 (4) | Schwannoma | 51 (5) | Sclerosing retroperitonitis | 7 (4) |
| | Other | 83 (25) | Other | 91 (12) | Other | 180 (19) | Other | 34 (20) |
| 46-65 | Lipoma | 76 (35) | Lipoma | 306 (46) | Lipoma | 290 (44) | Schwannoma | 33 (19) |
| | Myxoma | 36 (17) | Nodular fasciitis | 66 (10) | Fibromatosis | 63 (9) | Fibromatosis | 25 (14) |
| | Fibrous histiocytoma | 17 (8) | Hemangioma | 55 (8) | Nodular fasciitis | 44 (7) | Sclerosing retroperitonitis | 25 (14) |
| | Schwannoma | 17 (8) | Fibrous histiocytoma | 42 (6) | Hemangioma | 31 (5) | Hemangiopericytoma | 21 (12) |
| | Nodular fasciitis | 11 (5) | Neurofibroma | 30 (4) | Fibrous histiocytoma | 29 (4) | Angiomyolipoma Lipoma | 12 (7) |
| | Hemangiopericytoma | 11 (5) | Schwannoma | 25 (4) | Neurofibroma | 28 (4) | Paraganglioma | 10 (6) |

(*continued on the next page*)

(→ *cont.*) **Table 6.** Distribution of common benign soft tissue tumors by anatomic location and age

| Age (years) | Hip, groin and buttocks | No. (%) | Head and neck | No. (%) | Trunk | No. (%) | Retroperitoneum | No. (%) |
|---|---|---|---|---|---|---|---|---|
| | Hemangioma | 9 (4) | Myxoma | 23 (3) | Schwannoma | 28 (4) | Other | 9 (5) |
| | Other | 40 (18) | Other | 120 (18) | Other | 151 (23) | | 40 (23) |
| 66+ | Lipoma | 22 (21) | Lipoma | 158 (50) | Lipoma | 124 (42) | Schwannoma | 19 (26) |
| | Myxoma | 16 (15) | Hemangioma | 22 (7) | Fibromatosis | 26 (9) | Hemangiopericytoma | 14 (19) |
| | Neurofibroma | 13 (12) | Schwannoma | 18 (6) | Neurofibroma | 20 (7) | Lipoma | 6 (8) |
| | Schwannoma | 10 (9) | Fibrous histiocytoma | 17 (5) | Schwannoma | 18 (6) | Mesothelioma | 6 (8) |
| | Hemangiopericytoma | 10 (9) | Neurofibroma | 16 (5) | Elastofibroma | 17 (5) | Sclerosing retroperitonitis | 5 (7) |
| | Hemangioma | 8 (8) | Nodular fasciitis | 13 (4) | Myxoma | 16 (5) | Fibromatosis | 4 (6) |
| | Nodular fasciitis | 4 (4) | Myxoma | 12 (4) | Hemangioma | 14 (5; | Paraganglioma | 4 (6) |
| | Other | 23 (22) | Other | 58 (18) | Other | 61 (21) | Other | 14 (19) |

*GCT* giant cell tumor, *PVNS* pigmented villonodular synovitis

Based on an analysis of 18,677 cases seen in consultation by the Department of Soft Tissue Pathology (Armed Forces Institute of Pathology) over 10 years. Modified from [53]

a15(15) indicates there were 15 hemangiomas in the hand and wrist of patients 0-5 years, and this represents 15% of all benign tumors at this location in this age group

## Summary

Accurate diagnosis and staging of musculoskeletal tumors require an organized and integrated approach that involves the radiologist, pathologist and surgeon. Despite the wide variety of imaging modalities available today, radiographs remain the mainstay for the initial evaluation of suspected musculoskeletal neoplasms. Advanced imaging, using a combination of CT, MR, PET and/or scintigraphy will allow complete assessment for precise staging, biopsy planning and, in many cases, establishing or confirming a diagnosis.

## References

1. Hudson TM (1987) Radiologic-pathologic correlation of musculoskeletal lesions. Williams & Wilkins, Baltimore, pp 1-9
2. Madewell JE, Ragsdale BD, Sweet DE (1981) Analysis of solitary bone lesions. Part I. Internal margins. Radiol Clin North Am 19:715-748
3. Moser RP, Madewell JE (1987) An approach to primary bone tumors. Radiol Clin North Am 25:1049-1093
4. Ragsdale BD, Madewell JE, Sweet DE (1981) Analysis of solitary bone lesions. Part II. Periosteal reactions. Radiol Clin North Am 19:749-783
5. Sweet DE, Madewell JE, Ragsdale BD (1981) Analysis of solitary bone lesions. Part III. Matrix patterns. Radiol Clin North Am 19:785-814
6. Gartner L, Pearce CJ, Saifuddin A (2009) The role of the plain radiograph in the characterization of soft tissue tumours. Skeletal Radiol 38:549-558
7. Sundaram M, McGuire MH, Herbold DR (1988) Magnetic resonance imaging of soft tissue masses: an evaluation of fifty-three histologically proven tumors. Magn Reson Imaging 6:237-248
8. Dalinka MK, Zlatkin MD, Chao P et al (1990) The use of magnetic resonance imaging in the evaluation of bone and soft tissue tumors. Radiol Clin North Am 28:461-470
9. Pettersson H, Gillespy T, Hamlin DJ et al (1987) Primary musculoskeletal tumors: examination with MR imaging compared with conventional modalities. Radiology 164:237-241
10. Tehranzadeh J, Mnaymneh W, Ghavam C et al (1989) Comparison of CT and MR imaging in musculoskeletal neoplasms. J Comput Assist Tomogr 13:466-472
11. Ilaslan H, Wenger DE, Shives TC, Unni KK (2003) Unilateral hypertrophy of tensor fascia lata: a soft tissue tumor simulator. Skeletal Radiol 32:628-632
12. Panicek DM, Gatsonis C, Rosenthal DI et al (1997) CT and MR imaging in the local staging of primary malignant musculoskeletal neoplasms: Report of the Radiology Diagnostic Oncology Group. Radiology 202:237-246
13. Aisen AM, Martel W, Braunstein EM et al (1986) MRI and CT evaluation of primary bone and soft-tissue tumors. AJR Am J Roentgenol 146:749-756
14. Hudson TM, Hamlin DJ, Enneking WF et al (1985) Magnetic resonance imaging of bone and soft tissue tumors: early experience in 31 patients compared with computed tomography. Skeletal Radiol 13:134-146
15. Lang P, Johnston JO, Arenal-Romero F et al (1988) Advances in MR imaging of pediatric musculoskeletal neoplasms. Magn Reson Imaging Clin N Am 6:579-604
16. Rubin DA, Kneeland JB (1994) MR imaging of the musculoskeletal system: technical considerations for enhancing image quality and diagnostic yield. AJR Am J Roentgenol 163:1155-1163
17. Bhosale P, Ma J, Choi H (2009) Utility of the FIESTA pulse sequence in body oncologic imaging: review. AJR Am J Roentgenol 192:S83-93
18. Bydder GM (1992) Technical advances in magnetic resonance imaging. Curr Opin Neurol Neurosurg 5:854-858
19. Lee SS, Byun JH, Hong HS et al (2007) Image quality and focal lesion detection on T2-weighted MR imaging of the liver: comparison of two high-resolution free-breathing imaging techniques with two breath-hold imaging techniques. J Magn Reson Imaging 26:323-330
20. Rumboldt Z, Marotti M (2003) Magnetization transfer, HASTE, and FLAIR imaging. Magn Reson Imaging Clin N Am 11:471-492
21. Outwater EK (1999) Ultrafast MR imaging of the pelvis. Eur J Radiol 29:233-244
22. Van Epps K, Regan F (1999) MR cholangiopancreatography using HASTE sequences. Clin Radiol 54:588-594
23. Fuchs F, Laub G, Othomo K (2003) TrueFISP—technical considerations and cardiovascular applications. Eur J Radiol 46:28-32
24. Puderbach M, Hintze C, Ley S et al (2007) MR imaging of the chest: a practical approach at 1.5T. Eur J Radiol 64:345-355

25. Carr JC, Finn JP (2003) MR imaging of the thoracic aorta. Magn Reson Imaging Clin N Am 11:135-148

26. Mirowitz SA (1993) Fast scanning and fat-suppression MR imaging of musculoskeletal disorders. AJR Am J Roentgenol 161:1147-1157

27. Dwyer AJ, Frank JA, Sank VJ et al (1988) Short T1 inversion-recovery pulse sequence: analysis and initial experience in cancer imaging. Radiology 168:827-836

28. Shuman WP, Baron RL, Peters MJ et al (1989) Comparison of STIR and spin echo MR imaging at 1.5T in 90 lesions of the chest, liver and pelvis. AJR Am J Roentgenol 152:853-859

29. Cohen MD, Weetman RM, Provisor AJ et al (1986) Efficacy of magnetic resonance imaging in 139 children with tumors. Arch Surg 121:522-529

30. Sundaram M, McLeod RA (1988) Computed tomography or magnetic resonance for evaluation of solitary tumor and tumor-like lesions of bone. Skeletal Radiol 17:393-401

31. Bloem JL, Taminiau AHM, Eulderink F et al (1988) Radiologic staging of primary bone sarcoma: MR imaging, scintigraphy, angiography, and CT correlated with pathologic examination. Radiology 169:805-810

32. Seeger LL, Widoff BE, Bassett LW et al (1991) Preoperative evaluation of osteosarcoma: value of gadopentetate dimeglumine-enhanced MR imaging. AJR Am J Roentgenol 157:347-351

33. Benedikt RA, Jelinek JS, Kransdorf MJ et al (1994) MR imaging of soft-tissue masses: role of gadopentetate dimeglumine. J Magn Reson Imaging 4:485-490

34. Jordan RM, Mintz RD (1995) Fatal reaction to gadopentetate dimeglumine. AJR Am J Roentgenol 164:743-744

35. Tardy B, Guy C, Barral G et al (1992) Anaphylactic shock induced by intravenous gadopentetate dimeglumine. Lancet 339:494

36. Shellock FG, Hahn HP, Mink JH et al (1993) Adverse reaction to intravenous gadoteridol. Radiology 189:151-152

37. Prince MR, Zhang H, Morris M et al (2008) Incidence of nephrogenic systemic fibrosis at two large medical centers. Radiology 248:807-816

38. Wertman R, Altun E, Martin DR et al (2008) Risk of nephrogenic systemic fibrosis: evaluation of gadolinium chelate contrast agents at four American universities. Radiology 248:799-806

39. Weigle JP, Broome DR (2008) Nephrogenic systemic fibrosis: chronic imaging findings and review of the medical literature. Skeletal Radiol 37:457-464

40. Cowper SE, Robin HS, Steinberg SM et al (2000) Scleromyxoedema-like cutaneous diseases in renal-dialysis patients. Lancet 356:1000-1001

41. Lauenstein TC, Salman K, Morreira R et al (2007) Nephrogenic systemic fibrosis: center case review. J Magn Reson Imaging 26:1198-1203

42. Kanal E, Barkovich AJ, Bell C et al (2007) ACR guidance document for safe MR practices: 2007. AJR Am J Roentgenol 188:1447-1474

43. Costelloe CM, Murphy WA Jr, Haygood TM et al (2011) Comparison of half-dose and full-dose gadolinium MR contrast on the enhancement of bone and soft tissue tumors. Skeletal Radiol 40:327-333

44. Schulte M, Brecht-Krauss D, Werner M et al (1999) Evaluation of neoadjuvant therapy response of osteogenic sarcoma using FDG PET. J Nucl Med 40:1637-1643

45. Enneking WF, Spanier SS, Goodman MA (1980) A system for the surgical staging of musculoskeletal sarcoma. Clin Orthop 153:106-120

46. American Joint Committee on Cancer (AJCC) (2002) Staging Manual, 6th edn. www.cancerstaging.net

47. Unni KK (1996) Dahlin's bone tumors. General Aspects and data on 11,087 cases, 5th edn. Lippincott-Raven, Philadelphia, pp 1-9

48. Crim JR, Seeger LL, Yao L et al (1992) Diagnosis of soft-tissue masses with MR imaging: can benign masses be differentiated from malignant ones? Radiology 185:581-586

49. Kransdorf MJ, Jelinek JS, Moser et al (1989) Soft-tissue masses: diagnosis using MR imaging. AJR Am J Roentgenol 153:541-547

50. De Schepper A, Ramon F, Degryse H (1992) Statistical analysis of MRI parameters predicting malignancy in 141 soft tissue masses. Rofo Fortschr Geb Rontgenstr Neuen Bildgeb Verfahr 156:587-591

51. Gielen JL, De Schepper AM, Vanhoenacker F et al (2004) Accuracy of MRI in characterization of soft tissue tumors and tumor-like lesions. A prospective study in 548 patients. Eur Radiol 14:2320-2330

52. Kransdorf MJ (1995) Malignant soft-tissue tumors in a large referral population: distribution of diagnoses by age, sex, and location. Am J Roentgenol AJR 164:129-34

53. Kransdorf MJ (1995) Benign soft-tissue tumors in a large referral population: distribution of specific diagnoses by age, sex, and location. Am J Roentgenol AJR 164:395-402

# Arthritis

Charles S. Resnik[1], Andrew J. Grainger[2]

[1] Department of Diagnostic Radiology, University of Maryland School of Medicine, Baltimore, MD, USA
[2] Chapel Allerton Orthopaedic Center, Chapel Allerton Hospital, Leeds Teaching Hospitals, Leeds, UK

## Overview

Correct diagnosis of arthritis (Fig. 1) involves consideration of numerous factors, including clinical features [age and sex of the patient, duration of symptoms, clinical appearance of involved joint or joints, presence or absence of associated diseases (e.g., skin disease, uveitis, urethritis)], laboratory values (e.g., markers for inflammation, serum rheumatoid factor, serum uric acid level), and various imaging features. Radiographs represent the

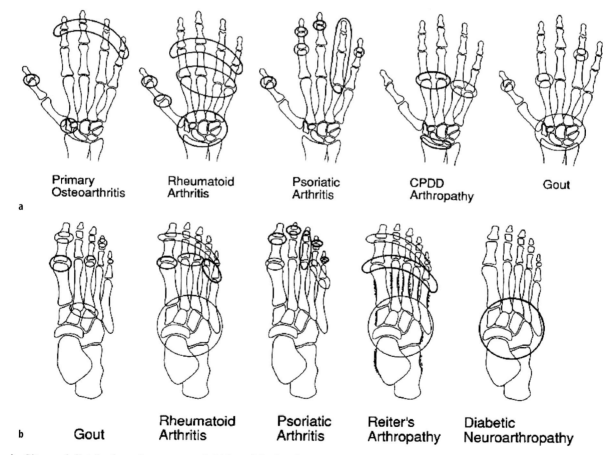

**Fig. 1 a, b.** Sites and distribution of common arthritides of the hand (**a**) and foot (**b**). The more common sites are encircled with *bold lines* and the less common sites with *lighter lines*. Note the periosteal reaction (new bone formation) classically identified in reactive arthritis (Reiter's arthropathy). Note also the potential for "sausage digit" distribution in psoriatic arthritis. When joints are encircled in isolation, the distribution is random and may be isolated to any joint (Courtesy of Lee F. Rogers, MD)

J. Hodler et al. (eds.), *Musculoskeletal Diseases 2013-2016,*
DOI: 10.1007/978-88-470-5292-5_12 © Springer-Verlag Italia 2013

mainstay for diagnosis and follow-up of joint damage, although magnetic resonance imaging (MRI) and sonography can be useful evaluation tools, especially in the early stages of disease. Many imaging features have to be systematically assessed to establish a correct diagnosis: (1) the distribution of joint involvement [monoarticular or polyarticular, symmetrical or asymmetrical, proximal or distal, associated axial involvement, associated enthesis (ligament and tendon attachment to bone) involvement]; (2) soft tissue swelling (periarticular, fusiform, nodular); (3) joint space narrowing (uniform, non-uniform, none); (4) bone erosion (marginal, central, periarticular, well-defined, none); (5) bone production (osteophytes, enthesophytes, periosteal new bone); (6) calcification (periarticular, chondrocalcinosis); (7) subchondral cysts; (8) periarticular osteoporosis.

In recent years, there has been a significant change in the management of the inflammatory arthritides, with the advent of powerful and effective biological therapies. The use of these drugs has led to a dramatic improvement in patient lifestyle and morbidity from this disease group, which previously resulted in relentless joint destruction. To achieve these outcomes, drug therapy must be initiated before irreversible joint damage has occurred. This requires early diagnosis, often before conventional radiographs show manifestations of the disease. This has led to increasing use of more advanced imaging techniques, principally MRI and ultrasound, to diagnose and manage these conditions. Intense research activity is currently centered on the use of these techniques to detect disease progression and remission; in the future they might become important tools in therapeutic decision-making.

## Rheumatoid Arthritis

Rheumatoid arthritis is characterized by proliferative, hypervascularized synovitis, resulting in bone erosion, cartilage damage, joint destruction and long-term disability. Diagnosis is based on clinical, laboratory and radiographic findings. The disease typically begins in the peripheral joints, usually the metacarpophalangeal (MCP) and proximal interphalangeal (PIP) joints, the wrists, and the metatarsophalangeal (MTP) joints, with a predominantly symmetrical distribution. As the disease progresses, it affects more proximal joints.

The initial radiographic manifestations are soft tissue swelling and periarticular osteoporosis. These features represent indirect evidence of synovial inflammation, and their assessment is quite subjective. More specific are marginal erosions of bone that occur at the so-called bare areas between the peripheral edge of the articular cartilage and the insertion of the joint capsule. In the early stages of the disease, these may occur at the radial aspect of the second and third metacarpal heads, at the ulnar styloid process, and at the metatarsal heads, especially at the lateral aspect of the fifth metatarsal head. This is followed by diffuse narrowing of PIP, MCP, MTP and wrist joints. Unfortunately, these features represent late consequences of synovitis. Characteristically, the distal interphalangeal (DIP) joints are spared. There is no osseous proliferation and no involvement of entheses.

The development of new, powerful, but expensive therapeutic agents for rheumatoid arthritis, such as the anti-tumor necrosis factor agents, has created new demands on radiologists to identify patients with aggressive rheumatoid arthritis at an early stage. MRI and sonography can be useful tools in evaluating these patients. Sonography is a quick and inexpensive way to detect synovitis and tenosynovitis, whereas MRI is a more global way to evaluate the small synovial joints of the appendicular skeleton, and is more sensitive than radiography in detecting synovitis, bone marrow edema and bone erosions. MRI is also an excellent means to assess spinal complications of rheumatoid arthritis, in particular subluxation at the atlantoaxial joint. Both MRI and sonography may be used to demonstrate the soft tissue changes of rheumatoid arthritis, such as tenosynovitis and rheumatoid nodules.

## Seronegative Spondyloarthropathies

The seronegative spondyloarthropathies are represented by ankylosing spondylitis, psoriatic arthritis, reactive arthritis (Reiter's syndrome), colitic arthritis and undifferentiated spondyloarthropathies. Affected persons usually have a negative serum rheumatoid factor, but a significant percentage has the HLA-B27 antigen. These diseases frequently cause symptoms in the axial skeleton, but the appendicular skeleton may also be affected, in isolation or in combination. Radiographically, these diseases differ from rheumatoid arthritis by the absence or mild nature of periarticular osteoporosis, the involvement of entheses with erosions and with new bone formation, and the asymmetrical involvement of the peripheral skeleton.

### Ankylosing Spondylitis

Involvement in ankylosing spondylitis starts and is most typical in the axial skeleton (spine and sacroiliac joints), but the appendicular skeleton may also be involved, especially the feet. Radiography may demonstrate arthritis and enthesitis with erosive changes and osseous proliferation. MRI is well suited for demonstrating the early spinal and sacroiliac changes of ankylosing spondylitis. High T2 signal change (edema like) seen at the corners of vertebral bodies and in the subchondral bone of the sacroiliac joints is a typical feature. Later, erosive change at the sacroiliac joints and ultimately fusion in the sacroiliac joints and spine may be seen. Costovertebral disease is a common finding on MRI. Sites of previous inflammatory change may be evident as fatty change within the bone marrow, typically seen at the corners of the vertebral bodies. At an early stage of the disease, sonography and MRI may be useful in showing peripheral inflammatory changes at the entheses, including extra-articular sites such as the calcaneal attachments of the Achilles tendon and plantar fascia. While sonography will show synovitis and erosive change along with enthesophytes, MRI will also demonstrate edema-like change within the bone marrow.

## Psoriatic Arthritis

The extent of arthritis does not correlate with the degree of psoriatic skin disease and, in some cases, the skin manifestations may follow the arthritis by several years or may never develop. Psoriatic arthritis tends to involve the small joints of the hands and feet. The process is characteristically asymmetrical. Involvement of the DIP joints of the hands and toes, usually in association with psoriatic changes of the nails, or involvement of one entire digit (MCP + PIP + DIP, "sausage digit"), is very suggestive of psoriatic arthritis. This arthritis is not necessarily associated with periarticular osteoporosis, and erosions are often small. In contrast, extensive osseous proliferation at entheses and periostitis are common.

At an early stage, sonography and MRI may show synovitis, tenosynovitis and bursitis that are similar to those seen in rheumatoid arthritis. In addition, MRI may demonstrate extensive signal abnormality in the bone marrow and soft tissues far beyond the joint capsule, related to enthesitis. These features may be useful in patients with inflammatory polyarthralgia of the hands for differentiating rheumatoid arthritis from psoriatic arthritis. Sacroiliitis is common and resembles that seen in ankylosing spondylitis, except that it is more often asymmetrical. Spinal involvement is less common, and the paravertebral ossification that occurs in psoriatic spondylitis is typically broad, coarse and asymmetrical in contrast to the symmetrical syndesmophytes of ankylosing spondylitis.

## Reactive Arthritis (Reiter's Syndrome)

Reactive arthritis is characterized by urethritis, conjunctivitis and mucocutaneous lesions in the oropharynx, tongue, glans penis and skin, as well as arthritis. In general, the radiographic manifestations are similar to those of psoriatic arthritis, except that the axial skeleton is not as commonly involved, and changes in the upper extremities are exceptional. The most prominent involvement is in the lower extremities, particularly the feet.

## Colitic Arthritis

Arthritis occurs in approximately 10% of patients with chronic inflammatory bowel disease, more commonly in ulcerative colitis than in Crohn's disease. The most common manifestation is sacroiliitis, which is similar to but not as extensive as that in ankylosing spondylitis, with bilateral symmetrical involvement. Patients are rarely symptomatic, and the radiographic findings of sacroiliitis are often noted incidentally on abdominal radiographs obtained as part of a small bowel or colon examination. Peripheral arthritis is uncommon.

## Degenerative Joint Disease (Osteoarthritis)

Osteoarthritis is characterized by degeneration and shredding of articular cartilage. It mainly affects the interphalangeal joints of the fingers (sparing the MCP joints) and the weight-bearing joints (hips and knees). Degenerative joint disease occurs in two major forms: a primary form, which is a generalized disease affecting all of the aforementioned joints, and a secondary form limited to joints affected by previous localized trauma or other joint disease. The radiographic and pathologic changes are similar in the two forms.

The general radiographic features of osteoarthritis are nonuniform joint space narrowing, subchondral sclerosis of bone, marginal osteophytes and subchondral cysts. Narrowing of the joint space in osteoarthritis is almost invariably uneven and more pronounced in that portion of the joint where weight-bearing stresses are greatest. In general, the greater the degree of narrowing, the more severe the associated findings of subchondral sclerosis and osteophytosis. Calcified or ossified fragments (loose bodies) may be identified within the joint and are particularly common in the knee.

Clinical and radiographic features are usually straightforward, and MRI is not used for primary diagnosis. It should be recognized that some MRI features may be misleading, including extensive edema of subchondral bone marrow, signal changes of subchondral bone located on only one side of a joint, enhancement of subchondral cysts after intravenous gadolinium administration, and heterogeneous signal intensity of joint fluid.

### Erosive Osteoarthritis

Erosive osteoarthritis is an inflammatory form of osteoarthritis that occurs primarily in postmenopausal women. It is usually limited to the interphalangeal joints of the hand. Clinically, the joints are acutely inflamed. Erosions of the central portion of articular surfaces are prominent and are superimposed on the standard radiographic features of osteoarthritis. They are often more pronounced at the PIP joints. Involved joints may eventually undergo osseous ankylosis, which does not occur in noninflammatory osteoarthritis. Inflammatory changes of these joints may also be demonstrated by MRI.

## Metabolic Joint Disease

### Gout

Gouty arthritis is characterized by recurring acute attacks of arthritis involving one or more joints, with an increase in the serum level of uric acid and resulting deposition of sodium urate. The first MTP joint is the joint most often affected. Involvement of the tarsometatarsal and carpometacarpal joints frequently occurs. Over time, chronic tophaceous gout develops with a typical asymmetrical joint involvement. The tophaceous deposits occur in periarticular soft tissues and sometimes in synovium and subchondral bone. These can produce hard masses that may cause ulceration of the overlying skin and extrusion of chalky material.

Radiographic features include eccentric nodular soft tissue swelling. Soft tissue masses are especially suggestive of tophi when they have high density on radiographs due to microcalcifications often related to chronic renal disease. Soft tissue tophi may produce erosion of subjacent bone, including deposition in the olecranon bursa that may be associated with erosion of the olecranon.

Erosions are suggestive of gout if they are located at a distance from any joint. In many cases, though, they may be intra-articular and may be marginal in location, mimicking rheumatoid arthritis. However, other features are helpful for the diagnosis of gout: erosions are often large in size (greater than 5 mm), they are frequently oriented along the long axis of the bone, they are characteristically surrounded by a sclerotic border due to the long duration of disease, and there may be an "overhanging edge" of new bone partially surrounding them. Also, there is commonly relative preservation of joint space, and there is not extensive osteoporosis.

Sonography may demonstrate soft tissue tophi before they are radiographically evident. They appear as hyperechoic or heterogeneous masses, sometimes with acoustic shadowing due to calcifications. They may demonstrate hyperemia on power Doppler evaluation. The double contour sign, which is a hyperechoic irregular band over the superficial margin of cartilage, and the presence of hypo- to hyperechoic inhomogeneous material surrounded by a small anechoic rim, might also be suggestive of gout. Sonography may also be used to guide aspiration of a joint. Computed tomography (CT) may be helpful to confirm the high density of a soft tissue tophus (often about 160 Hounsfield units), which is less than the density of hydroxyapatite deposits in calcific tendinitis. MRI features may be misleading, as there may be hypointense masses within the synovium on T2-weighted images, mimicking pigmented villonodular synovitis.

### Calcium Pyrophosphate Dihydrate Crystal Deposition Disease

Calcium Pyrophosphate Dihydrate (CPPD) crystal deposition disease is generally observed in middle-aged and elderly patients. It may be associated with two types of radiographic features, which are frequently combined: articular/periarticular calcification and arthropathy.

### Calcification

Chondrocalcinosis is the presence of intra-articular calcium-containing salts, most commonly CPPD, within hyaline cartilage and/or fibrocartilage. Calcium within the fibrocartilage is characteristically somewhat irregular, as seen in the menisci of the knee or the triangular fibrocartilage of the wrist. Calcification of hyaline cartilage along an articular surface appears as a fine, linear radiodensity closely paralleling the subjacent cortical margin. Capsular, synovial, ligament, and tendon calcifications are less frequent. Many affected persons are asymptomatic, but, in others, intermittent acute attacks of arthritis resemble gout (pseudogout). The correct diagnosis is established by the identification of typical CPPD crystals in synovial fluid. Sonography may also be helpful by demonstrating multiple sparkling hyperechoic dots without acoustic shadows in the joint fluid that are very suggestive of CPPD crystals.

### Pyrophosphate Arthropathy

The joints most commonly involved are the knee, the radiocarpal and midcarpal joints of the wrist, and the MCP joints of the hand, the shoulder and the hip. The joint changes that occur in this disorder resemble osteoarthritis, with joint space narrowing, bone sclerosis and subchondral cyst formation. The unusual distribution of these findings, the small size of the osteophytes contrasting with the severity of the arthropathy, and the presence of chondrocalcinosis allow a specific diagnosis to be made. Involvement of the MCP joints, particularly the second and third, is characteristic of this disorder. Hemochromatosis also affects the MCP joints in a similar fashion, but all MCP joints are characteristically affected, and there may be large "hook-like" osteophytes along the radial aspect of the metacarpal heads.

### Neuropathic Osteoarthropathy

Neuropathic osteoarthropathy has a variety of causes. Nowadays, this most frequently occurs in patients with diabetes mellitus. In these patients, findings are confined almost exclusively to the ankle and foot. Calcification of the smaller arteries of the foot is a frequent and important clue to the presence of underlying diabetes but may not always be evident. Fractures or fracture-dislocations of the tarsal bones or metatarsals are particularly common manifestations of diabetic neuropathic disease. Often such fractures or dislocations are incidental findings on radiographs obtained for the evaluation of infection of the foot or complaints of swelling without a history of trauma. Less commonly, the neuropathic process appears to be initiated by a traumatic event that results in a fracture or dislocation. CT may be useful to assess the extent of microtraumatic changes of joint surfaces. MRI may demonstrate extensive abnormal signal intensity changes of bone that may mimic infection, but the distribution of arthropathy is typically widespread, contrasted with the localized nature of osteomyelitis associated with adjacent soft tissue infection.

**Acknowledgment.** The authors would like to acknowledge the major contribution of material to this manuscript by Anne Cotten, MD, and Lee F. Rogers, MD.

## Suggested Reading

Aliabadi P, Nikpoor N, Alparslan L (2003) Imaging of neuropathic arthropathy. Semin Musculoskelet Radiol 7:217-225

Bennett DL (2004) Spondyloarthropathies: ankylosing spondylitis and psoriatic arthritis. Radiol Clin North Am 42:121-134

Bohndorf K, Imhof H, Pope TL (2001) Musculoskeletal Imaging: a concise multimodality approach. Thieme, pp 292-377

Buchmann RF (2004) Imaging of articular disorders in children. Radiol Clin North Am 42:151-168

Cotten A (2005) Imagerie Musculosquelettique – Pathologies Générales. Elsevier Masson

Greenspan A (2003) Erosive osteoarthritis. Semin Musculoskelet Radiol 7:155-159

Gupta KB (2004) Radiographic evaluation of osteoarthritis. Radiol Clin North Am 42:11-41

Klecker RJ, Weissman BN (2003) Imaging features of psoriatic arthritis and Reiter's syndrome. Semin Musculoskelet Radiol 7:115-126

Monu JU (2004) Gout: a clinical and radiologic review. Radiol Clin North Am 42:169-184

Rowbotham EL, Grainger AJ (2011) Rheumatoid arthritis: Ultrasound versus MRI. AJR Am J Roentgenol 197:541-546

Steinbach LS (2004) Calcium pyrophosphate dihydrate and calcium hydroxyapatite crystal deposition diseases: imaging perspectives. Radiol Clin North Am 42:185-205

Tehranzadeh J (2004) Advanced imaging of early rheumatoid arthritis. Radiol Clin North Am 42:89-107

# Metabolic Bone Disease I

Murali Sundaram

Diagnostic Radiology, Musculoskeletal Division, Cleveland Clinic Foundation, Cleveland, OH, USA

## Introduction

Metabolic bone disease may result from genetic, endocrine, nutritional or biochemical disorders, with variable and often inconsistent imaging findings. For the radiologist, the cornerstone of "metabolic bone disease" has been osteoporosis, osteomalacia, hyperparathyroidism and Paget's disease. Over the past three decades each of these diseases has undergone diagnostic and therapeutic changes influenced by biochemical discoveries, imaging advances and epidemiology that in turn have had an impact on current radiological practice.

## Osteoporosis

Osteoporosis remains the most common metabolic abnormality of bone. It has been described as "a silent epidemic" affecting one in two women and one in five men, older than 50 years of age, during their lifetime [1]. It is now defined as a systemic skeletal disease characterized by low bone mass and micro-architectural deterioration of bone resulting in little or no trauma [2]. Although long recognized as a quantitative abnormality of bone, it was the introduction of dual energy x-ray absorptiometry (DXA) in 1987 [3, 4], with its advantages of high precision, short scan times, low radiation dose and stable calibration, that has permitted quantification of osteoporosis (bone mineral density, BMD) in routine clinical practice to make the diagnosis and guide management. Prior to BMD measurements, it required the development of a fracture before a diagnosis of osteoporosis could be made. Following the routine clinical application of BMD measurements, it no longer requires an individual to have sustained a fracture for a diagnosis of osteoporosis and it has permitted the diagnosis to be made on the concepts of low bone mass, bone fragility and increased fracture risk.

Because trabecular bone comprises 20% of the skeleton and is highly responsive to metabolic stimuli, the assessment of trabecular bone alone, site specific, is felt to be important for assessing osteoporosis fracture risk and treatment response [5]. DXA measures cortical and trabecular bone. Considerable research effort is ongoing in assessing micro-trabecular architecture by computed tomography (CT) and magnetic resonance imaging (MRI) [5].

Vertebral compression fractures occur in 26% of women over 50 years of age [6]. They are not always symptomatic, and most fractures heal within a few weeks or months, although a minority do not respond to conservative measures [7]. Percutaneous vertebroplasty is now a widely used technique for the treatment of such patients to prevent further bone loss from prolonged bed rest.

Since the previous musculoskeletal course in Davos, the iatrogenic adverse effects of bisphosphonates on the skeleton have taken a new controversial twist. At that time the concern was mandibular necrosis. That controversy has been settled by evidence showing mandibular necrosis usually occurred following recent dental surgery and when bisphosphonates were administered in large doses, usually parenterally, for underlying malignancies and not in the doses recommended for osteoporosis.

The current controversy deals with atypical insufficiency fractures developing in patients on long-term oral bisphosphonates for osteoporosis. Rather than being drawn into the therapeutic controversies of the subject, radiologists should be aware of the potential for patients on oral bisphosphonates to develop atypical insufficiency fractures, and recognize them for what they are (Fig. 1). Because these fractures when untreated can result in a shattered bone they are treated by intramedullary nailing (Fig. 2).

### Osteoporosis in the First Three Decades

In 2000, Glorieux and co-workers described a subtype of osteogenesis imperfecta (OI) with a propensity to such

J. Hodler et al. (eds.), *Musculoskeletal Diseases 2013-2016*,
DOI: 10.1007/978-88-470-5292-5_13 © Springer-Verlag Italia 2013

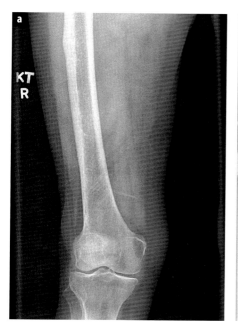
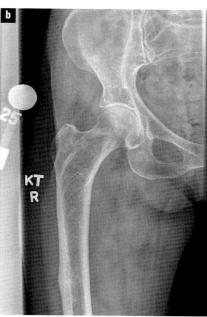

**Fig. 1 a, b.** A subtle cortical thickening of the distal lateral femoral cortex is evident on both radiographs, which display the knee joint and the hip joint, respectively. This highlights the importance of careful cortical scrutiny of the femoral cortex in patients radiographed for presumed articular disease

## Female Athlete Triad (Third Decade)

The female athlete triad comprises eating disorder such as anorexia nervosa, menstrual disorder (amenorrhea or oligomenorrhea) and osteopenia/osteoporosis [10]. "The female athlete triad" becomes a diagnostic consideration for the radiologist when stress fractures and serous atrophy of bone marrow are identified on MRI [11]. Serous atrophy of bone marrow on MRI demonstrates abnormal low signal in T1-weighted images, and high signal on T2-weighted or STIR images, and in advanced cases it can be associated with loss of subcutaneous fat and loss of fat in muscle septa. Stress fractures are usually an unequivocal finding on MRI, but might be difficult to identify in the presence of serous marrow change because the typical edema pattern silhouetting a fracture in normal bone marrow is masked by a serous marrow [12].

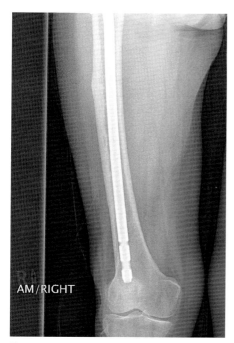

**Fig. 2.** Intramedullary nailing of the atypical femoral insufficiency from a shattered displaced fracture

## Osteomalacia and Rickets

Classically, the deficiency of vitamin D, essential for the absorption of calcium, has been the major cause of rickets in the child and osteomalacia in the adult, as a consequence of absence or delay in the mineralization of growth cartilage or newly formed bone collagen. Perhaps not as widely recognized is the development of rickets/osteomalacia as a consequence of a low serum phosphate and normal serum calcium. Two such conditions are X-linked hypophosphatemic rickets/osteomalacia and oncogenic osteomalacia. When present, the signs of rickets and osteomalacia in the low serum phosphate states are indistinguishable from the classic hypo-

abundant hyperplastic callus after fracture that it bore a strong resemblance to osteosarcoma. They designated this particular complication as type V OI and considered the hyperplastic exuberant callus formation to represent a new form of brittle bone disease [8]. This form of the disease with hyperplastic callus can also lead to significant long-term morbidity [9].

calcemic states, i.e., widened growth plate, metaphyseal cupping and fraying about joints in the child and Looser's zones (a lucency that runs perpendicular to the cortex of bone, and is indistinguishable from the frequently encountered stress fracture) in the adult [13, 14]. However, there are some distinctive imaging signs that have been recently emphasized and described in these two conditions, along with clinical, genetic and biochemical advances.

### X-linked Hypophosphatemic Osteomalacia

The condition is characterized by low tubular reabsorption of phosphate in the absence of secondary hyperparathyroidism. X-linked hypophosphatemia occurs in about 1 in 25,000 and is said to be the most common form of genetically induced rickets [15]. From an imaging standpoint, a curious and paradoxical finding in this condition is that in addition to Looser's zones and femoral bowing there may be striking extraskeletal ossifications at sites of enthesis (mimicking a seronegative spondylitis or fluorosis) and occasionally intraspinal ossifications [16, 17].

### Oncogenic Osteomalacia

Oncogenic osteomalacia, first described by Prader et al. in 1959 [18], is a paraneoplastic syndrome in which a bone or soft tissue tumor or tumor-like lesion induces hypophosphatemia and low vitamin D levels that reverse when the inciting lesion is resected.

### Imaging Considerations

As elusive as the diagnosis of oncogenic osteomalacia appears to be for the clinician, it is more so for the radiologist unaware of the critical biochemical abnormalities of hypophosphatemia and hyperphosphaturia. The radiologist may consider the diagnosis of oncogenic osteomalacia if radiographs demonstrate Looser's zones in adults or the classic signs of rickets in children in the absence of malnutrition or malabsorption. Once the presumptive clinical diagnosis of oncogenic osteomalacia is made, the search for the causative neoplasm begins. A recent review observed a range of 5 months to 14 years from the time of presentation to diagnosis [19]. Skeletal surveys and radioisotope bone scans have been the mainstays in the search for a clinically inapparent neoplasm. More recently, whole body MRI and indium III labeled octreotide scanning have been employed [20, 21]. Whatever the imaging modality used, any discovered lesion, however innocuous, should be considered causative of the syndrome and removed [22]. Tumors responsible for this syndrome may arise equally in bone or soft tissue with a predilection for the craniofacial region and extremities. A single case report and a single case from our institution has demonstrated cure being achieved by imaging-guided radiofrequency ablation of the suspected tumor, which pathologists now characterize as a phosphaturic mesenchymal tumor.

### Renal Osteodystrophy

The connection between renal glomerular disease and bone disease was made a little over a hundred years ago [23], and the term renal osteodystrophy to describe the musculoskeletal complications of chronic renal failure was introduced in 1943 [24]. Renal osteodystrophy is the result of two major pathological processes that vary in severity: hyperparathyroidism from an excess of parathyroid hormone, and rickets or osteomalacia from a deficiency of 1,25-dihydrocholecalciferol, the renal hormone of vitamin D [25]. Dialysis and renal transplantation, the only life-sustaining and life-saving therapeutic options for chronic renal failure, modify the natural history of renal osteodystrophy, i.e., hyperparathyroidism and osteomalacia. Worldwide there are over one million patients on maintenance hemodialysis [26]. Since hyperparathyroidism is universal in chronic renal failure irrespective of imaging findings, it may be assumed that these patients have renal osteodystrophy. The development of a new disease state, amyloidosis, is a direct consequence of long-term dialysis in chronic renal failure. The problem is unresolved and on the rise with patients kept alive by dialysis for long periods of time while awaiting renal transplantation. Cameron refers to this as the "rise and rise of amyloidosis" [27]. Amyloid deposition is a consequence of $B_2$ microglobulin, which is elevated to between 30 and 50 times the normal level in patients with chronic renal failure. The complication is almost universal in patients who have been on dialysis for 15 years or longer, tending to become evident after 8 years [27]. The most common location of these deposits is the carpal tunnel. Because primary hyperparathyroidism is diagnosed at a biochemical level, and more patients with renal failure are being sustained for longer periods of time on peritoneal or hemodialysis, brown tumors are now not uncommonly seen in poorly controlled patients on dialysis. Thus, in contradistinction to what was taught three decades ago, the practicing radiologist in the western world is more likely to encounter "brown" tumors more often as a manifestation of secondary rather than primary hyperparathyroidism.

Destructive discovertebral disease may on occasion be encountered in patients on long-term dialysis, and has been termed renal spondyloarthropathy. Its prevalence is unknown. Whether the destructive changes are due to amyloid, or they are multifactorial, is uncertain. The most pressing diagnosis to be excluded is discitis or osteomyelitis. Often this is resolved by an aspiration. However, in some of these patients the abnormality has a short T2 signal and in this circumstance may be considered to represent renal spondyloarthropathy rather than a discitis or discovertebral osteomyelitis [28], thus obviating a biopsy.

## Paget's Disease

There has been a significant decline in the prevalence of Paget's disease, both in severity and disease of young onset. Paget's disease remains mostly an asymptomatic and often incidental radiographic finding. MRI is employed when sarcoma is suspected and for staging prior to biopsy. An unexpected MRI finding of uncomplicated Paget's disease is the preservation of marrow fat, irrespective of the phase of the disease, in the appendicular skeleton on T1-weighted sequences [29, 30]. Paget's disease of the appendicular skeleton is one of those unusual disease processes where marrow fat may be diffusely preserved on T1-weighted MRI sequences in the presence of a diffuse radiographic abnormality. This has been attributed to a repopulation of fat within the marrow space. Osteolytic Paget's, the result of osteoclastic resorption, can radiographically mimic a malignant process. The presence of a fatty marrow signal should suggest the correct diagnosis. MRI can also serve to identify the so-called pseudosarcoma of Paget's disease, which clinically presents as a soft-tissue mass with or without erosion of the underlying cortex. Distinction from a sarcoma may be difficult, but preservation of a fatty marrow signal would indicate against a sarcoma.

## References

1. Sambrook P, Cooper C ((2006) Osteoporosis. Lancet 367:2010-2018
2. Consensus Development Conference (1993) Diagnosis prophylaxis and treatment of osteoporosis. Am J Med; 94:646-651
3. Genant HK, Engelke K, Fuerst T et al ((1996) Noninvasive assessment of bone mineral and structure: state of the art. J Bone Minor Res 11:707-730
4. Baran DT, Faulkner KG, Genant HK et al (1997) Diagnosis and management of osteoporosis – guidelines for the utilization of bone densitometry. Calcif Tissue Int 61:433-440
5. Majumdar S (2008) Magnetic resonance imaging for osteoporosis. Perspective. Skeletal Radiology 37:95-97
6. Melton LJ III (1997) Epidemiology of spinal osteoporosis. Spine 22(Suppl):S2-S11
7. Rapado A (1996) General management of vertebral fractures. Bone 18(Suppl):191S-196S
8. Glorieux FH, Rauch F, Plotkin H et al (2000) Type V Osteogenesis Imperfecta: a new form of brittle bone disease. J Bone Minor Res 15:1650-1658
9. Cheung MS, Azouz EM, Glorieux FH, Rauch F (2008) Hyperplastic callus formation in Osteogenesis Imperfecta Type V: follow up of three generation over ten years. Skeletal Radiol 37:465-467
10. Nattor A, Loucks AB, Manore MM et al; American College of Sports Medicine Position Stand (2008) The female athlete triad. Med Sci Sports Exerc 39:1867-1882
11. Vande Berg BC, Malghem J, Devuyst O et al (1994) Anorexia nervosa: correlation appearance between MR appearance of bone marrow and severity of disease. Radiology 193:859-864
12. Tins B, Cassar-Pullicino V (2006) Marrow changes in anorexia nervosa masking the presence of stress fractures on MR imaging. Skeletal Radiol 35:857-860
13. Harrison HE, Harrison HC (1975) Rickets then and now. J Pediatr 87:1144-1151
14. Pitt MJ (1991) Rickets and Osteomalacia are still around. Radiol Clin North Am 29:97-118
15. Weissman Y, Hochberg Z (1994) Genetic rickets and osteomalacia. Curr Ther Endocinrol Metab 5:492-495
16. Polisson RP, Martinez S, Khoury M et al (1985) Calcification of enthesis associated with x-linked hypophosphatemic osteomalacia. N Engl J Med 313:1-6
17. Adams JE, Davies M (1986) Intraspinal new bone formation and spinal cord compression in familial hypophosphatemic vitamin D resistant Osteomalacia. Am J Med 61:1117-1129
18. Prader VA, Inig R, Vehlinger E, Stalder G (1959) Rachitis Infolge, Knochen Tumors. Helv Pediatr Acta 14:554-565
19. Siegel HJ, Rock MG, Inwards C, Sim FH (2002) Phosphaturic mesenchymal tumor. Orthopedics 25:1279-1281
20. Avila NA, Skarulis M, Rubino DM, Doppmath JL (1996) Oncogenic osteomalacia: lesion detection by MR skeletal survey. AMJ Am J Roentgenol 167:343-345
21. Seufert J, Ebert K, Muller J et al (2001) Brief report: octreotide therapy for tumor induced osteomalacia. N Engl J Med 3451883-1888
22. Sundaram M, McCarthy EF (2000) Oncogenic osteomalacia. Skeletal Radiol 29;117-124
23. Lucas RC (1883) A form of late rickets associated with albuminuria: rickets of adolescents. Lancet 1:993.
24. Liu SH, Chu HI (1946) Studies of calcium and phosphorous metabolism with special reference to pathogenesis and effects of dihydrotachysterol and iron. Medicine 22:103
25. Parfitt AM (1976) The actions of parathyroid hormone on bone: relation to bone remodeling and turnover calcium homeostasis and metabolic bone disease. Metabolism 25:1157
26. Cameron JS (2002) Dialysis today and tomorrow: History of the treatment of renal failure by dialysis. Oxford University Press, Oxford, p 336
27. Cameron JS (2002) The rise and rise of dialysis amyloidosis. A history of the treatment of renal failure by dialysis. Oxford University Press, Oxford, p 263
28. Leone A, Sundaram M, Cerase A et al (2001) Destructive spondyloarthropathy of the cervical spine in long-term hemodialyzed patients: a five-year clinical radiological prospective study. Skeletal Radiol 30:431-441
29. Kaufmann GA, Sundaram M, McDonald DJ (1991) Magnetic Resonance imaging in symptomatic Paget's Disease. Skeletal Radiol 20:413-418
30. Sundaram M, Khanna G, El-Khoury G (2001) T1 weighted MR imaging for distinguishing large osteolysis of Paget's disease from sarcomatous degeneration. Skeletal Radiol 30:378-383

# Metabolic Bone Disease II

Bruno Vande Berg, Patrick Omoumi, Ahmed Larbi, Frédéric Lecouvet

Department of Radiology, Cliniques Universitaires Saint-Luc, IREC Institut de Recherche Clinique, Université catholique de Louvain, Louvain Academy, Brussels, Belgium

This chapter aims to provide an overview of important imaging features observed in metabolic bone diseases [1, 2]. Common and uncommon imaging findings observed in insufficiency stress fractures will also be reviwed and illustrated.

## Overview of Metabolic Bone Disorders

### Normal Bone Metabolism

Bone is a specialized connective tissue made up of a matrix of collagen fibers, mucopolysaccharides and inorganic crystalline mineral matrix (calcium hydroxyapatite) that is distributed along the length of the collagen fibers. Bone remains metabolically active throughout life (bone turnover), with bone being constantly resorbed by osteoclasts (osteoclastic activity) and accreted by osteoblasts (osteoblastic activity). Since bone turnover takes place mainly on bone surface, trabecular bone, which has a greater surface area to volume ratio than compact bone, is consequently some eight times more metabolically active than cortical bone. The strength of bone is related not only to its hardness and other physical properties, but also to its size, shape and architectural arrangement of the compact and trabecular bone.

Bone formation and bone resorption are linked in a consistent sequence under normal circumstances. Precursor bone cells are activated at a particular skeletal site to form osteoclasts, which erode a fairly constant amount of bone. After a period of time, the bone resorption ceases and osteoblasts are required to fill the eroded space with new bone tissue. This coupling of osteoblastic and osteoclastic activity constitutes the basal multicellular unit (BMU) of bone and is normally in balance, with the amount of bone eroded being replaced with new bone in about 3-4 months. At any one time, there are numerous BMUs throughout the skeleton at different stages of this cycle. The amount of bone in the skeleton at any moment is entirely dependent on peak bone mass attained during puberty and adolescence, and on the balance between bone resorption and formation. Bone turnover is under the influence of general factors, including age and hormones, but is also locally modified by many factors such as physical forces.

## Osteoporosis

### Definition

Osteoporosis, by far the most common metabolic disease in western countries, is a systemic skeletal disease with quantitative abnormality of bone, whereas in rickets/osteomalacia there is qualitative abnormality of bone (Fig. 1). Osteoporosis is characterized by reduction in bone mass (amount of mineralized bone per unit volume) and by altered trabecular structure due to a loss of trabeculae interconnectivity with a consequent increase in bone fragility (decrease in biomechanical strength) and susceptibility to fracture (insufficiency fractures) [3] (Fig. 2).

### Prevalence of Osteoporosis

Osteoporosis is a serious public health problem for which, over the past 20 years, there have been significant advances in knowledge of its epidemiology, pathophysiology and treatment. In the western world, osteoporosis is reported to affect one in two women and one in five men over the age of 50 years [4]. The risk of fracture increases with advancing age and progressive loss of bone mass, and varies with the population being considered. The incidence of hip fracture has doubled over the past three decades and is predicted to continue to grow beyond what one would predict from increased longevity. After hip or vertebral fracture, mortality rate is about 20% greater than that expected. At 1 year after hip fracture, 40% patients are unable to walk independently, 60% have difficulty with one essential activity of life, 80% are restricted in other life activity, and 27% will have been admitted to a nursing home for the first time [4].

J. Hodler et al. (eds.), *Musculoskeletal Diseases 2013-2016*,
DOI: 10.1007/978-88-470-5292-5_14 © Springer-Verlag Italia 2013

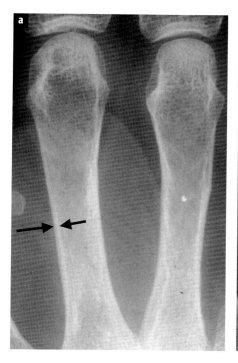 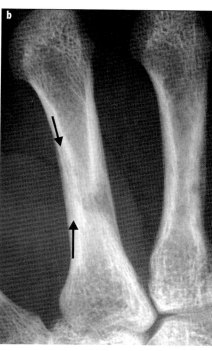

**Fig. 1 a, b.** Osteopenia and osteomalacia. **a** Osteopenia is characterized by quantitative bone abnormality with decreased bone density and cortical thinning (*arrows*). **b** Osteomalacia is characterized by qualitative bone abnormality with intracortical lucencies (*arrows*)

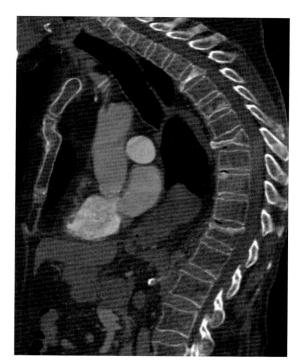

**Fig. 2.** Osteoporosis. Presence of multiple vertebral fractures with focal bone sclerosis superimposed on a background of hypertrophic osteoporosis. Note the sternal fracture associated with kyphosis

## Clinical Presentation and Etiology

Generalized osteoporosis is a chronic disease with late clinical consequence (low-energy insufficiency fractures) (Fig. 2). Vertebral fractures are the most commonly oc-

curring osteoporotic fracture. They occur as an acute event related to minor trauma or they occur spontaneously, and they can be accompanied by pain, which generally resolves spontaneously over 6-8 weeks. Vertebral fractures cause disability and limited spinal mobility and are associated within increased morbidity. They are powerful predictors of future fracture with a 12% increased risk of a future vertebral fracture within 12 months if a single vertebral fracture is present (22% increased risk in the presence of multiple fractures) [2]. Questionnaires are also available to evaluate fracture risk (FRAX). Consequently, the accurate identification and clear reporting of vertebral fracture by radiologists have vital roles to play in the diagnosis and appropriate management of patients with, or at risk of, osteoporosis. There is evidence that vertebral fractures are under-reported [European Society of Skeletal Radiology, Osteoporosis Group (ESSR.org); International Osteoporosis Foundation (www.osteofound.org)].

Generalized osteoporosis is the end-stage of several diseases and can be either primary or secondary (Boxes 1 and 2).

## Imaging Findings in Osteoporosis

Radiography is relatively insensitive in detecting early bone loss (less than 30-40% loss of bone tissue). In addition, radiographic bone density is affected by patient characteristics and radiographic factors used. The subjectivity of visual judgment of bone density on conventional radiographs supports the value of modern quantitative techniques such as bone densitometry.

The radiologic appearance of osteoporosis is essentially the same, irrespective of the cause (primary and sec-

**Box 1.** Causes of primary osteoporosis

- Idiopathic juvenile osteoporosis: self-limited (2- to 4-year duration) form of osteoporosis in pre-pubertal children. Acute course of the disease with growth arrest and fractures. Mild to severe forms. Differential diagnosis: osteogenesis imperfecta or other forms of juvenile osteoporosis, cortisolism and leukemia
- Post-menopausal (type I) osteoporosis: onset at the time of menopause but important bone loss during first 4 years after the menopause related to reduction in blood estrogen. Clinically significant in women 15-20 years after the menopause. Fractures in bones with high trabecular cortical ratio (vertebral bodies and distal forearm)
- Senile (type 2) osteoporosis: found in men and women 75 years or older and caused by age-related bone loss (age-related impaired bone formation associated with secondary hyperparathyroidism as a consequence of reduced calcium absorption from the intestine secondary to decreased production of the active metabolic vitamin D in the kidney). Reduction in both cortical and trabecular bone. Fractures in vertebrae but also in bones with low trabecular cortical ratio (tibia, humerus and pelvis)
- Osteogenesis imperfecta: congenital disorders due to gene mutation associated with osteoporosis of variable severity. Blue sclerae and occasional dental involvement

**Box 2.** Causes of secondary osteoporosis

- Endocrine: glucocorticoid excess, estrogen/testosterone deficiency, hyperthyroidism, hyperparathyroidism
- Nutritional: intestinal malabsorption, chronic alcoholism, chronic liver disease, partial gastrectomy, vitamin C deficiency
- Hereditary: homocystinuria, Marfan syndrome, Heler-Danlos syndrome
- Hematologic: sickle-cell disease, thalassemia, Gaucher disease, multiple myeloma
- Others: rheumatoid arthritis, hemochromatosis, long-term heparin therapy

ondary osteoporosis). The main radiographic features of generalized osteoporosis are decreased bone density and cortical thinning (Fig. 3). A decrease in radiographic bone density, in the absence of fractures, is termed osteopenia. It is caused by resorption and thinning of trabeculae. The process initially affects secondary (parallel to biomechanical forces) trabeculae; the primary (perpendicular to biomechanical forces) trabeculae can appear more prominent as they are affected at a later stage.

Cortical thinning occurs as a result of endosteal, periosteal or intracortical (cortical tunneling) bone resorption. Endosteal resorption is the least specific radiographic finding because it may be evident in metabolic disorders, including osteoporosis, and also in bone marrow

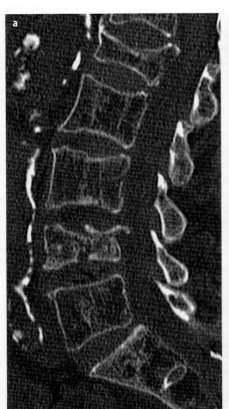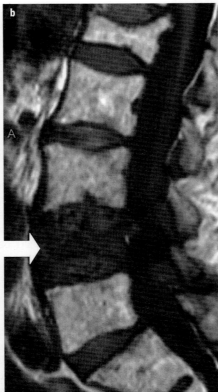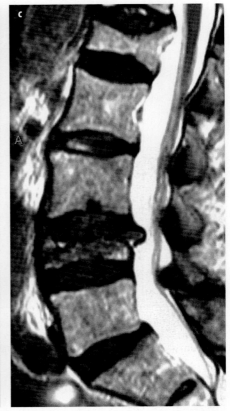

**Fig. 3 a-c.** Severe osteoporosis and vertebral fractures. **a** Sagittal computed tomography reformat of the lumbar spine shows reduced trabecular bone density and fractures. **b** Corresponding sagittal T1-weighted spin-echo image shows normal bone marrow except in a recent vertebral fracture (*arrow*). Altered trabecular bone pattern is not visible on a routine magnetic resonance image. **c** Corresponding sagittal SE T2-weighted spin-echo image shows intermediate to low signal intensity in recent L4 vertebral fracture

## Measurement of Osteoporosis

Several methods have been used to standardize measurements of cortical thickness (radiogrametry), trabecular pattern (Singh index) and vertebral deformity (morphometry) from radiographs (Box 3). None of these techniques is used currently because they lack accuracy and precision. Several quantitative techniques, including dual energy X-ray absorptiometry (DXA), quantitative computed tomography (QCT) and quantitative ultrasonography (QUS), have been developed to enable accurate and precise assessment of mineral bone density [2].

## Rickets and Osteomalacia

Rickets and osteomalacia are similar metabolic bone disorders characterized by inadequate or delayed mineralization of osteoid in cortical bone and trabecular bone in children and in adults, respectively [5].

Pseudofracture or Looser's zone is the radiological hallmark of osteomalacia, as it represents cortical fracture without a mineralized callus. Looser's zone corresponds to a linear cortical lucency frequently perpendicular to the cortex of the bone without periosteal reaction (Fig. 4). It typically involves the ribs, the superior and inferior pubic rami, and the inner margins of the proximal femora or lateral margin of the scapula. Widened physeal growth plate and metaphyseal cupping and fraying are the radiological signs of rickets that are best seen at rapidly growing ends of bone, such as distal femur and radius or anterior ends of ribs. Additional radiological findings of rickets/osteomalacia include bone deformities, osteopenia or a coarsened pattern of the cancellous bone [5].

There is no magnetic resonance (MR) hallmark of osteomalacia, but the presence of multiple trabecular bone

disorders. Intracortical tunneling is more specific, occurring mainly in disorders with rapid bone turnover such as diffuse osteoporosis and reflex sympathetic osteodystrophy. Subperiosteal resorption is the most specific finding, and is diagnostic of hyperparathyroidism.

Osteoporosis remains occult on magnetic resonance imaging (MRI) (Fig. 3), although a relationship between trabecular bone density and marrow fat has been reported. The presence of multiple vertebral fractures with different ages (increased amount of fat in old fractures, and marrow edema or infiltration in recent fractures) suggests increased bone fragility and, hence, osteoporosis.

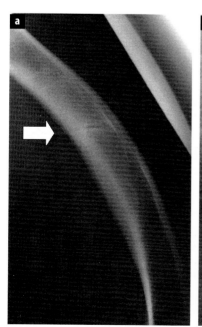 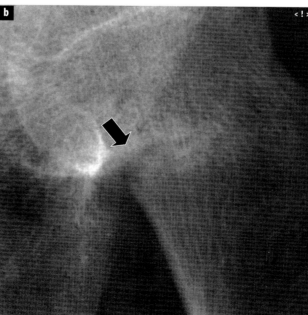

**Fig. 4 a, b.** Osteomalacia. **a** Lateral radiograph of a femur demonstrates bone deformity with anterior bowing of the femoral shaft and cortical fracture (*arrow*). **b** Close-up radiograph of another patient with osteomalacia demonstrates pseudofracture or Looser's zone with cortical discontinuity and bone resorption (*arrow*)

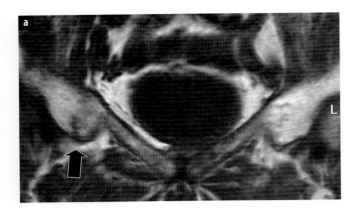
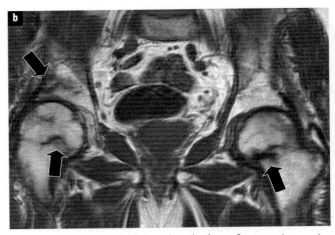

**Fig. 5.** Coronal T1-weighted image of the pelvis of a patient with osteomalacia demonstrates multiple trabecular bone fractures (*arrows*)

fractures with variable appearance at MRI (variable signal intensity on T2-weighted spin-echo images that are probably due to the various ages of the fractures) in a background of normal bone marrow should suggest the disease [6, 7] (Fig. 5). Fractures in osteomalacia can show a nonspecific bone marrow edema pattern or a more linear pattern with an occasional double line sign (probably due to the lack of adjacent edema). These fractures generally remain unchanged at short-term follow-up MRI, as osteomalacia is a disease in which the healing process is deficient. Typical cortical bone fractures or Looser's zones are barely visible at MRI as the cortical lesion is barely visible and the adjacent marrow and soft tissue changes are discrete due to the chronicity of the lesion.

### Renal Osteodystrophy and Hyperparathyroidism

The term renal osteodystrophy relates to all musculoskeletal manifestations of chronic renal failure [5]. Traditionally, renal osteodystrophy encompassed secondary hyperparathyroidism, osteomalacia, osteoporosis and soft tissue calcification. In fact, hyperparathyroidism and rickets or osteomalacia are the major pathologic processes of renal osteodystrophy. Primary hyperparathyroidism (generally related to the presence of a solitary adenoma in the parathyroid gland) and the classic radiographic changes of hyperparathyroidism are largely historical because diagnosis and treatment are based on serum calcium and parathyroid homone levels.

The radiographic signs of hyperparathyroidism that can appear in a patient with chronic renal failure (as in primary hyperparathyroidism) are phalangeal resorption in the hands and/or exclusive phalangeal tuft resorption (Fig. 6). The hands are the earliest and most sensitive sites for detection of hyperparathyroidism (other sites include the end of the clavicle, sacroiliac joint, and other periosteal surfaces, such as the proximal humeri or proximal femora).

Osteoclastoma or brown tumors occur in renal osteodystrophy and, in fact, are encountered more frequently

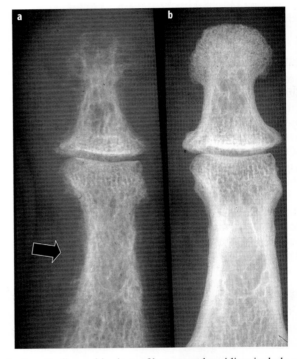

**Fig. 6 a, b. a** Radiographic signs of hyperparathyroidism include subperiosteal bone (*arrow*) and phalangeal tuft resorption. **b** After successful treatment, there is reappearance of woven (primary) bone

than in primary hyperparathyroidism, which is a rare condition. In the presence of brown tumors, there will almost always be phalangeal signs of hyperparathyroidism. Osteosclerosis can also be encountered in renal osteodystrophy. It is commonly appreciated in vertebrae, pelvis, ribs and metaphyses of long tubular bones. In vertebrae, sclerosis is frequently confined to the endplates, producing a characteristic appearance of alternating bands of different density (the so-called rugger jersey spine).

Marginal erosions at the periphery of articular surfaces in the peripheral joints have been reported with variable incidence. There are usually minor erosions that progress slowly and are not associated with loss of joint space.

Soft tissue calcifications can develop anywhere, in the vessels and also in the muscular or tendinous structures. Massive amorphous calcification can develop in the soft tissue around articulations and probably reflects poorly controlled renal osteodystrophy. Presence of chondrocalcinosis (knees and wrists) in patient younger than 50 years of age should indicate the possibility of a hypercalcemic state, but it should be kept in mind that hemochromatosis can also present with osteoporosis and chondrocalcinosis.

In mild hyperparathyroidism and renal osteodystrophy, DXA can appear normal because it assesses the amount of trabecular bone. The most reliable site for measuring bone loss in primary hyperparathyroidism is the distal part of the forearm, which contains proportionately a large content of cortical bone (bone loss in hyperparathyroidism predominantly involves the outer compact bone).

## Insufficiency Stress Fractures

### Definitions of Bone Fractures

Fractures can be classified according to the bone status before the fracture and the applied forces (Table 1). Traumatic fracture occurs as a response to an acute increase in biomechanical stress on normal bone. Fatigue fractures occur in response to a chronic repetitive increase in biomechanical stresses on normal bone. Insufficiency fracture occurs as a response to normal or slightly increased stress on diffusely weakened bones.

Medical imaging plays a crucial role in the diagnosis of insufficiency and pathological fractures because both lack a clinical history suggestive of these types of fracture [8-10]. Insufficiency stress fracture (ISF) of the cortical bone (femur, tibia, metatarsal bones) generally occurs in response to compression or traction stresses. ISF of the trabecular bone (vertebral body, long bone metaphysis, tarsal bone) generally occurs in response to compressive forces.

**Table 1.** Classification of bone fractures

| Type of fracture | Bone status | Applied forces | Clinical clues |
|---|---|---|---|
| Traumatic fracture | Normal | Increased | History |
| Fatigue fracture | Normal | Increased | History |
| Insufficiency fracture | Diffuse weakening | Normal | None |
| Pathological fracture | Focal weakening | Normal | None |

### Radiographic Findings in ISF

The spectrum of radiographic findings in ISF depends on the cortical/trabecular bone ratio of the involved bone and on the age of the fracture (Table 2). The radiological diagnosis of ISF is difficult both at an early stage (limit-ed alterations) and at a late stage (predominant healing-related changes).

ISF of trabecular bone is barely seen on radiographs because of the lack of visibility of trabecular bone interruption and of significant bone deformation. At a later stage, radiographs display trabecular bone sclerosis that is typically linear and perpendicular to the dominant trabeculae.

ISF of cortical bone can be recognized on plain films at an early stage if there is cortical bone discontinuity or bone deformity. After a few weeks, fractures become more obvious because of focal periosteal reactions, although the cortical discontinuity can be subtle.

**Table 2.** Radiologic appearance of trabecular and cortical insufficiency stress fractures

| Radiograph/CT | Acute ISF | Chronic ISF | Healed ISF |
|---|---|---|---|
| Trabecular bone | Normal | Mild sclerosis | Normal |
| Cortical bone | Cortical interruption | Periosteal reaction | Cortical thickening |

*CT* computed tomography, *ISF* insufficiency stress fracture

### MRI Findings in ISF

MR features of trabecular ISF include marrow edema or infiltration and intramedullary low signal intensity bands (impaction fractures) (Table 3). Marrow edema or infiltration could represent early marrow changes in response to increased biomechanical stress. Low signal intensity bands add specificity when present, because marrow infiltration or edema lacks specificity. Low signal intensity bands are best detected on T2-weighted spin-echo (SE), fat-saturated intermediate- or enhanced T1-weighted SE images (in an unpredictable manner). Some features may be subtle with respect to marrow changes and include altered bone shape, cortical interruption and periosteal reaction.

MR features of cortical ISF are misleading because of the lack of obvious cortical bone fracture. Extensive infiltration of the adjacent medullary cavity or of the adjacent soft tissue can be misleading.

A bone scan is useful to exclude the possibility of a fracture. It is sensitive for the detection of ISF but generally lacks specificity.

**Table 3.** Magnetic resonance appearance of trabecular and cortical insufficiency stress fractures

| MRI | Acute ISF | Chronic ISF | Healed ISF |
|---|---|---|---|
| Trabecular bone | Extensive edema | Band, edema | Normal |
| Cortical bone | Subtle marrow and soft tissue edema | Subtle marrow and soft tissue edema; periosteal callus | Normal |

*ISF* insufficiency stress fracture, *MRI* magnetic resonance imaging

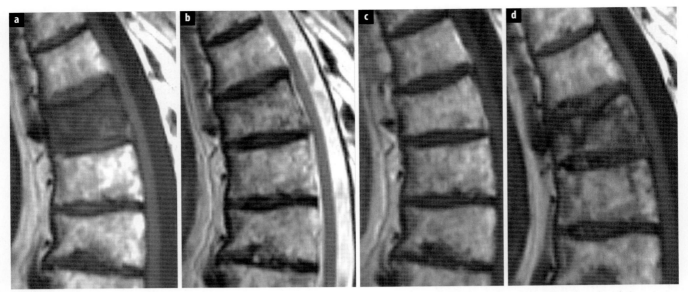

**Fig. 7 a-d.** Spontaneous insufficiency stress fractures of a thoracic vertebral body. **a** T1-weighted image of the thoracic spine demonstrates a vertebral body with decreased signal intensity. Corresponding T2-weighted (**b**) and enhanced T1-weighted (**c**) spin-echo (SE) images demonstrate a return to normal signal intensity, suggestive of a benign fracture. **d** Follow-up T1-weighted SE image obtained 2 months later demonstrates partial and spontaneous regression of the lesion with appearance of intravertebral bands of low signal intensity

## Common ISFs

### ISF of the Vertebral Body

Vertebral fractures are the most common osteoporotic fractures. The anterior and central midportion of the vertebrae withstand compression forces less well than the posterior and outer ring element of the vertebrae, resulting in wedge or endplate fractures or, less commonly, crush fractures. A good radiographic technique is required when imaging the spine, particularly in the lateral projection. The spine must be parallel to the radiographic table to prevent the vertebrae appearing to have an apparent biconcave endplate, which is a an artefact caused by tilting of the vertebrae or the divergence of the X-ray beam (beam cam effect). Scheuermann's disease also causes vertebral body deformities. Endplate irregularity, most commonly in the thoracic spine, involving several adjacent vertebrae generally enables the differentiation between vertebral fracture and growth-related bone deformities.

Typically, spinal ISF involves one or several vertebral bodies of the thoracolumbar junction and is not observed above the T4 level. Anterior wedge-shaped deformity is the most frequent pattern. There is extensive bone marrow edema on MRI that generally spares the posterior arch and the vertebral body opposite to the fracture vertebral end plate (differential diagnosis from disc-related marrow changes) (Fig. 7). The low signal bands are parallel to and located a few millimeters from the involved vertebral end plate.

### ISFs of the Pelvic Bones

ISFs of the pelvic ring involve pubic and ischiatic rami, supraacetabular area and lateral aspects of sacrum. There is an increased prevalence of these lesions in patients who have had previous radiation therapy (importance of differential diagnosis with metastases). Radiographs are rarely diagnostic except in pubic bones (cortical fracture). Computed tomography (CT) can contribute to the diagnosis by demonstrating cortical interruption or callus formation in trabecular bone (sacrum) [11]. MRI is the best imaging modality for sacral and supra-acetabular fractures. Pubic bone fractures are more difficult to recognize, but adjacent muscle infiltration on STIR images is suggestive.

### ISF of the Femoral Neck

Early recognition of femoral neck ISF is extremely important because of possible progression to displaced femoral neck fracture (if cortex is involved). Plain films obtained early might reveal cortical interruption with subtle periosteal reaction, but remain generally normal in trabecular bone fractures. MRI better displays associated marrow edema with intramedullary low signal intensity bands (Fig. 8).

### ISFs of the Tarsal Bones

Lower extremity ISF is frequent and involves the greater tuberosity of the calcaneus, the talar dome and neck, and the cuboid bone. Radiographs are generally normal (no deformity) except in calcaneum (callus formation). MRI

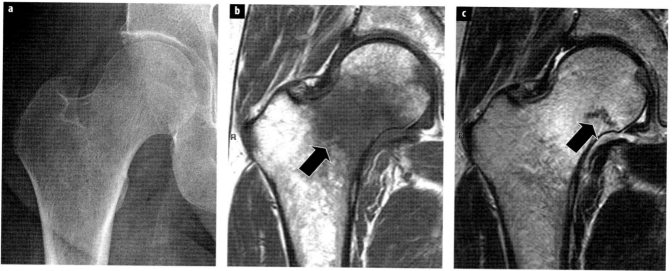

**Fig. 8 a-c.** Spontaneous femoral neck fracture in a patient with osteoporosis. **a** Normal radiograph. **b** Coronal spin-echo (SE) T1-weighted image with abnormal signal in femoral neck (*arrow*). **c** Coronal SE T2-weighted image shows marrow edema surrounding a low signal intensity line (*arrow*) suggestive of a trabecular bone fracture

is diagnostic, but confusion with acute reflex sympathetic dystrophy syndrome is possible. Bone scintigraphy may contribute to their recognition.

## Uncommon ISFs

Uncommon ISF can be related to characteristics intrinsic to the lesion (unusual topography or shape) or to patient characteristics (abnormal healing process).

### Uncommon ISF Appearance due to Unusual Topography or Shape

#### Epiphyseal Insufficiency Fractures

ISF can involve convex weightbearing epiphyses such as the femoral head, femoral condyles [12] and metatarsal heads [13] (Fig. 9). Radiographs are generally normal but may show subtle subchondral sclerosis. MRI shows extensive marrow edema and low signal intensity bands located a few millimeters from the subchondral bone plate, which is generally not deformed.

Until the early 1990s, epiphyseal ISF remained underdiagnosed and epiphyseal osteonecrosis was the unique epiphyseal condition associated with metabolic bone disorders. The concept of transient epiphyseal bone lesions corresponding presumably to fractures emerged progressively and is now widely accepted [9]. There is also general agreement on the fact that some patterns of epiphyseal osteonecrosis, such as spontaneous osteonecrosis of the medial condyles, represent irreversible fracture or pseudoarthrosis rather than primary ischemic osteonecrosis [10, 12].

#### Longitudinal Stress Fractures

Cortical ISFs are generally perpendicular to the cortical shaft. Rarely, longitudinal ISFs develop in the tibia but

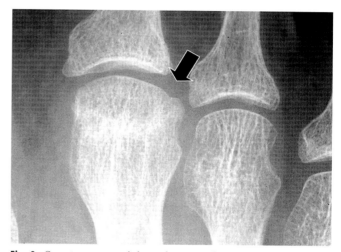

**Fig. 9.** Spontaneous epiphyseal stress fracture of the second metatarsal head. Radiograph shows mild flattening and deformity of the epiphyseal contour (*arrow*) with linear sclerosis of the metatarsal head

also in the femur or metatarsal bones [14, 15]. Cortical interruption is difficult to detect because it is parallel to the longitudinal axis of the bone. Axial CT images are important for the recognition of the cortical discontinuity (importance of bone settings window) [14]. The lesion may be confused with infection or tumor at MRI because of the longitudinal extent of marrow infiltration [15] (Fig. 10).

### Uncommon ISF Appearance due to Abnormal Healing Process

The healing process can be altered by various mechanisms (Box 4) that cause unusual features at imaging (Box 5). An imbalance in favor of bone destruction over

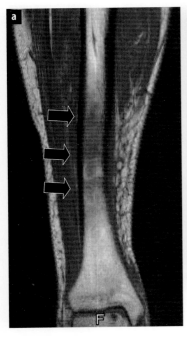

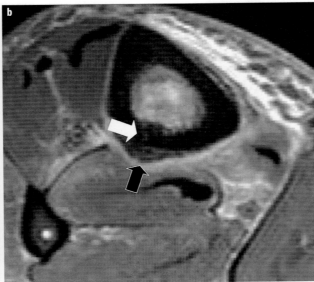

**Fig. 10 a, b.** Longitudinal insufficiency fracture of the tibia. **a** Coronal T1-weighted image demonstrates marrow infiltration in the distal third of the tibia (*arrows*). **b** Transverse fat-saturated proton density weighted image demonstrates marrow and soft tissue infiltration. Cortical discontinuity (*white arrow*) is barely visible. Periosteal (*black arrow*) and endosteal bone formation is visible

bone reconstruction is observed in fractures that are submitted to repetitive persistent stress due to reduced pain sensitivity (e.g., pelvic ring fractures in patients with steroids) or in bones with altered metabolism (e.g., after radiation therapy) [16] (Fig. 11).

---

**Box 4.** Causes of abnormal healing process

- Local causes: distraction stress (scaphoid); persistent mechanical stress due to topography of the lesions (pubis, epiphysis, rib) or altered threshold of pain (steroid, alcohol, neuropathy)
- Regional causes: radiation therapy, vascular disorders
- Diffuse causes: metabolic bone disease (osteomalacia, steroid or fluor therapy)

---

**Box 5.** Unusual features of insufficiency stress fracture related to altered healing process

- Increased amount of bone destruction (pubis bone, epiphysis, rib)
- Increased amount of callus formation
- Increased number of fractures (steroids, osteomalacia)

---

An imbalance in favor of bone sclerosis can be observed in chronic ISF in patients with steroids. Patients on steroid therapy can show a spectrum of changes that include a large number of spontaneous fractures with hypertrophic callus formation and unusual persistence of the lesions over time (Fig. 12) [17]. At MRI, ISFs show a wide spectrum of changes that range from marrow infiltration to focal lipomatosis in association with hypertrophic callus formation. Patients on long-term bisphosphonate therapy can show unusual fractures of the femurs that should be recognized [18].

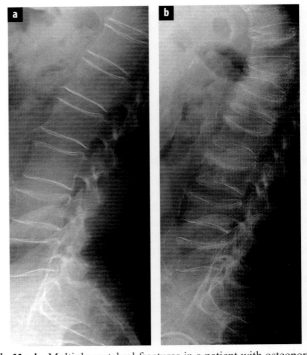

**Fig. 11 a, b.** Multiple vertebral fractures in a patient with osteoporosis and long-term steroid therapy. **a** Initial lumbar spine radiograph demonstrates osteoporosis with L4 fracture. **b** Same radiograph obtained 1 year later after an increase in steroid dosage demonstrates appearance of multiple fractures and trabecular bone sclerosis

## Take-Home Points

1. Metabolic disorders of the skeleton involve the mineralized components of the skeleton. Metabolic bone alterations can be depicted on radiographs and CT

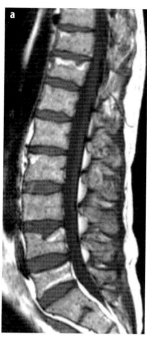 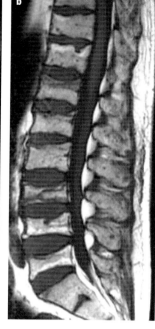 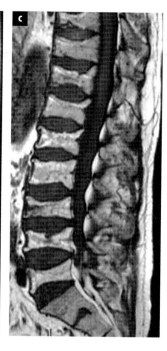

**Fig. 12 a-c.** Patient with multiple myeloma and chronic steroid treament. **a** Initial T1-weighted magnetic resonance image obtained during treatment demonstrates multiple areas of increased signal intensity (similar to Modic II changes) in vertebrae with abnormal shape but without disc disease. **b** Eight months later, there is appearance of multiple fractures and bands of low signal intensity. **c** Eighteen months later, there is partial regression of focal marrow changes. Steroid-related vertebral fractures often show a very slow pace of changes over time

images but remain occult on MR images because the bone marrow is spared in the vast majority of these disorders.

2. Metabolic disorders of the skeleton affect all bone components histologically, but involvement patterns may vary depending on the age of the patient (growing versus adult skeleton) as well as the type of bone (cortical versus trabecular bone). The importance of cortical and trabecular bone in each individual bone (high trabecular/cortical ratio in vertebral bodies, ribs and pelvis; low trabecular/cortical ratio in long bones and extremities) can influence the radiographic patterns of metabolic bone diseases.

3. Medical imaging (X-ray, CT, bone scintigraphy and MRI) plays a limited role in the detection and quantification of osteoporosis. Medical imaging contributes to the work-up of symptomatic patients with suspected fractures and occasionally contributes to the detection of patients at risk of vertebral fracture (old vertebral fractures). Accurate reporting of vertebral fracture is important.

4. A wide spectrum of marrow changes seen at MRI have been observed in insufficiency stress fractures. Bone marrow edema or infiltration is the most prominent feature of insufficiency fractures of the trabecular bone at MRI and the presence of low signal intensity bands (best seen on T2-weighted, fat saturated intermediate-, or enhanced T1-weighted images) adds specificity. In insufficiency stress fractures of the cortical bone, cortical discontinuity is best appreciated on CT images than on MR images. Bone marrow and adjacent soft tissue edema or infiltration is a subtle but occasionally misleading feature in cortical fractures.

5. Uncommon ISF can be related to characteristics intrinsic to the lesion (unusual topography or shape) or to patient characteristics (abnormal healing process because of persistent mobility, radiation therapy or osteomalacia and steroid therapy).

## References

1. Resnik D (1988) Diagnosis of bone and joint disorders. 4th volume, 2nd edn. WB Saunders, Philadelphia, pp 1983-1987; 2096-2099
2. Adams J (2008) Osteoporosis. In: Pope TL, Bloem HL, Beltran J et al (Eds) Imaging of the musculoskeletal system, 1st edn. WB Saunders, Philadelphia, pp 1489-1508
3. Bouxsein ML, Karasik D (2006) Bone geometry and skeletal fragility. Curr Osteoporosis Rep 4:49-56
4. Sambrook P, Cooper C (2006) Osteoporosis. Lancet 367:2010-2018
5. Sundaram M, Schils J (2008) Hyperparathyroidism, renal osteodystrophy, osteomalacia and rickets. In: Pope TL, Bloem HL, Beltran J et al (Eds) Imaging of the musculoskeletal system, 1st edn. WB Saunders, Philadelphia, pp 1509-1523
6. Kanberoglu K, Kantarci F, Cebi D et al (2005) Magnetic resonance imaging in osteomalacic insufficiency fractures of the pelvis. Clin Radiol 601:105-111
7. Ohashi K, Ohnishi T, Ishikawa T et al (1999) Oncogenic osteomalacia presenting as bilateral stress fractures of the tibia. Skeletal Radiol 28:46-48
8. Soubrier M, Dubost JJ, Boisgard S (2003) Insufficiency fracture. A survey of 60 cases and review of the literature. Joint Bone Spine 70:209-218
9. Vande Berg BC, Malghem J, Goffin EJ et al (1994) Transient epiphyseal lesions in renal transplant recipients: presumed insufficiency stress fractures. Radiology 1994 191:403-407
10. Vande Berg BC, Malghem J, Lecouvet FE, Maldague B (2001) Magnetic resonance imaging and differential diagnosis of epiphyseal osteonecrosis. Semin Musculoskelet Radiol. 5:57-67

11. Cabarrus MC, Ambekar A, Lu Y, Link TM (2008) MRI and CT of insufficiency fractures of the pelvis and the proximal femur. AJR Am J Roentgenol 191:995-1001

12. Lecouvet FE, Malghem J, Maldague BE, Vande Berg BC (2005) MR imaging of epiphyseal lesions of the knee: current concepts, challenges, and controversies. Radiol Clin North Am 43:655-672

13. Torriani M, Thomas BJ, Bredella MA, Ouellette H (2008) MRI of metatarsal head subchondral fractures in patients with fore-foot pain. AJR Am J Roentgenol 190:570-575

14. Feydy A, Drapé J, Beret E et al (1998) Longitudinal stress frac-tures of the tibia: comparative study of CT and MR imaging. Eur Radiol 8:598-602

15. Craig JG, Widman D, van Holsbeeck M (2003) Longitudinal stress fracture: patterns of edema and the importance of the nutrient foramen. Skeletal Radiol 32:22-27

16. Kwon JW, Huh SJ, Yoon YC et al (2008) Pelvic bone compli-cations after radiation therapy of uterine cervical cancer: eval-uation with MRI. AJR Am J Roentgenol 1914:987-994

17. Sidhu HS, Venkatanarasimha N, Bhatnagar G et al (2012) Imaging features of therapeutic drug-induced musculoskeletal abnormalities. Radiographics 32:105-127

18. Haworth AE, Webb J (2012) Skeletal complications of bispho-sphonate use: what the radiologist should know. Br J Radiol 85:1333-1342

# Spine Trauma

John A. Carrino[1], Murray K. Dalinka[2]

[1] Russell H. Morgan Department of Radiology and Radiological Science, Johns Hopkins Hospital, Baltimore, MD, USA
[2] Department of Musculoskeletal Radiology, Hospital of the University of Pennsylvania, Philadelphia, PA, USA

## Introduction

Spine trauma is not uncommon and can have devastating consequences if misdiagnosed. Most injuries are secondary to blunt trauma (motor vehicle accidents, falls, sports injuries), although penetrating trauma accounts for a substantial minority of cases. Spinal fractures represent 3-6% of all skeletal injuries. Spinal injuries can produce a neurologic deficit, sometimes severe or fatal. Spine trauma is a complex diagnostic area in which the imaging assessment is crucial. The overall goal of initial spine imaging is to detect potentially unstable fractures, to enable immobilization and/or stabilization, and prevent development and/or progression of neurological injury. Spinal injury can be divided into the segment of the spine that is affected: craniocervical, subaxial cervical or thoracolumbar. Injuries within these regions of the spine can be further subdivided based upon the mechanism of injury. Imaging examinations may be performed to inform prognosis and guide surgical intervention, particularly for unstable injuries. Radiography, computed tomography (CT) and magnetic resonance (MR) imaging are all applied to the traumatized patient depending on the circumstance. Pediatric and geriatric populations have some unique considerations. Underlying musculoskeletal disorders such as spondyloarthropathy or osteoporosis can affect the nature and pattern of spinal injuries.

## Classification

Spinal injuries frequently are subdivided into stable and unstable categories. An unstable spinal injury is one in which the mechanically unstable spine moves and undergoes potentially deleterious deformation in response to physiologic loading and a normal range of movement. The determination of spinal stability remains an important task, as treatment strategies rely heavily on this assessment. This determination remains challenging and continues to evolve. When a traumatic lesion is deemed unstable,

the patient's prognosis is less favorable, and treatment tends to be more aggressive. Stability is provided by intact osseous and ligamentous structures. Classification of injuries into stable and unstable categories depends on an understanding of which of these structures is injured and imaging provides important information. Ideally imaging of spine instability relies on both static anatomic imaging and functional assessment of spine motion. Numerous classification systems have been proposed.

White and Panjabi proposed a checklist point system to assess spinal stability (cervical, thoracic and lumbar) that remains one of the best recognized systems to date. This system uses a point system based on a combination of radiographic findings, neurologic examination and anticipated biomechanical demands of the patient [1]. Radiographic stability of the cervical spine is best assessed with a functional examination that includes flexion and extension views. Such an examination, however, should be reserved for alert, cooperative patients with a normal neurologic examination and without radiographic evidence of injuries that are almost certainly unstable. Because of pain and muscle spasm present at the time of acute injury, patient motion is often limited. As such, delayed flexion and extension views (obtained 7-10 days following the injury) may be more informative. In the acute setting, the theoretical risk of radiographically occult unstable ligamentous injury in subjects who are unexaminable due to head injury has led to a variety of imaging approaches using magnetic resonance imaging (MRI), and/or fluoroscopy; there is insufficient evidence to support any particular approach. However, a normal CT scan of the cervical spine in obtunded and/or "unreliable" patients with blunt trauma does exclude unstable injuries [2].

Denis proposed that spinal integrity depended on the three-column system (anterior, middle and posterior) and used it to describe thoracolumbar fractures [3]. The anterior column is defined as containing the anterior longitudinal ligament, the anterior half of the vertebral body, and the related portion of the intervertebral disc and its anulus

J. Hodler et al. (eds.), *Musculoskeletal Diseases 2013-2016*,
DOI: 10.1007/978-88-470-5292-5_15 © Springer-Verlag Italia 2013

fibrosus. The middle column contains the posterior longitudinal ligament, the posterior half of the vertebral body, and the intervertebral disc and its annulus fibrosus. The posterior column contains the osseous elements of the posterior neural arch and the ligamentous elements, which include the flavum, interspinous and supraspinous ligaments. The joint capsule of the intervertebral articulations is also part of the posterior column. When only one column is disrupted, the injury is considered mechanically stable. When two columns are disrupted, the injury is considered unstable. In general, this requires failure of the middle column with either the anterior or the posterior column. Imaging signs of instability include widening of the interspinous and interlaminar distance, >2 mm translation, >20 degrees of kyphosis, dislocation, >50% height loss, and articular process fractures. However, fractures may be unstable in the absence of these signs. Unrecognized supraspinous ligament disruption contributes to this instability.

Fractures of the spine can be classified based on the pattern of injury and the forces involved reflecting the mechanical mode of failure [4]:

- Flexion-compression mechanism (wedge or compression fracture): anterior column is compressed sparing the middle and posterior column.
- Axial-compression mechanism (burst fracture): most commonly found at the thoracolumbar junction characterized by a loss of height of the vertebral body. The fracture implicates the anterior and middle columns and thus is considered an unstable lesion.
- Flexion-distraction mechanism (Chance fractures): the posterior column is involved with injury to ligamentous components, bony components or both. Chance fractures are often associated with intra-abdominal injuries. The pathophysiology depends on the axis of flexion and several subtypes exist.
- Rotational fracture-dislocation mechanism: The resultant injury pattern is failure of both the posterior and middle columns with varying degrees of anterior column insult.

The majority of the classification systems currently in use in clinical practice are primarily descriptive and are based on presumed injury mechanisms. A spinal injury classification system should be clinically relevant, reliable and accurate [5]. Along these lines, new classification systems have been proposed by Patel et al., who based the system on three injury characteristics [6, 7]. These new classifications put greater focus on the posterior ligamentous complex and its integrity rather than on the middle column, and take into account the morphology of the injury and the clinical neurologic status of the patient, with each category being assigned points related to the severity of the findings. When combined, the clinical and radiologic findings generate a numeric score that can help predict the need for surgical intervention. These are known as the subaxial cervical spine injury classification system (SLIC) and thoracolumbar injury classification and severity score (TLICS).

## Cervical Spine

The imaging evaluation of adult patients following acute injury to the cervical spine has undergone major changes over the past 10-15 years. In the not so distant past, patients with even trivial trauma and minimum if any symptoms were subject to radiographic examinations of the cervical spine consisting of between three and seven views. In patients with severe injuries, the examinations were usually acquired with portable images beginning with a cross-table lateral view; occasionally this was the only radiograph obtained acutely. There was considerable controversy concerning the limitation of the cross-table lateral view and papers were written describing whether a three or five view portable study should be performed in acutely injured patients. When CT became available it was often utilized as a supplement to the radiographs to "clear" the cervical spine.

The issue of which patients require CT in addition to radiography is the subject of many good studies that created decision rules based upon clinical criteria and cost-benefit analysis [8]. Patients with a (potential) cervical spine injury can be subdivided into low-risk and high-risk patients. Cervical spine imaging is not necessary in subjects with all five of the following NEXUS (National Emergency X-Radiography Utilization Study) criteria [9]: (1) absence of posterior midline tenderness, (2) absence of focal neurological deficit, (3) normal level of alertness, (4) no evidence of intoxication, and (5) absence of painful distracting injury. CT scan of the cervical spine is cost-effective as the initial imaging strategy in subjects at high probability of fracture (neurological deficit, head injury, high energy mechanism) who are already to undergo head CT. However, no adequate data exist on the appropriate cervical spine evaluation in subjects who are unexaminable due to head injury.

Cervical spine CT is more sensitive than radiography, and more specific in subjects at high risk of fracture [10]. CT has higher direct costs than radiography. However, CT is cost-effective, and may actually be cost-saving from the societal perspective in subjects at high probability of fracture. Cost savings with CT are from a decreased number of second imaging examinations resulting from inadequate radiograph studies, and from the high cost in dollars and health for the rare fracture missed from radiography that leads to severe neurological deficit. A retrospective comparative effectiveness analysis supports that CT alone is sufficient to detect unstable cervical spine injuries in trauma patients. Adjuvant imaging is unnecessary when the CT scan is negative for acute injury. Results of meta-analysis strongly show that the cervical collar may be removed from obtunded or intubated trauma patients if a CT scan is negative for acute injury [11]. Another review concluded that it remains acceptable for clinicians to "clear" the spine of obtunded blunt trauma patients using CT alone or CT followed by MRI, with implications to either approach [12]. MRI following "normal" CT may detect up to 7.5% missed injuries with an operative fixation in 0.29% but with prolonged collar application in an additional 4.3%.

Whiplash injury is associated with chronic impairment in a substantial number of patients. High-resolution craniocervical MRI in symptomatic chronic whiplash syndrome shows structural changes (high-grade lesions felt to represent tears or partial tears) in the soft tissues, particularly the alar ligaments not present in controls, with correlation between clinical impairment and morphologic findings and certain lesions to specific structures could be linked with specific trauma mechanisms [13]. However, in acute whiplash-associated injury, bone and muscle injuries, occult vertebral body fracture, marrow contusion, strain, tear, or hematoma of muscle and perimuscular fluid are rarely evident [14].

The spectrum of cervical spine injuries with associated characteristics and imaging features are listed in Tables 1-7 categorized by mechanism, and detailed reviews are available [15]. When present, there is often multiple cervical spine fractures associated with a similar mechanism.

**Table 1.** Cervical spine: hyperflexion injuries

| Injury | Etiology | Characteristics | Imaging |
|---|---|---|---|
| Hyperflexion sprain (anterior subluxation) | • "Whiplash" | • Injury to PLC <br> • Posterior anulus fibrosis may also be disrupted <br> • 50% show delayed instability | • Radiography: abrupt focal kyphosis at injury level <br> • MRI: increased T2 signal in PLC and posterior anulus injury |
| Bilateral interfacetal dislocation (BID) | • Disruption of anterior longitudinal ligament, posterior longitudinal ligament, intervertebral disc and PLC | • Unstable with high risk of cord injury damage <br> • "Bilateral locked facets" <br> • Generally within low cervical spine | • Radiography: ≥50% anterior subluxation of vertebral body in complete dislocation; bilateral perched facets in partial facet joint displacement <br> • CT: detects subtle fractures; "inverted hamburger sign" of facet dislocation |
| Simple wedge compression | • Compressive forces affecting anterior superior endplate of vertebral body | • Anterior longitudinal ligament and disc intact <br> • Deformity of anterior superior endplate of affected vertebrae | • Radiography: loss of vertebral height; impacted superior endplate; angulated anterior cortical margin of vertebral body |
| Clay shoveler's fracture | • Forced flexion of head and upper cervical spine <br> • Downward traction on spinous processes by muscular attachments to scapulae while arms perform forceful lifting | • Avulsion fracture of C6, C7 or T1 spinous process <br> • Stable due to intact PLC <br> • Mimicked by unfused apophysis | • Radiography: shows avulsion fracture fragments |
| Flexion teardrop fracture | • Severe flexion with disruption of all ligaments and their stability | • Unstable: worst cervical spine injury compatible with life <br> • Comminuted anterior inferior vertebral body fracture with triangular fragment <br> • Posterior vertebral body retropulses into spinal cord with resultant injury to spinal cord (many patients present with acute anterior cord syndrome) | • Radiography: visualize kyphosis, "teardrop" fragment, retropulsed bone and significant prevertebral soft tissue swelling |

*CT* computed tomography, *MRI* magnetic resonance imaging, *PLC* posterior ligament complex

**Table 2.** Cervical spine: hyperflexion injuries with rotation

| Injury | Etiology | Characteristics | Imaging |
|---|---|---|---|
| Unilateral interfacetal dislocation (UID) | • Mechanism similar to BID except accompanied by rotation | • Most common at C5-6 and C6-7 <br> • Dislocation on opposite side of rotation <br> • Disruption of PLC and articular joint capsule <br> • 70% with impaction fracture <br> • "Unilateral locked facet" when stable | • Radiography: "bowtie sign" <br> • CT: required to detect subtle fractures |

*BID* bilateral interfacetal dislocation, *CT* computed tomography, *PLC* posterior ligament complex

**Table 3.** Cervical spine: vertical compression (axial load) injuries

| Injury | Etiology | Characteristics | Imaging |
|---|---|---|---|
| Jefferson fracture | • Force to top of skull, transmitted through occipital condyles to cervical spine at instant spine is straight | • Stability dependent on status of transverse ligament<br>• Ring of C1 fractured anteriorly and posteriorly<br>• Uni- or bilateral fractures<br>• 50% associated with C2 fracture | • Radiography: displacement of lateral C1 borders off C2 superior articular facet in odontoid view<br>• CT: multiple disruptions of atlas ring |
| Burst fracture | • Nucleus pulposus protrudes into vertebral body causing vertebral body rupture | • Common at C3-7 levels, usually involving cord injury | • Radiography: vertical fracture line best seen on AP view<br>• CT: evaluate fracture fragments<br>• MRI: evaluate cord, disc, and ligaments |

*AP* anteroposterior, *CT* computed tomography, *MRI* magnetic resonance imaging

**Table 4.** Cervical spine: hyperextension injuries

| Injury | Etiology | Characteristics | Imaging |
|---|---|---|---|
| Hangman's fracture ("traumatic spondylolisthesis of axis") | • Most common fracture in fatal auto accidents | • Bilateral fracture of C2 arch<br>• Neurologic involvement rare<br>• May involve transverse foramina<br>• Effendi classification | • Radiography: shows extent of anterior dislocation and involvement of transverse foramina<br>• CT: fracture lines and displacement |
| Hyperextension dislocation | • Direct blow to forehead or "whiplash" | • Unstable with significant soft tissue injury and ligament disruption<br>• Common in low cervical spine<br>• Paralysis, acute central cervical cord syndrome | • Radiography: "normal" but with prevertebral soft tissue swelling and ant. widening of disc space<br>• MRI: evaluate cord, soft tissues, and ligaments |
| Anterior arch avulsion of atlas | • Hyperextension | • Site at middle or inferior anterior arch of C1<br>• At attachments of longus colli muscles or atlantoaxial ligaments | • Radiography: prevertebral soft tissue swelling; facture line seen in odontoid view |
| Posterior arch atlas fracture | • Forceful hyperextension trapping posterior arch of C1 between occiput and spinous process of C2 | • Bilateral fractures of arches posterior to articular masses<br>• With significant prevertebral soft tissue swelling, Jefferson fracture considered<br>• Unstable when associated with C2 fracture (50%) | • Radiography: appears on lateral<br>• CT: fracture lines |
| Extension teardrop fracture | • Acute avulsion fracture caused by attachments of anterior longitudinal ligament | • Fragment originates from anterior inferior vertebral body, most commonly at C2<br>• Common in elderly with osteopenia | • Radiography/CT: vertical dimension > longitudinal dimension |
| Laminar fracture | • Compression between superior and inferior lamina in neck extension | • Stable<br>• Common in low cervical spine | • Radiography/CT: fracture line |

*CT* computed tomography

**Table 5.** Cervical spine: hyperextension injuries with rotation

| Injury | Etiology | Characteristics | Imaging |
|---|---|---|---|
| Pillar fracture | • Fracture through articular mass caused by impaction from superior articular process | • Vertical fracture line, may be comminuted<br>• Stable if isolated to articular mass<br>• Common patient presentation: radiculopathy, lateralizing neck and arm pain | • Radiography: AP, pillar, oblique to show fracture line<br>• CT: delineate extent |
| Pediculolaminar fracture (pedicolaminar fracture-separation injury) | • Similar to pillar fracture mechanism<br>• May also be result of a hyperflexion-lateral rotation injury | • Fracture through ipsilateral pedicle and lamina creating free floating lateral mass | • Radiograph: difficult to detect<br>• CT: fracture with/without displacement<br>• CT angiography: used if fracture extends to transverse foramina to asses vertebral artery |

*AP* anteroposterior, *CT* computed tomography

**Table 6.** Cervical spine: lateral flexion injury

| Injury | Etiology | Characteristics | Imaging |
|---|---|---|---|
| Host of injuries (fractures of occipital condyles, uncinate process, transverse process, lateral wedge compression, eccentric atlas burst fractures, odontoid fractures) | • Extreme lateral tilt in coronal plane | • Often involves transverse foramina thus associated with vertebral artery injury | • Best modalities are AP radiograph and CT to show fractures<br>• CT angiography: to asses vertebral artery |

*AP* anteroposterior, *CT* computed tomography

**Table 7.** Cervical spine: other injuries/fractures

| Injury | Etiology | Characteristics | Imaging |
|---|---|---|---|
| Rotatory atlantoaxial fixation - torticollis | • Secondary to mild trauma; can occur when sleeping in unusual position<br>• Torticollis results when symptoms not resolved within a few days | • Incongruity of C1 and 2 articular surfaces<br>• Asymmetry in distance between ring of C1 and dens<br>• Associated prevertebral soft tissue swelling (secondary to trauma) | • Radiography: odontoid view to visualize incongruity and asymmetry<br>• CT: further visualize facet joint disruption |
| Odontoid fractures | • Associated with Jefferson fractures and atlantoaxial dislocations | • May mimic a Mach line<br>• Classification: Anderson and D'Alonzo | • Radiography: II and III often visible in odontoid view<br>• CT: definitive diagnosis, and to exclude other bony injuries |
| Transverse atlantal ligament rupture | • Isolated tearing not involving dens or associated with dens fracture<br>• Trauma (blunt force to occiput) | • Unstable: anterior translation of skull and atlas<br>• Associations: Jefferson fractures | • Radiography/CT: widened atlanto-dental interval |
| Occipito-atlantal dissociation (OAD) | • Severe head trauma causing extensive ligamentous injury | • Often fatal if there is medullary transaction<br>• If incomplete, significant neurologic and vascular compromise | • Radiography: shows increase of over 12 mm in basion-dental |

*CT* computed tomography

## Craniocervical Junction (C0-C1-C2)

Occipital condylar fractures are frequently missed on standard radiographs and with the advent of CT imaging these fractures are more common than previously demonstrated. Three types have been described according to the classification system of Anderson and Montesano: type I is a comminuted fracture of the occipital condyle with minimal or no fragment displacement into the foramen magnum, type II is a basilar skull fracture extending into the occipital condyle, and type III is a fracture with a fragment displaced medially from the inferomedial aspect of the occipital condyle into the foramen magnum. Occipitoatlantal dislocation (OAD) is a rare devastating often fatal injury. Various radiographic criteria can be used to establish the diagnosis of OAD and direct measurement of occipitovertebral skeletal relationships altered by occipitoatlantal dissociation using the basion-axial and basion-dental intervals provides the most accurate imaging assessment of this injury. More survivors are reported because of improvements in diagnosis and treatment [16].

The unique anatomical relationship between the atlas and axis produces a variety of injury patterns not seen elsewhere in the spine. Injury to the C1/C2 complex accounts for about 25% of cervical spine injuries. Fractures of C2 occur most frequently, 55% of which involve the odontoid peg. Traumatic subluxation of C1 on C2 and rotatory fixation also occur with or without associated bone injury [17]. Atlantoaxial subluxation occurs when there is loss of integrity of the odontoid peg and/or the transverse ligament. Post-traumatic atlantoaxial subluxation is rare and even rarer without odontoid fracture.

Atlantoaxial dissociation is a general term used to encompass all types of atlantoaxial subluxation, dislocation and rotatory fixation. In the majority of atlantoaxial rotatory fixation (atlantoaxial rotatory subluxation, atlantoaxial dislocation), fixation occurs within the normal range of movement of the joint so the C1/C2 complex is not truly subluxed or dislocated. This entity is defined as persistent pathological fixation of the atlantoaxial joint in a rotated position such that the atlas and the axis move as a single unit rather than independently. It usually results from apparently insignificant cervical spine trauma. It is a rare condition occurring in children more than adults. Positional CT is required to differentiate atlantoaxial rotatory fixation from physiological atlantoaxial rotation and other causes of torticollis because these conditions can appear identical on static CT. CT is initially performed in the anatomical position. Further images are then obtained with the patient's head turned as much as they can to the right and then to the left; this determines whether the atlas and axis rotate independently of each other, as is normal.

Fractures of the atlas (C1) account for 2-13% of cervical spine fractures and are generally not associated with neurological deficit. C1 fractures are frequently associated with fractures elsewhere in the cervical spine particularly at the C2 and C7 levels. C1 fractures have been classified into five types including fractures of the anterior arch, posterior arch, lateral mass, transverse process and the burst type (Jefferson) fracture. This classification also describes the mechanism of injury and the stability of each fracture type.

Dens fractures of the axis (C2) are most commonly described by the Anderson-D'Alonzo classification system, with three types depending on location of the fracture plane and level of involvement (tip, base or C2 body), which has important therapeutic and prognostic implications. The mechanism of injury resulting in an odontoid process fracture involves a combination of extreme flexion, extension or rotation, plus a shearing force. The majority of cases have no neurological injury but deficit may develop later due to atlantoaxial subluxation. Fractures of the ring of the axis can occur through the laminae, the inferior articular facets, the pars interarticularis, the superior articular facets, the pedicles and the posterior wall of the vertebral body. These fractures are invariably bilateral but not symmetrical. Traumatic spondylolisthesis (neural arch avulsion from body) of C2, known as "hanged man's fracture", is a group of injuries with variable mechanisms accounting for 4-23% of cervical spine fractures. Effendi and coworkers [18] produced a classification of fractures of the ring of the axis according to radiological displacement and stability. The type and degree of displacement of the C2 vertebral body, the state of the C2/C3 disc space and articular facets of C2/C3 are considered. Extension teardrop fractures and hyperextension dislocations account for about 20% of C2 injuries. The teardrop fracture is caused by avulsion of the anterior longitudinal ligament off the anteroinferior endplate of the vertebral body; a variant, hyperextension strain is the same mechanism, but only involves soft tissue injury without the osseous avulsion. Hyperextension dislocation injury also involves a fracture of the anteroinferior corner of a vertebral body. It most frequently involves the lower cervical vertebra, but is not rare at the C2/C3 level. Fractures involving both C1 and C2 occur less frequently than isolated C1 and C2 fractures.

### Subaxial Cervical Spine

There are multiple types of subaxial cervical spine injury (i.e., below C2). These injuries are best classified by the mechanism of injury. The mechanism of injury is described by the vector of the force that causes the subsequent injury. Many patients with cervical spine trauma have more than one injury and they tend to occur in "families" based on the mechanism. Hyperflexion injuries are the most common injuries to the spine. Injuries from hyperflexion mechanisms include hyperflexion sprains, a purely ligamentous injury, bilateral facet dislocations, anterior wedge compressions of the vertebral body, clay shovelers fractures and flexion teardrop fractures. The "flexion teardrop" fracture is an unstable fracture, and is the most devastating cervical spine injury compatible with life. This injury is caused by severe flexion with resultant disruption of all ligaments and their associated stability. The anterior vertebral body is comminuted, with a triangular fragment or "teardrop," anteroinferiorly. The posterior portion of the vertebral body retropulses into the spinal canal causing injury to the spinal cord. Patients clinically present with acute anterior cord syndrome, characterized by complete paralysis, hypesthesia and hypalgesia to the level of injury, and preservation of dorsal column function. The addition of a rotational component and posterior distraction with hyperflexion injuries can result in unilateral facet dislocations. Axial loading and accompanying hyperflexion will lead to burst fractures. Forces acting along the coronal plane (i.e., a lateral flexion injury) give rise to lateral compression of the vertebral bodies. In general, hyperflexion injuries cause narrowing of the anterior interverterbal disc, with distraction of the posterior ligament complex and the posterior disc. Anterior translation of the vertebral body and posterior elements may also be present, distinguishing this injury from anterior subluxations caused by hyperextension injuries wherein the spinolaminar line is not usually displaced. Hyperextension injuries are more common in the cervical spine than in the thoracolumbar spine. Most of these fractures are due to hyperextension forces and are usually stable, such as the "extension teardrop" that classically occurs at the anteroinferior margin of C2.

### Vascular Injury in the Neck

Blunt carotid and vertebral arterial injuries are collectively known as blunt cerebrovascular injuries (BCI) and are the result of nonpenetrating trauma to the neck [10]. Motor vehicle accidents are the most common mechanisms (80%), with other less frequent causes including falls, diving injuries, chiropractic manipulation and assault. The incidence is about 1% of patients with blunt trauma. Screening criteria for BCI include skull base fractures (particularly those extending into the carotid canal), cervical spine fractures involving C1-3, foramen transversarium, cervical subluxation or dislocations, certain facial fractures (LeFort II or III), Glasgow Coma Scale score <6, and/or severe chest injuries.

Vertebral artery injury (VAI) can occur in association with cervical spine trauma and have the potential for neurological ischemic events. The overall incidence of VAI is about 0.5% in all trauma patients, with the incidence of VAI in patients who sustain cervical spine trauma reported to be between 15% and 45%; approximately 70% are associated with a fracture. VAI can occur as a result of direct trauma from bone fragments or from excessive stretch in fractures and dislocations, and is more frequent with multilevel foramina fractures and in patients with foramen transversarium comminuted fracture. Cervical spine translation injuries and transverse foramen fractures are most commonly cited as having a significant association with VAIs. VAIs associated with cervical spine fractures are most likely to occur in the foraminal (V2) segment, where

the artery is immediately adjacent to osseous structures. The incidence of neurologic deficits secondary to VAI ranges from 0% to 24% in reports that incorporate a screening protocol for asymptomatic patients. Treatment options include observation, antiplatelet agents, anticoagulation and endovascular treatments. Although some authors have advocated antithrombotic therapy for most asymptomatic VAIs, there is a lack of good evidence to support any strong guidelines for treatment [19].

Traditional imaging of BCI and VAI used catheter angiography. However, advanced imaging modalities may incorporate vascular assessment during the same setting as trauma imaging. CT angiography is emerging as an accurate, rapid, noninvasive diagnostic alternative in the initial evaluation of patients with possible BSI, effectively demonstrating carotid and vertebral injury. CT criteria for diagnosis of arterial injury include vessel irregularity, wall thickening secondary to mural hematoma, abrupt caliber change, raised intimal flap, intraluminal thrombus, pseudoaneurysm, occlusion, active extravasation and early venous filling (arteriovenous fistula). CT angiography may be preferable to MR angiography for evaluation of the vertebral arteries in a trauma setting in part because of convenience. However, arterial visualization can be limited if contrast bolus timing is suboptimal and if poor segmentation results from overlapping bony architecture. Differentiating minimal irregularity representing a low-grade dissection from artifact can be difficult, but this has lesser clinical import compared with the more severe injuries.

With regard to MRI, important information can also be obtained by careful observation of the major arterial structures in the neck. Standard MR sequences, T1-weighted and T2-weighted images should demonstrate flow void in the carotid and vertebral arteries, except when confounded by artefacts such as entry slice brightness of a nonmagnetized plug of blood, especially on T1-weighted sequences. Gradient echo T2*-weighted images of the cervical spine often show flow enhancement, so absence of this flow-related signal can be another clue. With the application of fat suppression to a T1-weighted axial sequence, an intramural hematoma can be made more conspicuous in cases of nonocclusive dissection. MR angiography of the neck may be performed without or with contrast enhanced techniques, with the hyperintense vessels displayed using image processing techniques such as maximum intensity projection (MIP) algorithms.

### Thoracolumbar Spine

Thoracolumbar spinal injuries have been variably reported in 2-20% of blunt trauma victims, with the majority at the thoracolumbar junction. Thoracolumbar spine fractures are more common than fractures of the cervical spine. Thoracolumbar spine fractures are associated with increasing severity of injury and often occur concurrently with other major organ, vascular or bone injuries in the head, chest, abdomen, pelvis and extremities. In 75-90%, these fractures occur without spinal cord injury. Injury to the cord or the cauda equina occurs in about 10-40% of adult thoracolumbar fractures, and in 50-60% of adult fracture-dislocations. Fractures of the thoracolumbar spine may be difficult to diagnose and completely characterize by radiography and can be time consuming; cross-sectional CT imaging is superior to projectional radiography and can be more expedient particularly when a patient is undergoing CT for other indications [20]. Missed, delayed or misclassified diagnosis contributes to an increased incidence of neurologic deficits (about 10.5% compared with 1.4%) when diagnosed at presentation.

While validated screening guidelines exist for traumatic c-spine injury, equivalent guidelines for thoracolumbar screening are lacking. Predictors of thoracolumbar injury with fracture in prospective studies include high-risk injury mechanism, symptoms or signs of vertebral injury, painful distracting injury, known c-spine fracture and any impairment in cognition [21]. Thus, CT screening the thoracolumbar spine of the trauma patient is indicated in the following circumstances: CT indicated for chest, abdomen or pelvis injury; neurological symptoms or deficit suggesting thoracolumbar or cervical spine injury; high velocity implicated (e.g., motor vehicle crash >60 kph/40mph, ejection from vehicle); abnormal sensorium - particularly Glasgow Coma Scale <14; hematoma over the spine or other clinical sign of a thoracolumbar spine fracture; severe back pain or spinal tenderness to palpation. Thoracolumbar spine screening may be accomplished using reformatted images acquired when scanning the chest/abdomen/pelvis or from direct/focused CT examinations of the spine if there are only spinal symptoms/indications. Accurate evaluation of the thoracolumbar spine is possible with targeted image reconstruction based on a standardized trauma protocol of the chest and abdomen, with attention to technical details [22]. The simultaneous assessment of organ and spinal injuries also results in a reduction in scanning time, which may be of paramount importance in maintaining the "golden hour" in the management of patients with multiple injuries. Absence of any the criteria stated above in a patient following blunt trauma implies a very low risk of thoracolumbar spine injury. If CT is not clinically indicated for investigation of other injuries, then radiography may be used as the initial imaging examination.

The spectrum of thoracolumbar spine injury patterns with associated characteristics and imaging features are listed in Table 8, and detailed reviews are available [15].

In terms of fracture classification, the Magerl (AO) scheme based on the pathomorphological characteristics of the injury is comprehensive and provides categories with subtypes for all possible injuries; however, no predictive validity studies have been performed [23]. Special mention should be made of burst fractures. Burst fracture is one of the most common injuries of the thoracolumbar spine. The characteristic finding of this type of injury,

**Table 8.** Thoracolumbar spine injury patterns

Axial load
- Force applied from superior direction
- Most common: fall from significant height
- Most common site: thoracolumbar junction
- Can produce two types of fracture: compression (stable) and burst (unstable)

Flexion/compression
- Anterior wedge and burst fractures
- Greater risk of posterior ligament disruption: >50% loss of vertebral body height, widening of interspinous distance
- MRI recommended to identify posterior ligament injury

Flexion/rotation
- Anterior wedge and burst fractures
- Rotation also causes posterior element fractures and posterior ligament injury, especially in dislocations
- Often at thoracolumbar junction
- Often severe neurologic damage

Flexion/distraction
- Common seat belt injuries
- Usually no neurologic damage
- Produce chance and chance variant fractures: chance (purely osseous), chance variant (osseous and ligamentous)

Lateral flexion/compression
- Loss of lateral vertebral body height
- Scoliosis deformity
- Posterior elements often fractured

Shear injury
- Upper and lower body drawn in different directions
- Severe ligamentous injury
- Can produce spondylolisthesis
- Neurologic impairment with fractures and dislocations

Extension
- Compression of posterior components, distraction of anterior components
- Possible injury to anterior longitudinal ligament and anterior anulus, and fractures of posterior spine elements

Transverse process fractures
- Common, present at multiple levels
- Often clue signifying more serious injury

*MRI* magnetic resonance imaging

caused by an axial compressive force, is a fracture involving the superior endplate and the posterior cortex with herniation of the intervertebral disc into the vertebral body, causing retropulsion of a bony fragment into the spinal canal. The thoracolumbar segment of spine is more frequently affected by this kind of fracture because of its anatomical characteristics and transition from thoracic kyphosis to lumbar lordosis. Special mention should also be made for stability evaluation. The posterior ligamentous complex (PLC) is thought to contribute significantly to the stability of thoracolumbar spine. Obvious translation or dislocation of an intervertebral space interspace denotes injury to the PLC. However, in the setting of normal-appearing radiographs, PLC injury is diagnosed by MRI as disruption of the ligaments (T1 and STIR weighted images) and diastasis of the facet joints (this latter feature may also be noted on CT imaging) [24].

Lumbosacral fracture dislocation, also called lumbosacral dissociation, is a very rare lesion relatively recently described (by Watson-Jones in 1940) representing an anatomic separation of the pelvis from the spinal column [25]. The key features of lumbosacral dislocations are a traumatic spondylolisthesis of the lumbosacral junction, with or without fractures of the zygapophyseal joints or the pars interarticularis. The fracture type is characterized by an antero- or retrolisthesis or a lateral translation of the lowest lumbar vertebra in relation to the sacrum. Most patients suffer from a high-energy trauma with concomitant severe injuries. There is a high rate of additional neurological deficits. Fractures of the transverse process are thought to be sentinel fractures. MRI and CT scans are essential to detect the whole extent of the lesion. A relative increase in these injuries has been seen in young healthy combat casualties subjected to high-energy blast trauma [26].

## Spinal Cord Injury

Trauma to the spinal cord involves either true cord injury or compression with secondary cord damage. Spinal cord dysfunction occurs in about 25% of patients with thoracolumbar injury. Thoracic spinal cord injury (SCI) is more likely to be complete than injury at other spinal levels. It is important to understand that imaging is of particular importance in evaluating these patients since clinical evaluation can be difficult. The American Spinal Injury Association publishes the "Standards for Neurological Classification of Spinal Cord Injured Patients" known as the ASIA classification. Cord injuries can be divided into complete or incomplete lesions on the basis of the extent of motor and sensory function. In patients with pre-existing spondylosis or spinal canal stenosis, hyperextension injuries are more likely to injure the spinal cord, particularly in the cervical spine with a poorer prognosis. At any level, the cord is vulnerable to transection if the applied forces are sufficient; however, cord transection cannot be presumptively diagnosed based on fracture dislocation pattern.

Imaging the spinal cord is a challenge because of small size and the magnetic susceptibility changes caused by surrounding bone and nearby cerebrospinal fluid (CSF) flow and vascular pulsations. Sagittal turbo spin-echo T2-weighted images, sagittal SE T1-weighted images and axial TSE T2-weighted images are part of the protocol for evaluation of cervical and thoracic spine trauma. Axial gradient echo T2* is also employed, particularly in the cervical and thoracic segments. This sequence can be acquired with thin sections (two-dimensional or three-dimensional), has almost no CSF pulsation artefacts and is sensitive to early blood products (deoxyhemaglobin) because of the susceptibility artefact generated that is more prominent on a gradient echo based sequences. The spectrum of MRI manifestations of acute SCI is: swelling defined as a smooth enlargement of the cord contour (typically on T1-weighted images); edema, where internal signal demonstrates T1 and T2 prolongation (low and high signal respectively); and

hemorrhage, where the signal alteration can be complex. Acute intramedullary hemorrhage is seen as a focus of T2 shortening (hypointensity) [15].

Four prognostication patterns are predictive of neurological outcome (normal, single-level edema, multi-level edema, and mixed hemorrhage and edema) [27]. Patients with a partial cord syndrome and normal MRI tend to make full recoveries. Up to 75% of patients with cord edema will have recovered motor function. Cord contusion carries a worse prognosis since it may evolve into cyst formation, but recovery may occur in 70% of patients with incomplete spinal cord syndromes. The presence of abnormalities on MRI in a patient with a complete cord syndrome is generally a bad prognostic sign. The presence and extent of spinal cord hematoma are each significantly associated with poor long-term neurological outcomes. Cervical cord intramedullary hematomas have a strong correlation with a complete neurologic deficit and irreversible spinal cord injury. Complete cord transections and penetrating injuries do not fall within this classification because of their different and easily differentiated patterns on MRI. Those injuries are also associated with quite different prognoses.

A recent systematic review and meta-analysis weakly recommended that MRI be done in all patients with acute SCI (when feasible, to direct management), strongly recommended that an MRI be done in the acute period following a spinal cord injury for prognostication, and strongly recommended that a sagittal T2 pulse sequence be obtained to prognosticate neurological outcome [28]. It is generally recommended that the first MRI be performed 24-72 h post trauma. In addition to a SCI, the presence of an epidural haematoma or a post-traumatic disc herniation may warrant immediate surgery.

## Special Circumstances/Conditions

### Pediatric

Pediatric spine injuries are not in the purview of this chapter. In general, spine injuries in children are much less common than in adults, the criteria for imaging and screening are different and less well defined (in part related to less evidence), and a guiding principle should be very judicious use of ionizing radiation imaging modalities because of potential downstream consequences of neoplasm.

### Geriatric

The incidence and type of cervical spinal injury in the elderly patient (older than 65 years) differs from those in younger patients because spondylosis (degenerative changes) and/or decreased bone mineralization (osteoporosis) predisposes to vulnerability of low-velocity injuries (such as a fall from standing height) [29]. These features of the senescent spine make imaging of the spine, particularly cervical spine, more difficult. Typically, upper cervical spine injuries, especially at C2, are caused by hyperextension in patients with degenerative changes [30].

## Pseudofractures

There are many normal anatomical variants that can simulate disease, including some that can be confounded for spinal trauma [31]. These are often related to developmental anomalies [32]. The craniocervical junction and upper cervical spine have a number of these, owing to the unique transitional aspects of this anatomy.

In some people, nonfusion of the atlas (C1) ossification centers results in a cleft that persists into adulthood showing smooth corticated margins, which helps distinguish it from a fracture. Clefts of the atlas most commonly occur at the posterior synchondrosis, but may occur anywhere within the C1 ring, including rarely anteriorly (0.1%). In response there may be overgrowth of the neural arches at the margins of the cleft as they attempt to fuse. The atlantooccipital membrane may become partially or completely ossified (latter resulting in an arcuate foramen). The odontoid process of C2 may have a persistent os terminale (small summit ossification center) or os odontoideum (larger fragment which may involve the base and extend into the body of C2). These may be a post-traumatic phenomenon that occurred during childhood. When an os odontoideum is developmental it may have a dysplastic appearance and be associated with a hypertrophic anterior arch of C1. A remnant of subdental synchondrosis of C2 often persists into adulthood, appearing as a sclerotic line surrounded by lucency at the base of the dens.

Clefts may have multiple locations in verterbrae involving the subaxial portions of the spine. Spina bifida occulta results from failed osseous fusion of the posterior synchondrosis. A cleft may also occur within the pars interarticularis (spondylolysis), pedicle (retrosomatic cleft) or lamina (retroisthmic cleft). An isolated defect within the bony wall of the transverse foramen is a very uncommon variant that is unlikely to represent a fracture (the latter of which is characterized by disruptions in two locations with displacement of the fragment). Anterior wedging of the vertebral bodies can also be a normal finding in adults at the thoracolumar junction. Occasionally, a Schmorl node might be initially confused with an acute fracture, particularly if there is associated physiologic wedging of the vertebral body. Occasionally, secondary ossification centers may remain unfused later into adulthood (beyond 16-25 years). The margins will be smooth and corticated as opposed to acute fractures, which are irregular and noncorticated.

## Spondyloarthropathy

Conditions such as diffuse idiopathic skeletal hyperostosis (DISH) and ankylosing spondylitis (AS) cause alterations in biomechanics because of fused spinal segments that predispose to superimposed acute fractures [33]. DISH (Forestier disease) is a common disorder of unknown cause often diagnosed by radiographic criteria of (1) flowing mineralization of the anterior longitudinal ligament along the anterolateral aspect of at least four contiguous vertebral bodies, (2) absence of degenerative disc disease in the involved vertebral segment, and (3) the absence of spondylitis features (apophyseal/costovertebral joint ankylosis and sacroilitis/ankylosis). The association of ossification of the posterior longitudinal ligament (OPLL) in up to 50% and ossification of the ligamentum flavum with DISH may explain, in part, the occasional presence of neurologic findings in patients with DISH. Acute spinal fractures associated with DISH are not common but can lead to serious complications, including nonunion, deformity, neurologic injury and death.

The ankylosed spine is more prone to fracture than a normal spine, and this has been reported in both DISH and AS. These fractures can occur after even minor trauma. Spinal fractures in AS are more common than those in DISH, probably because of the more extensive segments involved and the associated osteoporosis. Fractures in DISH typically occur in patients with moderate to severe disease in which there is osseous fusion of the long spinal segments, similar to AS. They are more common in the thoracic and cervical spine than in the lumbar region. Hyperextension is the most common mechanism of injury. Acute spinal fractures that occur in DISH may be mistaken for or misinterpreted as those of AS. Fractures in DISH tend to occur through the vertebral body within the ankylosed segment or may occur close to the endplate as opposed to the fractures in AS which tend to be trans-discal. Different patterns of spinal fractures in patients with DISH and in those with AS can be explained by differences in the pathomechanics of these diseases (longitudinal ligament mineralization versus syndesmophyte formation).

## Conclusion

The main objectives of imaging patients with spinal trauma are: rapid and accurate depiction of the spinal axis, identification of (potentially) unstable injuries, and assisting decision making for surgical treatment. Radiologists who interpret trauma images should have basic concepts of spinal instability because the lack of detection and characterization of these injuries places the patient at risk of pain and neurological dysfunction. While the exact classification or specific nomenclature can be important to facilitate uniform communication, the critical element is identifying this as an unstable lesion. CT has become an integral part of the initial assessment of many injured patients, and the spine is easily included in the total body screening performed in patients with severe blunt polytrauma. Radiography now has a more limited, adjunctive role. The application of validated clinical prediction rules dramatically decreases the rate of unnecessary imaging to clear the cervical spine in adults. While CT scanning has assumed a significant role as a primary screening modality, radiologists must be conscious of the increased radiation dose that accompanies it, particularly when children are being imaged. Cervical spine trauma in children is rare and the diagnosis can be challenging due to anatomical and biomechanical differences as compared with adults. Recognition of the normal developing spine and variants can prevent misdiagnoses of injury. Vascular injuries have been increasingly recognized in association with cervical spinal trauma and CT angiography, MR angiography and catheter angiography may have roles in their detection. MRI is the method of choice for assessing spinal cord lesions, ligamentous injury, discal pathology and vertebral bone marrow edema. MRI is employed to direct clinical decision making for spinal cord injury. Patients with advanced DISH or AS may sustain acute spinal fractures even after minor trauma and occur in typical distinguishing patterns.

## References

1. White AA 3rd, Johnson RM, Panjabi MM, Southwick WO (1975) Biomechanical analysis of clinical stability in the cervical spine. Clin Orthop Relat Res 109:85-96
2. Hogan GJ, Mirvis SE, Shanmuganathan K, Scalea TM (2005) Exclusion of unstable cervical spine injury in obtunded patients with blunt trauma: is MR imaging needed when multi-detector row CT findings are normal? Radiology 237:106-113
3. Denis F (1984) Spinal instability as defined by the three-column spine concept in acute spinal trauma. Clin Orthop Relat Res 189:65-76
4. Parizel PM, van der Zijden T, Gaudino S et al (2010) Trauma of the spine and spinal cord: imaging strategies. Eur Spine J 19 (Suppl 1):S8-17
5. van Middendorp JJ, Audigé L, Hanson B et al (2010) What should an ideal spinal injury classification system consist of? A methodological review and conceptual proposal for future classifications. Eur Spine J 19:1238-1249
6. Patel AA, Dailey A, Brodke DS et al; Spine Trauma Study Group (2008) Subaxial cervical spine trauma classification: the Subaxial Injury Classification system and case examples. Neurosurg Focus 25:E8
7. Patel AA, Dailey A, Brodke DS et al; Spine Trauma Study Group ((2009) Thoracolumbar spine trauma classification: the Thoracolumbar Injury Classification and Severity Score system and case examples. J Neurosurg Spine 10:201-206
8. Blackmore CC, Ramsey SD, Mann FA, Deyo RA (1999) Cost-effectiveness of cervical spine CT in trauma patients. Radiology 212:117-125
9. Hoffman J, Mower W, Wolfson A et al (2000) Validity of a set of clinical criteria to rule out injury to the cervical spine in patients with blunt trauma. N Eng J Med 343:94-99
10. Munera F, Rivas LA, Nunez DB Jr, Quencer RM (2012) Imaging evaluation of adult spinal injuries: emphasis on multidetector CT in cervical spine trauma. Radiology 263:645-660
11. Panczykowski DM, Tomycz ND, Okonkwo DO (2011) Comparative effectiveness of using computed tomography alone to exclude cervical spine injuries in obtunded or intubated patients: meta-analysis of 14,327 patients with blunt trauma. J Neurosurg 115:541-549
12. Plumb JO, Morris CG (2012) Clinical review: Spinal imaging for the adult obtunded blunt trauma patient: update from 2004. Intensive Care Med 38:752-771
13. Krakenes J, Kaale BR (2006) Magnetic resonance imaging assessment of craniovertebral ligaments and membranes after whiplash trauma. Spine (Phila Pa 1976) 31:2820-2826
14. Anderson SE, Boesch C, Zimmermann H (2012) Are there cervical spine findings at MR imaging that are specific to acute symptomatic whiplash injury? A prospective controlled study with four experienced blinded readers. Radiology 262:567-575
15. Looby S, Flanders A (2011) Spine trauma. Radiol Clin North Am 49:129-163
16. Garrett M, Consiglieri G, Kakarla UK et al (2010) Occipitoatlantal dislocation. Neurosurgery 66(3 Suppl):48-55
17. Pratt H, Davies E, King L (2008) Traumatic injuries of the c1/c2 complex: computed tomographic imaging appearances. Curr Probl Diagn Radiol 37:26-38
18. Effendi B, Roy D, Cornish B et al (1981) Fractures of the ring of the axis. A classification based on the analysis of 131 cases. J Bone Joint Surg Br 63-B:319-327
19. Fassett DR, Dailey AT, Vaccaro AR (2008) Vertebral artery injuries associated with cervical spine injuries: a review of the literature. J Spinal Disord Tech 21:252-258
20. Bernstein M (2010) Easily missed thoracolumbar spine fractures. Eur J Radiol 74:6-15
21. O'Connor E, Walsham J (2009) Review article: indications for thoracolumbar imaging in blunt trauma patients: a review of current literature. Emerg Med Australas 21:94-101
22. Roos JE, Hilfiker P, Platz A et al (2004) MDCT in emergency radiology: is a standardized chest or abdominal protocol sufficient for evaluation of thoracic and lumbar spine trauma? AJR Am J Roentgenol 183:959-968
23. Chapman JR, Dettori JR, Norvel DC (2009) Spine classifications and severity measures.Thieme, Stuttgart
24. Lee JY, Vaccaro AR, Schweitzer KM Jr et al (2007) Assessment of injury to the thoracolumbar posterior ligamentous complex in the setting of normal-appearing plain radiography. Spine J 7:422-427
25. Schmid R, Reinhold M, Blauth M (2010) Lumbosacral dislocation: a review of the literature and current aspects of management. Injury 41:321-328.
26. Helgeson MD, Lehman RA Jr, Cooper P et al (2011) Retrospective review of lumbosacral dissociations in blast injuries. Spine (Phila Pa 1976) 36:E469-75
27. Andreoli C, Colaiacomo MC, Rojas Beccaglia M et al (2005) MRI in the acute phase of spinal cord traumatic lesions: relationship between MRI findings and neurological outcome. Radiol Med 110:636-645
28. Bozzo A, Marcoux J, Radhakrishna M et al (2011) The role of magnetic resonance imaging in the management of acute spinal cord injury. J Neurotrauma 28:1401-1411
29. Liebermann H, Webb JK (1994) Cervical spine injuries in the elderly. J Bone Joint Surg Br 76:877-881
30. Walid MS, Zaytseva NV (2009) Upper cervical spine injuries in elderly patients. Aust Fam Physician 38:43-45
31. Keats T, Anderson M (2013) Atlas of normal Roentgen variants that may simulate disease, 9th edn. Elsevier, Philadelphia, in print
32. Jinkins JR (2000) Atlas of Neuroradiologic embryology, anatomy, and variants. LWW, Baltimore
33. Taljanovic MS, Hunter TB, Wisneski RJ et al (2009) Imaging characteristics of diffuse idiopathic skeletal hyperostosis with an emphasis on acute spinal fractures: review. AJR Am J Roentgenol 193(3 Suppl):S10-19

# Inflammatory Disorders of the Spine

Victor N. Cassar-Pullicino

Department of Radiology, The Robert Jones and Agnes Hunt Orthopaedic Hospital, Oswestry, UK

## Introduction

The underlying pathology of target organs in spinal inflammatory disorders dictates the imaging appearances throughout the natural history of the disease processes. Although overlap exists, inflammatory disorders can predominantly affect the synovial articulations of the spine (rheumatoid disease) or primarily the enthesis of ligaments and intervertebral discs (seronegative spondyloarthropathies). The various disease states are not static but rather need to be viewed as dynamic and progressive, usually resulting in complications. In rheumatoid disease it is primarily the cervical spine that is involved, but it is very rare that the rheumatoid arthritis patient presents with cervical spine manifestations as the first mode of presentation. On the other hand seronegative spondyloarthropathies usually present with axial manifestations of enthesitis as the first mode of presentation, and these are easily overlooked.

Synovial involvement of the cervical spine in seropositive inflammatory states has a predilection for the facet joints, and in particular the C1-C2 articulations. In seronegative spondyloarthropathy, the inflammatory site is the enthesis where the collagen of the ligaments or intervertebral disc annulus enters bone directly. The cause of the inflammatory process is the generation of cytokines, which results in edema, bone erosion, disorganization of bone and ligament structure, which promotes a reactive osteitis and eventually ossification of the ligaments commencing at the enthesis interface. Histologically, the inflammatory enthesitis reveals a macrophage-predominant cellular infiltrate consistent with the knowledge that tumor necrosis factor (TNF)-α, which is a pro-inflammatory cytokine produced by macrophages, plays a key role in the inflammatory spondyloarthropathies. The seronegative spondyloarthropathies can be further categorized based on the imaging findings equated to the clinical features and laboratory findings. Although multiple modalities such as radiography, computed tomography (CT) and scintigraphy can be employed to assess the inflammatory sites within the axial and the appendicular skeleton, it is primarily

magnetic resonance imaging (MRI) that is the optimal imaging modality to assess inflammatory disorders of the spine because of its high sensitivity and specificity. Although contrast-enhanced magnetic resonance (MR) studies are not usually required for diagnosis, they can distinguish between active and inactive disease and also help in assessing the response to anti-inflammatory therapy.

## Clinical Features

The etiology of the inflammatory spondyloarthropathies is still unknown, although the human leukocyte antigen (HLA-B27) is found to be present in 90% of patients suffering from ankylosing spondylitis, 50% patients with reactive arthritis (previously known as Reiter's syndrome) and only 20% of patients with psoriasis. Inflammatory back pain that is worse at night and in the early morning is the key clinical hallmark of inflammatory spondyloarthropathy. Ankylosing spondylitis usually presents with early morning stiffness that is eased by movement and exercise. However the onset is usually insidious allied with multiple relapsing episodes of back pain that usually starts in the lumbar spine. The condition can remain undiagnosed for years, resulting in fusion of the spine, which renders the condition painless. Although classification subtypes have evolved over the last 30-40 years, the main challenge facing the radiologist is the early diagnosis of inflammatory spinal disorders because the early institution of therapy can limit disability and diminish disease progression. MRI has not only helped in the early detection of disease, but also is increasingly being employed in scoring mechanisms that without doubt will be incorporated in time in decision-making therapeutic protocols.

## Sacroiliitis

Sacroiliitis is the hallmark of all spondyloarthropathies. It is a fundamental component required in establishing

J. Hodler et al. (eds.), *Musculoskeletal Diseases 2013-2016,*
DOI: 10.1007/978-88-470-5292-5_16 © Springer-Verlag Italia 2013

the diagnosis of ankylosing spondylitis, but it is also relevant to the other spondyloarthropathies. In ankylosing spondylitis it is bilateral and symmetrical, while in psoriatic spondyloarthropathy and reactive arthritis it can be bilateral or unilateral. Involvement of the axial skeleton is unusual and indeed rare in the absence of sacroiliitis.

Conventional radiography remains the initial diagnostic imaging modality recommended despite its low sensitivity and relatively high false-negative rate in early disease. There are inherent limitations to the proper radiographic assessment of the sacroiliac joints; these arise because the joints themselves are divergent in the anteroposterior projection, which is why a posteroanterior projection is usually a better option of assessing the sacroiliac joints. It is also well known that conventional radiography can miss advanced sacroiliitis. Early inflammatory sacroiliitis can result in a loss of the sharpness of the subchondral bone outline of the joint; this then progresses to becoming irregular due to the presence of erosions, and this in turn produces an appearance of localized joint widening. Sclerosis of the subchondral bone on either side of the joint is fairly diagnostic in established disease, especially when it involves the inferior and middle portion of the joint and is more pronounced on the iliac side. However, in established disease, the sacroiliac joint can also exhibit loss of sharpness due to ossification across the joint leading to ankylosis. The modified New York criteria have identified five radiographic stages of sacroiliac joint involvement:

Grade 0: no abnormality
Grade 1: suspicious changes
Grade 2: sclerosis with early erosions
Grade 3: severe erosions, pseudo joint widening and partial ankylosis
Grade 4: complete ankylosis.

In practice, however, radiological detection of these changes is challenging with poor interobserver and intraobserver reliability for the changes in early disease, namely stages 1 and 2.

The relatively late development of radiographic changes in ankylosing spondylitis is undeniably one of the factors that can delay the diagnosis. However, MRI has revolutionized the early diagnosis of sacroiliitis. This is primarily dependent on the pericartilage osteitis, which is an important feature of ankylosing spondylitis and produces bone marrow edema that is well picked up on the edema-sensitive sequences such as T2-weighted sequences with fat suppression or the short tau inversion recovery (STIR) sequence. T1-weighted spin-echo sequences are, however, better at depicting articular erosions. The degree of the edema can vary, ranging from florid, fairly extensive areas of periarticular edema to more focal and localized zones of edema paralleling the joint line. It is usually the inferior iliac portion of the joint that is involved in the early stages of sacroiliac inflammatory change. Gadolinium-enhanced MR studies have been advocated in active disease, as there is a rise in the MR signal at the point of enhancement in the joint space

and periarticular tissues in the first 2 min. However, contrast enhancement is particularly useful if the edema-sensitive sequence (STIR) is equivocal. Using contrast enhancement, MRI can not only distinguish active from inactive disease, but it can also monitor the treatment response where a decrease in the enhancement even in the persistent presence of bone marrow edema has been shown to be strongly correlated with a good clinical response to treatment. There are various ways of utilizing post-contrast MRI in the assessment of sacroiliac disease. They are particularly helpful in determining whether the instituted drug regime is working, identifying a need to alter the drug regime, and deciding to stop drug regimes if they are not working in view of the significant side-effects and high cost.

Although the edema-sensitive sequences, in particular the T2 sequences with fat suppression, are very sensitive and specific in visualization of bone marrow edema, joint widening and joint fluid, they are not as good in identifying subtle erosions because of the relatively low spatial resolution compared with CT. The high spatial resolution inherent in CT identifies subtle erosions and subchondral sclerosis in sacroiliac joint involvement. CT indeed is the preferred modality for the detection of very early erosions of the sacroiliac joints and their early ankylosis. However, one needs to bear in mind that sclerosis on its own can have a similar appearance in both active disease and in burnt-out inflammation.

## Axial Skeleton

Ankylosing spondylitis is the seronegative spondyloarthropathy prototype. It is primarily a disease of the axial skeleton involving the sacroiliac joints and the spine. The primary target organ is the enthesis where the spinal longitudinal ligaments and annulus fibrosus merge directly with the bone. In the early manifestations of inflammation an osteitis is produced by the inflammatory response, and this leads to bone marrow edema and then subsequently this is followed by reactive sclerosis and eventually ossification of the involved ligaments. There is usually an orderly progression of involvement of the spine commencing first in the thoracolumbar and lumbosacral regions, and then advancing to the midlumbar, midthoracic and eventually the cervical spine.

### Spondylitis

Spondylitis occurs in about 50% of ankylosing spondylitis patients, although females are relatively less affected. The earliest changes are caused by enthesitis at the insertion of the outer fibers of the annulus fibrosus on the ring apophysis of the vertebral end plate. Although this occurs circumferentially, it is predominantly the anterior attachment that usually produces the more florid manifestations. Subtle erosions with reactive sclerosis in the vertebral corners are seen, and radiographically these have been referred to as Romanus lesions when viewed as erosions, and "shiny corners" when the erosion is associated with sclerosis due to the reactive osteitis. The Romanus erosive disease can also produce an apparent squaring of the anterior outline of the vertebral body. However, the Romanus lesions are short lived and resolve by producing resultant syndesmophyte formation. The syndesmophytes represent the ossification of the outer fibers of the annulus fibrosus in ankylosing spondylitis. They are seen radiographically as very fine and symmetric in appearance, bridging the intervertebral space. This may initially appear at a single disc level, but usually progresses to involve multiple segments producing the so-called characteristic "bamboo spine". The same inflammatory process results in ossification of the longitudinal ligaments, which insert onto the vertebral bodies producing squaring of the vertebral body appearance as the fusion progresses.

MRI is the most sensitive diagnostic tool for the identification of discovertebral inflammatory disease. The Romanus lesions are identified on the sagittal sequences and characterized by a triangular pattern of bone marrow edema at the corners of the vertebral end plates highlighted by low T1 signal and high T2 fat-saturated and STIR sequence appearance. The small erosion can be overlooked when compared with the areas of edema. After the acute Romanus lesion phase subsides, the chronic lesions are identified by a fatty marrow replacement at the sites of enthesis inflammation within the vertebral bodies, highlighted by a high T1 signal and a low signal on STIR and T2 fat-saturated sequences. Multiple contiguous areas of high T1 signal can be seen in vertebral bodies and in particular at their corners in segments of the spine that have undergone extensive fusion. The intervertebral disc in cases of long-term spinal fusion can also undergo changes producing a high T1 inherent MR signal. This has been related to the presence of calcification or alternatively the presence of marrow within mature transdiscal ankylosis.

Contrast-enhanced MR studies and diffusion-weighted MR sequences have also been employed in the detection of inflammatory disease of the spine. They can be useful in the acute phase of inflammatory change, particularly in the early manifestations of the disease. In acute Romanus lesions, contrast medium injection usually renders the erosions more clearly defined. However, comparative studies with STIR sequences have concluded that there is very little advantage as both have high intraobserver and interobserver reliability and more active lesions are seen on the STIR sequences. In cases where the STIR sequence is equivocal, dynamic gadolinium diethylenetriaminepentaacetate dextran (DTPA) studies have been found useful.

Although there is no doubt that MRI has revolutionized the role of imaging in the early and active phases of inflammatory disorders of the spine, one also needs to bear in mind that it does have a particular drawback in identifying the syndesmophytes that are the hallmark of established disease. Syndesmophytes are not well seen by MRI and easily overlooked because the low signal of the syndesmophyte is similar to the low signal of the normal anterior longitudinal ligament and annulus fibrosus. Similarly MRI can overlook ossification and fusion of other spinal elements, namely the apophyseal joints, paraspinal ligaments and interspinous ligaments. It is still the case that radiographic diagnosis is very easy when compared with MRI in the chronic case where there is established soft tissue ossification.

## Spondylodiscitis

There are two types of spondylodiscitis that can be detected within the discovertebral junction. Primary spondylodiscitis, or as it is sometimes known Andersson type A lesions, resembles Schmorl's nodes exhibiting a rim of edema within the vertebral body, a focal endplate defect and enhancement of the marrow edema. The primary spondylodiscitis is usually a sign of early discovertebral involvement with a stable spinal status. In the secondary spondylodiscitis, or as it sometimes known Andersson type B lesions, there is more extensive and florid discovertebral disease and destruction. These are particularly well demonstrated on CT and MRI. The degree of vertebral destruction is usually mild, but there is often extensive bony edema and bony sclerosis, and in long established cases the endplates can be completely destroyed on both sides of the intervertebral disc. In Andersson type B lesions the spine is unstable at the site of involvement because of increased mobility. This increased mobility could be at a level between fused segments or be associated with deficiency of the posterior elements where there is a pseudoarthrosis due to a fracture. It is therefore imperative that the posterior elements are assessed assiduously to differentiate type A from type B Andersson lesions, as the latter are associated with pain and instability and can give rise to neurological dysfunction.

## Costovertebritis

This is the hallmark of spondyloarthropathy, and usually starts in the lower thoracic spine.

## Complications

The most important spinal complications in ankylosing spondylitis include osteoporosis, fracture, instability, cauda equine syndrome and spinal stenosis.

### Osteoporosis

Osteoporosis increases in prevalence directly with increased patient age, increased severity of spinal involvement, increased disease duration and peripheral arthritis. The vertebral marrow signal is usually increased on the T1 sequences as a result of the osteoporosis. The osteoporosis obviously increases the chances of vertebral compression fractures, posterior element fractures, pseudoarthrosis and unstable fractures from relatively minor trauma.

## Fractures

Fractures of the cervical spine can occur after a minor fall or injury to the head and neck. Typically the conventional radiographs show a chalk-stick type of break either through the disc or the vertebral body anteriorly and horizontally through the posterior fused elements. A common spinal location for fracture is the thoracolumbar and cervicothoracic and lastly the lumbosacral junction. By definition all three columns of the spine are involved in this type of fracture. There is a high risk of missing the fracture at the time of initial evaluation particularly if radiographic techniques are not optimal. A delayed diagnosis can lead to the development of a true pseudoarthrosis resulting in instability and cord injury. Increasingly it has been shown that conventional radiography is not sufficient in excluding a fracture complicating a fused spine in ankylosing spondylitis. Any ankylosing spondylitis patient suffering minor trauma who complains of pain should have advanced imaging preferably by CT, as this will show the full extent of the fracture in both the axial and the reconstructive sagittal and coronal images. If the patient has neurological deficit, MR is essential in assessing the status of the cord and in particular whether there is an epidural hematoma or disc/bone fragment compressing the cord.

## Cauda Equina Syndrome

Cauda equina syndrome is a rare but specific complication following long-standing ankylosing spondylitis. It invariably occurs in a fused spine and is most common in the lumbar region. Dural ectasia producing leptomeningeal sacculations is common, resulting in erosions of primarily the posterior neural arch. This is best evaluated with CT or MRI. MR will show enlargement of the spinal canal with arachnoid diverticulae, erosion of the laminae and adherent nerve roots.

## Spinal Stenosis

It is important that one remembers that the ligamentous ossification that takes place as a result of the chronic in-

flammatory reactive process can also involve the ligaments within the spinal canal, namely the longitudinal ligaments and the ligamentum flavum. As a result of this ossification there can be encroachment onto the contents, namely the cord and nerve roots. Neurological deficit in patients with ankylosing spondylitis could have a number of causes but C1-C2 subluxation, fracture, pseudoarthrosis, ligamentous ossification and cauda equina syndrome would tend to be the most common list that one needs to remember in directing imaging to the spine to assess the underlying reason for the neurological deficit.

## Suggested Reading

Amrami KK (2012) Imaging of seronegative spondyloarthropathies. Radiol Clin N Am 50:841-854

Braun J, Bollow M, Eggens U et al (1994) Use of dynamic magnetic resonance imaging with fast imaging in the detection of early and advanced sacroiliitis in spondyloarthropathy patients. Arthritis Rheum 37:1039-1045

Dougados M, Baeten D (2011) Spondyloarthritis. Lancet 377:2127-2137

El-Khoury GY, Kathol MH, Brandser EA (1996) Seronegative spondyloarthropathies. Radiol Clin North Am 34:343

Fam A, Rubenstein J, Chin-Sang H et al (1985) Computed tomography in the diagnosis of early ankylosing spondylitis. Arthritis Rheum 28:930-937

Forrester D, Hollingsworth P, Dawkins RL (1983) Difficulties in the radiographic diagnosis of sacroiliitis. Clin Rheum Dis 9:323-332

Hollingsworth P, Cheah P, Dawkins RL et al (1983) Observer variation in grading sacroiliac radiographs in HLA-B27 positive individuals. J Rheumatol 10:247-254

Kurugoglu S, Kanberoglu K, Kanbergolu A et al (2002) MRI appearances of inflammatory osteitis in early ankylosing spondylitis. Paediatr Radiol 32:191-194

Toussirot E (2010) Late-onset ankylosing spondylitis and spondyloarthritis: and update on clinical manifestations, differential diagnosis and pharmacological therapies. Drugs Aging 27:523-531

Van Der Linden S, Valkenburg H, Cats A (1984) Evaluation of diagnostic criteria for ankylosing spondylitis. A proposal for modification of the New York criteria. Arthritis Rheum 27:361-368

Weber U, Ostergaard M, Lambert RG et al (2011) The impact of MRI on the clinical management of inflammatory arthritides. Skeletal Radiol 40:1153-1173

Yu W, Feng F, Dion E et al (1998) Comparison of radiography, computed tomography and magnetic resonance imaging in the detection of sacroiliitis accompanying ankylosing spondylitis. Skeletal Radiol 27:311-320

# Imaging of Degenerative Disorders of the Spine

David Wilson

Oxford University Hospitals, and St Luke's Radiology, St Luke's Hospital, Oxford, UK

## Introduction

Degenerative disease of the spine affects all humans. The consequences are disabling and can potentially become the major factor in an individual's life. There is a definite genetic influence on the form and nature of degeneration and particular types are seen in family groups. There is evidence that patients with harder collagen tend to form spondylitic changes, whilst those with softer collagen are more likely to develop disc degeneration and intervertebral disc prolapse. Physical activity is a risk factor that may accelerate the onset of degenerative changes and therefore occupation has a significant influence. Smoking is also an accelerant of degenerative changes. Disc degeneration is particularly common and changes that are observed on imaging are almost universal in the adult population. Asymptomatic disc prolapse affects approximately three-quarters of the adult population and over 70% of adults have experienced an episode of low back pain. Root compression due to herniated intervertebral discs affects only 1% of the population (Fig. 1).

Patients present in a variety of ways and the interpretation of imaging is based very much on the clinical pattern. The syndromes that may be considered are: (1) postural low back pain, (2) nerve root pain (sometimes called sciatica), (3) spinal claudication, (4) cauda equine syndrome and myelopathy, (5) mechanical pain, and (6) difficulty in maintaining sagittal balance.

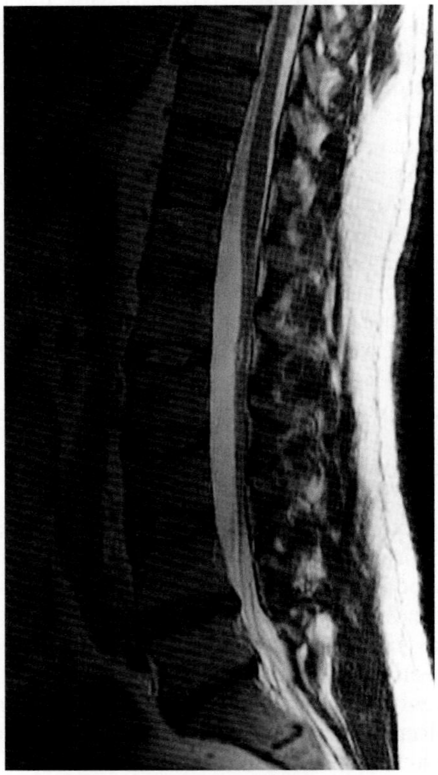

**Fig. 1.** Asymptomatic degenerate disc disease in a patient aged 45 years

## Specific Patterns of Degeneration

### Intervertebral Disc Degeneration

Disc degeneration is signified by tears within the annulus fibrosus. Disruption of the normal contour of the annulus leads to disc bulges and substantial tears lead to disc herniation. There is debate over the significance of hydration of the nucleus. Some studies have shown that there is little change in the hydration and that the signal changes observed on magnetic resonance imaging (MRI) may be regarded as fibrotic changes occurring with annular tears. However, there is up to a 20% decrease in hydration by the third decade of life. The annulus does not normally contain substantial vessels or large numbers of nerve fibres; those who undertake discographic procedures are aware that the periphery of the annulus is a very sensitive area. During the degenerate process there is increasing vascularization and an increasing number of nerve fibres

J. Hodler et al. (eds.), *Musculoskeletal Diseases 2013-2016,*
DOI: 10.1007/978-88-470-5292-5_17 © Springer-Verlag Italia 2013

within the degenerate material. In the late stages of degeneration, tears may allow extrusion of nucleus pulposus material into a hernial sac. Disc herniation is very common and may be confined to the region deep within the longitudinal ligament, or may herniate into the spinal canal, or at any point around the periphery of the vertebral disc. The majority of disc hernias are asymptomatic; however, those that cause compression of nerve roots may produce leg pain and neurological deficit.

There is considerable evidence that the acute disc herniation releases a number of chemicals that exacerbate the symptoms. These include prostaglandins, tumor necrosis factor and interleukin.

Annular tears may be associated with a small high-intensity zone within the margins of the tear. The so-called high-intensity zone has been associated with increased incidence of pain arising from the affected disc. There is evidence from a comparison of lumbar discography with the high-intensity zone seen on MRI showing that there is a strong association. However, this is not a universal finding and there are patients who will have asymptomatic high-intensity zones.

## Joint Degeneration

Facet joint arthropathy follows a similar pattern to osteoarthritis elsewhere in the body. Cartilage fragmentation and thinning is associated with the formation of marginal osteophytes. Bone edema deep to the articular surface resolves. Hypertrophy of the margins of the joint leads to osteophytes that may in turn compress adjacent nerve roots. Mechanical instability of the facet joints arises due to disruption of the normal attachment of the capsule of the joints. Subchondral cysts may form within the facet joints leading to further structural collapse.

The disc space is not a synovial joint; however, osteophytes may form at the insertion of the longitudinal ligaments. Traction osteophytes are associated with mechanical segment instability and may in turn lead to nerve root compression.

Osteophyte formation is more common in the areas of maximum mobility, including the lower lumbar region and the mid-cervical region.

Ligamentous trauma may lead to premature degeneration resulting in an unstable segment.

Although not a direct result of degeneration, osteoporosis may lead to fractures, which in turn cause mechanical instability of the segment and accelerate degenerative changes. In many, the pain associated with vertebral fractures is difficult to disassociate from that resulting from facet joint overload in the same area. Facet joint overload is due to mechanical changes in the shape and structure of the spine.

The combination of facet joint instability and disc degeneration with reduction in vertebral height of the disc will lead to shortening of the spinal column, which in turn may lead to additional mechanical instability and nerve root entrapment.

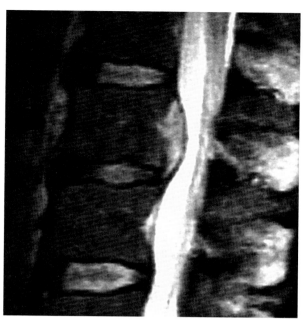

**Fig. 2.** Intervertebral disc prolapse with sequestration; note the increased signal in the disc fragment indicating separation from the parent disc (for color reproduction p 306)

## Nerve Compression and Spinal Claudication

In younger patients, the commonest cause of nerve root compression is disc prolapse. Some patients with lytic spondylolisthesis may also show entrapment of the exiting nerve roots. Older patients with disc space narrowing, facet joint osteoarthritis and facet joint synovial cysts are more likely to have bony entrapment in the narrow exit foramina. In many patients, the nerve compression is multifactorial [1, 2].

Osteophyte formation, loss of height and buckling of the ligament and flavum may cause further narrowing of the spinal canal. This may be associated with disc prolapse, which may worsen or could be the primary cause of the narrowing or stenosis. Spinal stenosis crowds the blood supply to the cauda equina and may cause claudication symptoms, with back pain and leg symptoms associated with walking, which is then relieved by rest. Spinal stenosis of this nature tends to be progressive and it is unusual to see spontaneous improvement. Clinical examination of the peripheral blood supply is important to differentiate spinal from vascular causes. Lateral recess stenosis without central canal stenosis may also cause claudicant symptoms, but is often confined to one side or limited segmental innervation regions [3] (Fig. 2).

## Sagittal Imbalance

Osteoporosis is normally considered a metabolic disorder and not a degenerative disease. However the very high incidence of insufficiency fractures in the aging population

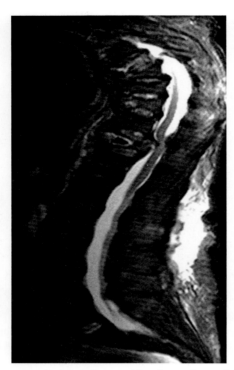

**Fig. 3.** Severe sagittal imbalance with advanced spondylosis and multiple insufficiency fractures

is linked to symptoms associated with degenerative disease. Fractures are most often asymptomatic or minimally symptomatic and therefore occur insidiously in older individuals [4]. The structural change due to vertebral collapse increases load on adjacent segments and the overall deterioration in sagittal balance causes pain in remote parts of the spine. Therefore, those with insufficiency fractures old or new will have a predisposition to postural pain resulting from what may be termed "adult spinal deformity". The concept of sagittal balance is useful. When standing, the center of the C7 vertebral body should be vertically above the centre of the S1 vertebral body. With worsening kyphosis, the first compensation to prevent losing balance is to rotate the pelvis with the iliac crests more posterior and the acetabulae more anterior. When this compensation is exhausted some increase in the cervical and lumbar lordotic curves will occur, and this leads to extra load on the facet joints and may cause impingement of the spinous processes (Baarstrup's disease). These are common causes of pain on standing. Eventually even these compensations are insufficient and walking is only possible leaning on a walking frame or sticks (Fig. 3).

## Role of Imaging

The goals of imaging and assessing patients with symptoms related to degenerative disease are as follows. (1) To exclude other diseases that may mimic degenerative

symptoms; this includes tumor, infection and fracture. (2) To determine the site and nature of nerve root compression and to plan potential surgical intervention. (3) To assess the extent of spinal stenosis to plan surgical intervention. (4) To assess the nature of the disc degeneration to plan percutaneous or surgical intervention.

## Investigations

Imaging investigations that may be used include conventional radiographs, MRI, computed tomography (CT), bone scintigraphy, pain provocation and diagnostic anesthetic blocks. Imaging may also be used to guide percutaneous treatment methods.

### Conventional Radiographs

Conventional radiographs have been largely supplanted by the use of MRI as a primary technique. The radiograph is useful in judging the height and shape of vertebral bodies and the integrity of the pedicles on the anterior view. Osteophytes, disc space narrowing and disc calcification may be observed. Fractures may be assessed or excluded. Congenital anomalies, including transitional vertebrae, can be assessed, and this is particularly useful prior to surgery.

Currently, standing radiographs are the principal means of imaging problems of adult spinal deformity and sagittal balance. However, those who are imbalanced may not be able to stand unaided, and in moderate to severe cases the need to hold onto a support while being examined may give misleading results.

### Computed Tomography

Combining bone and soft tissue windows on CT images will allow a moderate assessment of the integrity of the intervertebral discs, as well as a measurement of the diameter of the bony spinal canal. Prior to the use of magnetic resonance, CT was useful in the assessment of disc herniation and nerve root compression, and therefore provides an alternative to magnetic resonance examination in patients who are unable to enter a magnetic resonance scanner for reasons of claustrophobia or contraindications such as an implanted electronic device. Lesions that destroy bone, such as tumors or infection, are particularly well imaged using CT where the structure and integrity of the spine is well demonstrated by sagittal and coronal reconstructions.

If there is doubt regarding root compression and the patient is not suitable for MRI, then contrast-enhanced CT especially CT myelography can be employed.

### Magnetic Resonance Imaging

MRI is the mainstay of imaging of the spine.

Images should be acquired in sagittal and axial planes using sequences that will assess the anatomy, the

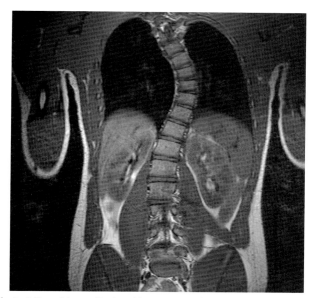

**Fig. 4.** Idiopathic scoliosis with no congenital vertebral anomalies

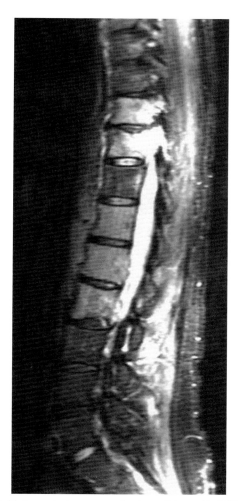

**Fig. 5.** Multiple metastases seen best on this sagittal FSTIR sequence; sclerotic metastases from breast or prostate cancer can only be seen on T1-weighted images

fatty content of bone marrow and edema in soft tissues and bone. Occasionally, coronal images are useful, especially in those with scoliosis or other spinal deformities (Fig. 4).

MRI can be used to assess the bone content, exclude tumors, infection and fracture, assess for disc herniation, nerve root compression and spinal stenosis. In the majority of patients MRI of the spine will be the only imaging required to make a reasonable diagnosis as the cause of the patient's symptoms.

For the exclusion of metastatic disease it is important to combine both fat imaging sequences with water imaging sequences. Sclerotic metastases are best seen on the former, and soft metastases on the latter (Fig. 5).

Newer techniques, including functional imaging, show promise in monitoring the outcome of treatment [5, 6].

With the exception of detailing the nature of a fracture, MRI will achieve all the imaging roles listed above.

## Review of an Imaging Investigation

In all imaging, the important approach is to have a structured review of the examination. A useful template for reviewing the spine is to assess:

- the discs
- height of the interspaces
- the bones
- the facet joints
- the vertebral endplates
- the cross section of each level examination by axial imaging
- the presence or absence of tumor, infection or fracture
- the integrity of the structures adjacent to the spine, including lymph nodes, vessels, paravertebral soft tissues, kidneys and liver
- alignment and sagittal balance.

Probably the most difficult issue is to recognise degenerative lesions that are symptomatic. Conventional radiography, CT and MRI cannot image pain and most individuals over 35 years of age have clearly apparent but asymptomatic degenerative disease of discs, joints and ligaments [7, 8]. Careful correlation between symptoms, clinical signs and the imaging appearances is essential. When there is doubt, pain blocking or provocation procedures will assist in the diagnosis.

### Pain Provocation

The placement of needles or injections of fluid into facet joints or the intervertebral discs may be used to assess the potential sources of pain. This depends on the patient being sufficiently conscious to give a response to the injection process. Imaging may be used to position the needles and this may either be fluoroscopy or CT.

Anesthetic blocks of nerve roots, the facet joints or the paravertebral muscles may be used for diagnostic purposes. Injection into the discs (discography) is used, but

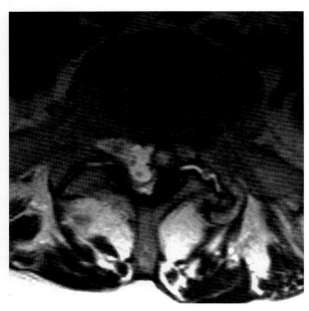

**Fig. 6.** A synovial cyst arising from the left facet joint is causing root compression

the interpretation of findings is complex and controversial [9].

The interpretation of the outcome of such procedures is difficult as it depends very much on the symptoms of the patient. A particular problem is that the pain can often arise from more than one structure.

Cysts arising from the intervertebral facet joints may cause nerve root compression. These may be readily identified on cross-sectional imaging. Treatment by a percutaneous aspiration or percutaneous pressure rupture may be an effective management to avoid the need for surgery (Fig. 6).

The therapeutic potential of nerve root blocks, epidural injections and facet joint injections will not be discussed further in this syllabus.

## Conclusion

The key to the use of imaging in spinal degeneration is to have a careful correlation between the symptoms, signs and imaging findings. In general, maximum importance should be placed on the patient's symptoms rather than the imaging findings given the very high incidence of asymptomatic degenerative change. Care should be taken to recognize asymptomatic degeneration.

The role of imaging in excluding sinister disease such as tumor [10], infection or fracture is pivotal in management. In particular, MRI is sensitive to all of these conditions and a normal study will be reassuring and will assist both the patient and the clinician.

## References

1. Issack PS, Cunningham ME, Pumberger M et al (2012) Degenerative lumbar spinal stenosis: evaluation and management. J Am Acad Orthop Surg 20:527-535
2. Wassenaar M, van Rijn RM, van Tulder MW et al (2012) Magnetic resonance imaging for diagnosing lumbar spinal pathology in adult patients with low back pain or sciatica: a diagnostic systematic review. Eur Spine J 21:220-227
3. Maus TP (2012) Imaging of spinal stenosis: neurogenic intermittent claudication and cervical spondylotic myelopathy. Radiol Clin North Am 50:651-679
4. Griffith JF, Genant HK (2012) New advances in imaging osteoporosis and its complications. Endocrine 42:39-51
5. Lotz JC, Haughton V, Boden SD et al (2012) New treatments and imaging strategies in degenerative disease of the intervertebral disks. Radiology 264:6-19
6. Wald JT (2012) Imaging of spine neoplasm. Radiol Clin North Am 50:749-776
7. Bogduk N (2012) Degenerative joint disease of the spine. Radiol Clin North Am 50:613-628
8. Del Grande F, Maus TP, Carrino JA (2012) Imaging the intervertebral disk: age-related changes, herniations, and radicular pain. Radiol Clin North Am 50:629-649
9. Maus TP, Aprill CN (2012) Lumbar diskogenic pain, provocation diskography, and imaging correlates. Radiol Clin North Am 50:681-704
10. Thakur NA, Daniels AH, Schiller J et al (2012) Benign tumors of the spine. J Am Acad Orthop Surg 20:715-724

# Imaging of Musculoskeletal Infections

Florian M. Buck[1], Klaus Bohndorf[2]

[1] Radiology, University Clinic Balgrist, University of Zurich, Zurich, Switzerland
[2] Department of Diagnostic Radiology and Neuroradiology, Klinikum Augsburg, Augsburg, Germany

## Introduction

Acute infections of bones, joints and soft tissues are a common clinical problem in children and adults, and considered therapeutic emergencies. Their manifestations are variable and influenced by many circumstances, such as patient age, acute or chronic nature of the infection, infecting organism (bacteria, mycobacteria, fungus), location (bone marrow, bony cortex, periosteum, soft tissue, synovial joint, intervertebral disc), route of infection (hematogenous seeding, contiguous spread, direct traumatic or iatrogenic implantation), and pre-existing predisposing pathologies (immunocompromising diseases, bone diseases, implants).

In the following text, a brief review of some of the concepts of musculoskeletal infection is provided. Imaging of osteomyelitis is frequently discussed along its time course (acute, subacute, chronic). This structure is also adopted in this text. The authors would like to emphasize that no definite distinction exists between one stage and another, nor do all patients go through all of these stages.

## Terminology

*Osteomyelitis*, better called bacterial or infective osteomyelitis, is defined as an infection of bone marrow, whereas the term *spondylitis* is used if the bone marrow of a vertebral body is affected. *Infective osteitis* implies involvement of the bony cortex. In surgical usage the term is related to an exogenous route of infection. Infection of the periosteum is called *infective periostitis*. *Soft tissue infection* is a general term for infections of cutaneous and subcutaneous tissues as well as *myositis*, *fasciitis*, *bursitis* and contamination of tendons and ligaments. The term *septic arthritis* indicates infection of a joint originating from the synovial membrane, whereas the term *septic spondyloarthritis* is appropriate for the facet joints of the spine. *Infective discitis* means contamination of an intervertebral disc whereas *infective spondylodiscitis* implies infection of a vertebral body and an adjacent intervertebral disc.

These types of infection can develop separately or in various combinations, generally evolving in a typical sequence over time depending on the route of infection. *Inside-out infection* is typically initiated by osteomyelitis due to hematogenous seeding of the infecting organism to the bone marrow, and may be followed by infective osteitis, periostitis, soft tissue infection, abscess formation and sinus formation to the skin in that order if not treated correctly [1]. *Outside-in infection* can be caused by a soft tissue infection due to a skin lesion in a patient suffering from diabetes. Abscess formation, infective periostitis, infective osteitis and osteomyelitis may follow in that order.

## Etiology and Pathogenesis

Depending on the route of infection and comorbidity of the patient, different infecting organisms are typically found in patients suffering from osteomyelitis.

The most common route of infection is hematogenous seeding and the most commonly encountered infecting organisms in endogenous hematogenous osteomyelitis are Gram-positive bacteria, in the majority of cases staphylococci (e.g., *Staphylococcus aureus*) and streptococci in infants. Osteomyelitis following direct traumatic or iatrogenic inoculation is more commonly caused by Gram-negative bacteria. Superimposed infections of feet in diabetic patients with reduced peripheral blood supply are commonly caused by anaerobic bacteria or have a polymicrobial composition. A large variety of mycobacteria and fungi can also be the cause of osteomyelitis and spondylodiscitis.

## Acute Osteomyelitis

Symptoms of acute osteomyelitis turn up within days. Early treatment of osteomyelitis is crucial to prevent

J. Hodler et al. (eds.), *Musculoskeletal Diseases 2013-2016*,
DOI: 10.1007/978-88-470-5292-5_18 © Springer-Verlag Italia 2013

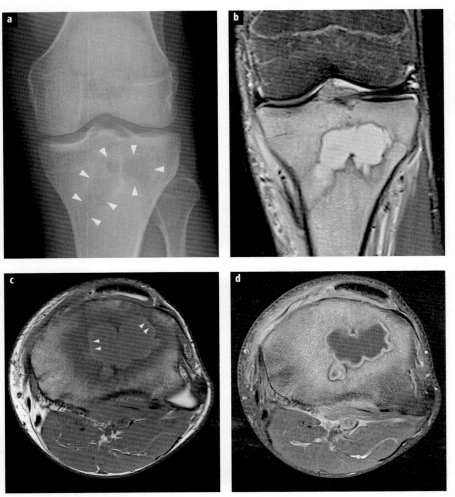

**Fig. 1 a-d.** Osteomyelitis and bone abscess in the left tibial head of a 24-year-old man. **a** Anteroposterior radiograph of the left knee shows focal trabecular lysis involving the tibial head (*arrowheads*). **b** Coronal STIR image shows an osteolytic area with marked perifocal bone marrow edema and reactive periosteal and soft tissue edema at the medial aspect of the tibial head. **c** On the axial T1-weighted turbo spin-echo image there is a barely visible thin hyperintense line ("penumbra sign") at the border of the abscess (*arrowheads*). **d** The corresponding T1-weighted fat-suppressed post-contrast image shows linear peripheral contrast enhancement of the abscess and lack of central enhancement. There is also contrast enhancement of the periosteal membrane and adjacent soft tissue at the anteromedial aspect of the tibial head

complications. Long bones (femur, tibia, humerus) are most commonly affected. Depending on changes to the vascular anatomy of long bones during growth, hematogenous osteomyelitis typically affects the metaphysis or epiphysis of a bone. In infants up to approximately 1 year, fetal vascular blood supply connecting the metaphysis and epiphysis enables epiphyseal involvement of osteomyelitis. In children (1-year-old until closure of growth plate), the metaphyseal growth plate acts as a barrier for the blood flow [2]. Therefore, the epiphysis is locked and the physis prevents spreading of osteomyelitis from the metaphysis to the epiphysis. In adults, closure of the growth plate and restoration of nutrient vessels connecting metaphysis and epiphysis permit epiphyseal involvement of osteomyelitis.

Plain radiographs are generally the first imaging modality employed if osteomyelitis is suspected. However, because it can take several days to some weeks for radiography to be positive, radiography is not particularly suited to diagnose acute osteomyelitis. It has its benefits to supervise response to therapy [3]. Soft tissue swelling and blurring of adjacent fat planes, periosteal

reaction, osteolysis and cortical erosions are typical findings (Fig. 1).

A fluid-sensitive STIR-sequence or fat-suppressed intermediate or T2-weighted turbo spin-echo sequence is the mainstay of magnetic resonance (MR) imaging in the evaluation of suspected osteomyelitis. Acute osteomyelitis can be excluded in the absence of an abnormal high signal in fluid-sensitive sequences [4]. An additional T1-weighted spin-echo sequence is acquired to evaluate the extent and location of osteomyelitis. T1-weighted fat-suppressed spin-echo sequences after intravenous administration of gadolinium-bearing contrast media is the sequence of choice to distinguish abscesses or necrotic tissue from inflammatory edema [5, 6]. On MR images, an ill-defined area within the bone marrow, which is hyperintense on fluid-sensitive sequences and hypointense on T1-weighted sequences, is the typical presentation of acute osteomyelitis [7]. Generally, the size of the lesion is smaller on T1-weighted sequences than on fluid-sensitive sequences or contrast-enhanced fat-suppressed T1-weighted sequences [8]. Perifocal edema is a hallmark of acute osteomyelitis. Without its presence or if the perifocal edema is very thin, the diagnosis of osteomyelitis has to be questioned. Edema in the adjacent periosteal membrane, soft tissue edema and reactive synovitis of adjacent joints may be present. A bone abscess is defined as a circumscribed site of active infection surrounded by sclerotic bone and granulation tissue. Abscesses typically occur in a subperiosteal location in children or in the bone marrow in adults. Both, abscesses and reactive edema are characterized by hyperintense signal on fluid-sensitive sequences. Peripheral enhancement and lack of central enhancement on gadolinium-enhanced sequences is diagnostic of an abscess. Occasionally, a hyperintense rim at the margin of an abscess can be seen on T1-weighted images, which is called "penumbra sign" (Fig. 1c) [9]. The penumbra sign is highly specific for musculoskeletal infection and helpful in differentiating neoplasm from infection [10]. Secondary septic arthritis in osteomyelitis located within the epiphysis is difficult to differentiate from reactive joint effusion and contrast media enhancement of the synovial membrane. In the course of disease there is often a smooth transition from reactive changes in a joint to septic arthritis. Joint effusion and mild synovitis are compatible with reactive changes, whereas septic arthritis is characterized by marked synovitis and enhancement of the adjacent soft tissue. The spectrum of imaging findings in patients with acute osteomyelitis, neoplastic bone disease and stress fractures sometimes overlap. Biopsy may be needed to rule out bone tumors or to identify the causing organism. The latter only makes sense if there was no previous antibiotic therapy.

## Chronic Osteomyelitis

Long-standing osteomyelitis over at least 4-6 weeks is defined as chronic osteomyelitis. Clinically less severe, non-septic disease is sometimes termed subacute osteomyelitis.

Brodie's abscess is the classical form of a clinically less severe osteomyelitis. In around 50% of cases *Staphylococcus aureus* can be cultivated. Brodie's abscess is characterized by a sharply delineated focus of infection.

Chronic osteomyelitis in almost all cases occurs due to nonhematogenous route of infection (chronic exogenous osteomyelitis). Primary chronic osteomyelitis initiated by hematogenous seeding is possible but rare [11]. These cases mostly represent acute osteomyelitis with inadequate antibiotic therapy, which turn to chronicity.

The classical route of infection in chronic exogenous osteomyelitis is by direct inoculation of pathogens into the soft tissues and/or bone (traumatic or iatrogenic). The other route is penetration of injured barriers (skin, teeth). Chronic osteomyelitis in the majority of cases shows an acute onset, followed by a chronic course of disease with a strong tendency to relapse. Chronic osteomyelitis is a long-standing disease.

Signs of relapse in the time course of chronic osteomyelitis are destruction of infected bone and formation of new bone, presence of an abscess, sequestrum or involucrum. Formation of a sinus tract, cloaca or fistula may ensue. An abscess in primary chronic osteomyelitis is typically caused by low-virulence organisms and is generally large in size. The term sequestrum indicates a piece of necrotic bone located in the bone marrow or soft tissue without connection to living bone. Sequestra may embody infective organisms and therefore constitute a source of recurrent disease. A sequestrum is characterized by signal-void on fluid-sensitive sequences and lack of contrast enhancement. Bony substance around a sequestrum exhibits hyperintense signal on fluid-sensitive sequences. Reactive, mostly periosteal, new bone formation encapsulating a sequestrum is called an involucrum. An involucrum can completely surround a sequestrum or become perforated by sinus tracts depending on immune competence of the patient and the aggressiveness of the infective organism. A sinus tract increasing in size and forming a gap in the periosteum/involucrum through which pus may discharge is called a cloaca (Fig. 2). Fistulation denotes sinus tracts connecting two internal organs or an internal organ with the skin surface [1].

MR imaging of chronic osteomyelitis follows the same principles as described for acute osteomyelitis. Infection of the bone marrow is characterized by low signal intensity on T1-weighted images and high signal on fluid-sensitive sequences when compared with unaffected bone marrow. On gadolinium-enhanced sequences, granulation tissue and the membrane of an abscess typically enhance, whereas the center of an abscess does not. On diffusion-weighted images, the center of an abscess typically demonstrates high diffusivity [high signal on diffusion-weighted images and low signal on apparent diffusion coefficient (ADC) maps] [12]. This enables identification of pus formations and differentiation from cystic lesions [13, 14]. During the first months after trauma/surgery, osteomyelitis is difficult to distinguish from nonspecific postoperative/post-traumatic changes such as edema, granulation tissue and fibrosis on MR images [15, 16]. Therefore, an abscess or fistula needs to be present to justify the diagnosis of bacterial osteomyelitis. In later stages, marked remodeling processes, such as osteosclerosis, persistent callus and soft tissue fibrosis, may be impressive.

Susceptibility artifacts due to metallic implants may considerably lessen image quality and necessitate adaptation of the imaging protocol. Measures to reduce susceptibility artifacts are: using a scanner with lower magnetic field strength, increasing receiver band-width, reducing echo time, reducing slice thickness, using fast spin-echo sequences instead of spin-echo sequences, using STIR-sequences instead of frequency-selective fat saturation, or utilizing novel sequences combining in-plane and through-plane correction for metallic artifacts (e.g., view-angle tilting, VAT, or slice encoding for metal artifact correction, SEMAC, technique) [17].

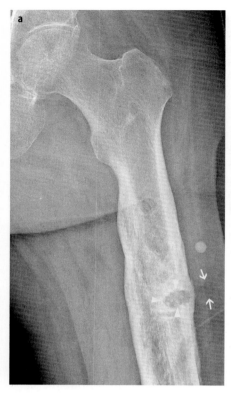
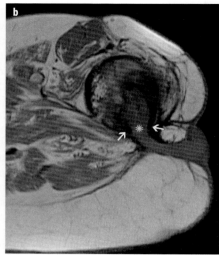
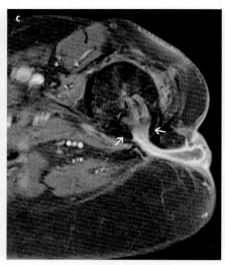

**Fig. 2 a-c.** Chronic post-traumatic osteomyelitis and cloaca in a 64-year-old man 1 year after a compound femoral fracture. **a** Anteroposterior radiograph of the left femur demonstrates marked post-traumatic remodeling and a solitary soft tissue calcification at the lateral aspect of the femoral shaft. There is a well-defined osteolytic area (*arrowheads*) and peripheral osteosclerosis. In the adjacent lateral soft tissues, a barely visible hypodense area (*arrows*) raises suspicion for soft tissue involvement. On the axial T1-weighted turbo spin-echo image (**b**) and the corresponding T1-weighted fat-suppressed post-contrast image (**c**), there is a wide cortical defect (*) with adjacent periosteal new bone formation (involucrum) (*arrows*). Pus discharges in the adjacent soft tissue forming an abscess without visible fistulation through the skin but marked subcutaneous edema

## Septic Arthritis

Septic arthritis is a medical emergency. Hematogenous spread to the synovial membrane and subsequent infection of the joint fluid is the most common route of infection. Otherwise spreading from adjacent (epiphyseal) osteomyelitis or soft tissue infection, post-traumatic direct implantation, postoperative septic arthritis following injections, surgery or arthroplasty is possible. The diagnosis is generally made by joint aspiration. On radiographs, the first signs of septic arthritis are periarticular soft-tissue swelling, joint effusion with articular distention, and fuzziness of periarticular fat planes. In pyogenic infections, proteolytic enzymes released by leukocytes and lysosomes based in the synovial membrane rapidly degrade joint cartilage. Therefore, joint space narrowing, bony erosions and juxta-articular osteoporosis are early changes. In tuberculous arthritis, periarticular osteopenia is the main feature, whereas joint space narrowing and bony erosions occur late in the course of the disease.

On MR images, joint effusion and a markedly thickened synovial membrane with contrast enhancement are mandatory for the diagnosis of septic arthritis. Without their presence septic arthritis can be excluded [18]. However, differentiation from reactive changes due to adjacent infection, rheumatoid arthritis or sterile synovitis (e.g., coxitis fugax) may be difficult.

In primary septic arthritis, contrast enhancement of adjacent bone and increased signal intensity on fluid-sensitive sequences are common findings and do not necessarily represent osteomyelitis [19]. Adjacent osteomyelitis may be difficult to differentiate from reactive bone changes. The presence of bone marrow changes isolated to one side of the infected joint, obvious bone erosions and periosteal reaction suggests osteomyelitis [1].

## The Diabetic Foot

In the diabetic foot, peripheral neuropathy and reduced trophic conditions due to peripheral arterial occlusive disease promote diabetic neuroarthropathy ("Charcot foot") and ulceration at the sole of the foot [20]. Wound healing and infection defense are hampered.

The route of infection in the majority of cases of osteomyelitis in patients suffering from diabetes is direct inoculation through soft-tissue infection and ulceration at the sole of the foot (exogenous chronic osteomyelitis) [21]. Ulcers are typically located at the plantar aspect of the forefoot (metatarsal heads, phalanges) and the hindfoot (calcaneus) where increased pressure prevails. Diabetic neuroarthropathy mostly affects midfoot joints, leading to collapse of the longitudinal arc of the foot. In advanced collapse the cuboid achieves a weight-bearing position ("rocker bottom deformity") and subjacent ulcers may develop [22]. Therefore, superinfection of advanced diabetic neuroarthropathy often occurs plantar to the midfoot.

Both osteomyelitis and acute stage neuroarthropathy may develop rapidly and are characterized by bone marrow edema on fluid-sensitive sequences. Bone marrow edema in osteomyelitis is characterized by a confluent pattern of decreased T1 marrow signal intensity in a geographic medullary distribution [7]. The high signal intensity bone marrow in T1-weighted spin-echo images is generally less reduced in case of reactive bone marrow edema compared with the very low signal in osteomyelitis due to residual fat within the marrow of noninfected bones [23]. The presence of an abscess and cortical destruction is indicative of osteomyelitis. The "ghost sign" is a typical sign of cortical destruction [20]. It is characterized by almost imperceptible margins of a bone on T1-weighted images, which become visible after application of contrast media. In the absence of an ulcer and in the presence of sclerosis without significant edema osteomyelitis is unlikely.

## Chronic Recurrent Multifocal Osteomyelitis

Chronic recurrent multifocal osteomyelitis (CRMO) is not caused by an infective organism, but it is an inflammatory bone disease of unknown etiology. Because of some similarities with SAPHO (synovitis, acne, pustulosis, hyperostosis and osteitis) syndrome, CRMO and SAPHO may be manifestations of the same underlying disease [24]. Children and young adults are mostly affected with a peak incidence at 4-14 years. Typically there are multiple lesions, but only one being symptomatic [25]. Fluid-sensitive sequences are helpful in finding additional lesions. 99mTc bone scans or whole body MR imaging may be useful to identify additional foci. The metaphyses of long bones are mostly affected, and symmetrical involvement has been described in many cases.

Differentiation of CRMO and infective osteomyelitis may be challenging. Imaging characteristics are comparable to those of acute or chronic osteomyelitis. However, fistula or abscess formation does not exist in CRMO. Clinical history (slow onset, vague pain), laboratory findings (no or minimal erythrocyte sedimentation rate, ESR, and C-reactive protein, CRP, elevation) and the multiplicity of the lesions allow distinction from bacterial osteomyelitis in most of the cases, making biopsy and antibiotic therapy unnecessary. Histology reveals an nonspecific chronic inflammatory response, and cultures are usually negative unless there was contamination during biopsy procedure.

## Infectious Spondylitis and Spondylodiscitis

Four different manifestations of spinal infections can be distinguished: spondylitis, discitis, spondylodiscitis and spondyloarthritis.

Spinal infections in children and adolescents are rare. In adults, however, spondylitis is the most common form of hematogenous osteomyelitis. Secondary invasion of the adjacent intervertebral disc causes infectious discitis. Most frequently found infecting organisms are *Staphylococcus aureus* and *Mycobacterium tuberculosis*.

Isolated discitis is rare. In adults, inciting events are surgical interventions with direct inoculation of infective organisms into the disc. Hematogenous discitis is only possible in children, where nutrient vessels supply the growing disc, and degenerative disc disease, where secondary vessel ingrowth occurs in the otherwise not perfused mature intervertebral disc. Spondyloarthritis usually follows therapeutic interventions, but may also be caused by adjacent spondylodiscitis.

Although MR imaging is the imaging method of choice for vertebral osteomyelitis and discitis in the early stages, it may show subtle, nonspecific endplate subchondral changes and a repeat examination may be required to show the typical features [26]. MR imaging characteristics of acute spondylitis are the same as those of acute osteomyelitis. The same applies for intraosseous abscesses. A T1-weighted sagittal sequence to depict endplate destruction and a fluid-sensitive sagittal sequence to visualize bone marrow edema are the cornerstones in the evaluation of suspected spondylodiscitis. Additional contrast-enhanced sequences are most sensitive for early infection. Involvement of the adjacent disc is generally seen early and characterized by a reduction of disc height, T2-hyperintense signal changes and contrast enhancement within the disc. In contrast to early loss of disc height and destruction of vertebral endplates in acute spondylodiscitis, tuberculosis is characterized by bone destruction with maintained disc height and no substantial changes to the endplates until late in the course of the disease.

Epidural and paravertebral abscess formation are often encountered complications. Abscesses may spread over a long distance in a craniocaudal direction, which is why at least one fluid-sensitive or contrast-enhanced fat-saturated sequence should be acquired using the widest field of view possible. Compared with cerebrospinal fluid, an abscess is a slightly more hyperintense on T1-weighted images and less hyperintense on T2-weighted images. To reliably differentiate diffuse soft tissue infection from an abscess, transverse contrast-enhanced images are recommended. Soft tissue infection typically enhances uniformly, whereas an abscess is void of contrast enhancement centrally. Contrast enhancement within the myelon is suggestive of direct spread into the myelon (infective myelitis).

The differential diagnosis of spondylodiscitis includes edematous degenerative signal changes in the vertebral endplates due to disc degeneration (Modic type I changes) and metastatic disease [27, 28]. In the postoperative setting, it may be impossible to differentiate spondylodiscitis from postoperative edema and granulation tissue unless there is an abscess. The diagnosis may only become apparent in the course of the disease.

# References

1. Resnick D (2007) Infectious disorders of bones, joints, and soft tissues. In: Resnick D, Kang HS, Pretterklieber ML (Eds) Internal derangements of joints, 2nd edn. Saunders Elsevier, Philadelphia, pp 371-393

2. van Schuppen J, van Doorn MMAC, van Rijn RR (2012) Childhood osteomyelitis: imaging characteristics. Insights imaging 3:519-533

3. Jaramillo D (2011) Infection: musculoskeletal. Pediatr Radiol 41 Suppl 1:S127-134

4. Wunsch R, Darge K, Rohrschneider W et al (2001) Acute hematogenous osteomyelitis-exclusion with Turbo-STIR sequence? Radiologe 41:439-441

5. Hopkins KL, Li KC, Bergman G (1995) Gadolinium-DTPA-enhanced magnetic resonance imaging of musculoskeletal infectious processes. Skeletal Radiol 24:325-330

6. Kan JH, Young RS, Yu C, Hernanz-Schulman M (2010) Clinical impact of gadolinium in the MRI diagnosis of musculoskeletal infection in children. Pediatr Radiol 40:1197-1205

7. Howe BM, Wenger DE, Mandrekar J, Collins MS (2012) T1-weighted MRI imaging features of pathologically proven non-pedal osteomyelitis. Acad Radiol Sep 2012 [epub ahead of print]

8. Jones KM, Unger EC, Granstrom P et al (1992) Bone marrow imaging using STIR at 0.5 and 1.5 T. J Magn Reson Imaging 10:169-176

9. Grey AC, Davies AM, Mangham DC et al (1998) The 'penumbra sign' on T1-weighted MR imaging in subacute osteomyelitis: frequency, cause and significance. Clin Radiol 53:587-592

10. McGuinness B, Wilson N, Doyle AJ (2007) The "penumbra sign" on T1-weighted MRI for differentiating musculoskeletal infection from tumour. Skeletal Radiol 36:417-421

11. Munoz P, Bouza E (1999) Acute and chronic adult osteomyelitis and prosthesis-related infections. Baillieres Best Pract Res Clin Rheumatol 13:129-147

12. Bitzer M, Schick F, Hartmann J et al (2002) MRI of intraosseous fistulous systems and sequesters in chronic osteomyelitis with standard spin echo sequences, highly selective chemical-shift imaging, diffusion weighted imaging, and magnetization-transfer. Rofo 174:1422-1429

13. Unal O, Koparan HI, Avcu S et al (2011) The diagnostic value of diffusion-weighted magnetic resonance imaging in soft tissue abscesses. Eur J Radiol 77:490-494

14. Harish S, Chiavaras MM, Kotnis N, Rebello R (2011) MR imaging of skeletal soft tissue infection: utility of diffusion-weighted imaging in detecting abscess formation. Skeletal Radiol 40:285-294

15. Bohndorf K (1996) Diagnostic imaging of acute and chronic osteomyelitis. Radiologe 36:786-794.

16. Ledermann HP, Kaim A, Bongartz G, Steinbrich W (2000) Pitfalls and limitations of magnetic resonance imaging in chronic posttraumatic osteomyelitis. Eur Radiol 10:1815-1823

17. Sutter R, Ulbrich EJ, Jellus V et al (2012) Reduction of metal artifacts in patients with total hip arthroplasty with slice-encoding metal artifact correction and view-angle tilting MR imaging. Radiology 265:204-214

18. Karchevsky M, Schweitzer ME, Morrison WB, Parellada JA (2004) MRI findings of septic arthritis and associated osteomyelitis in adults. AJR Am J Roentgenol 182:119-122

19. Graif M, Schweitzer ME, Deely D, Matteucci T (1999) The septic versus nonseptic inflamed joint: MRI characteristics. Skeletal Radiol 28:616-620

20. Toledano TR, Fatone EA, Weis A et al (2011) MRI evaluation of bone marrow changes in the diabetic foot: a practical approach. Semin Musculoskelet Radiol 15:257-268

21. Donovan A, Schweitzer ME (2010) Use of MR imaging in diagnosing diabetes-related pedal osteomyelitis. Radiographics 30:723-736

22. Schoots IG, Slim FJ, Busch-Westbroek TE, Maas M (2010) Neuro-osteoarthropathy of the foot-radiologist: friend or foe? Sem Musculoskelet Radiol 14:365-376

23. Johnson PW, Collins MS, Wenger DE (2009) Diagnostic utility of T1-weighted MRI characteristics in evaluation of osteomyelitis of the foot. AJR Am J Roentgenol 192:96-100

24. Schmit P, Glorion C (2004) Osteomyelitis in infants and children. Eur Radiol 14 Suppl 4:L44-54

25. Iyer RS, Thapa MM, Chew FS (2011) Chronic recurrent multifocal osteomyelitis: review. AJR Am J Roentgenol 196(6 Suppl):S87-91

26. Dunbar JAT, Sandoe JAT, Rao AS et al (2010) The MRI appearances of early vertebral osteomyelitis and discitis. Clin Radiol 65:974-981

27. Pruthi S, Thapa MM (2009) Infectious and inflammatory disorders. Radiol Clin North Am 47:911-926

28. Mellado JM, Pérez del Palomar L, Camins A et al (2004) MR imaging of spinal infection: atypical features, interpretive pitfalls and potential mimickers. Eur Radiol 14:1980-1989

# Ultrasonography: Sports Injuries

Stefano Bianchi[1], Jon A. Jacobson[2]

[1] Cabinet Imagerie Médicale SA, Geneva, Switzerland
[2] Department of Radiology, University of Michigan, Ann Arbor, MI, USA

## Upper Extremity

### Introduction

Musculoskeletal ultrasound (MSUS) is today considered to be one of the most efficient imaging modalities in the assessment of most sport injuries [1, 2]. MSUS is economic, dynamic, noninvasive and patient-friendly. Color Doppler allows accurate assessment of inflammation. A variety of procedures, including hematoma or seroma aspiration and local therapeutic injections, are easily performed under real-time MSUS guidance, thus reducing the risk of injuries to adjacent structures and allowing a more precise and less painful injection. The aims of this chapter are to discuss the role of MSUS in the assessment of sport injuries and to present the sonographic appearances of the main disorders affecting the upper and lower limbs.

## Shoulder

Rotator cuff tears frequently affect sportsmen as the end result of chronic subacromial impingement or acute trauma. Dynamic MSUS, realized during active movements of the arm, can help in the diagnosis of subacromial impingement. Coronal oblique sonograms allow simultaneous assessment of the coracoacromial ligament, subacromial synovial bursa and supraspinatus tendon. Real-time examination during active abduction and antepulsion of the arm can detect subacromial impingement and easily correlate the findings with clinical data, thus confirming the origin of the patient's pain. Subacromial bursitis appears as thickening of the bursa wall that can be associated to an internal effusion or hypervascular changes at color Doppler (Fig. 1). When there is an associated tendinopathy, the tendon is thickened and irregularly hypoechoic. Tears of the rotators tendons are easily detected.

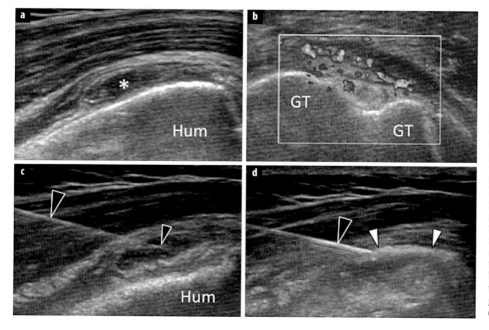

**Fig. 1 a-d.** Subacromial bursitis. Coronal oblique (**a**) and axial (**b**) sonograms show the subacromial synovial bursa presenting a thick hypervascularized wall and some fluid content (*asterisk*). **c** MSUS-guided intrabursal injection. Note the needle (*black arrowheads*) correctly positioned under the real-time guidance of ultrasound. The tip of the needle (*small black arrowhead*) lies inside the bursa. **d** After injection of a small amount of steroid-lidocaine, note the drug (*white arrowheads*) filling the bursa. No injection into the surrounding tissues is noted. *Hum* humerus, *GT* greater tuberosity of the humeral head (for color reproduction see p 302)

J. Hodler et al. (eds.), *Musculoskeletal Diseases 2013-2016*,
DOI: 10.1007/978-88-470-5292-5_19 © Springer-Verlag Italia 2013

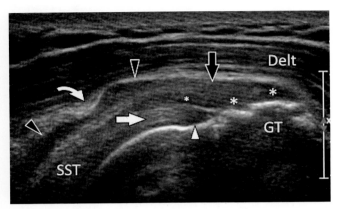

**Fig. 2.** Supraspinatus tendon partial tear. Coronal oblique sonogram obtained over the axis of the supraspinatus tendon (*SST*) at the anterior third. Sonogram shows an avulsion (*asterisks*) of the bursal two-thirds (*black arrow*) of the supraspinatus tendon associated with a horizontal tear (*small asterisk*). The deep third of the tendon (*white arrow*) is continuous. Note the hypoechoic appearance of its preinsertional part (*white arrowhead*) due to anisotropy. The subacromial synovial bursa (*black arrowheads*) presents an internal fluid effusion. Note the coracoacromial ligament (*curved arrow*). *Delt* deltoid muscle, *GT* greater tuberosity of the humeral head

MSUS can evaluate the involved tendons (subscapularis, supraspinatus, infraspinatus or teres minor), and appreciate the tear size (partial or full thickness tear, complete tear) and its location (anterior, middle or posterior part of the involved tendon) [3] (Fig. 2). In addition, MSUS can evaluate atrophy and fat infiltrations of the muscle, thus helping with the therapeutic decision [4] (Fig. 3).

MSUS plays only a minor role in the assessment of glenohumeral instability, because it cannot assess accurately the glenoid labrum because of its deep location. MSUS can detect a Hill-Sachs fracture and evaluate its size. In posterior shoulder dislocation, which can go undiagnosed at radiography in nearly 50% of cases, MSUS can detect the posterior displacement of the humeral head in relation to the glenoid in axial sonograms, obtained over either the anterior or the posterior aspect of the joint. MSUS-guided injection of the acromioclavicular joint can be performed if pain persists after joint instability.

Spinoglenoid and supraglenoid notch ganglia, caused by degeneration or trauma of the glenoid labrum, can be associated with sports that use a repetitive overhead action. As a result of their location, they can compress the suprascapular nerve and lead to ill-defined shoulder pain and muscle fat degeneration and atrophy. They appear on MSUS as well-marginated hypoanechoic masses with no internal flow signals at color Doppler. The relation with the nerve can seldom be demonstrated because of the small size of the nerve. Sometimes, a labrum tear can be visualized at MSUS. Muscle edema, the first manifestation of nerve denervation, cannot be assessed by MSUS. Hypotrophy is detected as a decrease of the size of the muscle and is usually more visible in axial sonograms. Fat infiltration starts at the myotendinous junction and presents as an increased echogenicity of the muscle.

MSUS can accurately assess the extra-articular portion of the long head of the biceps tendon (LHBT). Most tears of LHBT are easily diagnosed clinically in the presence of a local post-traumatic pain and lump in the anterior aspect of the lower arm corresponding to the displaced muscle belly. MSUS is only indicated when the clinical findings are not diagnostic, such as in obese patients in whom the palpation of the retracted muscle can be difficult. MSUS shows absence of the tendon inside the humeral sulcus with concomitant inferior muscle retraction. The injured tendon and muscle can be surrounded by a hematoma in acute cases. MSUS can accurately show fat infiltrations of the muscle by comparing it with the normal short head of the biceps in axial images. LHBT instability is associated with rotator cuff interval or subscapularis tears. Its recognition can be difficult clinically. MSUS easily demonstrates the medial displacement of the tendon in axial images. In subluxation, the tendon is located over the anterior aspect of the lesser tuberosity, while in tendon dislocation it lies completely outside the sulcus. A careful scanning technique is necessary to detect the intra-articular displacement of the LHBT (Fig. 4).

MSUS allows accurate, safe and quick injections of subacromial bursa, glenohumeral and acromioclavicular

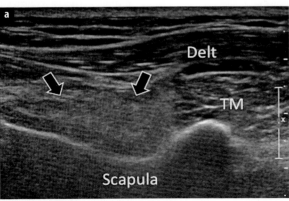
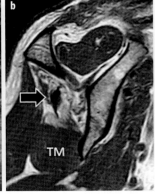

**Fig. 3 a, b.** Infraspinatus muscle fat degeneration due to chronic tendon tear. **a** Sagittal oblique sonogram obtained over the posterior aspect of the scapula. **b** Corresponding sagittal oblique T1-weighted magnetic resonance image. The hypotrophic infraspinatus muscle (*arrows*) shows a hyperechogenic appearance due to fat infiltration. Note the slightly hypertrophic teres minor muscle (*TM*) presenting a normal echogenicity. *Delt* deltoid muscle

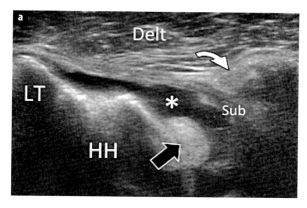

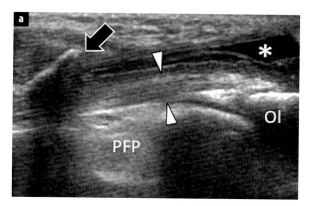

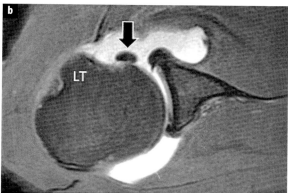

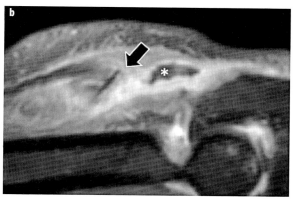

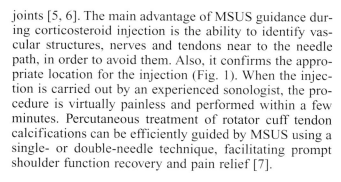

**Fig. 4 a, b.** Dislocation of the long head of the biceps tendon. **a** Axial sonogram obtained over the anterior aspect of the humeral head (*HH*). **b** Corresponding axial T1-weighted fat-saturated image after intra-articular injection of gadolinium contrast. The sonogram shows a full-thickness avulsion of the subscapularis tendon (*Sub*) that is retracted at the level of the short head of the biceps muscle (*curved arrow*). A reactive joint fluid effusion (*asterisk*) is evident. The long head of the biceps tendon (*black arrow*) is dislocated inside the glenohumeral joint. *LT* lesser tuberosity, *Delt* deltoid muscle

**Fig. 5 a, b.** Partial tear of the triceps tendon at the elbow. **a** Sagittal sonogram obtained over the distal triceps tendon. **b** Corresponding sagittal T1-weighted fat-saturated image after intravenous injection of gadolinium contrast. The sonogram shows a partial-thickness avulsion of the triceps tendon with presence of an avulsed osseous fragment (*arrow*) retracted proximally. A reactive local fluid effusion (*asterisk*) is evident. The deep portion (*arrowheads*) of the tendon is continuous. Note absence of articular effusion. *Ol* olecranon, *PFP* posterior fat pad of the elbow joint

joints [5, 6]. The main advantage of MSUS guidance during corticosteroid injection is the ability to identify vascular structures, nerves and tendons near to the needle path, in order to avoid them. Also, it confirms the appropriate location for the injection (Fig. 1). When the injection is carried out by an experienced sonologist, the procedure is virtually painless and performed within a few minutes. Percutaneous treatment of rotator cuff tendon calcifications can be efficiently guided by MSUS using a single- or double-needle technique, facilitating prompt shoulder function recovery and pain relief [7].

### Elbow

Tendinopathy, and partial and complete tears of the triceps are not uncommon in athletes, particularly weightlifters. MSUS can diagnose tears and accurately differentiate partial tears from complete tears. Partial tears typically affect the superficial layer of the tendon, arising from the fusion of the long and lateral heads of the tendons, and they are frequently associated with bony avulsion [8] (Fig. 5).

Distal biceps tendonitis is usually caused by chronic overuse. MSUS can show a hypoechoic swelling and irregular fibrillar pattern of the tendon. Differentiating a chronic tendinopathy from a partial tear is difficult because their sonographic appearances can be very similar. In these situations, correlation of the MSUS data with clinical findings is very helpful. Clinical signs and symptoms of complete tears are acute antecubital pain, elbow supination and flexion weakness, and proximal retraction of the muscle from its insertion at the radial tuberosity. A local ecchymosis is usually present. These tears typically result from a powerful eccentric contraction of the biceps. The amount of muscle retraction depends mainly on the integrity of the lacertus fibrosus, the integrity of which needs to be substantially altered to cause a significant retraction. On MSUS, complete tears appear as complete interruption of the tendon usually by an avulsion from the radial tuberosity. If the lacertus fibrosus remains continuous, there is usually a 1-2 cm tendon retraction. In a significant tear of the lacertus fibrosus, the tendon can retract as far as the distal $^{1}/_{3}$ of the arm and is often

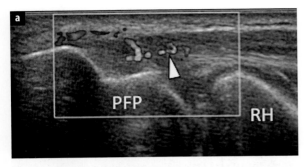

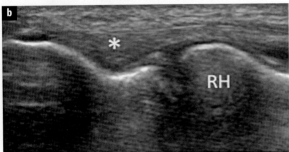

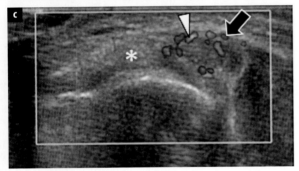

**Fig. 6 a-c.** Tendinopathy of the common extensor tendon at the elbow. All sonograms were obtained over the common extensor tendon. **a** Coronal color Doppler sonogram obtained over the anterior part of extensor. **b** Coronal sonogram obtained over the posterior part of the tendon. **c** Axial color Doppler sonogram. Note swelling, irregular hypoechoic appearance and hypervascular changes (*arrowheads*) limited to the anterior part (*arrow*) of the common extensor tendon. The posterior part (*asterisk*) of the tendon is normal. *RH* radial head, *PFP* posterior fat pad of the elbow joint (for color reproduction see p 303)

surrounded by a hematoma. Bicipitoradial bursitis lesions are caused by overuse, and they present as hypoechoic fluid collections located between the distal biceps tendon and the radius. In severe cases, the tendon can be surrounded by fluid, mimicking tenosynovitis [9].

The common extensor tendinopathy at the lateral epicondyle (tennis elbow), and the common flexor tendinopathy at the medial epicondyle (golfer's elbow,) are frequent and related to local repeated mechanical trauma. In both cases, MSUS can show the thickened and irregularly hypoechoic tendon. Presence of intratendinous calcifications (hyperechoic spots), their size and exact location can also be accurately determined. Color Doppler can show the presence of neovascularization of the tendon

(Fig. 6). Small tears are usually horizontal and located in the middle third of the tendon. Severe full-thickness tears affect mainly the anterior third of the tendon and are more common in patients treated previously by local steroid injections [10]. Dry needling and/or therapeutic local injections can, when needed, be effectively guided by MSUS.

## Wrist and Hand

A wide variety of tendinopathies at the wrist and hand can affect the sportsman, and they are usually caused by repetitive microtrauma. On the posterolateral side of the wrist, the tendinopathy of the extensor carpi ulnaris (ECU) can cause chronic pain in sportsmen, particularly tennis players [11]. A predisposing factor of this pathology may be recurrent subluxation of the ECU tendon. Clinical findings are usually not specific and may mimic disorders of the distal radioulnar joint. MSUS can determine the presence of tendinopathy and/or tenosynovitis by showing the ECU tendon size, identifying the presence of irregular hypoechoic changes, detecting intrasubstance longitudinal splits commonly related to its instability, and by showing synovial hypertrophy, sheath effusion or local hypervascularization. Associated retinaculum tears are not infrequent and can cause instability of the tendon. Tears usually follow acute traumas, such as powerful pronation from a supinated position when playing tennis. This causes the ECU to dislocate anteriorly. Dynamic ultrasound scanning performed during pronation-supination movements is ideal to depict this condition.

Detection of some wrist fractures can be difficult by plain radiographs because of the superposition bony structures, and, because of its tomographic capabilities, MSUS can aid in their diagnosis. MSUS can help in identifying the scaphoid and hook of hamate fractures. It can also detect dorsal avulsion of the triquetrum.

Tears of the scapholunate ligament are frequent in sports trauma. MSUS accurately shows the dorsal band of the ligament [12]. Tears appear as swelling and interruption of the ligament that can be associated with widening of the scapholunate space during dynamic examination performed in radial and ulnar deviation of the hand.

In acute complete tears of annular pulleys, MSUS shows palmar subluxation of the flexor tendons, which are no longer retained against the anterior aspect of the phalanges [13]. Longitudinal static sonograms obtained with the fingers extended adequately show tendons bowstringing in patients where a complete tear is present. During forced flexion, the gap between the flexor tendons and the phalanx increases proportionally to the number of disrupted pulleys. Partial tears appear as thickened and hypoechoic pulleys without subluxation of the flexor tendons.

"Jersey finger" is a traumatic flexor digitorum profundus (FDP) tendon avulsion that most frequently affects the ring finger. It is commonly caused when an active flexion of the distal interphalangeal joint is countered by a sudden and powerful external extension force such as when a player grabs another player's jersey during a tackle. MSUS clearly shows the relation between the avulsed hyperechoic fragment and the retracted FDP tendon. The size and location of the fragment, as well as its relationship with the annular pulleys, can be assessed. The empty distal tendon sheath and the irregular appearance of the base of the distal phalanx are also evident.

Ultrasound can accurately assess the presence of tears of the UCL, and help distinguish between partial and complete tears [14]. In partial tears, the ligament is swollen, irregular and hypoechoic. Full-thickness tears are visualized on MSUS as complete discontinuity of the ligament fibers. The interruption is frequently noted at the distal attachment, although injury can also occur in the middle third. Local hypervascular changes on color Doppler are frequent in acute cases. MSUS can accurately assess the presence of an interposition of the aponeurosis of the adductor brevis muscle between the torn ligament ends (Stener's lesion), which frequently requires surgical treatment. In this event, the torn swollen ligament appears retracted proximally and separated from the distal stump by the thin hyperechoic adductor aponeurosis. Passive flexion of the interphalangeal joint during MSUS examination helps to distinguish the aponeurosis, which moves simultaneously with the extensor pollicis longus tendon from the underlying UCL. An avulsion fracture at the insertion of UCL onto the proximal phalanx is also well visualized on MSUS, revealing the bony fragment as a hyperechoic structure with posterior acoustic shadowing.

The volar plate and collateral ligaments of the proximal interphalangeal joints are well visualized on MSUS, which can confirm the presence of a rupture. In bony avulsion of the distal insertion of the palmar plate, MSUS allows detection of the fragment, its size and amount of displacement. Complete tears are shown as avulsions and proximal displacement of the plate. In partial tears, the ligament is thickened, irregular and hypoechoic. In acute injury, color Doppler shows increased vascular signals resulting from hypervascularity. In complete tears, MSUS can show a gap in the ligament filled by synovial fluid. Gentle stress can increase the gap, thus confirming the diagnosis of a complete interruption of the ligament.

## Lower Extremity

### Introduction

Ultrasound can be an effective imaging tool to evaluate sports injuries of the lower extremity; however, ultrasound is most effective when performed by an experienced sonographer for a focused or precise indication [15]. For example, the scenario of "evaluate for Achilles tendon tear" is preferred over an indication such as "hip pain." As a general rule, ultrasound performs best when assessing superficial structures, where resolution is optimized with higher frequency transducers (greater than 10 or 12 MHz). Resolution and accuracy decreases with

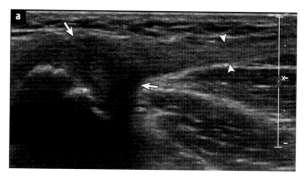

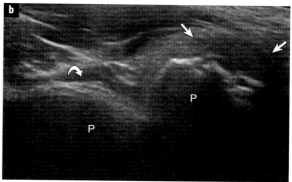

**Fig. 7 a, b.** Common aponeurosis injury at pubis ("sports hernia"). Ultrasound images of the long axis (**a**) and short axis (**b**) to the proximal adductor longus tendon show (*arrows*) abnormal hypoechoic tendinosis and bone irregularity involving common aponeurosis between rectus abdominis and adductor longus over pubis (*P*). Note normal contralateral common aponeurosis (*curved arrow*), and normal distal adductor longus tendon (*arrowheads*)

deeper structures, such as about the hip, where magnetic resonance imaging (MRI) is often indicated, especially when there is a negative ultrasound examination. Ultrasound does have the advantages of portability and accessibility, and the ability to correlate directly with patient symptoms and compare with the contralateral asymptomatic side. The purpose of this section is to briefly review the ultrasound findings of some of the more common lower extremity sports injuries.

### Hip

Ultrasound can be effective to evaluate the tendons about the hip, although there is limited evaluation of deeper structures that may require further imaging with MRI. One such indication is evaluation of the adductor tendons at the pubic symphysis for injury. Findings include hypoechoic tendinosis, cortical irregularity and calcification, anechoic interstitial tears, and complete retracted full-thickness tendon tear. In the athlete, groin pain may be related to the proximal adductor tendons. While the exact cause of "sports hernia" is often multifactorial, a proposed theory includes hypoechoic injury to the common aponeurosis over the pubis between the rectus abdominis and adductor longus tendon [16] (Fig. 7). Abnormalities of the pubic symphysis, such as joint fluid and cortical irregularity, can also be seen.

Other tendon abnormalities of the hip region resulting from sports injuries include the rectus femoris anteriorly and the hamstring origin posteriorly. An additional tendon that can be effectively evaluated with ultrasound is the iliopsoas, specifically including dynamic evaluation for iliopsoas tendon snapping. The cause of iliopsoas snapping is temporary entrapment of the medial aspect of the iliacus between the psoas major tendon and the superior pubic ramus, lateral to the iliopectineal eminence [17]. Moving the patient from a flexed, externally rotated and abducted hip position to full extension is one maneuver that often produces the abnormal finding of abrupt snapping of the iliopsoas tendon. In addition, the patient can be simply asked to reproduce the symptoms while imaging under ultrasound. Another form of snapping hip syndrome involves abrupt movement of the iliotibial band (or tract) and/or gluteus maximus over the greater trochanter. Ultrasound evaluation of this condition involves placing the probe short axis to the femur directly over the greater trochanter with the patient laying on the side while flexing and extending the hip.

Ultrasound can also effectively evaluate the hip joint for effusion and other intra-articular processes. While evaluation of the labrum is limited due to depth of this structure and inability to comprehensively assess it, ultrasound can show a labral tear as a well-defined hypoechoic or anechoic cleft within or at the base of the normal hyperechoic fibrocartilage labrum. The finding of an anterior labrum tear and abnormal bone contour at the femoral head-neck can indirectly suggest a diagnosis of femoroacetabular impingement. A paralabral cyst may also be identified with ultrasound, and this commonly appears as multilocular and hypoechoic in direct connection with the acetabular labral tear [18].

## Knee

Ultrasound evaluation of the knee is primarily limited to the superficial tendons and ligaments, as well as joint effusion and various bursa about the knee [19]. While the peripheral aspects of the menisci can show anechoic or hypoechoic tears similar to the hip labrum, a comprehensive evaluation is not possible. In addition, sports injuries of the knee often involve an array of structures, many of which are not adequately assessed with ultrasound (such as the anterior cruciate ligament and posterior cruciate ligament), and therefore MRI is typically indicated; nonetheless, ultrasound can be effective in evaluation of many structures, such as the extensor mechanism of the knee.

A common pathology that involves the extensor mechanism of the knee is termed Jumper's knee, where the proximal patellar tendon can show hypoechoic tendinosis, anechoic interstitial or partial-thickness tears, and potential neovascularity on color and power Doppler imaging (Fig. 8). Various bursa, such as the prepatellar, superficial infrapatellar, deep infrapatellar and pes anser-

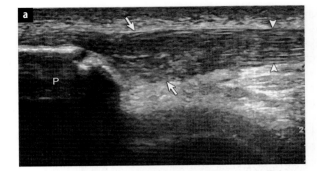
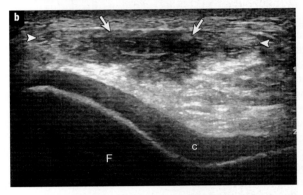
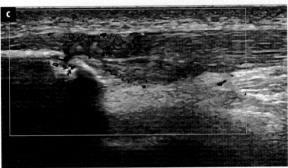

**Fig. 8 a-c.** Patellar tendon tendinosis (Jumper's knee). Ultrasound images of the long axis (**a**) and short axis (**b**) to the patellar tendon (*arrowheads*) show hypoechoic tendinosis (*arrows*) and bone irregularity of the patella (*P*). **c** Note hyperemia from neovascularity on the color Doppler image. *F* femur, *c* articular cartilage (for color reproduction see p 303)

inus bursa, can be evaluated with ultrasound, which may show distention with anechoic fluid and heterogeneous complex fluid or synovial proliferation. In the older athlete, distention of the semimembranosus-medial gastrocnemius bursa, or Baker cyst, can be identified by ultrasound, with its characteristic neck extending to the knee joint between the tendons of the semimembranosus and medial head of the gastrocnemius. Ultrasound can also evaluate for Baker cyst rupture and other causes of calf symptoms, such as deep venous thrombosis.

## Ankle and Foot

Ultrasound is an ideal imaging method to evaluate various structures about the ankle and foot given the superficial

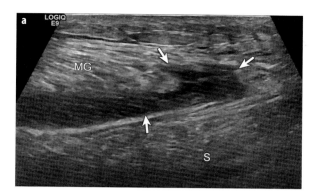

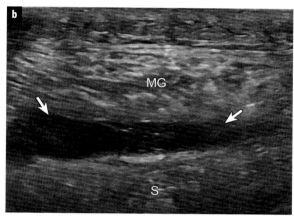

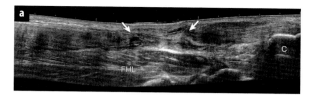

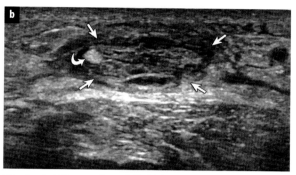

**Fig. 10 a, b.** Achilles tendon: full-thickness tear. Ultrasound images of the long axis (**a**) and short axis (**b**) to the Achilles tendon show heterogeneous hypoechoic tendon disruption with tendon retraction (between the *arrows*). Note the intact plantaris tendon (*curved arrow*) at the medial aspect. *FHL* flexor hallucis longus, *C* calcaneus

**Fig. 9 a, b.** Medial gastrocnemius tear ("tennis leg"). Ultrasound images of the long axis (**a**) and short axis (**b**) to the distal medial head of gastrocnemius (*MG*) show a hypoechoic tear at the distal aponeurosis (*arrows*). *S* soleus

location of many structures [20]. Ultrasound performs well in evaluation of structures such as tendons and ligaments, whereas MRI is required to evaluate bone marrow and the articular surfaces of the ankle joint. There are several structures of the calf and posterior ankle that are commonly involved with sports injuries. Injury of the distal medial head of the gastrocnemius, also termed tennis leg, appears as hypoechoic or anechoic disruption of the distal tendon at its aponeurosis attachment (Fig. 9). Injury to the plantaris tendon will appear as a tubular sagitally oriented fluid collection in the expected location of the plantaris tendon located between the muscle bellies of the medial head of the gastrocnemius and soleus muscles. Injuries to the plantaris and medial head of the gastrocnemius commonly coexist. While injury and hematoma to the soleus may occur with sports injuries, the finding of an isolated hematoma in the soleus muscle should raise concern for potential underlying malignant tumor in the absence of a bleeding disorder or anticoagulants.

Injuries may involve tendons about the foot and ankle, which commonly include the Achilles, tibialis posterior and peroneal tendons. With respect to the Achilles, abnormalities commonly involve a segment of tendon 2-6 cm proximal to its calcaneal attachment, although distal abnormalities at the calcaneus may also

occur [21] (Fig. 10). Potential findings at ultrasound include hypoechoic tendinosis, anechoic interstitial tears, partial-thickness tears and full-thickness tears. Since there is no surrounding synovial sheath, the term peritendinitis is often used to describe abnormal hypoechoic injury or inflammation surrounding the Achilles tendon. Distention of the retrocalcaneal or retro-Achilles bursa may also be seen. In evaluation for Achilles tendon tear, the use of dynamic imaging with dorsiflexion and plantar flexion of the foot will help differentiate a partial-thickness from a full-thickness tendon tear. A partial-thickness tear shows tendon fiber continuity, with movement of the entire tendon during dynamic imaging, while a full-thickness tear shows lack of tendon translation across the abnormal tendon segment and retracted torn tendon stump. Other tendons about the ankle may also show tenosynovitis, tendinosis and various types of tendon tears, usually where a tendon changes course near an osseous structure, such as the malleoli. With regard to the peroneal tendons, a common tear is the longitudinal split of the peroneus brevis. Dynamic imaging with the foot in dorsiflexion and eversion is helpful to demonstrate possible peroneal tendon subluxation and dislocation in the setting of a peroneal retinaculum tear or fibula avulsion.

The ligaments of the ankle can be visualized with ultrasound [22]. Laterally, the anterior talofibular ligament is most commonly injured, followed by the calcaneofibular ligament. An abnormal ligament can appear as hypoechoic swelling or frank discontinuity with possible hyperechoic avulsion fracture fragment. Evaluation of the anterior inferior tibiofibular ligament is important in the setting of high ankle sprain, where further evaluation of the interosseous membrane and proximal fibula is important to exclude Maisonneuve injury. Medially, the deltoid ligament can also be evaluated for injury. Lastly, a fracture can be identified by ultrasound as a cortical step-off that correlates with point tenderness, with variable echogenic callous depending on the chronicity of the injury.

# References

1. Bianchi S, Martinoli C (2007) Musculoskeletal ultrasound. Springer, Berlin Heidelberg New York
2. Jacobson JA (2007) Fundamentals of musculoskeletal ultrasound. Saunders, Philadelphia, PA, 2007
3. Smith TO, Back T, Toms AP et al (2011) Diagnostic accuracy of ultrasound for rotator cuff tears in adults: a systematic review and meta-analysis. Clin Radiol 66:1036-1048
4. Wall LB, Teefey SA, Middleton WD et al (2012) Diagnostic performance and reliability of ultrasonography for fatty degeneration of the rotator cuff muscles. J Bone Joint Surg Am 94:e83
5. Peng PW, Cheng P (2011) Ultrasound-guided interventional procedures in pain medicine: a review of anatomy, sonoanatomy, and procedures. Part III: shoulder. Reg Anesth Pain Med 36:592-605
6. Daley EL, Bajaj S, Bisson LJ et al (2011) Improving injection accuracy of the elbow, knee, and shoulder: does injection site and imaging make a difference? A systematic review. Am J Sports Med 39:656-62
7. Serafini G, Sconfienza LM, Lacelli F et al (2009) Rotator cuff calcific tendonitis: short-term and 10-year outcomes after two-needle MSUS-guided percutaneous treatment—nonrandomized controlled trial. Radiology 252:157-164
8. Downey R, Jacobson JA, Fessell DP et al (2011) Sonography of partial-thickness tears of the distal triceps brachii tendon. J Ultrasound Med 30:1351-1356
9. Chew ML, Giuffrè BM (2005) Disorders of the distal biceps brachii tendon. Radiographics 25:1227-1237
10. Poltawski L, Ali S, Jayaram V et al (2011) Reliability of sonographic assessment of tendinopathy in tennis elbow. Skeletal Radiol 2012 41:83-89
11. Montalvan B, Parier J, Brasseur JL et al (2006) Extensor carpi ulnaris injuries in tennis players: a study of 28 cases. Br J Sports Med 40:424-429
12. Jacobson JA, Oh E, Propeck T et al (2002) Sonography of the scapholunate ligament in four cadaveric wrists: correlation with MR arthrography and anatomy. AJR Am J Roentgenol 179:523-527
13. Klauser A, Frauscher F, Bodner G et al (2002) Finger pulley injuries in extreme rock climbers: depiction with dynamic MSUS. Radiology 222:755-761
14. Ebrahim FS, De Maeseneer M, Jager T et al (2006) MSUS diagnosis of UCL tears of the thumb and Stener lesions: technique, pattern-based approach, and differential diagnosis. Radiographics 26:1007-1020
15. Jacobson JA (2002) Ultrasound in sports medicine. Radiol Clin North Am 40:363-386
16. Robinson P, Bhat V, English B (2011) Imaging in the assessment and management of athletic pubalgia. Semin Musculoskelet Radiol 15:14-26
17. Guillin R, Cardinal E, Bureau NJ (2009) Sonographic anatomy and dynamic study of the normal iliopsoas musculotendinous junction. Eur Radiol 19:995-1001
18. Mervak BM, Morag Y, Marcantonio D et al (2012) Paralabral cysts of the hip: sonographic evaluation with magnetic resonance arthrographic correlation. J Ultrasound Med 31:495-500
19. Lee MJ, Chow K (2007) Ultrasound of the knee. Semin Musculoskelet Radiol 11:137-148
20. Khoury V, Guillin R, Dhanju J, Cardinal E (2007) Ultrasound of ankle and foot: overuse and sports injuries. Semin Musculoskelet Radiol 11:149-61
21. Calleja M, Connell DA (2010) The Achilles tendon. Semin Musculoskelet Radiol 14:307-322
22. Peetrons P, Creteur V, Bacq C (2004) Sonography of ankle ligaments. J Clin Ultrasound 32:491-499

# Cartilage: How Do We Image It? From Basic to Advanced MRI Protocols

Daniel Geiger[1], Eric Y. Chang[2], Christine B. Chung[2]

[1] Department of Radiological, Oncological and Pathological Sciences, Sapienza University of Rome, Rome, Italy
[2] Department of Radiology, University of California-San Diego, San Diego, CA, USA

## Introduction

In the last 40 years, the general interest in imaging evaluation of articular cartilage has significantly increased.

Early imaging of cartilage was indirect and achieved through standard radiographic methods and low-resolution radioisotope bone scans [1]. In fact, prior to the advent of cross-sectional imaging, radiographic evaluation [2] of joint space width [3] was considered the noninvasive reference standard to stage osteoarthritis. At that same time, radiographic arthrography [4, 5] was investigated for the same purpose and later improved with computed tomography (CT) [6]. Pioneering investigations also contemplated the value of ultrasound in the direct assessment of articular cartilage [7]. In 1984, magnetic resonance imaging (MRI) appeared on the scene and quickly demonstrated its superiority for the noninvasive evaluation of tissue [8], revolutionizing the practice of medicine. In the 21st century, MRI is considered the technique of choice for direct noninvasive articular cartilage evaluation. It is able to exquisitely assess cartilage injuries, both qualitatively and quantitatively, along with an overall evaluation of joint damage. CT arthrography has proven to be a valid option for patients with higher grade chondral lesions who are unable to undergo MRI, but it suffers from lack of soft tissue contrast and is minimally invasive. Ultrasound is still considered a potential research tool for cartilage evaluation [9] and is highly operator dependent.

We will therefore focus our discussion on MRI techniques, describing basic and advanced sequences, as useful tools in our armamentarium to assess articular cartilage.

## Basic Magnetic Resonance Sequences

Since the introduction of MRI evaluation of joints, there has been a quest for MRI sequences that optimize articular cartilage evaluation. Over time, increased signal-to-noise ratio (SNR), contrast-to-noise ratio (CNR) and acquisition speeds have become available, along with coil and scanner improvements. Despite this, there is currently no single specific sequence that allows for one-stop shopping evaluation of this complex tissue. It is generally accepted that a combination of sequences is necessary for comprehensive morphologic and quantitative evaluation. Essential requirements for evaluation of hyaline cartilage include high in-plane and through-plane resolution and optimal SNR and CNR, thereby avoiding partial-volume artifacts and allowing differentiation from surrounding fluid and tissues. To this end, utilization of high field strength scanners and dedicated coils is strongly advised [10].

Various pulse sequences have been investigated over time and different acquisitions techniques compared [11, 12]. Historically, better results were obtained from the family of gradient recalled echo (GRE) sequences, including: fast low angle shot (FLASH), spoiled gradient echo (SPGR), fast field echo (FFE) along with steady-state free precession techniques (SSFP), fast imaging with steady state precession (FISP) and gradient recalled acquisition in the steady state (GRASS). Other acquisition techniques such as dual echo steady state (DESS) [13], magnetization transfer [14] and pulse transfer [15] have been investigated in order to improve cartilage-bone and cartilage-fluid image contrast. Three-dimensional (3D) acquisitions have demonstrated a reduction in partial volume artifacts while maintaining optimal SNR [16]. Specifically, 3D T1 fat-saturated GRE sequences (FLASH and SPGR) have proven to be very accurate in cartilage evaluation with stark contrast between high-signal (bright) cartilage on a background of suppressed fat, fluid and bone marrow (dark). In comparison, with DESS and other more fluid-sensitive GRE acquisitions, cartilage signal is lower than fluid highlighting defects and fissures, which appear as bright alterations on a darker background. More recent sequences include the family of steady-state free precession techniques such as fluctuating equilibrium MR (FEMR), linear-combination steady-state free precession (LCSSFP) and vastly undersampled isotropic projection (VIPR), and the balanced variants including true fast imaging with steady-state precession (True FISP), fast imaging employing steady-state acquisition (FIESTA) and balanced fast field echo (b-FFE). Unfortunately many of these sequences suffer from off

J. Hodler et al. (eds.), *Musculoskeletal Diseases 2013-2016,*
DOI: 10.1007/978-88-470-5292-5_20 © Springer-Verlag Italia 2013

resonance artefacts, RF transmit coil profile sensitivity and require multiple averages. Despite some advantages of using the GRE-family sequences for articular cartilage evaluation, the assessment of other articular structures (ligaments, menisci and bone marrow) is less optimal in comparison with fast spin-echo techniques (FSE) [17]. As a result, two-dimensional (2D) FSE techniques are the most commonly used sequences for global joint evaluation, but are not without limitations, which include blurring with longer echo trains and the necessity of anisotropic voxels. Traditional 3D FSE techniques were limited due to prolonged acquisition times and high specific absorption rate; however, the new generation of 3D FSE with flip angle modulation have overcome such limitations, allowing for one high-resolution acquisition with submillimeter isotropic voxels and multiplanar reconstruction in any desired plane. However, persistent limitations include blurring and contrast that differs from 2D FSE imaging, somewhat limiting evaluation of noncartilaginous structures. Despite this, current-generation 3D FSE sequences (including XETA, SPACE, CUBE and VISTA) provide a useful alternative for 3D GRE techniques [18]. There is yet insufficient evidence to entirely replace existing 2D protocols, and for this reason 2D FSE remains strongly preferred in clinical practice.

3D pseudo-arthrogram images with T1/T2 contrast are also made possible using short TR and short TE acquisitions, with an additional 90 degree pulse used to return residual transverse magnetization to the longitudinal axis, known under the names of driven equilibrium Fourier transform (DEFT), fast recovery FSE (FRFSE) and driven equilibrium (DRIVE) [19, 20]. Fat suppression techniques are routinely applied in articular cartilage imaging protocols to improve dynamic range. Frequency selective fat saturation, selective water excitation, short TI inversion recovery (STIR) imaging and iterative decomposition of water and fat with echo asymmetry and least-squares estimation (IDEAL) are among the applicable techniques [9, 10, 20].

## Advanced Magnetic Resonance Sequences (Compositional Imaging)

Advanced magnetic resonance (MR) sequences for cartilage evaluation are focused on the assessment of articular cartilage biochemical composition, more specifically to the collagen and glycosaminoglycan content. Hyaline cartilage is in fact a macromolecular network that supports mechanical loads. Three-quarters of its weight is composed of water and the rest is a molecular mesh composed of collagen and proteoglycans. Collagen accounts for one-fifth of its volume, with aggrecan as the most abundant proteoglycan. Proteoglycans have glycosaminoglycans (GAGs) attached as side chains that are negatively charged. The preservation of proteoglycan is directly assessed by the distribution pattern of associated positively charged sodium (Na$^+$). Similarly, regions lacking proteoglycan cause negatively charged gadolinium-based contrast (Gd-DTPA$^{2-}$) agents to accumulate [9, 10], as will be further discussed below.

## Mapping

T2 is defined as the decay of transverse magnetization, reflecting interactions between macromolecules and water [21]. Multi-echo spin-echo or gradient-echo sequences are used to measure T2 or T2* values, respectively, that are plotted into one or more decay exponentials, with a single exponential usually preferred for the TE values applied in clinical practice (Fig. 1). Post-processing of the images acquired at various echo times is then performed to generate a color-map that displays the spatial distribution of T2 values. Cartilage degeneration is associated with a regional increase in T2 relaxation time (high signal) and also heterogeneous T2 values, due to loss of collagen integrity and increased total water. Decrease in proteoglycan has much less impact on cartilage T2 values. T2 mapping has proven useful in iden-

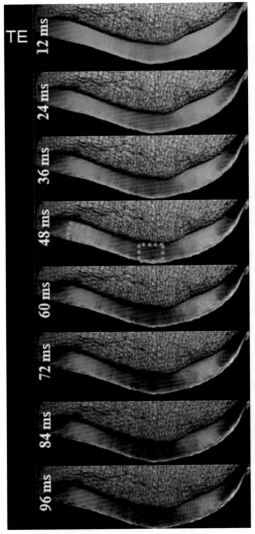

**Fig. 1.** Multi-echo T2 images at the level of the osteochondral junction (patellar specimen). Post-processing of the following images allows generation of corresponding T2 maps (for color reproduction see p 304)

tification of early stage cartilage degeneration and for monitoring the effectiveness of cartilage repair over time. Multi-echo sequences, along with specific software packages for post-processing, are offered by most vendors and are able to be implemented on most clinical MRI scanners [9, 10].

### Delayed Gadolinium-Enhanced MR Imaging of Cartilage

Delayed gadolinium-enhanced MR imaging of cartilage (dGEMRIC) technique is based upon the fact that ions distribute in cartilage following the concentration of the negatively charged GAG molecules [22]. Negatively charged Gd-DTPA$^{2-}$ anionic molecules will be repulsed by preserved cartilage. Conversely, if Gd-DTPA$^{2-}$ is present in the hyaline cartilage, concentration can be assumed to be in regions where glycosaminoglycan is relatively depleted. Therefore the T1 values of hyaline cartilage assessed after Gd-DTPA$^{2-}$ intravenous administration will quantitatively reflect GAG concentration. For a typical dGEMRIC protocol, a double or triple dose of Gd-DTPA$^{2-}$ is usually administered intravenously and joint range of motion is performed for 10 min. T1-weighted images are acquired after 30 min to 3 h (usually at least a 90 min delay is preferred) and color maps can be generated based on per-pixel calculation. Different parameters have been proposed to acquire the data based on T1-weighting such as STIR imaging, saturation recovery, fast mapping, Look-Locker and driven equilibrium single pulse observation (DESPOT). T1 maps are then generated using specific curve-fitting software and values are defined as a dGEMRIC index. Notably, due to variations in intra-articular distribution of gadolinium in vivo, an equilibrium state is never reached. Therefore GAG concentration as measured with dGEMRIC must be considered an estimate. Areas with a low dGEMRIC index (low T1 values) reflect high gadolinium concentration and low GAG concentration (abnormal cartilage). Conversely, areas with a high dGEMRIC index (high T1 values) demonstrate low gadolinium distribution and normal GAG concentration (preserved cartilage). dGEMRIC can be implemented on clinical high-field-strength MRI systems, but requires upgrading to specific software packages in order to post-process the T1 acquired data. The dGEMRIC index has a low inter- and intraobserver variability and presently is one of the most specific noninvasive techniques to evaluate hyaline cartilage GAG concentration [9, 10].

### T1ρ (T1-Rho)

T1ρ is defined as the spin-lattice relaxation time in the rotating frame and is measured using a spin-lock. It reflects the interaction between motion-restricted water molecules and the macromolecular environment. Therefore it can describe changes in the extracellular matrix of cartilage (macromolecular environment), which includes alterations to proteoglycans. T1ρ measurements appear less sensitive in the identification of collagen changes than proteoglycans. Although T1ρ mechanisms are still not fully understood, variations in measurements have been observed depending

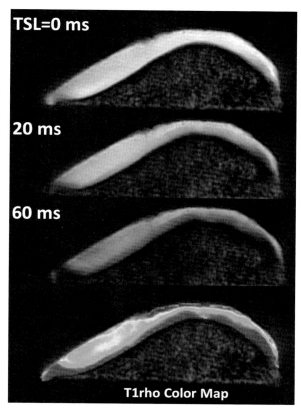

**Fig. 2.** Patellar T1ρ (*T1-Rho*) images acquired using different spin lock times (*TSL*) and corresponding T1ρ map (for color reproduction see p 304)

on cartilage depth, corresponding to known GAG concentration gradients. T1ρ measurements show promising results in the assessment of damaged cartilage (high T1ρ values) and in early stage osteoarthrosis when compared with T2 imaging [9, 10, 23, 24]. T1ρ of cartilage involves a specific pulse sequence with multiple acquisitions at varying spin-lock times (Fig. 2). Presently the technique is typically performed in the research setting and is still under extensive investigation.

### Na$^+$ Imaging

The rationale for Na$^+$ imaging of cartilage relies in the previously described concept that GAGs carry negative charges from their sulfate and carboxyl groups. In accordance to Donnan equilibrium theory and electroneutrality principles, the negative charges are counterbalanced by positive charges in cartilage extracellular matrix. Sodium (Na$^+$), a positive ion, is present in cartilage and can be measured by means of MR due to its nuclear spin momentum, which is characterized by a measurable specific resonance frequency ($\omega$=11.262 MHz/T). Therefore healthy cartilage, rich in GAGs, presents a normal amount of Na$^+$, while damaged areas (poor in GAGs) demonstrate a decreased amount of Na$^+$. Na$^+$ imaging is technically challenging and requires an MR system with multinuclear capabilities and dedicated sodium

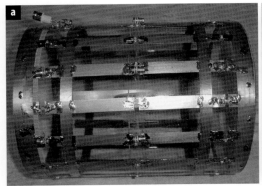
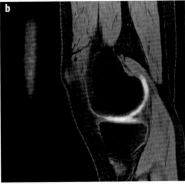

**Fig. 3 a, b. a** Dedicated dual tuned 23 Na$^+$/$^1$H magnetic resonance imaging (MRI) coil. **b** 3T Na$^+$ MRI sagittal image of the knee, directly measuring cartilage glycosaminoglycan content. (Courtesy of Professor Garry Gold, Stanford University USA) (for color reproduction see p 304)

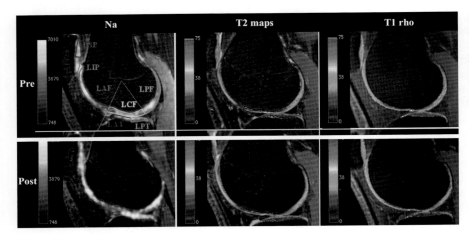

**Fig. 4.** Na$^+$, T2 and T1-rho knee cartilage maps from the Stanford basketball study. Post-season degenerative changes of the patellofemoral joint cartilage are demonstrated, in keeping with higher rates of injury at this level in jumping athletes. (Courtesy of Professor Garry Gold, Stanford University, USA) (for color reproduction see p 305)

coils (Figs. 3, 4). High field strength is required for sufficient SNR since in vivo Na$^+$ NMR signal is ~22,000 times smaller than that of hydrogen. Additionally, Na$^+$ has very fast biexponential transverse relaxation decay, necessitating the use of ultrashort TE sequences and is therefore still used as a research tool [9, 10, 25].

## Ultra-Short Echo Time

Ultra-short echo time (UTE) imaging has its rationale in the application of specific MRI sequences with ultra-short echo times (on the order of microseconds or less) to evaluate tissues presenting a majority of short T2 components. While these tissues are hypointense on clinical imaging sequences, UTE allows abundant signal detection (Figs. 5, 6). Among these tissues are the calcified layer of cartilage, aponeuroses, menisci, tendon and bone [26]. Alteration of T2 relaxation times in these now visible tissues is associated with pathology, as is the case with conventional MRI of long T2 tissues. With the acquisition of several echoes, UTE T2 maps can be generated [9]. Recent literature has demonstrated the effectiveness of UTE MRI in the evaluation of the osteochondral junction [27]. Additionally, UTE T2 maps of articular cartilage have been used to evaluate matrix degeneration [28]. UTE MRI is presently used as a research

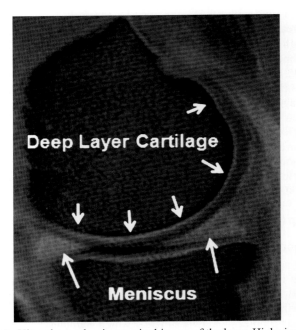

**Fig. 5.** Ultra-short echo time sagittal image of the knee. High signal is observed within the articular cartilage and meniscus (*arrows*). Note the elegant depiction of the deep articular cartilage layer (*small arrows*) along with the osteochondral junction area (for color reproduction see p 305)

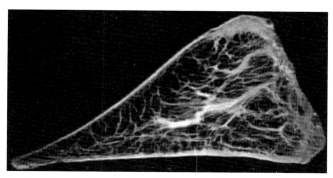

**Fig. 6.** Ultra-short echo time high-resolution image of a knee meniscus (specimen) demonstrates its fine anatomic details

tool and demands high performance MR hardware and specific sequence design. In the near future, we expect widespread implementation on high-field-strength clinical scanners, thereby improving their diagnostic potential.

### Diffusion Weighted Imaging and Diffusion Tensor Imaging

Diffusion weighted imaging (DWI) is based on the random Brownian motion of water molecules and its dependence on the intra- and extracellular surrounding environment. The macromolecular environment affects the magnitude and direction of the diffusing bulk water. Intact extracellular matrix restricts the motion of bulk water and normal cartilage demonstrates more restriction of diffusion at the deeper layers. DWI is able to provide quantitative information on cartilage structural integrity by means of diffusion rates of water expressed by apparent diffusion coefficient (ADC) values. The ADC values in healthy cartilage are lower in comparison with damaged cartilage, where increased water diffusion and therefore increased ADC values are observed. Although DWI is a technique readily implemented on clinical scanners for long T2 tissues [9], many challenges exist with regards to implementation in short T2 structures such as articular cartilage including poor spatial resolution (large field of view and slice thicknesses) and low SNRs.

Diffusion tensor imaging (DTI) measures the direction of water diffusion and can be used to evaluate cartilage in terms of collagen structural organization and proteoglycan content to assess cartilage structural degenerative changes, as recently demonstrated in literature [29].

### Conclusion

Various modalities have been proposed for articular cartilage evaluation, with MRI presently appearing as the champion of the noninvasive methods. Many sequence types and variants have been investigated in order to define a best one-stop shop evaluation. Although there exist many techniques to depict cartilage injury, at present a perfect sequence does not exist. Many compromises are required, with the specific compromise depending on the clinical question and the

effect on clinical management. Advanced sequences described above allow evaluation of the molecular structure of cartilage, although many are presently restricted to research environments or advanced musculoskeletal clinical units. Novel technical developments and application to cartilage imaging continues to occur. It is exciting to witness the new horizon with concurrent advances in orthopaedic surgery and regenerative medicine.

### References

1. Darracott J, Vernon-Roberts B (1971) The bony changes in "chondromalacia patellae". Rheumatol Phys Med 11:175-179
2. Pogrund H, Bloom R, Mogle P (1983) The normal width of the adult hip joint: the relationship to age, sex, and obesity. Skeletal Radiol 10:10-12
3. Buckland-Wright JC, Macfarlane DG, Lynch JA et al (1995) Joint space width measures cartilage thickness in osteoarthritis of the knee: high resolution plain film and double contrast macroradiographic investigation. Ann Rheum Dis 54:263-268
4. Horns JW (1972) Single contrast knee arthrography in abnormalities of the articular cartilage. Radiology 105:537-540
5. Hall FM, Wyshak G (1980) Thickness of articular cartilage in the normal knee. J Bone Joint Surg Am 62:408-413
6. Vande Berg BC, Lecouvet FE, Poilvache P et al (2002) CT arthrography of the knee: technique and value in the assessment of internal derangement of the knee. Eur Radiol 12:1800-1810
7. Aisen AM, McCune WJ, MacGuire A et al (1984) Sonographic evaluation of the cartilage of the knee. Radiology 153:781-784
8. Li KC, Henkelman RM, Poon PY, Rubenstein J (1984) MR imaging of the normal knee. J Comput Assist Tomogr 8:1147-1154
9. Winalski CS, Rajiah P (2011) The evolution of articular cartilage imaging and its impact on clinical practice. Skeletal Radiol 40:1197-1222
10. Crema MD, Roemer FW, Marra MD et al (2011) Articular cartilage in the knee: current MR imaging techniques and applications in clinical practice and research. Radiographics 31:37-61
11. Konig H, Sauter R, Deimling M, Vogt M (1987) Cartilage disorders: comparison of spin-echo, CHESS, and FLASH sequence MR images. Radiology 164:753-758
12. Reiser MF, Bongartz G, Erlemann R et al (1988) Magnetic resonance in cartilaginous lesions of the knee joint with three-dimensional gradient-echo imaging. Skeletal Radiol 17:465-471
13. Hardy PA, Recht MP, Piraino D, Thomasson D (1996) Optimization of a dual echo in the steady state (DESS) free-precession sequence for imaging cartilage. J Magn Reson Imaging 6:329-335
14. Wolff SD, Chesnick S, Frank JA et al (1991) Magnetization transfer contrast: MR imaging of the knee. Radiology 179:623-628
15. Peterfy CG, van Dijke CF, Janzen DL et al (1994) Quantification of articular cartilage in the knee with pulsed saturation transfer subtraction and fat-suppressed MR imaging: optimization and validation. Radiology 192:485-491
16. Tyrrell RL, Gluckert K, Pathria M, Modic MT (1988) Fast three-dimensional MR imaging of the knee: comparison with arthroscopy. Radiology 166:865-872
17. Potter HG, Linklater JM, Allen AA et al (1998) Magnetic resonance imaging of articular cartilage in the knee. An evaluation with use of fast-spin-echo imaging. J Bone Joint Surg Am 80:1276-1284
18. Subhas N, Kao A, Freire M et al (2011) MRI of the knee ligaments and menisci: comparison of isotropic-resolution 3D and conventional 2D fast spin-echo sequences at 3 T. AJR Am J Roentgenol 197:442-450

19. Hargreaves BA, Gold GE, Lang PK et al (1999) MR imaging of articular cartilage using driven equilibrium. Magn Reson Med 42:695-703

20. Recht MP, Goodwin DW, Winalski CS, White LM (2005) MRI of articular cartilage: revisiting current status and future directions. AJR Am J Roentgenol 185:899-914

21. Mosher TJ, Dardzinski BJ (2004) Cartilage MRI T2 relaxation time mapping: overview and applications. Semin Musculoskelet Radiol 8:355-368

22. Williams A, Gillis A, McKenzie C et al (2004) Glycosaminoglycan distribution in cartilage as determined by delayed gadolinium-enhanced MRI of cartilage (dGEMRIC): potential clinical applications. AJR Am J Roentgenol 182:167-172

23. Regatte RR, Akella SV, Wheaton AJ et al (2004) 3D-T1rho-relaxation mapping of articular cartilage: in vivo assessment of early degenerative changes in symptomatic osteoarthritic subjects. Acad Radiol 11:741-749

24. Link TM, Stahl R, Woertler K (2007) Cartilage imaging: motivation, techniques, current and future significance. Eur Radiol 17:1135-1146

25. Gold GE, Chen CA, Koo S et al (2009) Recent advances in MRI of articular cartilage. AJR Am J Roentgenol 193:628-638

26. Robson MD, Gatehouse PD, Bydder M, Bydder GM (2003) Magnetic resonance: an introduction to ultrashort TE (UTE) imaging. J Comput Assist Tomogr 27:825-846

27. Bae WC, Dwek JR, Znamirowski R et al (2010) Ultrashort echo time MR imaging of osteochondral junction of the knee at 3 T: identification of anatomic structures contributing to signal intensity. Radiology 254:837-845

28. Williams A, Qian Y, Chu CR (2011) UTE-T2 * mapping of human articular cartilage in vivo: a repeatability assessment. Osteoarthritis Cartilage 19:84-88

29. Raya JG, Melkus G, Adam-Neumair S et al (2011) Change of diffusion tensor imaging parameters in articular cartilage with progressive proteoglycan extraction. Invest Radiol 46:401-409

# Magnetic Resonance Imaging of Articular Cartilage

Michael P. Recht

Department of Radiology, NYU Langone Medical Center, New York, NY, USA

Magnetic resonance (MR) imaging has proven to be an accurate noninvasive method for the evaluation of articular cartilage [1-13], demonstrating morphologic changes as well as biochemical and structural changes. This chapter will concentrate on the morphologic imaging of articular cartilage and articular cartilage repair procedures using MR. Multiple MR pulse sequences have been used to evaluate the morphology of articular cartilage, but the most widely used clinically are proton density or T2-weighted fast spin-echo (FSE, TSE) sequences with or without fat suppression.

Fast spin-echo sequences employ multiple refocusing pulses that allow high-resolution images to be acquired in a relatively short time period. In addition, the multiple refocusing pulses produce a magnetization transfer effect within articular cartilage, which decreases its signal intensity. There is no corresponding effect within joint fluid, and therefore the magnetization transfer effect increases the contrast between articular cartilage and joint fluid, and improves the conspicuity of chondral defects. Studies have shown both proton density and T2-weighted fast spin-echo images with and without fat suppression to be accurate in the detection of chondral abnormalities. On fast spin echo images, cartilage has intermediate signal intensity tissue and is outlined by high signal intensity joint fluid providing excellent depiction of surface morphology as well as intrinsic signal changes potentially reflective of intrasubstance pathology. Chondral lesions appear as focal areas of increased signal intensity compared with normal surrounding cartilage. Although images without fat suppression have been shown to be accurate, the addition of fat suppression improves the ability to detect underlying subchondral bone marrow signal changes, which have been shown to be an important indicator of overlying articular cartilage defects. Studies have demonstrated a sensitivity of 86-94%, specificity of 94-99%, and accuracy of 81-98% for the detection of cartilage abnormalities on fast spin-echo techniques.

Over the past several years, three-dimensional (3D) fast spin-echo sequences have been developed, and these offer the promise of isotropic resolution and multiplanar reconstructions without loss of resolution while maintaining the excellent contrast of two-dimensional (2D) fast spin-echo sequences with reasonable times of acquisition (6-8 min) [14-16]. Initial studies have demonstrated equivalent diagnostic performance with 2D fast spin-echo sequences. 3T MR imaging and multichannel coils have also been utilized in cartilage imaging to take advantage of the potential advantages of imaging with relative increased image signal-to-noise or higher spatial resolution at similar imaging acquisition times, compared with 1T or 1.5T imaging (albeit with somewhat increased sensitivity to postoperative metal-related artifacts) [17, 18].

## Clinical MR Imaging of Articular Cartilage

### Degenerative Cartilage Disease

Degenerative cartilage disease or osteoarthritis is the most common form of arthritis, with symptomatic disease affecting 6-10% of all adults greater than 30 years of age, and illustrating a steep increase in prevalence with increasing age [19]. Early changes of osteoarthritis may be detected as areas of surface irregularity and fibrillation, as well as small focal defects presenting as focal areas of increased signal intensity on proton density or T2-weighted fast spin-echo images. More advanced changes of osteoarthritis include large areas of chondral thinning, often on apposing surfaces of the joint, and multiple focal defects of varying size. The focal defects tend to have obtuse margins as opposed to the sharply angled margins of traumatic chondral lesions. There is frequently increased signal abnormality subjacent to the focal defects within the subchondral bone marrow representing cysts and/or subchondral bone marrow edema like changes, and/or low signal representing subchondral fibrosis or trabecular sclerosis. The presence of additional secondary features of degenerative disease, such as osteophytes, and synovitis are also frequently identified on MR imaging.

J. Hodler et al. (eds.), *Musculoskeletal Diseases 2013-2016*,
DOI: 10.1007/978-88-470-5292-5_21 © Springer-Verlag Italia 2013

## Traumatic Cartilage Injury

Traumatic articular cartilage injuries are well recognized sequella of acute or repetitive impact or twisting injuries to a joint and are a significant source of patient morbidity. Surgical studies have highlighted that cartilage lesions are common, with an incidence ranging from 63% to 66% in patients undergoing arthroscopic surgery [20, 21]. Traumatic chondral lesions typically present as solitary lesions with acutely angled margins. The lesions usually result from shearing, rotational or tangential impaction forces, and can occur at the surface or in the deeper layers of articular cartilage. Traumatic lesions are often full thickness or high-grade partial thickness tears, and can frequently involve the underlying subchondral bone with either subchondral bone marrow edema like changes, contusions or frank fractures. Chondral fractures may remain in situ or become displaced, and present as intraarticular chondral or osteochondral bodies, which may cause locking of the knee and masquerade as a bucket handle meniscal tear.

## Imaging of Cartilage Repair Procedures

Increased awareness of the prevalence and significance of articular cartilage lesions, coupled with the limited natural capacity of cartilage for effective intrinsic repair, has contributed to growing interest in surgical techniques for the treatment of articular cartilage lesions. There are several techniques used to treat cartilage lesions; these techniques can be grouped into three main categories: local stimulation, autologous transplantation of cartilage, and allograft transplantation of osteochondral grafts. The most commonly used techniques are those of local stimulation, but these typically lead to formation of fibrous repair tissue rather than hyaline cartilage. Therefore, there has been great interest and increased use of autologous transplantation techniques, including autologous osteochondral transplantation and autologous chondrocyte implantation, because of their potential for providing hyaline or "hyaline-like" repair tissue and the promise of better functional results. In addition to a routine assessment of joint anatomy, a complete MR imaging evaluation of cartilage repair procedures should include specific assessment of the following. (a) Repair tissue: defect fill, surface morphology, MR signal characteristics. (b) Adjacent cartilage and bone: repair tissue integration to native cartilage and subchondral bone, MR signal characteristics subchondral bone. (c) The articulation: joint effusion, synovitis, adhesions, loose bodies.

## Local Stimulation for Cartilage Repair

The most commonly used surgical procedure for local stimulation is microfracture, which relies on bleeding from the penetration of the subchondral bone to form a fibrin clot containing pleuripotent stem cells. This clot differentiates and remodels leading to the formation of fibrocartilaginous repair tissue. With microfracture, a pick instrument is used to penetrate the subchondral bone multiple times about 4 mm in depth and approximately 3-4 mm apart from each other [22].

In the first few months following the microfracture procedure, repair tissue forms that is typically thinner than the adjacent native articular cartilage and is of intermediate signal intensity [23]. Over time, the amount of repair tissue increases with the optimal result being 100% defect fill with a congruent articular surface and repair tissue of similar signal intensity compared with native articular cartilage. It is common to see edema-like signal change within the subchondral bone following the procedure, though this usually resolves over several months [23]. Failure of the microfracture procedure is demonstrated as poor fill of repair tissue, often with fissuring and chondral flaps.

## Autologous Osteochondral Transplantation

Autologous osteochondral transplantation involves the harvesting and reimplantation of osteochondral plugs to repair chondral defects. The osteochondral plugs are harvested from a relative non-weight-bearing area of the joint, typically the intercondylar notch region or the borders of the femoral trochlea. The chondral defect being repaired is debrided and the osteochondral plugs are transplanted into the defect site. The orientation, position and number of osteochondral plugs are important determinants of the outcome of the procedure. The goal of the procedure is to create a congruent cartilage surface and therefore the plugs need to be placed perpendicular to the surface. Because the plugs typically come from a region of the knee joint where the articular cartilage is thinner than the recipient site, in order to have a flush articular surface there is often an incongruent bone-bone interface. Histologic evaluation of autologous osteochondral transplants has shown viable graft hyaline cartilage with the interstices between graft plugs filled with fibrocartilage-like repair tissue [24, 25]. Therefore, it is desirable to fill as much of the defect as possible with the plugs. However, the number of plugs that can be used is limited by the availability of donor sites and the need to limit morbidity at the donor sites.

Autologous osteochondral transplantation is primarily recommended for small lesions, 1-2 cm$^2$ in size, though lesions as large as 8 cm$^2$ have been treated with this procedure. Theoretical advantages of osteochondral transplantation include the ability to provide hyaline cartilage repair tissue, the ability to perform the technique with one procedure, the possibility of bone to bone healing of the grafts, and the ability to add bone to an osteochondral lesion such as osteochondritis dissecans. Potential disadvantages include the need to use a portion of the articular surface, though not a major weight-bearing surface, as a donor site, the creation of an irregular bone/cartilage interface and possible resultant irregular "tidemark" and the technical difficulty of the procedure especially in the accurate placement of the plugs. MR imaging following autologous osteochondral transplantation is used to evaluate: graft incorporation, graft congruity, repair tissue characteristics and donor site appearance.

## Autologous Chondrocyte Implantation

Autologous chondrocyte implantation (ACI) is a two-stage procedure primarily indicated for repair of symptomatic medium to large chondral lesions [26-28]. In the first stage, cartilage is harvested from the intercondylar notch or trochlear border. This cartilage is cultured and grown "ex vivo" for 4-6 weeks to produce a suspension of approximately 12 million cells. In the second stage, an open arthrotomy, the chondral defect is debrided to subchondral bone and all unstable margins are removed. A periosteal flap is taken from the ipsilateral femur or tibia and used to cover the cartilage defect. The periosteal patch is sewn to the margins of the defect and made water tight with fibrin glue except for one corner. Through this open corner, the cartilage suspension is injected, after which the open corner is stitched and glued. Advantages of ACI are the limited disruption to the joint and the potential to reform hyaline or hyaline-like cartilage. Potential disadvantages are the need for a two-step procedure and the expense of the procedure. Histologic studies following ACI have demonstrated hyaline or hyaline-like cartilage in 75-80% of the grafts and clinical studies have shown 80-90% improved outcomes [27, 29].

The MR imaging characteristics of cartilage following ACI vary, depending on the age of the tissue [30]. In the early phases, the transplanted cartilage has heterogeneous signal intensity but is typically intermediate on proton density and T1-weighted images, and hyperintense, similar to fluid, on T2-weighted images. There is prominent enhancement following intravenous contrast injection of this immature tissue. As the graft matures, the signal intensity of the graft tissue becomes more similar to the native articular cartilage, but frequently remains heterogeneous in signal intensity. The significance of the different signal intensity patterns of the graft tissue is uncertain at this time. Over time, the amount of enhancement of the graft decreases.

The goal of ACI is to restore the articular surface, and therefore the optimal result is 100% fill of the defect. Subchondral bone marrow edema like signal intensity is typically present immediately following ACI and can be intense. Over time this diminishes, though the exact time course of the resolution is uncertain. However, persistence of significant edema-like signal changes after 1 year has been reported as a worrisome finding for potential complications [30].

## Allograft Osteochondral Transplantation

Allograft osteochondral transplantation is a salvage procedure reserved for lesions that are too large for autologous transplantation procedures and which typically have failed less-invasive procedures [30]. Fresh frozen or fresh cadaveric osteochondral grafts are harvested en bloc, and then transplanted into the defect site.

In the early postoperative period, the graft is usually well demarcated with a large amount of edema-like signal change in the adjacent native bone marrow. Over time the signal intensity of both the graft and the host bone marrow returns to that of fatty marrow with integration of the graft and resultant poor definition of the interfaces between the graft and host bone. MR imaging can be used to assess the integrity of the articular cartilage of the allograft as well as the adjacent native cartilage. In addition, complication of the procedure including graft collapse, graft migration and progressive osteoarthritis can be assessed on MR images.

## References

1. Disler DG, McCauley TR, Kelman CG et al (1996) Fat-suppressed three-dimensional spoiled gradient-echo MR imaging of hyaline cartilage defects in the knee: comparison with standard MR imaging and arthroscopy. AJR Am J Roentgenol 167:127-132
2. Yao L, Gentili A, Thomas J (1996) Incidental magnetization transfer contrast in fast spin-echo imaging of cartilage. J Magn Reson Imaging 1:180-184
3. Potter HG, Linklater JM, Allen AA et al (1998) MR imaging of articular cartilage in the knee: a prospective evaluation utilizing fast spin-echo imaging. J Bone Joint Surg Am 80:1276-1284
4. Broderick LS, Turner DA, Renfrew DL et al (1994) Severity of articular cartilage abnormality in patients with osteoarthritis: evaluation with fast spin-echo MR vs. arthroscopy. AJR Am J Roentgenol 162:99-103
5. Bredella MA, Tirman PFJ, Peterfy CG et al (1999) Accuracy of T2-weighted fast spin-echo MR imaging with fat saturation in detecting cartilage defects in the knee: comparison with arthroscopy in 130 patients. AJR Am J Roentgenol 172:1073-1080
6. Recht MP, Piraino DW, Paletta GA et al (1996) Accuracy of fat-suppressed three-dimensional spoiled gradient-echo FLASH MR imaging in the detection of patellofemoral articular cartilage abnormalities. Radiology 198:209-212
7. Disler DG, McCauley TR, Wirth CR, Fuchs MD (1995) Detection of knee hyaline articular cartilage defects using fat suppressed three dimensional spoiled gradient-echo MR imaging: comparison with standard MR imaging and correlation with arthroscopy. AJR Am J Roentgenol 165:377-382
8. Konig H, Sauter R, Deimling M, Vogt M (1987) Cartilage disorders: comparison of spin-echo, CHESS, and FLASH sequence MR images. Radiology 164:753-758
9. Chandnani VP, Ho C, Chu P et al (1991) Knee hyaline cartilage evaluated with MR imaging: a cadaveric study involving multiple imaging sequences and intraarticular injection of gadolinium and saline solution. Radiology 178:557-561
10. Bashir A, Gray M, Boutin RD, Burstein D (1997) Glycosaminoglycan in articular cartilage: in vivo assessment with delayed Gd(DTPA)2–enhanced MR imaging. Radiology 205:551-558
11. Rubenstein JD, Kim JK, Morava-Protzner I et al (1993) Effects of collagen orientation on MR imaging characteristics of bovine articular cartilage. Radiology 188:219-226
12. Nieminen MT, Rieppo J, Toyras J et al (2001) T2 relaxation reveals spatial collagen architecture in articular cartilage: a comparative quantitative MRI and polarized light microscopy study. Magn Reson Med 46:487-493

13. Link TM, Stahl R, Woertler K (2007) Cartilage imaging: motivation, techniques, current and future significance. Eur Radiol 17:1135-1146

14. Duc SR, Pfirrmann CWA, Schmid MR et al (2007) Articular cartilage defects detected with 3D Water excitation true FISP: Prospective comparison with sequences commonly used for knee imaging. Radiology 245:216-223

15. Gold GE, Busse RF, Beehler C et al (2007) Isotropic MRI of the knee with 3D fast spin echo extended echo train acquisition (XETA): initial experience. AJR Am J Roentgenol 188: 1287-1293

16. Kijowski R, Lu A, Block W, Grist T (2006) Evaluation of the articular cartilage of the knee joint with vastly undersampled isotropic projection reconstruction steady-state free precession imaging. JMRI 24:168-175

17. Kladny B, Bluckert K, Swoboda B et al (1995) Comparison of low-field (0.2 Tesla) and high-field (1.5 Tesla) magnetic resonance imaging of the knee joint. Arch Orthop Trauma Surg 114:281-286

18. Vahlensieck M, Schneiber O (2003) Performance of an open low-field MR unit in routine examination of knee lesions and comparison with high field systems. Orthopade 32:175-178

19. Felson DT, Lawrence RC, Dieppe PA et al (2000) Osteoarthritis: New insights. Part 1: the disease and its risk factors. Ann Intern Med 133:635-646

20. Curl WW, Krome J, Gordon ES et al (1997) Cartilage injuries: a review of 31,516 knee arthroscopies. Arthroscopy 13:456-460

21. Aroen A, Loken S, Hei S et al (2004) Articular cartilage lesions in 993 consecutive knee arthroscopies. Am J Sports Med 32:211-215

22. Steadman J, Rodkey W, Singleton S, Briggs K (1997) Microfracture technique for full-thickness chondral defects: technique and clinical results. Oper Tech Ortho 7:300-304

23. Alparslan L, Winalski CS, Boutin RD, Minas T (2001) Postoperative magnetic resonance imaging of articular cartilage repair. Sem Musculoskel Radiol 5:345-363

24. Hangody L, Kish G, Karpati Z, Eberhardt R (1997) Osteochondral plugs: autogenous osteochondral mosaicplasty for the treatment of focal chondral and osteochondral articular defects. Operative Techniques in Orthopaedics 7:312-322

25. Pearce SG, Hurtig MB, Clarnette R et al (2001) An investigation of 2 techniques for optimizing joint surface congruency using multiple cylindrical osteochondral autografts. Arthroscopy 17:50-55

26. Peterson L (1996) Articular cartilage injuries treated with autologous chondrocyte transplantation in the human knee. Acta Orthop Belg 62:196-200 (suppl 1)

27. Peterson L, Minas T, Brittberg M (2000) Two- to 9-year outcome after autologous chondrocyte transplantation of the knee. Clin Orthop & Rel Res 374:212-234

28. Minas T, Chiu R (2000) Autologous chondrocyte implantation. Am J Knee Surg 13:41-50

29. Peterson L, Brittberg M, Kiviranta I et al (2002) Autologous chondrocyte transplantation: biomechanics and long term durability. AM J Sports Med 30:2-12

30. Recht, M, White LM, Winalski C et al (2003) MR imaging of cartilage repair procedures. Skeletal Radiol 32:185-200

# Magnetic Resonance Imaging of Muscle

Robert D. Boutin[1], Mini N. Pathria[2]

[1] Department of Radiology, University of California Davis, Sacramento, CA, USA
[2] Department of Radiology, University of California San Diego, San Diego, CA, USA

## Introduction

Muscles – you use them every time you climb stairs, lift a suitcase, hug a loved one, play sports, or do an infinite number of other activities. And yet – as long as our muscles are healthy and free of pain – we take this "miraculous machinery" for granted. Muscle, however, can be affected by all the usual categories of disease, including inherited and developmental conditions (e.g., anomalous muscles), trauma (e.g. strain, contusion), ischemia and necrosis (e.g., compartment syndrome, myonecrosis), inflammation (e.g., infection, autoimmune), neurological derangements (e.g., denervation), neoplasms and various other disorders (e.g., iatrogenic) [1-3].

This review takes a systematic approach to aid in diagnosing muscle derangements with magnetic resonance imaging (MRI) in adults, with four steps to achieving success for the practical radiologist: (1) know the clinical context; (2) understand normal muscle anatomy; (3) be familiar with common pathological conditions; and (4) know the differential diagnostic possibilities when you see a mass, edema or fatty infiltration in muscle.

## Clinical Context

Step number 1 for interpreting MRI exams is knowing the "clinical context" (i.e., patient demographics combined with a targeted medical history and anatomic localization). Relevant clinical information significantly improves the accuracy of imaging interpretations. Ideally, a detailed history is provided by the referring clinician; if a detailed history is not available, we advocate a proactive approach to obtaining a targeted medical history directly from the patient at the time of the MRI exam (e.g., with a questionnaire). Placing a skin marker over the area of maximal symptoms is also helpful, allowing correlation of clinical complaints with imaging abnormalities.

## Muscle Anatomy

For interpreting imaging exams of muscle, the second step is understanding normal muscle anatomy. Skeletal muscle is the single largest tissue in the body by weight, and some scholars spend a lifetime dedicated to studying its anatomy. When it comes to muscle anatomy and interpreting MRI exams, three practical highlights are: (1) be familiar with compartmental anatomy (that's the "big picture"!); (2) for the anatomic details, have easy access to a reliable anatomic atlas; and (3) recognize that anatomic variations in certain muscles are common (though compartmental anatomy remains constant).

First, the easiest way to conceptualize the location and function of the hundreds of muscles in the body is to become familiar with compartmental anatomy. Most muscles are arranged into compartments that are bounded by connective tissue termed fascia (or epimysium). This muscular fascia plays a fundamental role in the pathogenesis of certain muscle disorders (e.g., compartment syndrome, muscle herniation) and influences the extent of others (e.g., spread of tumor and infection). In musculoskeletal imaging, the most common compartments of interest reside in the upper and lower extremities. In the upper extremity, both the arm and the forearm can be thought of simply as having two major compartments each (i.e., anterior and posterior). In the lower extremity, the thigh is divided into three compartments: anterior (containing the quadriceps and sartorius), posterior (containing the hamstrings), and medial (containing the adductors and gracilis). The lower leg has four compartments: anterior, lateral, superficial posterior and deep posterior.

Second, have easy access to a reliable anatomic reference. There are several excellent resources available as reference books and online [4-5]. Even the best radiologists can benefit from an anatomic atlas. For example, even if you remember the compartments of the thigh, you might forget their motor innervations, which is often a key to unlocking the diagnosis of denervation-related muscle abnormalities. In the thigh, the medial

J. Hodler et al. (eds.), *Musculoskeletal Diseases 2013-2016*,
DOI: 10.1007/978-88-470-5292-5_22 © Springer-Verlag Italia 2013

compartment is supplied mostly by the obturator nerve (L2-4, anterior division), the anterior compartment is supplied by the femoral nerve (L2-L4, posterior division), and the posterior compartment is supplied by the sciatic nerve (L5-S2).

Third, be aware that muscle variations are common [6]. Although most anatomic variations are incidental and asymptomatic, they can be significant, particularly when a palpable mass mimics a neoplasm clinically or when mass effect causes a compressive neuropathy [7]. Muscle variations can be easily overlooked on MRI exams, because these "anomalies" are camouflaged amid other muscles with the same signal intensity. Although muscle variations may occur virtually anywhere, they are particularly common in the upper extremity near the wrist and in lower extremity near the ankle. Specific examples of "anomalous" muscles variations that potentially may be clinically significant include: the anconeus epitrochlearis at the elbow (impinging on the ulnar nerve), the extensor digitorum brevis manus at the wrist (mimicking tenosynovitis or a mass clinically), the third head of the gastrocnemius at the knee (causing popliteal artery entrapment syndrome), and the flexor digitorum accessorius longus at the ankle (causing tarsal tunnel syndrome).

## Common Muscle Disorders

The next step, number 3, is a big one: recognizing the many maladies affecting muscle. The most common derangements evaluated by MRI are reviewed here, including traumatic insults, ischemic changes, inflammatory disorders and denervation.

### Traumatic Injuries to the Muscle-Tendon-Bone Complex

In the acute setting, a feathery appearance of high T2 signal in muscle is common, owing to interstitial hemorrhage and edema. In the chronic setting, low T2 signal is characteristic, due to hemosiderin, fibrosis and/or heterotopic ossification. The most common types of injuries to the muscle-tendon-bone complex are the focus here: strains, avulsions and contusions. Less common traumatic derangements include laceration, muscle herniation and delayed-onset muscle soreness.

### Strain

Strain injuries result from excessive stretch or tension on myotendinous fibers, usually during eccentric muscle contraction. Eccentric contraction refers to the muscle lengthening during contraction (e.g., lowering a dumbbell weight), which generates more tension than when a muscle is allowed to shorten with (concentric) contraction (e.g., curling a dumbbell weight). Strains tend to occur in muscles that cross two joints, have a high proportion of fast-twitch fibers, and undergo eccentric contraction.

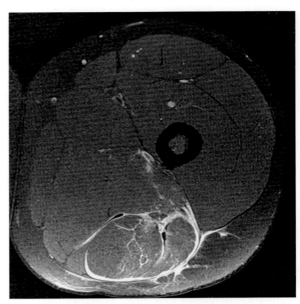

**Fig. 1.** Grade 2 muscle strain. 26-year-old man injured playing soccer 4 days prior to magnetic resonance imaging. Axial PD-weighted fat-suppressed image of the left thigh shows peritendinous and epimyseal fluid involving the hamstring musculature. Note the relative preservation of the muscle architecture

The degree of strain may be graded along a spectrum of injury – from-mild (grade 1, microscopic injury) to moderate (grade 2, partial tear) to severe (grade 3, complete tear):

• Grade 1 strains are typically displayed on MRI as edema-like signal at the myotendinous junction (which is commonly intramuscular) or the junction of the muscle with the overlying epimysium, without macroscopic discontinuity of fibers; muscle morphology is preserved.

• Grade 2 strains are defined by partial discontinuity of muscle fibers, with edema and blood in the acute setting that is associated with a tear at the myotendinous or subfascial region. With these tears, the epimysium is commonly disrupted, which allows hemorrhage to escape the injured muscle and track more superficially along the adjacent fascia (preferentially into a more dependent position). Such perifascial fluid-like signal occurs in the vast majority of athletes with acute partial tears (Fig. 1).

• Grade 3 strains are the least common type of injury. These complete ruptures are usually characterized by retraction and waviness of torn fibers, as well as substantial hemorrhage in the acute setting. With MRI, the injury grade (as well as the length and cross-sectional area of edema signal) often correlate with rehabilitation time.

The age of a patient influences the location of injury along the biomechanical chain formed by the linkage of muscle to tendon and tendon to bone:

• In older adults (or others with tendinopathy), the "weak link" is the degenerated tendon. Tendinopathy becomes more prevalent with advancing age, and so do tendon tears (e.g., rotator cuff tears through pre-existing tendinopathy).

• In adolescents, the weakest link in the chain tends to be the physis, and therefore apophyseal avulsions are common.

• In young adults (who have healthy tendons and closed apophyses), strains characteristically target the junction of muscle and tendon tissue (myotendinous junction), because strong muscles generate particularly high "strain" forces where these tissues with different physical properties interface. There are three locations for these interfaces: the classic myotendinous junction (where tendons emerge from muscle proximally and distally), the intramuscular myotendinous junction (along tendon slips that run within the muscle), and the myofascial junction (at the periphery of the muscle).

In one study of young athletes, acute hamstring injuries occurred at the myotendinous junction in diverse locations: the proximal myotendinous junction (33%), the intramuscular myotendinous junction (53%), and the distal myotendinous junction (13%) [8]. Note that this is in contradistinction to older adults; their hamstring injuries occur most commonly at the proximal tendon attachments, owing to underlying tendinopathy. Although the vast majority of *muscle* strains resolve with only nonoperative management, a common operative indication is an avulsion and a tear in the *tendon*, which are amenable to treatment with suture anchors and direct suture repair, respectively.

The most commonly strained muscles in the extremities include the rectus femoris, hamstrings, adductors and gastrocnemius muscles [9].

### Rectus Femoris Strain

The proximal rectus femoris has two heads. The direct (or "straight") head arises from the anterior-inferior iliac spine, and contributes to the anterior fascia of the muscle. The indirect (or "reflected") head arises from the superior acetabular ridge and hip capsule, contributing to a long musculotendinous junction within the muscle [10]. Rectus femoris strains targeting this deep intramuscular musculotendinous junction (sometimes referred to as the central tendon or aponeurosis) can result in a "bull's-eye sign" on MRI, and have a longer rehabilitation time than strains located at the muscle periphery [11].

### Hamstring Strain

The hamstrings are composed of the semimembranosus, semitendinosus and biceps femoris [12-14]. The semimembranosus origin is the superolateral facet of the ischial tuberosity. The semitendinosus and biceps femoris long head originate from a conjoint tendon at the inferomedial facet of the ischial tuberosity. High-grade or complete tendon rupture (or bony avulsion) at the proximal hamstring complex is considered an indication for surgical repair in active young adults, with better results in the acute setting [13].

The hamstrings are the most commonly injured muscles in sprinting and jumping athletes. Of the three hamstring components, the biceps femoris long head is the most commonly injured in the classic abrupt-onset hamstring strain. Less commonly, in some sports (e.g., dance), the onset of a stretching injury may occur more slowly, target the proximal semimembranosus *tendon*, and take much longer to heal [15]. Rehabilitation time may be suggested by the extent of hamstring injury seen by MRI. Convalescence periods reportedly vary widely from 2 weeks to 1.5 years before patients can return to vigorous activities. Recurrent injuries are common, occurring in one-quarter of athletes. Even minor hamstring injuries may double the risk of a more severe injury within 2 months.

### Calf Muscle Strain

Several muscles and tendons at the posterior aspect of the knee and calf may be subjected to strain injuries, including the gastrocnemius, soleus, plantaris, and popliteus muscles. "Tennis leg" may be defined clinically as the sudden onset of sharp pain in the mid-calf while participating in athletics (e.g., racket sports, running), typically in middle-aged persons [16]. Most commonly, these injuries are partial tears involving the (fast-twitch) medial head of the gastrocnemius muscle. Isolated strain of the (slow-twitch) soleus muscle is less common, usually occurring with endurance activities [17]. Treatment is almost always conservative, typically with relief of pain within 2 weeks and return to sports after at least 3 weeks. Clinical differential diagnosis may include a ruptured Baker's cyst, overuse "tendinitis", stress fracture, chronic exertional compartment syndrome, fascial herniation, venous thrombosis, nerve entrapment and popliteal artery entrapment syndrome.

### Avulsion

Given that the physis is a weak link in the biomechanical chain for skeletally immature patients, we commonly see apophyseal avulsion fractures in adolescent athletes. The pelvis, with its many apophyses, is a common site for such avulsions. In one study of 203 adolescent athletes with acute pelvic avulsion fractures, the most common sites were: (1) the ischial tuberosity (origin of the hamstrings), (2) the anterior-inferior iliac spine (origin of the rectus femoris), and (3) the anterior-superior iliac spine (origin of the sartorius) [18]. Such avulsions generally are treated conservatively and have a good prognosis, although nonunions can occur. The imaging appearance of osseous avulsion injuries may be mistaken for a neoplastic or infectious process, especially in the nonacute setting when no history of trauma is provided. Knowledge of the major tendinous attachments to bone is indispensable in arriving at a correct diagnosis – and avoiding misdiagnosis of an osteochondroma or osteosarcoma.

## Contusion

Unlike muscle strains caused by indirect (noncontact) injury, contusions are caused by direct concussive trauma, usually by a blunt object. The resultant interstitial edema and hemorrhage correspond to the site of impact (rather than being localized to the myotendinous junction). Hemorrhage can be seen in the muscle, intermuscular fat planes or the subcutaneous tissues. Soft tissue hemorrhage can collect focally, resulting in a hematoma.

## Sequelae of Musculotendinous Injury

Several sequelae of musculotendinous injury may be observed, including hematoma, heterotopic ossification, fibrosis and atrophy. These sequelae are not specific to the post-traumatic setting, but rather reflect the limited pathological responses that muscle has when confronted with a wide array of insults.

## Hematoma

Intramuscular hematomas evaluated between 5 days and 5 months after injury commonly display characteristics of methemoglobin, with increased signal intensity on both T1- and T2-weighted images. Most intramuscular hematomas tend to diminish in size over a period of 6-8 weeks. Differentiation between a simple hematoma and a hemorrhagic neoplasm may be difficult in some patients both clinically and with imaging. Administration of contrast material aids in excluding a neoplasm when the lesion in question shows no enhancement. Conversely,

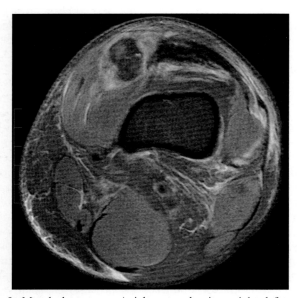

**Fig. 2.** Muscle hematoma. Axial proton-density-weighted fat-suppressed image of the left thigh obtained 1 day after a direct blow to the medial knee shows an acute hematoma in the vastus medialis muscle, with surrounding edema. Note signal heterogeneity, with some regions of higher signal representing early methemoglobin formation

the presence of an enhancing nodule in a muscle lesion may suggest the diagnosis of a neoplasm rather than a hematoma (Fig. 2). When the diagnosis of a probably benign hematoma is in doubt, clinical correlation and a follow-up MRI examination are indicated to confirm lesion stability or resolution. In the chronic setting, serous-appearing fluid may linger within a connective tissue sheath, creating an intramuscular pseudocyst or "seroma". Heterotopic ossification also may occur.

## Heterotopic Ossification

The most common type of heterotopic ossification occurs in muscle, and commonly is referred to as myositis ossificans. Risk factors for heterotopic ossification include traumatic insults (e.g., contusion, surgery, burns), neurological insults (e.g., paraplegia, traumatic brain injury, stroke), or bleeding dyscrasias (e.g., hemophilia). In the clinical and radiological arenas, three typical phases of evolution occur: (1) an acute or pseudo-inflammatory phase; (2) a subacute or pseudotumoral phase; and (3) a chronic, self-limited phase that may (or may not) undergo spontaneous healing. In the acute and subacute stages of myositis ossificans, imaging examinations have a notoriously nonspecific appearance. CT is the single best imaging examination for showing the characteristic ossific matrix. In the final stage, the imaging findings that permit confident differentiation of myositis ossificans from neoplasm are: (1) the ossific mass is well-defined, sharply marginated, and appears more mature peripherally than centrally with architecture that approximates native bone (an area of cancellous bone centrally surrounded by compact bone peripherally); (2) the lesion generally decreases in size with the passage of time; and (3) there is no destruction in the underlying bone.

Imaging findings evolve over time, and are typically nonspecific in the acute and subacute stages. The involved muscle is enlarged and underlying periostitis is common. With MRI, the muscle exhibits nonspecific intermediate T1 and high T2 signal intensity. As the lesion matures, T2 hyperintensity and contrast enhancement progressively decrease. The signal intensity of the lesion may remain inhomogeneous, although areas of signal intensity equivalent to marrow fat and cortical bone increase [19]. Mature myositis ossificans is easiest to recognize when there is a low signal rim and fat signal centrally, although persistent granulation-type tissue may make the diagnosis difficult by MRI.

Myositis ossificans has been designated a "don't touch" lesion that should not be biopsied injudiciously. Treatment for myositis ossificans may include physical therapy, nonsteroidal antiinflammatory agents, bisphosphonates, low-dose irradiation therapy and, in uncommon cases, surgical resection for a bulky area of ossification that causes nerve entrapment or limits range of motion. Surgical resection of myositis ossificans traditionally is performed after the mass "matures" in the hopes of minimizing the risk of recurrence.

## Fibrosis

Fibrosis is characteristically displayed as low signal intensity tissue in muscle on T2-weighted images after a nonacute insult. Recognized sites of muscle fibrosis include the deltoid, gluteus maximus and the vastus lateralis. Evaluation of the clinical impact and treatment of fibrosis is an active area of research.

## Atrophy

Muscle atrophy may occur after certain musculotendinous injuries, disuse or other insults. The cardinal feature of muscle atrophy is decreased muscle volume, which is often accompanied by fatty infiltration. The most frequent site of muscle atrophy is in the shoulder girdle after a rotator cuff tear. After a supraspinatus tendon tear, adjacent muscle atrophy is recognized as a negative prognostic factor for patients undergoing cuff repair. Atrophy of other shoulder girdle muscles also can occur, even when the rotator cuff tendons are intact. Muscle atrophy begins to develop within 10 days after immobilization. After bed rest for 20 days, the muscle cross-sectional area decreases approximately 10% in healthy men [20]. Muscle atrophy may be partially irreversible by 4 months.

## Muscle Ischemia and Myonecrosis

### Compartment Syndrome

Compartment syndrome is defined as elevated pressure in a relatively noncompliant anatomic space that is associated with ischemia, and may result in neuromuscular injury, including myonecrosis and rhabdomyolysis [21]. Risk factors for compartment syndrome include a history of trauma, external compression, systemic hypotension, increased intracompartmental volume (e.g., hemorrhage, edema, poor venous return, muscle hypertrophy), and loss of compartment elasticity (e.g., fibrotic or constricted fascia). Compartment syndrome can occur at virtually any location, most commonly in the leg and less commonly in other sites such as the thigh, forearm and paraspinal musculature (Fig. 3).

Patients initially complain of painful aching, tightness, or pressure that worsens with palpation and passive stretching of the affected muscles.

Compartment syndrome is generally classified as acute or chronic:

- Acute compartment syndrome is a surgical emergency treated by fasciotomy, which decompresses the hypertensive muscle and improves perfusion. Although most cases of acute compartment syndrome are associated with fractures, the second most common cause is injury to soft tissues (e.g., contusion) without fracture. The definitive diagnosis is made with direct percutaneous compartment pressure measurements that may be aided by near infrared spectroscopy.

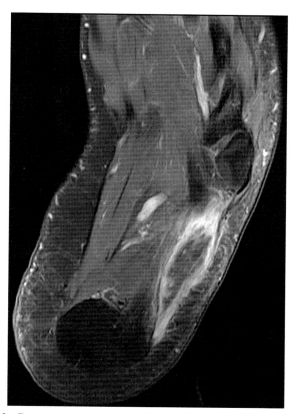

**Fig. 3.** Compartment syndrome. 40-year-old man with foot pain following prolonged surgical procedure of pelvis done with patient in lithotomy position with foot blocks. Axial T1-weighted fat-suppressed magnetic resonance image following intravenous contrast enhancement shows intense peripheral enhancement limited to the periphery of the abductor digiti quinti muscle. Similar changes were present in the contralateral foot (not illustrated) related to compression-induced compartment syndrome

- Chronic compartment syndrome may occur as a result of exertional causes (e.g., exercise, occupational overuse) or, less commonly, "non-exertional" causes (e.g., a mass lesion, infection). The most common type of chronic exertional compartment syndrome, for example, occurs in the legs of running athletes. The thigh, forearm and foot are the next most common sites in athletes, depending on the muscles used in their chosen sport.

Although imaging is not the primary technique for diagnosing compartment syndrome, MRI may be used to display the location and extent of high T2 signal associated with muscle ischemia in the nonacute setting. Familiarity with the imaging appearance of compartment syndrome is important, given that imaging may be performed for assessment of pain that initially is thought to be due to other causes (e.g., stress fracture, myotendinous strain, soft-tissue tumor). Imaging also assists in evaluation for an underlying lesion (e.g., hematoma, neoplasm) that may contribute to intracompartmental hypertension and needs to be addressed at surgery.

With MRI, the most common findings are non-specific T2 hyperintensity and increased muscle volume (due to muscle hypertrophy, edema or both), occasionally with fascial perforation or fascial thickening. Muscle herniation (protrusion of muscle tissue through a focal fascial defect, most commonly in the leg) also may be observed in patients with compartment syndrome. Although controversial, gadolinium-enhanced MRI may be helpful in distinguishing muscles that are still perfused from those with grossly devitalized areas. (The rate of contrast material "washout" may be prolonged in muscles affected by compartment syndrome.) The change of T2 signal intensity between pre-exercise and postexercise images is significantly greater in compartments with postexercise hypertension.

### Calcific Myonecrosis

Calcific myonecrosis refers to liquefied necrotic muscle and dystrophic calcification that occurs as an uncommon late complication of compartment syndrome. Patients typically are diagnosed decades after a traumatic event. MRI demonstrates a fusiform, cystic-appearing (necrotic) mass of heterogeneous signal intensity, most commonly in the anterior compartment of the leg.

### Rhabdomyolysis

Rhabdomyolysis refers to the breakdown of skeletal muscle and leakage of muscle contents into the circulation [22]. Clinically, rhabdomyolysis is defined as muscle pain or weakness associated with high creatine kinase levels (10 times higher than normal) and myoglobinuria (classically producing dark brown urine). Damaged muscle releases myoglobin and other metabolites that can potentially result in acute kidney injury (previously termed acute renal failure) in 15-30% of patients, electrolyte imbalance with cardiac arrest, or disseminated intravascular coagulation. The causes of rhabdomyolysis are numerous, including trauma (e.g., crush injury, electrical injury), prolonged compression of muscle due to immobilization, untreated compartment syndrome, excessive muscle activity, myositis and drugs (e.g., statin medications). MRI is considered the most sensitive imaging test to evaluate the location and extent of rhabdomyolysis. The principal MRI finding is hyperintense T2 signal within muscle (due to the presence of edema, hemorrhage and necrosis), typically with a paucity of mass effect.

### Diabetic Myopathy

In patients with diabetes, thrombosis may occur in arterioles due to diseased vascular endothelium and relative hypercoagulability. Diabetic myopathy may take the form of diabetic muscle infarction, typically in patients who also have other complications from poorly controlled or chronic diabetes (e.g., neuropathy, retinopathy, nephropathy). Multiple muscles are usually involved, often bilater-

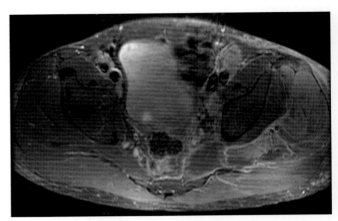

**Fig. 4.** Diabetic myopathy. Elderly man with poorly controlled diabetes with buttock pain. Axial T1-weighted fat-suppressed magnetic resonance image following intravenous contrast enhancement image of the pelvis demonstrates mild swelling and abnormal enhancement within the majority of the left hip buttock musculature due to diabetic myopathy. There were no clinical indications of infection. Symptoms and imaging findings resolved in 3 weeks with conservative management

ally. The most commonly affected muscles are in the thigh and calf. With MRI, fluid-sensitive images show diffuse edema-like signal in the areas involved by diabetic muscle infarction (Fig. 4). Contrast enhancement can be diffuse, often with focal areas of nonenhancement corresponding to macroscopic areas of muscle infarction. MRI is considered 100% sensitive for the detection of diabetic muscle infarction, although the findings are not specific. Depending on the clinical context, the imaging differential diagnosis may include trauma, pyomyositis and noninfectious forms of myositis.

### Inflammatory Myopathies – Infectious and Idiopathic

Myositis is defined as inflammation of muscle. Infectious causes of myositis include a wide variety of bacterial, viral, parasitic and fungal pathogens. Noninfectious inflammation of muscle may be caused by autoimmune or idiopathic mechanisms, including sarcoid myopathy, polymyositis, dermatomyositis and inclusion body myositis.

### Pyomyositis

Primary pyomyositis is an acute or subacute bacterial infection of skeletal muscle that usually results after an episode of transient bacteremia [23, 24]. Common risk factors for pyomyositis include immunosuppression (e.g., HIV infection), malnutrition, diabetes, malignancy, intravenous drug use and trauma (e.g., muscle contusion). Primary pyomyositis is most common in the largest muscle groups in the pelvis and lower extremities. Pyomyositis evolves over time through three general stages: (1) insidious onset of poorly localized diffuse inflammation, often

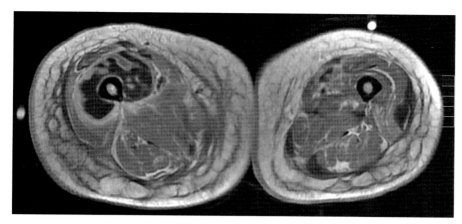

**Fig. 5.** Pyomyositis. 46-year-old woman with history of Behçet's syndrome presented with fever and intense thigh pain. Axial T1-weighted magnetic resonance image following intravenous contrast shows bilateral widespread muscle enhancement with numerous collections of non-enhancing fluid. Note the thickening of the deep subcutaneous tissues and overlying fascia. Surgical debridement was performed showing widespread muscle infection complicated by myonecrosis and abscess formation

over a period of 1-2 weeks; (2) focal muscle abscess formation; and (if untreated) (3) extension of infection and systemic sepsis. Laboratory analysis reveals leukocytosis in approximately 75% of patients. The most commonly identified bacterium is *Staphylococcus aureus* (77%). Cultures of blood and purulent material are positive in only approximately one-third of cases. Consequently, the diagnosis of pyomyositis is based commonly on clinical and imaging findings.

With MRI, areas affected by pyomyositis demonstrate hyperintense signal on fluid-sensitive pulse sequences, muscle enlargement, effacement of intramuscular and intermuscular fat, enhancement in the inflamed region after contrast administration, and focal collection of fluid that may contain septations. A purulent fluid collection usually is detected, but this is not invariably the case (Fig. 5). MRI also may show abnormal signal in the adjacent bone marrow, owing to either the presence of reactive inflammatory changes or the presence of coexisting osteomyelitis. Occasionally, soft tissue gas or lymph node enlargement is observed.

## Sarcoid Myopathy

Sarcoidosis is a systemic inflammatory disease characterized by the presence of noncaseating granulomas, most commonly in the lungs, skin, eyes, liver and musculoskeletal systems [25]. The diagnosis of sarcoid myopathy is made most commonly in young to middle-aged adult women, peaking in the third decade through to fifth decade. On MRI, sarcoid myopathy can have a variety of appearances. The nodular subtype is regarded as the most important, because it can be mistaken for a soft-tissue neoplasm. These focal, intramuscular masses may be multiple and bilateral, typically with central areas of low signal intensity on T1- and T2-weighted images. Less commonly, sarcoid myopathy presents as the myopathic subtype. MRI in these patients shows nonspecific, diffusely hyperintense signal in muscle (without a mass) on fluid-sensitive images in the acute phase. In the chronic setting, muscle atrophy and fatty infiltration can be observed.

## Idiopathic Inflammatory Myopathies

Idiopathic inflammatory myopathies are a heterogeneous group of diseases characterized by idiopathic nonsuppurative inflammation in muscle [26, 27]. The three most common forms of idiopathic inflammatory myopathies in adults are polymyositis, dermatomyositis and sporadic inclusion body myositis. All three are associated with an increased likelihood of autoimmune-related connective tissue diseases (e.g., scleroderma, systemic lupus erythematosis) and a variety of malignancies. Polymyositis and dermatomyositis preferentially target women, whereas sporadic inclusion body myositis is more common in men. Dermatomyositis is differentiated from polymyositis by the presence of a dermatologic exanthema and the presence of soft-tissue calcifications. The immune-mediated muscle damage results in progressive bilateral muscle weakness of the proximal muscles around the hip and shoulder in patients with polymyositis and dermatomyositis, but involves more distal muscles in patients with sporatic inclusing body myositis. Sporadic inclusion body myositis is differentiated most commonly by its insidious onset in adults older than age 50 years, distinctive biopsy findings, and incomplete, inconsistent response to treatment.

MRI may be indicated for patients with idiopathic inflammatory myopathies for aiding early diagnosis, determining disease activity, documenting disease extent, assessing therapeutic response, directing biopsy and narrowing the differential diagnosis. With respect to determining disease activity, the cardinal feature of active myositis is diffuse T2 hyperintensity in muscle, commonly referred to as "muscle edema". This T2 hyperintensity actually may be due to accumulation of extracellular water, an inflammatory cell infiltrate, or recent microinfarction. With active myositis, edema-like signal also may be present adjacent to muscle along the fascia or in the subcutaneous soft tissue (Fig. 6). Chronic disease characteristically is muscle atrophy manifested by fatty replacement and decreased muscle girth.

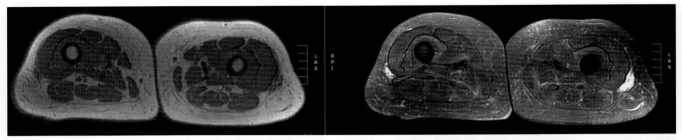

**Fig. 6.** Inflammatory polymyositis. Axial T1-weighted (*left*) and T2-weighted (*right*) images of the thighs in a middle-aged female with in-flammatory polymyositis demonstrate symmetrical mild muscle edema of both thighs. The T1-weighted image shows preservation of nor-mal muscle architecture

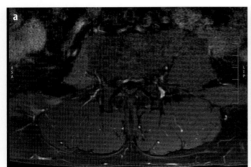
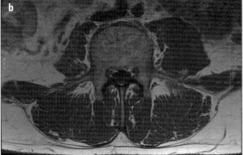

**Fig. 7 a, b.** Psoas denervation. Axial T2-weighted (**a**) and T1-weighted (**b**) images of the spine in a middle-aged man with back pain demonstrate loss of volume of the right psoas muscle. The T2-weighted image shows mild signal increase without fluid accumulation at the right psoas, with very subtle changes also seen at the right quadratus lumborum. There was a large lateral disk impinging on the L2 nerve root accounting for these denervation changes

## Muscle Denervation

Denervation of muscle can be associated with pain, weakness, atrophy and disability. Muscle denervation may be caused by various insults to nerves, including: entrapment, trauma, inflammation, infection, vascular compromise and idiopathic causes. MRI and MR neurography are used to diagnose the presence of muscle denervation, as well as its cause and location [28, 29]. With denervation, the signal intensity and morphology of muscle undergo characteristic changes with MRI.

Depending on the severity of a neurological insult, the onset of hyperintense T2 signal changes is reported from a few days to a few weeks. Three MRI features may help distinguish the hyperintense T2 signal in denervated muscles from that seen with strained muscles: (1) unlike strain injury, the hyperintense T2 signal in denervated muscles is not associated with perifascial edema; (2) the pattern of muscle involvement may suggest a specific nerve territory responsible for the denervation changes; and (3) abnormally hyperintense T2 signal in peripheral nerves is a hallmark of many neuropathies (Fig. 7).

With chronic denervation, diminished bulk and fatty infiltration occur in muscle. Atrophic changes are best displayed on T1-weighted MR images. Whereas the signal intensity changes of acute muscle denervation are reversible, profound fatty atrophic changes seen late in the course of denervation may be irreversible. The atrophic changes

from denervation are not specific, and may be seen with conditions as diverse as motor neuron diseases (e.g., poliomyelitis) and demyelination (e.g., hereditary motor and sensory neuropathies). Although chronic denervation usually results in atrophy, pseudohypertrophy and true hypertrophy have been reported in affected extremities.

## Differential Diagnosis

MRI facilitates the diagnostic process primarily by detecting alterations in muscle size or signal intensity. Although skeletal muscle may be afflicted by a spectacular array of disorders, only a limited number of biologic responses ("MRI patterns") are possible [3]. In other words, similar gross pathologic features may be caused by many different disorders. Given that the potential causes for abnormal signal intensity in muscle are diverse, the MRI differential diagnosis may be simplified by recognizing one of three basic patterns [30].

### Three Basic Patterns of Abnormal Signal Intensity in Muscle

The "mass lesion pattern" can be seen with traumatic injuries (e.g., myositis ossificans), as well as with neoplasm, infection (e.g., pyomyositis, parasitic infection), muscular sarcoidosis and anomalous muscles (Fig. 8).

The "muscle edema pattern" may be seen with recent trauma (e.g., strain injury), as well as with recent micro-

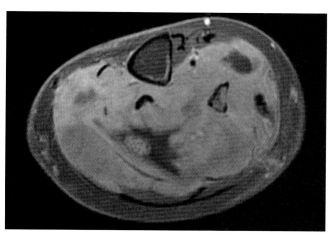

**Fig. 8.** Lymphoma. 84-year-old woman complaining of progressive left calf swelling for 6 months. Axial T1-weighted fat-suppressed MR following intravenous contrast enhancement shows near complete replacement of the muscles by enhancing tissue. Note the enhancing marrow at the fibula and the enlarged infiltrated tibial nerve at the posterior calf. Biopsy revealed B-cell lymphoma

trauma (e.g., delayed onset muscle soreness), subacute denervation, infectious or autoimmune myositis, rhabdomyolysis, vascular insult (e.g., diabetic muscle infarction, deep venous thrombosis) or recent iatrogenic insults (e.g., surgery, radiation therapy).

The "fatty infiltration pattern" may be observed in the chronic setting after a substantial myotendinous injury, as well as with other insults causing chronic muscle disuse or chronic denervation.

## Summary

Muscle disorders have a wide variety of causes, treatments and prognoses. Given that the cause and severity of these disorders may sometimes be difficult to determine clinically, MRI can be used to narrow the differential diagnosis and pinpoint the appropriate pain generator. Consequently, MRI can often help establish an appropriate prognosis, direct intervention (e.g., biopsy or surgery), monitor treatment response objectively, and diagnose possible complications associated with a disorder.

## References

1. Boutin RD (2002) Muscle Disorders. In: Resnick D (Ed) Diagnosis of bone and joint disorders, 4th edn. WB Saunders, Philadelphia, PA, pp 4696-4768
2. Boutin RD (2008) Radiologic perspective: magnetic resonance imaging of muscle. In: Pedowitz R, Chung C, Resnick D (Eds) Magnetic resonance imaging in orthopedic sports medicine. Springer, New York, NY, pp 1-20
3. Costa AF, Di Primio GA, Schweitzer ME (2012) Magnetic resonance imaging of muscle disease: a pattern-based approach. Muscle Nerve 46:465-481
4. Manaster BJ et al (Eds) (2006) Diagnostic and surgical imaging anatomy: musculoskeletal. Amirsys Publishing, Salt Lake City, UH
5. Richardson M (2008) Muscle Atlas. UW Radiology. http://www.rad.washington.edu/academics/academic-sections/msk/muscle-atlas
6. Bergman RA (2012) Anatomy Atlases: a digital library of anatomy information. http://www.anatomyatlases.org
7. Sookur PA, Naraghi AM, Bleakney RR et al (2008) Accessory muscles: anatomy, symptoms, and radiologic evaluation. Radiographics 28:481-499
8. De Smet AA, Best TM (2000) MR imaging of the distribution and location of acute hamstring injuries in athletes. AJR Am J Roentgenol 174:393-399
9. Ekstrand J, Hägglund M, Waldén M (2011) Epidemiology of muscle injuries in professional football (soccer). Am J Sports Med 39:1226-1232
10. Gyftopoulos S, Rosenberg ZS, Schweitzer ME, Bordalo-Rodrigues M (2008) Normal anatomy and strains of the deep musculotendinous junction of the proximal rectus femoris: MRI features. AJR Am J Roentgenol 190:W182-6
11. Cross TM, Gibbs N, Houang MT, Cameron M (2004) Acute quadriceps muscle strains: magnetic resonance imaging features and prognosis. Am J Sports Med 32:710-719
12. Rubin DA (2012) Imaging diagnosis and prognostication of hamstring injuries. AJR Am J Roentgenol 199:525-533
13. Harris JD, Griesser MJ, Best TM, Ellis TJ (2011) Treatment of proximal hamstring ruptures – a systematic review. Int J Sports Med 32:490-495
14. Miller SL, Webb GR (2008) The proximal origin of the hamstrings and surrounding anatomy encountered during repair. Surgical technique. J Bone Joint Surg Am 90 Suppl 2 Pt 1:108-116
15. Askling CM, Malliaropoulos N, Karlsson J (2012) High-speed running type or stretching-type of hamstring injuries makes a difference to treatment and prognosis. Br J Sports Med 46:86-87
16. Delgado GJ, Chung CB, Lektrakul N et al (2002) Tennis leg: clinical US study of 141 patients and anatomic investigation of four cadavers with MR imaging and US. Radiology 224:112-119
17. Balius R, Alomar X, Rodas G et al (2012) The soleus muscle: MRI, anatomic and histologic findings in cadavers with clinical correlation of strain injury distribution. Skeletal Radiol [Epub ahead of print]
18. Rossi F, Dragoni S (2001) Acute avulsion fractures of the pelvis in adolescent competitive athletes: prevalence, location and sports distribution of 203 cases collected. Skeletal Radiol 30:127-131
19. Ledermann HP, Schweitzer ME, Morrison WB (2002) Pelvic heterotopic ossification: MR imaging characteristics. Radiology 222:189-195
20. Kawakami Y, Muraoka Y, Kubo K (2000) Changes in muscle size and architecture following 20 days of bed rest. J Gravit Physiol 7:53-59
21. Verleisdonk EJ, van Gils A, van der Werken C (2001) The diagnostic value of MRI scans for the diagnosis of chronic exertional compartment syndrome of the lower leg. Skeletal Rad 30:321-325
22. Moratalla MB, Braun P, Fornas GM (2008) Importance of MRI in the diagnosis and treatment of rhabdomyolysis. Eur J Radiol 65:311-315
23. Gordon BA, Martinez S, Collins AJ (1995) Pyomyositis: characteristics at CT and MR imaging. Radiology 197:279-286
24. Chiedozi LC (1979) Pyomyositis. Review of 205 cases in 112 patients. Am J Surg 137:255-259
25. Moore SL, Teirstein AE (2003) Musculoskeletal sarcoidosis: spectrum of appearances at MR imaging. Radiographics 23:1389-1399
26. Schulze M, Kötter I, Ernemann U et al (2009) MRI findings in inflammatory muscle diseases and their noninflammatory mimics. AJR Am J Roentgenol 192(6):1708-1716

27. Del Grande F, Carrino JA, Del Grande M et al (2011) Magnetic resonance imaging of inflammatory myopathies. Top Magn Reson Imaging 22:39-43

28. Kamath S, Venkatanarasimha N, Walsh MA, Hughes PM (2008) MRI appearance of muscle denervation. Skeletal Radiol 37:397-404

29. Viddeleer AR, Sijens PE, van Ooyen PM et al (2012) Sequential MR imaging of denervated and reinnervated skeletal muscle as correlated to functional outcome. Radiology 264:522-530

30. May DA, Disler DG, Jones EA et al (2000) Abnormal signal intensity in skeletal muscle at MR imaging: patterns, pearls, and pitfalls. RadioGraphics 20:295-315

# Neuropathies of the Upper Extremity

Gustav Andreisek[1], Jenny T. Bencardino[2]

[1] Department of Radiology, University Hospital Zurich, Zurich, Switzerland
[2] Department of Radiology, NYU Hospital for Joint Diseases, NYU Langone Medical Center, New York, NY, USA

## Introduction

A spectrum of pathologies can affect peripheral nerves causing peripheral neuropathies. Traditionally, their evaluation relies on clinical history and clinical examination, including electrodiagnostic testing (e.g., nerve conduction studies, electromyography). However, clinical information is often insufficient as it does not provide spatial information regarding the nerves or their surrounding structures, i.e., innervated muscles [1]. Imaging provides important morphological information and thereby often helps in localization and characterization of these pathologies. Imaging using either ultrasound or magnetic resonance imaging (MRI) also can exclude neuropathies by demonstrating normal nerves and muscles. Although morphological assessment is the mainstay of nerve imaging, recent developments such as diffusion-weighted and diffusion tensor MRI may additionally allow functional assessment of nerves in the future [2].

To understand the imaging findings in peripheral neuropathies, deeper knowledge of nerve anatomy, underlying pathophysiology, technical requirements and individual pathologies is important. This syllabus outlines the anatomy of peripheral nerves and relevant pathophysiology. It discusses technical requirements, commonly imaged pathologies at the upper extremity, and provides an outlook on future developments.

## Peripheral Nerve Anatomy and Pathophysiology

### Nerve Anatomy

Understanding peripheral nerve anatomy is relevant for detection of subtle and gross deviations from the normal morphology. The axon is the basic unit of a peripheral nerve. It is surrounded by periaxonal supporting structures, which include the Schwann cells and connective tissue stroma. Axons can be myelinated or unmyelinated. The myelin sheath of myelinated nerves is formed by the Schwann cells, whereas unmyelinated nerves usually invaginate into the grooves of the Schwann cell cytoplasm [3]. The connective tissue stroma forms the endoneurium that surrounds the axons. Multiple axons form a fascicle. Fascicles are typically surrounded by perineurium. Multiple fascicles are arranged to form the peripheral nerve and are surrounded by the epineurium (Fig. 1).

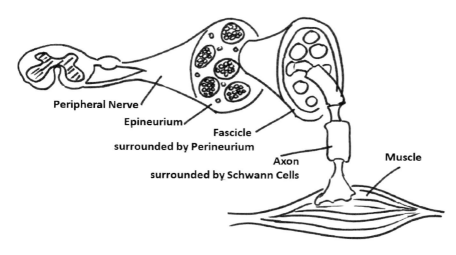

**Peripheral Nerve**
**Epineurium**
**Fascicle**
**surrounded by Perineurium**
**Axon**
**surrounded by Schwann Cells**
**Muscle**

**Fig. 1.** Structure of a peripheral nerve (type: myelinated axon)

J. Hodler et al. (eds.), *Musculoskeletal Diseases 2013-2016*,
DOI: 10.1007/978-88-470-5292-5_23 © Springer-Verlag Italia 2013

## Pathophysiology and Classification System

Several categorizations of peripheral neuropathies exist, including one that is based on the underlying etiology. It distinguishes between entrapment and nonentrapment neuropathies. Nerve entrapment syndromes at the upper extremity typically affect the median, radial and ulnar nerves at anatomic locations where the nerve courses through nerve fibro-osseous or fibromuscular tunnels or penetrates a muscle. In cases of nerve thickening, narrowing of the tunnel or hypertrophy of the muscles, the nerve might be entrapped. Nonentrapment neuropathies include all other etiologies such as traumatic nerve injuries, inflammatory conditions, polyneuropathies and mass lesions [1, 3].

Other categorizations distinguish systemic diseases from local as well as functional diseases. Systemic diseases include ischemia, vasculitis, toxic, endocrine and metabolic disorders (e.g., diabetes), motorsensory neuropathies, amyloidosis, hyperlipidemia, multifocal motor neuropathies and inflammatory neuropathies. MRI is not expected to establish these diagnosis but may help to confirm the clinical suspicion, to show the abnormality of the involved nerves and muscles, and to document the distribution/pattern of the neuropathy [3]. Local diseases include all local abnormalities such as masses, nerve injuries, entrapment neuropathies, infections and adhesive changes following surgery. MRI has a major role in these conditions as it adds morphological information to clinical information. Imaging can show the exact localization of the lesion, and detect the underlying nerve or other pathology [3]. Functional diseases such as traction or compression mononeuritis due to habitual leg crossing or repeated typing/exercise are difficult to evaluate by MRI, as in most cases only indirect signs are visible. Dynamic assessment of peripheral nerves by the means of MRI is often not conclusive. However, ultrasound can then be an important tool to evaluate, for example, functional compressive neuropathies, since it allows dynamic or functional nerve assessment during exercise.

Peripheral nerve injuries are typically classified according to the Seddon and Sunderland classification system. In this classification system three different types of nerve injury are described, namely: neuropraxia, axonotmesis and neurotmesis [3].

Neuropraxia is the least severe type of injury. It is characterized by a predominant loss of motor function due to a temporary block of the nerve conduction. Usually there is also some degree of loss of sensory function. Neuropraxia often is associated with blunt trauma where the myelin sheaths are injured. Wallerian degeneration (a process in which the part of the axon separated from the neuron's cell body degenerates distal to the injury) does not occur in neuropraxia. The electromyogram is usually negative. This type of injury is relatively mild and MRI of the peripheral nerve may show some abnormal increased nerve signal on fat suppressed T2-weighted magnetic resonance (MR) images, but typically no muscle denervation changes are seen [3]. Usually, there is no disruption, effacement or enlargement of the involved nerves.

Axonotmesis is a more severe type of injury and leads to axonal injury and Wallerian degeneration distal to the site of injury. Loss of both sensory and motor function occurs. Axonotmesis is characterized by axonal discontinuity and damage to the covering endoneurium. However, it is important to remember that the remaining connective tissue framework of the nerve (epineurium and perineurium) is usually preserved. As a consequence, axonotmesis injuries have the potential to recover spontaneously because the surrounding myelin sheaths remain intact. Typical clinical findings include decreased or absent evoked muscle and sensory action potentials. Electrodiagnostic tests are therefore useful for distinguishing the lower grade of injury (neuropraxia) from the more severe grade of injury (axonotmesis) [3]. Typical MRI findings include signs of muscle denervation as well as increased T2 signal intensity of the nerve on fat-suppressed images. Morphological changes can also be detected. The latter include fascicular enlargement, disruption and/or nerve effacement. Axonal regeneration occurs slowly at a rate of approximately 1 mm per day from the proximal to the distal nerve segment [3]. With advancing nerve regeneration, normalization of the abnormal T2-hyperintensity of the nerve can be seen on MR images. The typical time frame for meaningful functional recovery is several weeks to months.

Neurotmesis is the most severe type of nerve injury, resulting from severe contusion, crush, stretch or lacerations [3]. Axonal lesions, with complete disruption of the surrounding perineurium and epineurial layers, cause complete loss of motor, sensory (and autonomic) function. In most cases, neurotmetic injuries cannot be differentiated from axonotmetic injures by means of electrodiagnosis or clinical examination. They usually do not recover because of a complete disruption of axons and connective tissue, as this makes spontaneous functional regrowth virtually impossible [3, 4]. Imaging has the potential to show a complete nerve transection in acute cases or neuroma formation in chronic cases. Although nerve conspicuity is somewhat hampered in the acute phase by hemorrhage, imaging is usually able to differentiate neurotmetic from axonotmetic injures. Longstanding muscle denervation often results in severe fatty muscle infiltration and atrophy, which severely limits the success of surgery.

Other classification systems, such as those from Sunderland et al. and Mackinnon et al., exist but discussion is beyond the scope of this syllabus.

Peripheral nerves affected by entrapment syndromes are typically compressed along their course at predisposed anatomic locations, i.e., tunnels. The floor of these tunnels usually consists of bone, whereas the roof is usually made up of focal transverse thickenings of the deep fascia, retinaculae and muscle aponeurosis [1, 3-6]. Pathophysiology of entrapment syndrome is different from other acute nerve injuries, as the development of compressive neuropathy depends on the pressure within these tunnels and the fact that nerves typically can withstand only little pressure. At more than 15 mmHg, the venous supply to the nerves is increasingly hampered, and at over 40 mmHg the arterial blood supply is affected. Irreversible structural nerve damage begins at pressures of around 80 mmHg [3]. Typical MR findings of compressed nerves include increased signal intensity on T2-weighted MR images. Recent studies have demonstrated that the large myelinated axons at the outer portions of the nerve are most affected. This relative sparing of the fibers in the central portion of the nerve supports the theory that the primary mechanism of injury is shear forces; therefore, ischemia appears to be a secondary mechanism [3]. In the early stages, symptoms can be intermittent or even disappear spontaneously. As the disease progresses, fibrotic nerve changes can occur causing further nerve impingement. In chronic cases, severe axonal degeneration and myelin loss are common histological findings. Clinically, there is a permanent loss of nerve function. Long-standing disease causes fatty infiltration and atrophy of the denervated muscles. The abnormal T2 hyperintensity of the nerve, along with proximal enlargement, angulation and displacement, are characteristic findings of nerve entrapment. Regional muscle denervation changes on MR images support the diagnosis of neuropathy.

## Technical Considerations and Normal Appearance of Nerves*

MR neurography is a tissue-specific imaging technique optimized for evaluating peripheral nerves, their internal fascicular morphology (see above), alteration in neural signal and caliber, and associated space occupying and other compressive lesions [7]. Three-dimensional (3D) imaging is of critical importance in tracing the course of peripheral nerves, in identifying points of compression or disruption, and for preoperative planning. In general, MR neurography can be either T2 based or diffusion based. Diffusion-based MR imaging, especially diffusion tensor imaging, allows functional assessment of the nerves, but as yet remains a novel technique, with specific hardware and software requirements in an attempt to enhance the otherwise low signal-to-noise ratio (SNR) from these small nerves, limiting its application in routine clinical practice.

### The Magnet

The strength of the magnet is an important consideration, with impact on both image quality and speed of acquisition [8]. In general, there is superior performance of MR neurography at 3 Tesla (3T) compared with 1.5T. In our institutions, we perform the technique using 3T platforms only. In fact, it is the advent of high Tesla imaging and its

widespread availability that has facilitated the development of state of the art MR neurography and made it a reality in daily clinical practice. Compared with 1.5T MRI, 3T MRI provides increased (nearly double) SNR, which in part is related to improved coil design, better gradient performance and wider bandwidths. This translates into higher spatial resolution and thinner slice sections with improved fluid conspicuity, as well as superior contrast-to-noise ratio, which improves anatomic characterization and lesion detection [2]. Increased conspicuity of fluid and more uniform fat-suppression techniques result in better depiction of fascicular appearance of the nerves. There is also less inhomogeneity of the magnetic field. More robust hardware facilitates the application of multiple radiofrequency saturation pulses required for adequate vascular suppression. Furthermore, the application of parallel imaging allows faster acquisition times. It is difficult to produce quality T2-weighted 3D images on lower field strength magnets because of time and hardware limitations. 3D gradient echo sequences often have to be employed, and images thus generated are frequently nonisotropic with poor SNR and soft tissue contrast, and are prone to susceptibility artefacts [2]. In contrast, high-quality isotropic 3D proton density and T2-weighted images can be acquired with relative ease and speed at 3T, and serve as an invaluable adjunct to two dimensional (2D) images.

### MR Protocol

#### T1-Weighted Imaging

High-resolution T1-weighted imaging is excellent for depicting normal anatomy of the peripheral nerves and surrounding structures. Thin sections (maximum slice thickness of 4 mm) are necessary for adequate resolution of anatomic detail and fascicular morphology. Peripheral nerves appear as linear T1 hypointense structures, following an expected anatomical distribution. Differentiation from adjacent vessels is often possible, especially with the larger nerves, with arteries appearing as flow voids and veins appearing T1 hyperintense due to inflow phenomenon [9]. With larger nerves or at higher resolution imaging, the individual fascicles may be resolved [7]. Peripheral nerves are outlined by T1 hyperintense perineural fat, with a characteristic reverse tram track appearance of alternating T1 hyperintense and T1 hypointense signal that increases their conspicuity. Infiltration of the perineural fat and soft tissues is often best depicted on T1-weighted imaging. The presence of muscle fatty replacement in the setting of long-standing denervation is also seen to best advantage on this imaging sequence.

#### T2-Weighted Imaging

Pathological changes within the nerve are seen to best advantage on T2-weighted images [10]. In addition, many mass lesions and pathological processes that commonly result in neural compression (e.g., paralabral and ganglion

---

* The author of the section is Prof. J.T. Bencardino.

cysts, peripheral nerve sheath tumors, fluid-filled bursae) are best characterized and are most conspicuous on T2-weighted images. With standard fast spin-echo, (non fat suppressed) T2-weighted imaging, it is difficult to discern abnormal increased T2 signal from perineural and intraneural fat, therefore fat-suppressed T2-weighted imaging is the optimal sequence for detecting neural pathology. This imaging sequence is also most sensitive for early changes of muscle denervation signal alterations. However, there are drawbacks to fat-suppressed T2-weighted imaging, with more artefacts from hyperintense vascular structures and partial volume averaging [11]. Vascular structures, which typically accompany the nerve, appear hyperintense and can be confused with neural signal abnormality or perineural edema.

Dedicated MR neurography utilizes increased T2 weighting with thinner slices, to increase conspicuity of T2 signal change and achieve higher spatial resolution [11]. Maximizing the conspicuity of increased T2 signal in nerves is achieved in three ways: (1) utilizing sequences with long echo times (90-130 ms), (2) applying radiofrequency saturation pulses to suppress signal from adjacent vessels, and (3) utilizing frequency selective or adiabatic inversion recovery imaging type fat suppression [10]. This is best achieved at higher field strength, emphasizing the importance of technological advances in the development of high-resolution neural imaging. This results in increased T2 weighting while minimizing spurious signal from adjacent vessels and fat, and it is more sensitive for demonstrating neural signal abnormality [12]. Newer techniques employed in 3D imaging, namely steady state free precession and diffusion techniques, result in superior suppression of vascular signal in T2-weighted sequences, particularly when imaging the extremities [13].

### 3D Imaging

Isotropic 3D imaging is an essential component of state of the art MR neurography. Nerves often follow oblique courses and are not seen to best advantage on standard axial, coronal and sagittal imaging planes. 3D multiplanar reconstructed (MPR), curved planar reconstructed (CPR) and maximal intensity projected (MIP) images greatly facilitate the visualization of nerves and are particularly useful for preoperative planning. Decreased magic angle artefact and partial volume averaging on 3D imaging allow for more accurate depiction of pathology. Furthermore, caliber and signal change in nerves, which may be subtle or attributed to volume averaging on axial imaging, are seen to better advantage in the longitudinal plane, allowing better assessment of the true extent of the abnormality. Certain pathologies, such as plexiform neurofibromata, particularly lend themselves to 3D imaging for depiction of the entire disease burden in one image (Fig. 1). Compression of peripheral nerves by disc protrusions, space occupying lesions and anatomical fibro-osseous tunnels is also more accurately delineated on 3D imaging. Focal interruption of a nerve can be particular-

ly challenging to demonstrate on axial imaging, and 3D reconstructions may prove to be crucial in this scenario. Variations in muscular volume and anatomy may also be better assessed on 3D imaging.

A number of techniques can be employed in 3D imaging. SPACE (sampling perfection with application optimized contrasts by using different flip angle evolutions; Siemens, Erlangen, Germany) sequence is an isotropic single slab acquisition, mainly spin-echo type sequence, which allows MPR, CPR and MIP reconstructed images to map out the peripheral nerves and associated pathology in the longitudinal plane. This may be obtained in SPAIR (spectral adiabatic inversion recovery) or STIR (short tau inversion recovery sequence) contrasts, thus providing T2 weighting and optimizing sensitivity for detecting neural pathology. STIR imaging is preferred for imaging of the lumbosacral and brachial plexus due to superior fat suppression, while SPAIR imaging is preferred for imaging of the extremities. More recent developments include the 3D diffusion-weighted reversed fast imaging with steady state free precession (3D DW-PSIF) sequence, which is a heavily T2-weighted technique, combining selective suppression of vascular flow signal with multiplanar capabilities. The PSIF sequence holds great promise, particularly in the imaging of the extremities. Attempts to suppress vascular flow signal with the application of saturation bands usually fail in peripheral locations, due to the slow or in-plane flow within the peripheral vessels, or due to the variable oblique courses of peripheral neurovascular bundles. PSIF, because of its sensitivity to flow-related dephasing of the transverse magnetization, causes vessels in the imaging field of view to lose their signal intensity. Vascular signal suppression is also enhanced by the small diffusion moment applied to this sequence [13].

### The Field of View

Large field of view is most commonly utilized in pelvic neurography protocols. This occurs at the expense of resolution, but allows side to side comparison and evaluation of multiple nerve distributions on a single study. In our experience, the nerves most commonly affected in pelvic neuropathy can be reliably demonstrated when a dedicated MR neurography protocol is performed. In larger patients, and when a particularly large field of view is required, 3D STIR-SPACE might be preferable to 3D SPAIR-SPACE imaging given the superior and more robust fat suppression.

### Pitfalls and Technical Limitations

Magic angle effect, a well-described phenomenon in imaging of tendons, also occurs when imaging peripheral nerves. This results in spurious increased signal when the nerve lies in a plane 55 degrees to the main vector of the magnet. However, unlike tendons, this effect may persist in nerves, even at longer TE (>66 ms), and therefore higher TEs must be utilized to overcome it [14, 15]. Traditionally, the interpreting radiologist was advised to be particularly aware of this phenomenon when reporting increased intraneural T2 signal in MR neurography studies; however, more recently published literature concludes that magic angle effect is in reality a rare source of false-positive interpretation on MR neurography, particularly in nerves that run parallel to the main vector of the magnet [3].

Despite the use of suppressive radiofrequency pulses, hyperintense vascular signal is often present on MR neurography examinations, especially at high TE. This is a particular source of confusion in smaller nerves, when it occurs in the accompanying vascular bundle, and might be misinterpreted as neural or perineural signal abnormality. Inhomogeneous fat suppression is another potential source of error, which is particularly true in the pelvis, given the large field of view and the high number of patients who have hip or lumbar instrumentation, which further degrades the local magnetic field, thus worsening fat suppression. Increased susceptibility and chemical shift artefact, also seen at 3T, can be counteracted by shortening the echo time, performing parallel imaging and increasing the bandwidth. Nonetheless, 1.5T imaging might be preferable when evaluating nerves in close proximity to a metal prosthesis. Specific absorption rate limits are reached earlier at 3T compared with 1.5T, as there is increased energy deposition for radiofrequency excitation at 3T. However, this is usually balanced by faster image acquisition and shorter examination time and does not usually pose a clinical problem. Other potential drawbacks of 3D imaging include longer imaging times, and time spent producing and interpreting multiplanar reformatted images.

## Commonly Imaged Pathologies at the Upper Extremity

MR neurography is often used for the evaluation of entrapment syndromes at the upper extremity. These can affect the median and radial nerves, as well as the ulnar nerve. Detailed knowledge of the anatomy of the individual nerves is important for image interpretation, and a good text book showing the innervated muscles helps to indirectly localize the site of the nerve lesion based on the pattern of involved muscles in cases where direct visualization of the pathology is not feasible.

Several good review articles on MR neurography at the upper extremity have been published in the recent years. The following articles can be recommended for further reading: Andreisek et al. [16], Bordalo-Rodrigues et al. [17], and Kim et al. [18]. The following sections provide a brief overview.

### Median Nerve

### Anatomy

The median nerve arises from the medial and lateral cords of the brachial plexus (C6-T1). It follows the axil-

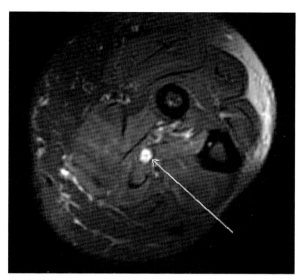

**Fig. 2.** Abnormal signal intensity of the enlarged median nerve (*arrow*) in the forearm of a 54-year-old man with nerve ischemia. Note the loss of fasculations (Courtesy of Prof. A. Chhabra) (for color reproduction see p 306)

lary artery superficial to the brachial muscle in the upper arm distally to the elbow where it courses between the two heads of the pronator teres muscles. Distal to this first anatomic bottleneck it gives off the anterior interosseous (antebrachial) nerve and then lies between the flexor digitorum superficialis muscle and profundus muscle (Fig. 2). The median nerve enters the wrist by passing under the flexor retinaculum. This second anatomic bottleneck is referred to as "carpal tunnel". Distal to it, it gives off the superficial palmar and the digital and muscular branches [1, 18].

### Supracondylar Process Syndrome

Supracondylar process (spur) syndrome is a very rare entity where an osseous structure at the anteromedial surface of the distal humerus (the so-called supracondylar process or spur) causes compression or irritation of the median nerve. This osseous process can be connected with the medial epicondyle by a fibrous band, which is known as the ligament of Struthers. Patients complain of paresthesia and numbness of the affected hand. Local pain following trauma might be associated with a fracture of the osseous process. As a result of the advance of MR neurography, is has become more likely that patients with supracondylar process syndrome will undergo MRI as the first imaging modality. Thus, the presence of a process is often not known in advance. Whereas the process itself is usually well visible on MR images, detection of the ligament of Struthers can be challenging, i.e., when it is very thin. MRI typically reveals median nerve signal abnormalities on T2-weighted fat-suppressed images, and might also be used to confirm an occult fracture of the process [1, 18, 19].

## Pronator Syndrome

In pronator syndrome, the median nerve is entrapped or compressed at the level of the pronator teres muscle, either between the humeral (superficial) and the ulnar (deep) muscle heads, at the bicipital aponeurosis (lacertus fibrosus), or at the arch of the origin of the superficial flexor digitorum muscle [1, 18]. Predisposing factors or causes for pronator syndrome include post-traumatic hematoma, soft tissue masses, prolonged external compression, fracture of the elbow (e.g., Volkman's fracture), hypertrophy of the pronator teres muscle bellies, or an aponeurotic prolongation of the biceps brachii muscle. Many of the latter conditions might not be clinically evident for years and then suddenly may become symptomatic in patients with repetitive pronation/supination stress [17]. Patients suffer from pain and numbness at the volar aspect of the elbow and forearm, as well as in the hand. Muscle strength is usually preserved. MRI of pronator syndrome is challenging because the normal median nerve at the elbow and forearm is surrounded by only minimal perifascial fat. It is therefore poorly visible. In addition, the nerve might not be enlarged at the site of the entrapment. However, thickening or nerve signal abnormalities can occur proximally or distally. Since direct assessment of the nerve remains challenging, evaluation of innervated muscles is important in pronator syndrome. The typical muscle denervation pattern with signal changes on T2-weighted fat-suppressed, STIR or T1-weighted sequences is then key to making the diagnosis [16, 18].

## Anterior Interosseous Nerve Syndrome

Distal to the pronator teres muscle, the median nerve gives off the anterior interosseus nerve. Entrapment or compression of this branch is called anterior interosseous nerve syndrome (AINS) or Kiloh-Nevin syndrome. Typical causes for this neuropathy are direct traumatic damage as a result of surgery, venous puncture, injection or cast pressure, as well as external compression mostly by anatomic variants including a bulky tendinous origin of the ulnar (deep) head of the pronator teres muscle, accessory muscles, fibrous bands originating from the superficial flexors, vascular abnormalities or soft-tissue masses such as lipoma or ganglia [16, 18]. Symptoms of AINS include dull pain in the volar aspect of the forearm and muscle weakness affecting the thumb, the index finger and occasionally the middle finger. Isolated weakness of the thumb can occur as a variant in cases where the particular nerve fascicle that supplies the flexor pollicis longus is affected. The anterior interosseus nerve does not have sensory function. Thus, numbness is not a symptom.

The anterior interosseous nerve can be best seen between the flexor digitorum superficialis and profundus muscles on axial MR images. Fat-suppressed T2-weighted or STIR images display increased signal intensity in the flexor digitorum profundus, flexor pollicis longus and pronator quadratus muscles. Since the ring and little finger are not involved in patients with AINS, the MR signal of the corresponding flexor muscles is normal [16, 18, 20]. As with other neuropathies, recognition of the pattern of involved muscles is an important part of image interpretation, as the underlying pathology is often not directly visible on MR images. Depending on the etiology, scar tissue or masses might be present. However, narrowing down the possible differentials as well as specifying the exact site of the lesion can aid surgeons in avoiding long incisions crossing the antecubital fossa and thereby minimizing invasiveness of surgery [18].

## Carpal Tunnel Syndrome

Carpal tunnel syndrome (CTS) is probably the most common peripheral neuropathy. It results from compression of the median nerve beneath the transverse carpal ligament. Etiology includes congenital, traumatic, metabolic/endocrine (e.g., diabetes, pregnancy), inflammatory, infectious or idiopathic conditions, as well as mass lesions (e.g., ganglion, lipoma, neurofibroma, fibrolipomatous hamartoma) [21]. Symptoms are well known and include burning wrist pain, paresthesia or numbness in the thumb, index and middle finger, as well as in the radial aspect of the ring finger. Clinical history is usually the key for diagnosis. In unclear cases, electrodiagnostic testing as well as imaging might help to establish the diagnosis or to evaluate the degree of muscle atrophy. Focal nerve enlargement, flattening at the level of the pisiform, and increased nerve signal on fat-suppressed T2-weighted or STIR images can be seen on MR images. Other findings, such as bowing of the flexor retinaculum at the level of the hook of the hamate might be associated with CTS, but they are rather nonspecific signs. In recent years, multiple articles in favor of or against MR imaging (as well as ultrasound) have been published. Extensive discussion of the literature is beyond the scope of this syllabus, but it might be worth mentioning that reported sensitivity and specificity for MRI remain pretty low in certain studies (sensitivity, 23-96%; specificity, 39-87%). Therefore, MRI does not usually play an important role in the routine assessment of CTS. Nevertheless, imaging might be used in recurrent or persistent disease or in cases of neoplasm (e.g., neurofibroma), arthritis (e.g., gouty tophi, rheumatoid tenosynovitis) or congenital anomalies (e.g., aberrant lumbrical muscles). Future developments using diffusion-based MRI techniques might help overcome the current limitations, since recent studies have shown that diagnosis of CTS is possible with relatively high accuracy based on quantitative diffusion parameters (fractional anisotropy and apparent diffusion coefficient; see below "Future Developments").

## The Radial Nerve

### Anatomy

The radial nerve arises from the posterior cord of the brachial plexus (C5-C8, Th1) and twists around the humerus diaphysis, crosses under the teres major muscle and then descends between the medial and lateral bellies of the triceps muscle [1]. The nerve courses from the dorsal compartment to the volar compartment just above the elbow. Therefore, it has to penetrate the intermuscular septum. The radial nerve then gives off a deep motor as well as a superficial sensory branch. The motor branch penetrates the supinator muscle at the beginning of its course, where it is then called the posterior interosseous nerve. The superficial sensory branch follows the radial artery and innervates the dorsal aspect of the thumb as well as the index and middle fingers [1]. Multiple muscles, including the triceps, anconeus, brachioradialis, extensor carpi radialis longus, extensor carpi radialis brevis, extensor digitorum, extensor carpi ulnaris, extensor digiti minimi, abductor pollicis longus, extensor pollicis brevis, extensor pollicis longus, extensor indicis muscles and the supinator muscle, are innervated by the radial nerve (please see textbooks for details and anatomic variants).

## Posterior Interosseous Nerve Syndrome

Posterior interosseous nerve syndrome (PINS) is also referred to as deep radial nerve or supinator syndrome. The latter indicates its characteristic etiology, namely the compression or entrapment of the nerve by the supinator muscle that it penetrates. Other etiologies include: nerve compression due to an anatomical variant of a fibrous adherence between the brachioradialis and the brachialis muscle (known as the Arcade of Frohse), fibrous adhesions at the radiohumeral joint capsule, abnormal recurrent blood vessels that cross the posterior interosseous nerve (leash of Henry), an intermuscular septum between the extensor carpi ulnaris and the extensor digitorum minimi muscle, as well as a fibrous adhesion at the margin of the extensor carpi radialis brevis muscle and the distal margin of the supinator muscle [1]. Pain and muscle weakness are the leading symptoms [18]. The radial nerve is usually very conspicuous on T1-weighted MR images, where it appears as a low signal intensity structure when it courses between the brachialis and the brachioradialis muscles [3]. The posterior interosseous nerve can also easily be detected on axial images when it penetrates the supinator muscle. Abnormalities to the nerves appear – similar to other neuropathies – as increased signal intensity on T2-weighted fat-suppressed or STIR weighted images. In the experience of the author, it is rarely possible to detect the anatomic structure that causes PINS. Occasionally, the Arcade of Frohse is seen (Fig. 3), but in most cases the diagnosis of PINS is primarily based on the muscle denervation pattern, which might indicate the level of the nerve lesion. Theoretically, a proximal lesion will affect all muscles innervated by the radial nerve, whereas a more distally located lesion might spare respective muscles that are innervated by motor branches that are given off proximal to the lesion [1, 18].

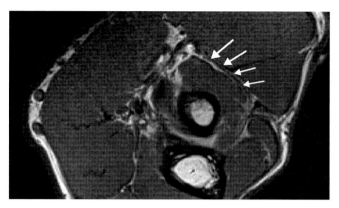

**Fig. 3.** A 32-year-old man with posterior interosseous nerve syndrome. The nerve is entrapped at the Arcade of Frohse (*arrows*) (Courtesy of Prof. A. Chhabra) (for color reproduction see p 306)

## The Ulnar Nerve

### Anatomy

The ulnar nerve arises from the medial cord of the brachial plexus (C8 and T1) and courses along the arteries downwards to the humerus where it penetrates the medial intermuscular septum. It then courses along the triceps muscle beneath the cubital tunnel retinaculum (also known as the epicondylo-olecranon ligament or the Osborne band) into the cubital tunnel, which is located at the mediodorsal side of the elbow. At the forearm, the ulnar nerve is positioned between the two heads of the flexor carpi ulnaris muscle. It courses at the volar aspect and enters the Guyon canal of the wrist where it divides into the superficial and the deep motor branches. Several muscles are innervated by the ulnar nerve; however, none is innervated at the upper arm (see anatomic textbooks for details) [1, 18]. Sensory function is provided to the distal forearm and ulnar aspect of the dorsum of the hand.

### Cubital Tunnel Syndrome

The ulnar nerve is frequently affected at the level of the elbow. Within the cubital tunnel, the nerve is often exposed to pathologic compression following overuse, chronic external compression (e.g., "sleepy palsy"; perioperative damage), trauma (using jackhammers), compression by a thickened retinaculum of the flexor carpi ulnaris muscle (also referred to as arcuate ligament in the literature), subluxation due to congenital laxity of fibrous tissue, humeral fracture (e.g., loose bodies, callus formation), arthritic spurs arising from the epicondyle or olecranon, muscle anomalies, soft tissue masses, ganglia, osteochondroma, synovitis secondary to rheumatoid arthritis, infection and hemorrhage [1, 18].

Typically, patients complain of local pain that increases during elbow motion. Paresthesia or numbness at the ulnar aspect of the palm and fingers is another typical sign in ulnar neuropathy, as well as weakness of innervated muscles. On MR images, the ulnar nerve can be easily depicted within the cubital tunnel. It usually has a round to oval structure, is surrounded by fat, and can be followed downwards into the forearm. It is usually isointense on both T1-weighted and fat-suppressed T2-weighted MR images. Recently, however, a study by Husarik et al. revealed that increased signal intensity on T2-weighted or STIR sequences was also typical in up to 60% of normal subjects [22]. Thus, in contrary to other nerves and locations, T2-hyperintensity of the ulnar nerve at the elbow does not necessarily correspond to a pathologic condition. Based on the findings of that study, increased signal intensity on fluid-sensitive MR images should not be used as the sole criterion for the presence of ulnar neuropathy. Evidence of other additional neuropathy criteria, such as qualitative changes in nerve diameter, should be present [22]. Overall, Husarik et al. found considerable variability in the elbow nerves and features that, in the literature, are considered to be related to compression neuropathy.

## Guyon Canal Syndrome

Guyon canal syndrome is characterized by ulnar neuropathies located at the level of the Guyon canal (also called pisohamate tunnel). This anatomic space is formed by various carpal ligament, tendons and muscles of the hand, as well as the pisiform bone and hook of hamate. The Guyon canal begins at the proximal edge of the volar carpal ligaments and ends at the fibrous arch of the hypothenar muscles [1, 23].

A very frequent cause of Guyon canal syndrome is chronic repetitive trauma in cyclists (i.e., "handlebar palsy"). During cycling, cyclists usually support themselves by tightly grasping the handlebars. The point of maximum pressure is usually at the level of the pisiform and hamate bone – exactly the region where the ulnar nerve passes through. Therefore, almost all protective cycling gloves have a cushion inserted to reduce the pressure on the ulnar nerve. Other repetitive stresses can have the same effect.

MR imaging can add important information in Guyon canal syndrome [i.e., to exclude causes other than chronic repetitive stress to the nerve; other causes include occult fracture of the hamate, masses (e.g., fibrolipoharmatoma) or compression by anomalous and accessory muscles and fibrous bands]. The normal size of the nerve is around 3-4 mm at the pisiform level and any enlargement or abnormally increased T2-signal intensity should raise suspicion of Guyon canal syndrome. Indirect signs such as acute muscle denervation might also help to establish the diagnosis.

## Nonentrapment Neuropathies

Nonentrapment neuropathies occur at any site along the course of the median, ulnar or radial nerve. They are usually not related to a predisposing anatomical location. Nonentrapment neuropathies include all other etiologies, such as traumatic nerve injuries, inflammatory conditions, polyneuropathies and mass lesions [1, 3].

### Nerve Injuries

Nerve injuries are frequent in many major trauma cases. However, the majority of patients with an acute peripheral nerve injury are not referred to MRI, as immediate surgery is often indicated. However, sometimes it is difficult for clinicians to distinguish between nerve lesions that might recover on their own (neuropraxia and axonotmesis according to Seddon's classification) and nerve lesions that will not recover, and therefore will need immediate surgery (neurotmesis). MRI has the potential to distinguish between the two entities, as axonotmetic and neurotmetic lesions exhibit different nerve and muscle signal characteristics. Transiently increased nerve signal on T2- and STIR-weighted images distal to the site of injury, followed by normalization with axonal regeneration as well as transient muscle denervation signs that occur as early as 24-48 h after the injury and which normalize with muscle re-innervation, are typical finding for axonotmetic injuries. In neurotmetic lesions, the increased nerve signal on T2- and STIR-weighted images disappears very late and transient neurogenic muscle edema is typically followed by muscle volume reduction and fatty muscle atrophy [1].

The increased signal seen in injured peripheral nerves on T2 and STIR pulse sequences might reflect endoneurial or perineurial edema as a result of changes in the blood-nerve barrier, changes in water content due to altered axoplasmatic flow, inflammation (as evidenced by a macrophage response), and/or presence of axonal and myelin breakdown products [1].

### Infectious Neuropathies

Various viral and bacterial infectious agents can cause an infectious neuropathy. Imaging does not usually play a role in the evaluation of these diseases. Rarely, MR neurography is performed for follow-up and therapy monitoring purposes.

### Inflammatory Demyelinating Polyradiculoneuropathies

This heterogeneous group of immune-mediated neuropathies [e.g., Guillain-Barré syndrome, chronic inflammatory demyelinating polyradiculoneuropathy (CIDP)] is characterized by demyelinating processes. Axonal degeneration often also occurs [1]. MRI is sometimes performed in acute stages to demonstrate the pattern of affected nerves. On T2-weighted or STIR images, diffuse nerve swelling, abnormal signal intensity and contrast enhancement after the intravenous administration of gadolinium chelates has been described. The pathological substrate of these MRI findings is not known, but signal abnormalities might result from demyelination and/or increased permeability of the blood-nerve barrier, while inflammation and edema might lead to the nerve swelling. In classic CIDP, onion bulb type hypertrophic changes caused by repetitive demyelination and remyelination may be revealed additionally along the course of the median, radial or ulnar nerves [1].

## Polyneuropathies

Various conditions can result in polyneuropathies. These include: diabetes mellitus, ethanol intoxication, uremia, deficiencies of thiamine and pyridoxine, and abnormalities to the nerve sheaths (e.g., seen in sphingolipidosis, paraproteinemia, and certain types of hereditary neuropathies such as Charcot-Marie-Tooth disease) or the soft tissue that surrounds the peripheral nerves (e.g., caused by vasculitis and metabolic diseases). In patients with polyneuropathies, MRI of the brain or the spine should be performed to assess central nervous system involvement [1]. MRI of the peripheral nerves is not well established.

## Mass Lesions

A mass lesion of a peripheral nerve can originate from the nerve or its nerve sheath cells. Benign and malignant neurogenic tumors should be distinguished. The former include schwannomas (also called neurilemomas), neurofibromas, fibrolipomatous hamartomas, traumatic neuromas and nerve sheath ganglions. The latter include malignant schwannomas, malignant triton tumors, malignant neurilemmomas, neurilemmosarcomas, neurofibrosarcomas, neurogenic sarcomas and neurosarcomas [24]. In addition, mass lesions can originate from surrounding soft tissue. Possible entities include ganglions, cysts, enlarged lymph nodes, lipomas, hemangiomas, and all other benign and/or malignant soft tissue tumors, as well as metastases, such as from malignant melanoma or breast cancer. A detailed description of individual characteristics of these masses and their associated diseases (e.g., neurofibromatosis 1 and 2) is beyond the scope of this syllabus and has been provided elsewhere [3].

## Future Developments

MR neurography using high-resolution 3T imaging has been successfully introduced into the clinical routine in recent years. To identify possible future developments in MR imaging of the peripheral nervous system, current research literature should be evaluated. One important topic for which an increasing number of articles has been published in the past 2 years is diffusion tensor imaging (DTI). DTI is a diffusion-weighted MRI technique that allows quantitative and functional assessment of peripheral nerves. This technique is basically well known from imaging the central nervous system, but its application to peripheral nerves has been hampered in the past because of technical constraints. However, these technical limitations are now being solved, as recent literature shows [25-28].

The basic principle of DTI is simple. Diffusion of protons along the peripheral nerve is three times greater than across the nerve because of restrictions posed by myelin sheaths. Dedicated MRI sequences using single-shot echo-planar-imaging sequences are used to visualize the main vector of diffusion using diffusion-sensitizing gradients. Multiple acquisitions are used to fill a matrix, which can be used – by mathematical calculations – to calculate diffusion parameters (e.g., fractional anisotropy, apparent diffusion coefficient, mean diffusivity). Peripheral nerve pathology causes changes to these parameters, such as a decrease in fractional anisotropy values and an increase in the apparent diffusion coefficient in tumors. Data gained from DTI studies can also be used to reconstruct 3D tractograms of individual peripheral nerves. However, these tractography images should not be considered as high-resolution anatomic images of a nerve. Rather, they mirror the diffusion properties of a nerve. As such, they allow direct conclusions regarding the nerve function.

Very recently, Guggenberger et al. published results from a study where the diagnosis of CTS was solely based on quantitative diffusion parameters of the median nerve [26]. Sensitivity and specificity were each up to 83%. Thus, it might be realistic to say that in 10 years, for example, standard MR evaluation of peripheral nerves in the daily routine practice will include quantitative data.

## Conclusions

There is a wide variety of peripheral neuropathies that may affect the nerves at the upper extremity. This syllabus has provided a short overview of the anatomy of peripheral nerves and their relevant pathophysiology. Moreover, it has discussed technical requirements, normal appearance of nerves and commonly imaged pathologies at the upper extremity. For further reading, the list of references might be a good guide.

## References

1. Andreisek G, Burg D, Studer A, Weishaupt D (2008) Upper extremity peripheral neuropathies: role and impact of MR imaging on patient management. Eur Radiol 18:1953-1961
2. Chhabra A, Andreisek G, Soldatos T et al (2011) MR neurography: past, present, and future. AJR Am J Roentgenol 197:583-591
3. Chhabra A, Andreisek G (2012) Magnetic resonance neurography. Jaypee Brothers Medical Publishers, New Dehli
4. Chhabra A, Subhawong TK, Williams EH et al (2011) High-resolution MR neurography: evaluation before repeat tarsal tunnel surgery. AJR Am J Roentgenol 197:175-183
5. Khachi G, Skirgaudes M, Lee WP, Wollstein R (2007) The clinical applications of peripheral nerve imaging in the upper extremity. J Hand Surg [Am] 32:1600-1604

6. Weishaupt D, Andreisek G (2007) Diagnostic imaging of nerve compression syndrome. Radiologe 47:231-239

7. Chhabra A, Faridian-Aragh N (2012) High-resolution 3-T MR neurography of femoral neuropathy. AJR Am J Roentgenol 198:3-10

8. Chhabra A, Lee PP, Bizzell C, Soldatos T (2011) 3 Tesla MR neurography – technique, interpretation, and pitfalls. Skeletal Radiology 40:1249-1260

9. Filler AG, Maravilla KR, Tsuruda JS (2004) MR neurography and muscle MR imaging for image diagnosis of disorders affecting the peripheral nerves and musculature. Neurol Clin 22:643-682, vi-vii

10. Filler AG (2009) MR Neurography and diffusion tensor imaging: origins, history & clinical impact. Neurosurgery 65(4 Suppl):A29-43

11. Lewis AM, Layzer R, Engstrom JW et al (2006) Magnetic resonance neurography in extraspinal sciatica. Archives of Neurology 63:1469-1472

12. Chhabra A, Soldatos T, Subhawong TK et al (2011) The application of three-dimensional diffusion-weighted PSIF technique in peripheral nerve imaging of the distal extremities. J Magn Reson Imaging 34:962-967

13. Chappell KE, Robson MD, Stonebridge-Foster A et al (2004) Magic angle effects in MR neurography. AJNR Am J Neuroradiol 25:431-440

14. Kastel T, Heiland S, Baumer P et al (2011) Magic angle effect: a relevant artifact in MR neurography at 3T? AJNR Am J Neuroradiol 32:821-827

15. Petchprapa CN, Rosenberg ZS, Sconfienza LM et al (2010) MR imaging of entrapment neuropathies of the lower extremity. Part 1. The pelvis and hip. Radiographics 30:983-1000

16. Andreisek G, Crook DW, Burg D et al (2006) Peripheral neuropathies of the median, radial, and ulnar nerves: MR imaging features. Radiographics 26:1267-1287

17. Bordalo-Rodrigues M, Amin P, Rosenberg ZS (2004) MR imaging of common entrapment neuropathies at the wrist. Magn Reson Imaging Clin N Am 12:265-279, vi

18. Kim S, Choi JY, Huh YM et al (2007) Role of magnetic resonance imaging in entrapment and compressive neuropathy – what, where, and how to see the peripheral nerves on the musculoskeletal magnetic resonance image: part 2. Upper extremity. Eur Radiol 17:509-522

19. Sener E, Takka S, Cila E (1988) Supracondylar process syndrome. Arch Orthop Trauma Surg 117:418-419

20. Spratt JD, Stanley AJ, Grainger AJ et al (2002) The role of diagnostic radiology in compressive and entrapment neuropathies. Eur Radiol 12:2352-2364

21. Jarvik JG, Yuen E, Kliot M (2004) Diagnosis of carpal tunnel syndrome: electrodiagnostic and MR imaging evaluation. Neuroimaging Clin N Am 14:93-102

22. Husarik DB, Saupe N, Pfirrmann CW et al (2009) Elbow nerves: MR findings in 60 asymptomatic subjects – normal anatomy, variants, and pitfalls. Radiology 252:148-156

23. Kim DH, Han K, Tiel RL et al (2003) Surgical outcomes of 654 ulnar nerve lesions. J Neurosurg 98:993-1004

24. Murphey MD, Smith WS, Smith SE et al (1999) From the archives of the AFIP. Imaging of musculoskeletal neurogenic tumors: radiologic-pathologic correlation. Radiographics 19:1253-1280

25. Guggenberger R, Eppenberger P, Markovic D et al (2012) MR neurography of the median nerve at 3.0T: optimization of diffusion tensor imaging and fiber tractography. European Journal of Radiology 81:e775-782

26. Guggenberger R, Markovic D, Eppenberger P et al (2012) Assessment of median nerve with MR neurography by using diffusion-tensor imaging: normative and pathologic diffusion values. Radiology 265:194-203

27. Skorpil M, Engstrom M, Nordell A (2007) Diffusion-direction-dependent imaging: a novel MRI approach for peripheral nerve imaging. Magn Reson Imaging 25:406-411

28. Sugiyama K, Kondo T, Higano S et al (2007) Diffusion tensor imaging fiber tractography for evaluating diffuse axonal injury. Brain Inj 21:413-419

# Entrapment Neuropathies of the Lower Extremity

Jenny T. Bencardino[1], Holly Delaney[2]

[1] Department of Radiology, NYU Hospital for Joint Diseases, NYU Langone Medical Center, New York, NY, USA
[2] Department of Radiology, AMNCH Tallaght Hospital, Tallaght, Dublin, Ireland

## Key Points

The diagnosis of entrapment neuropathy is challenging for both radiologists and clinicians alike. Detailed knowledge of neural anatomy and of clinical syndromes and denervation patterns that commonly affect the lower extremity is crucial to the correct interpretation of nerve imaging studies. Advances in magnetic resonance (MR) technology now enable high-resolution imaging of the deeply seated lumbosacral plexus and its pelvic neural branches, with reliable visualization of many of the nerves commonly implicated in pelvic neuropathy.

It must also be emphasized that the diagnostic performance of some of the MR findings indicative of neuropathy is yet to be established. Interpretation of MR neurography findings is best performed in conjunction with the clinical picture and in collaboration with the referring physician.

## Summary

Recent advances in magnetic resonance imaging (MRI) have revolutionized the field of peripheral nerve imaging and made high-resolution acquisitions a clinical reality. Neurogenic pain arising from the nerves of the pelvis, lumbosacral plexus and peripheral nerves of the lower extremity poses a particular diagnostic challenge for the clinician and radiologist alike, given the complexity of the anatomy, the common presence of coexistent pathology and potential symptom generators, and the difficulty in obtaining high-resolution imaging. In this article, a review of the complex neural anatomy of the lumbosacral plexus, pelvic branches and peripheral nerves of the lower extremity will be performed in a systematic fashion, followed by detailed description of the pathologic processes that may affect them.

## Introduction

Neurogenic pain arising from lumbosacral plexus and lower extremity poses a particular diagnostic challenge for the clinician and radiologist alike, given the complexity of the anatomy, the frequent coexistent pathology and potential symptom generators, and the difficulty in obtaining high-quality imaging. Classic symptoms of pain corresponding to a particular nerve distribution are not always present and patients may have vague clinical presentations that can be attributed to a multitude of other pathologies [1-3]. The picture becomes even more confusing with involvement of multiple nerves, as seen in lumbar plexopathy. Lumbar discogenic pain and other pathologies, such as hip osteoarthrosis, commonly coexist.

Until recently, imaging of peripheral nerves was limited from a technical standpoint, with no established gold standard imaging method to reliably visualize peripheral nerves and demonstrate pathology. With the advent of dedicated high-resolution magnetic resonance (MR) neurography, small caliber peripheral nerves and their associated pathology can now be reliably demonstrated.

## Anatomy

### Lumbosacral Plexus

The lumbosacral plexus is composed of a lumbar and sacral plexus (Fig. 1). The lumbar plexus is formed from the ventral rami of L1-L4 and a small contribution from the 12th thoracic nerve. The plexus descends dorsal or within the psoas muscle. Branches emerging from the lateral border of the psoas muscle include the iliohypogastric, ilioinguinal, genitofemoral, lateral femoral cutaneous and femoral nerves, while branches emerging from the medial border of the psoas muscle include the obturator nerve and lumbosacral trunk. A minor branch of L4

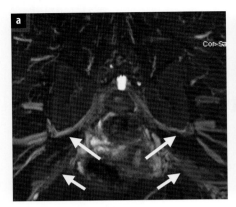 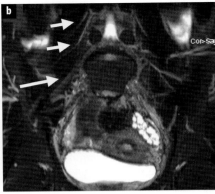

**Fig. 1 a, b. a** Coronal reformatted maximal intensity projection (MIP) image of a three-dimensional (3D) SPACE sequence demonstrates normal appearance of the bilateral sciatic nerves (*short arrows*) and superior gluteal nerves and associated vessels (*long arrows*) exiting the greater sciatic foramen. **b** Coronal reformatted MIP image of a 3D SPACE sequence demonstrates the exiting right L3 and L4 lumbar nerve roots (*short arrows*) as well as the lumbar contribution of the femoral nerve (*long arrow*). Note that the vessels are also projected in the reformatted MIP images

**Table 1.** Lumbosacral plexus muscular innervations by nerve root

|                     | T12 | L1 | L2 | L3 | L4 | L5 | S1 | S2 | S3 | S4 | S5 |
|---------------------|-----|----|----|----|----|----|----|----|----|----|----|
| Obturator internus  |     |    |    |    |    | *  | *  |    |    |    |    |
| Obturator externus  |     |    | *  | *  | *  |    |    |    |    |    |    |
| Pectineus           |     |    | *  | *  | *  |    |    |    |    |    |    |
| Psoas major         | *   | *  | *  | *  | *  |    |    |    |    |    |    |
| Iliacus             | *   | *  | *  | *  | *  |    |    |    |    |    |    |
| Iliopsoas           |     |    | *  | *  | *  |    |    |    |    |    |    |
| Gluteus minimus     |     |    |    |    |    | *  | *  |    |    |    |    |
| Gluteus medius      |     |    |    |    |    | *  | *  |    |    |    |    |
| Gluteus maximus     |     |    |    |    |    | *  | *  |    |    |    |    |
| Piriformis          |     |    |    |    |    | *  |    | *  |    |    |    |
| Adductor brevis     |     |    | *  | *  | *  |    |    |    |    |    |    |
| Adductor longus     |     |    |    | *  | *  |    |    |    |    |    |    |
| Adductor magnus     |     |    |    | *  | *  |    |    |    |    |    |    |
| Levator ani         |     |    |    |    |    |    |    | *  | *  | *  |    |

combines with the ventral ramus of L5 to form the lumbosacral cord or trunk. The latter descends over the sacral ala and joins the S1-S3 nerve roots on the anterior aspect of the piriformis muscle to form the sacral plexus [4]. Thus the sacral plexus is formed from L4-S4 ventral contributions. The sciatic, inferior and superior gluteal and pudendal nerves constitute its sacral branches. Lumbosacral plexus muscular innervations by nerve root are outlined in Table 1, and the most clinically important motor and sensory innervations of multiple peripheral nerves of the lower limb and pelvis are outlined in more detail below.

## Sciatic Nerve

The sciatic nerve is the largest peripheral nerve in the body and is reliably demonstrated on computed tomography (CT) and MRI [5]. It is formed from the L4-S3 nerve roots and most often descends anterior to the piriformis muscle. After exiting the pelvis through the infrapiriformis greater sciatic foramen, it descends in the thigh between the adductor magnus and the gluteus maximus muscles (Fig. 2). The sciatic nerve is composed of the medial tibial and the lateral common peroneal divisions, which provide motor innervation to the posterior thigh muscles, and all motor function below the knee

(anterior, lateral, posterior and deep muscular compartments). It gives all sensory innervation to the lower limb with the exception of medial sensory innervation of the thigh and leg, which is provided by the obturator and femoral nerves.

## Superior and Inferior Gluteal Nerves

The superior gluteal nerve is formed from the posterior roots of L4, L5 and S1. It exits the pelvis, through the suprapiriformis greater sciatic notch, and then passes between the gluteus minimus and gluteus medius muscles before giving off superior and inferior branches (Fig. 3). The superior branch terminates in the gluteus minimus muscle and the inferior branch terminates in the tensor fascia lata. The superior gluteal nerve acts to abduct the thigh at the hip by providing motor innervation to the gluteus minimus, gluteus medius and tensor fascia lata muscles.

The inferior gluteal nerve formed from the posterior roots of L5, S1 and S2 provides motor innervations to the gluteus maximus, which with the aid of the hamstrings, acts to extend the thigh. It exits the pelvis through the infrapiriformis sciatic notch and lies medial to the sciatic nerve before its terminal branch provides motor innervation to the gluteus maximus muscle. The superior and inferior gluteal nerves have no sensory contribution.

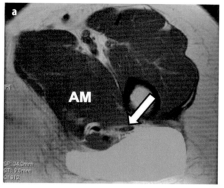

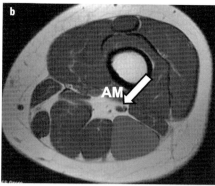

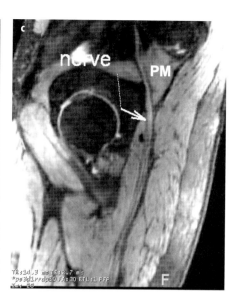

**Fig. 2 a-c.** Normal sciatic nerve. Axial T1 magnetic resonance images, just below the lesser trochanter (**a**) and at the proximal thigh (**b**), demonstrate the sciatic nerve (*arrow*) descending in the thigh between the adductor magnus (*AM*), gluteus maximus (*green*) and biceps femoris long head (*blue*) muscles. **c** Sagittal maximal intensity projection three-dimensional PSIF (pre-excitation refocused steady-state sequence) image depicts the sciatic nerve (*arrow*) exiting the pelvis at the level of the greater sciatic notch beneath the piriformis muscle (*PM*) (for color reproduction see p 306)

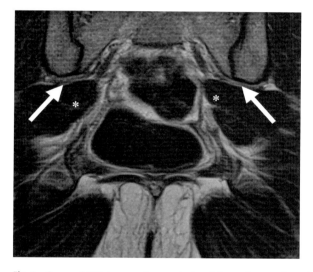

**Fig. 3.** Coronal T2 image demonstrates bilateral superior gluteal nerves (*arrows*) curving under the roof of the greater sciatic foramen above the piriformis muscles

## Lateral Femoral Cutaneous Nerve

The lateral femoral cutaneous nerve arises from L2 and L3, descends lateral to the psoas muscle, crosses the iliacus muscle deep to its fascia, and passes either through or underneath the lateral aspect of the inguinal ligament to the lateral thigh where it divides into anterior and posterior branches (Fig. 4). It innervates the skin on the lateral aspect of the thigh, and as its name implies is purely sensory.

## Femoral Nerve

The femoral nerve is formed by the L2, L3 and L4 nerve roots and descends between the iliacus and psoas muscles before exiting the pelvis under the inguinal ligament, in a canal between the iliopsoas muscle and the iliopectineal fascia (Fig. 5). It gives off a motor branch to the iliacus and the psoas muscles before dividing into anterior and posterior divisions and forming the saphenous nerve. The femoral nerve controls hip flexion and knee extension by

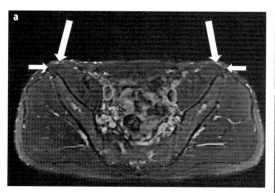

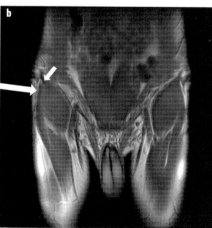

**Fig. 4 a, b.** Normal lateral femoral cutaneous nerve. **a** Axial T2 fat-saturated image demonstrates the bilateral lateral femoral cutaneous nerves (*long arrows*) adjacent to the anterior superior iliac spine origin of the sartorius (*short arrows*). **b** Coronal proton density image demonstrates the right lateral femoral cutaneous nerve (*long arrow*) at the level of the anterior superior iliac spine. Note the close relationship with the origin of the sartorius muscle (*short arrow*)

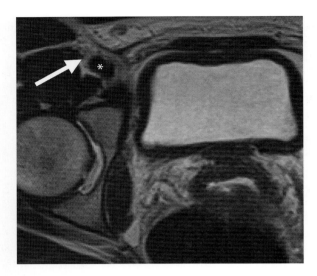

**Fig. 5.** Axial T2 image depicts the relationship of the femoral nerve (*arrow*), artery (*) and vein in the groin, going from lateral to medial. The femoral nerve can be difficult to visualize in the pelvis

providing motor innervation to the iliacus, psoas, pectineus, sartorius and quadriceps femoris muscles. Sensory innervation is of the medial thigh, anteromedial knee, medial leg and foot.

## Obturator Nerve

The obturator nerve is formed by the L2-L4 ventral rami. It descends into the pelvis, running along the iliopectineal line, exiting the pelvis via the obturator canal, at the superior aspect of obturator foramen. Within the pelvis, it assumes a near vertical orientation anterior to the psoas muscle and is well demonstrated on coronal imaging. It divides into an anterior branch, which passes anterior to adductor brevis and supplies the hip, and a posterior branch, which passes within the obturator externus muscle, and between adductor brevis and magnus muscles. The anterior branch gives motor innervation to

the hip, gracilis, adductor brevis and longus muscles and occasionally the pectineus muscle, while the posterior branch supplies the obturator externus and a portion of the adductor magnus muscles. Sensory innervation is to the medial thigh and knee.

## Pudendal Nerve

The pudendal nerve is formed by the ventral rami of S2, and all of the rami of S3 and S4. It passes between the piriformis and the coccygeus muscles and leaves the pelvis through the greater sciatic foramen. After crossing the ischial spine, it re-enters the perineum through the lesser sciatic foramen and travels in Alcock's canal along the lateral wall of the ischiorectal fossa (Fig. 6). The major branches are the inferior rectal nerve, the perineal nerve and the dorsal nerve of the penis or clitoris. Motor innervation is of the bulbospongiosus and ischiocavernosus muscles and the external urethral and rectal sphincters, while sensory innervation is of the perineum, scrotum and anus.

## Iliohypogastric Nerve

The iliohypogastric nerve is formed mainly from the anterior division of L1 with a small contribution from T12, and runs anteriorly and inferiorly along the lateral border of the psoas major and quadratus lumborum muscles. It pierces the transversus abdominus muscle and runs within the lateral abdominal wall, above the iliac crest, before dividing into its lateral and anterior cutaneous branches. Its terminal branch runs parallel to the inguinal ligament and exits the aponeurosis of the external oblique muscle. The nerve provides motor innervation to the abdominal wall musculature, and sensory innervation to the skin above the inguinal ligament and superior lateral gluteal region.

## Ilioinguinal Nerve

The ilioinguinal nerve is formed from the anterior division of L1, sometimes with a small contribution from

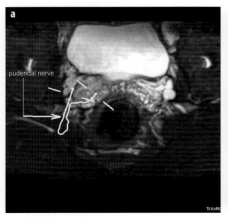
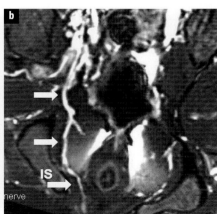

**Fig. 6 a, b.** Normal pudendal nerve. **a** Axial three-dimensional (3D) SPACE STIR image demonstrates mapping of the pudendal nerve on consecutive overlapped images. **b** Maximal intensity projection 3D SPACE STIR demonstrates the normal course of the right pudendal nerve and vessels (*arrows*) posterior and medial to the ischial spine (*IS*)

T12. It runs a similar course to the iliohypogastric nerve, running inferiorly along the quadratus lumborum before piercing the lateral abdominal wall and running medially to the inguinal ligament. It contributes to motor innervations of the abdominal wall musculature, and gives sensory branches to the pubic symphysis, femoral triangle, labia majora or root of the penis and scrotum.

### Genitofemoral Nerve

The genitofemoral nerve is formed by the anterior divisions of L1 and L2 nerve roots and pierces the psoas major muscle at the L3/L4 level before dividing into two branches which run along the anterior margin of the psoas muscle. The medial, genitalis or external spermatic, branch in males enters the inguinal canal and runs along with the spermatic cord to supply the cremaster muscle, spermatic cord, scrotum and adjacent thigh, and is responsible for the cremasteric reflex. In females, it runs with the round ligament of the uterus and gives sensory innervations of the labia majora and adjacent thigh. The lateral, or femoral, branch runs lateral to the femoral artery and posterior to the inguinal ligament into the proximal thigh, where it pierces the sartorius muscle and supplies the proximal lateral aspect of the femoral triangle. It is a purely sensory nerve.

### Imaging Findings

MRI plays a crucial role in evaluating patients with neurogenic pain and in characterizing potential etiologies. With recent technical advances in MRI, and particularly the advent of MR neurography, direct and indirect signs of neuropathy can be demonstrated even in the absence of a detectable compressive etiology. Diagnostic criteria for neural pathology include increased size of the nerve (larger than the adjacent artery), increased intraneural T2 signal and abnormal fascicular morphology, including focal enlargement or loss of definition of the internal fascicles. Nerves might have an abnormal course, with infiltration of the perineural fat when involved in scarring, and abnormal shape when focally enlarged or involved by tumor. Normal nerves should not enhance, except in those locations where the blood-nerve barrier is absent (dorsal root ganglion). Enhancement is most commonly seen in the setting of tumor or inflammation [3].

Indirect signs of neuropathy, particularly muscle denervation patterns, are also a very useful secondary sign of pelvic neuropathy. Increased T2 signal in the setting of muscular denervation does not represent true edema, and is best termed 'edema-like signal' or denervation signal alteration. This can progress to muscular fatty replacement, which is best detected on T1 weighted imaging, and eventually to muscle atrophy. Edema-like signal without fatty replacement is potentially reversible, if the underlying neuropathy resolves. There are multiple differential considerations for increased intramuscular T2

signal. Denervation edema-like signal is characterized by diffuse homogeneous involvement of the entire muscle, sharp margins, lack of associated fascial and perifascial fluid or inflammation, and conformation to a particular nerve distribution. Occasional variant innervation configurations and plexopathy can, however, confuse the pattern of muscle denervation changes.

### Pathology: General Concepts

A wide variety of pathology can result in abnormal imaging findings of the pelvic nerves and musculature, ranging from infectious and inflammatory lesions, systemic diseases such as polymyositis to benign and malignant space occupying processes. Pathology, which tends to result in painful neuropathic symptomatology, is usually due to local causes, and can be divided into three major categories: (1) space occupying lesions, (2) post-traumatic lesions, and (3) iatrogenic lesions. Space occupying lesions can be benign or malignant. Almost any pelvic mass can potentially result in neural compression; however certain lesions have a predilection for causing neural compression because of their anatomical location. Certain pelvic nerves can be susceptible to compression at particular anatomical bony or fibrous canals. Other nerves can be placed at risk during certain surgical procedures, or can be susceptible to traumatic injury because of their proximity to commonly fractured or avulsed osseous or tendinous structures. Relatively common benign lesions that can potentially cause a compressive neuropathy include, ganglion cysts, perineural cysts and fluid filled bursae. Para labral cysts of the hip should be specifically noted, as they might decompress anteriorly resulting in obturator nerve compression, or posteriorly compromising the sciatic or superior gluteal nerve [6, 7] (Fig. 7). Communication with the hip joint should always be considered when a cystic lesion in these locations is encountered, particularly as paralabral cysts may grow to a very large size and appear to be remote from the hip. Malignant lesions encompass any malignant pelvic soft tissue masses, including gynecological and rectal tumors, bone and lymph node metastases. Nerve sheath tumors may be benign or malignant, but are more commonly benign, and have quite characteristic imaging appearances, manifested by markedly hyperintense T2 signal, sometimes associated with a target sign, and avid enhancement [8]. The orientation along the long axis of a peripheral nerve and the presence of distal muscular atrophy are other useful signs suggestive of a neurogenic tumor [9]. Post-traumatic lesions include direct traumatic injury, where the more superficially located femoral and sciatic nerves are at greater risk. Nerve impingement may also occur in the setting of healed fractures, remote avulsion injuries and heterotopic ossification. The obturator nerve is particularly susceptible in the setting of pubic rami and pelvic fractures while the superior gluteal nerve may be injured after hip fracture [10]. Traumatic hamstring

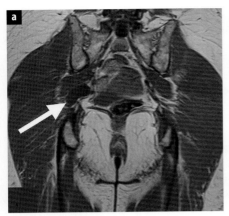 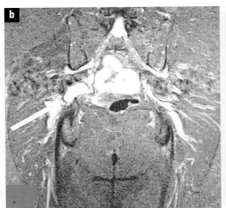 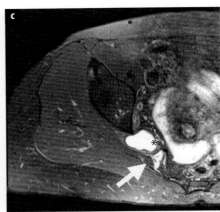

**Fig. 7 a-c.** Sciatic nerve compression. **a**, **b** Large field of view coronal T1 and STIR images show lobulated cystic structure in the region of the right sciatic notch (*arrows*). **c** Axial T2 fat-saturated image depicts intimate relationship with the right sciatic nerve, which is displaced posteriorly (*arrow*). Note the cystic structure (*) also abuts the posterior acetabulum

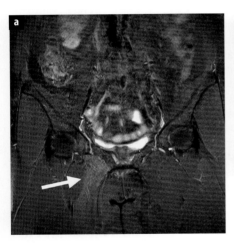 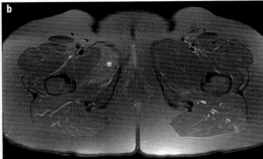

**Fig. 8 a, b.** Female patient status post hysterectomy. **a** Coronal large field of view STIR image of the pelvis demonstrates edema within the right adductor longus muscle (*arrow*). **b** Axial T2 fat-saturated image shows edema within the adductor longus and brevis muscles (*). There was also edema within the obturator externus muscle, in a pattern consistent with obturator nerve denervation. This may have been a manifestation of an iatrogenic injury of the obturator nerve

tendon avulsion from the ischial tuberosity may result in sciatic neuropathy. The anterior branch of the obturator nerve may be affected by adductor brevis tendinopathy [11]. Traction related indirect nerve injury, particularly to the sciatic, femoral and obturator nerves, during abdominal, hip and genitourinary surgery might range from subclinical to clinical but often resolves spontaneously. Direct iatrogenic injury of pelvic nerves can also occur during pelvic surgery, with the obturator nerve being particularly susceptible during genitourinary surgery (e.g., hysterectomy and prostatectomy) [12] (Fig. 8). The femoral nerve might be injured following vascular intervention in the groin, either directly while accessing the femoral artery, or indirectly by hematoma or pseudoaneurysm complicating the procedure. Neuropathy of the superior gluteal nerve is a recognized, relatively common, complication of total hip arthroplasty [13, 14], and there have been case reports of femoral and obturator neuropathy due to cement extrusion [15]. Like any peripheral nerve, the nerves of the pelvis and lumbosacral plexus may also become affected by neuritis or neuropathy in the absence of a compressive lesion or injury. This may be infectious

or inflammatory in origin, and is most commonly seen in the setting of systemic disease, following viral infections (chronic inflammatory demyelinating polyradiculoneuropathy) and pelvic irradiation. Neuropathy with secondary muscular denervation in the clinical setting of diabetes mellitus is a well-recognized phenomenon (diabetic amyotrophy), and has a particular predilection for the lumbosacral plexus [3]. Hereditary neuropathies can also occur, most notably Charcot-Marie-Tooth disease or hereditary motor and sensory neuropathy (HMSN).

## Lumbosacral Neuropathic Syndromes

### Lumbosacral Plexus

Lumbosacral plexopathy can be subdivided into structural causes such tumor, hemorrhage, postsurgical, traumatic and iatrogenic, and nonstructural causes such as amyotrophic neuralgia, radiation, vasculitis, diabetes, infections and hereditary pressure palsies. It can result, like any plexopathy, in a confusing clinical picture. Symptoms and objective clinical signs are often related to multiple spinal levels and multiple nerve distributions and do not conform to any recognizable syndrome. This may result in delayed diagnosis. Trauma, commonly secondary to high-speed deceleration, with pelvis or hip fractures and dislocation, typically causes stretch or traction related partial plexopathy and, less commonly, nerve avulsions. The lumbar component of the lumbosacral plexus may be involved in retroperitoneal pathology, including psoas abscess and hematoma. Inflammatory conditions such as retroperitoneal fibrosis, and malignant disease such as lymphoma or retroperitoneal lymph node metastases, can infiltrate the lumbosacral plexus. Radiation plexopathy is not often seen with current standard external beam pelvic irradiation regimens, but can be seen in the setting of brachytherapy or intraoperative radiation therapy. Unlike tumor-related plexopathy, which usually causes severe pain, radiation plexopathy is often painless and progresses slowly, appearing 5 years (on average) after the initial insult. The sacral distribution of the lumbosacral plexus may be involved in pathology of the sacroiliac joints such as inflammatory arthritis, or of the sacrum and presacral space including primary and secondary bone tumors (metastases, chordoma) or rectal carcinoma. Hereditary neuropathies can affect the lumbosacral plexus. Charcot-Marie-Tooth disease or HMSN is a rare disease that most commonly affects the brachial and lumbosacral plexuses, resulting in degeneration and marked enlargement of the affected nerves, and presenting clinically with sensory loss and muscle wasting and weakness of the distal extremities [13]. While this is a clinical diagnosis, MR neurography demonstrates moderate to marked nerve enlargement and can help direct site of biopsy. Symmetric or asymmetric diabetic neuropathy or plexopathy (diabetic amyotrophy), presenting in older patients with long-standing disease, is a common cause of lumbosacral plexopathy. It typically presents with proximal muscle weakness and atrophy. Pain, when severe, will often resolve within a few months, but is often mild or absent. Sensory loss is less severe than with peripheral neuropathy [3]. Denervation muscle signal alteration patterns in lumbosacral plexopathy, if present, are not particularly helpful and may correspond to multiple muscle groups related to multiple peripheral nerves. This can result in diagnostic confusion with a systemic or primary myopathic pathology such as polymyositis.

## Peripheral Neuropathic Syndromes of the Pelvis and Hip

### Superior and Inferior Gluteal Nerves

The clinical syndrome of superior gluteal nerve injury is manifested by weakness in abduction, with a gait limp and a positive Trendelenburg sign. The superior gluteal nerve is relatively commonly injured following pelvic orthopedic surgery [16]. The superior branch can be injured or compressed following placement of iliosacral screws, while the inferior branch can be injured during a lateral or anterolateral approach to hip replacement. Electromyography abnormalities are demonstrated in 77% of patients post total hip arthroplasty (THA), but usually resolve within 1 year [3]. Muscle denervation related signal alterations and end stage muscle atrophy can be seen within the gluteus minimus, medius and tensor fascia lata muscles and following THA. The inferior gluteal nerve can also be injured during THA and iliosacral screw placement, and results in weakness in thigh extension. Injury often occurs in conjunction with superior gluteal nerve injury [13]. Denervation edema-like pattern and atrophy can be seen within the gluteus maximus muscle. Both the superior and the inferior gluteal nerves can also be entrapped secondary to infectious or inflammatory processes, fracture or post-traumatic productive changes related to the greater sciatic notch, sacrum and sacroiliac joints.

### Lateral Femoral Cutaneous Nerve

Entrapment of the lateral femoral cutaneous nerve classically results in the clinical syndrome of meralgia paresthetica, characterized by burning, numbness, pain and paresthesias down the proximal lateral aspect of the thigh. The following are causes of meralgia paresthetica: (1) avulsion fracture of the anterosuperior iliac spine; (2) pelvic and retroperitoneal tumors; (3) stretching of the nerve due to prolonged leg and trunk hyperextension; (4) leg length discrepancy; (5) iatrogenic; (6) prolonged standing; and (7) external compression by belts, weight gain or tight clothing [17]. Injury during elective spine surgery is a recognized complication in up to 20% of patients, and is caused by compression of the nerve against the anterior iliac spine, traction of the psoas muscle or harvesting of iliac crest bone graft material [18]. MRI can have difficulty following the nerve along its course, except when surrounded by large amount of fat, but it can help to identify focal thickening, perineural scarring, mass effect from space occupying lesions or osseous deformity at the site of entrapment, typically following avulsion injury of the sartorius muscle at its origin from the anterosuperior iliac spine. The differential diagnosis includes lumbar discogenic disease.

### Femoral Nerve

Injury to the femoral nerve results in weakness of knee extension (quadriceps muscle) and hip flexion (iliopsoas muscle) as well as sensory loss of the anteromedial knee, medial leg and foot. The nerve is commonly injured in the iliacus compartment secondary to iliopsoas muscular pathology, or at the groin. Iatrogenic causes are most common and include femoral artery puncture for catheterization or bypass surgery, with compression of the nerve by hematoma or pseudoaneurysm [19], pelvic, hip and gynecological surgery. Hysterectomy is a well-known cause of femoral nerve injury. Other common causes include

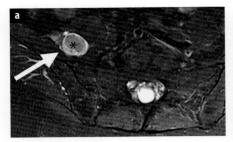

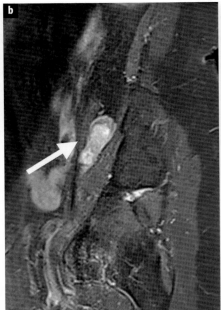

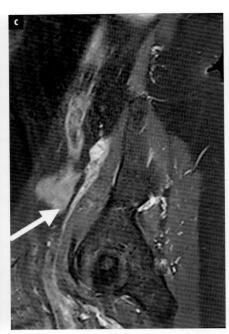

**Fig. 9 a-c.** Female patient presenting with right hip and thigh pain. **a** Axial T2 fat-saturated (FS) image through the right hemipelvis demonstrates multiple lobular T2 hyperintense structures (*arrow*) extending along the expected course of the femoral nerve contribution of the lumbrosacral plexus posterior to the psoas and anterior to the iliacus muscles. Note central hypointensity consistent with a target sign (*), highly suggestive of peripheral nerve sheath tumor. **b, c** Sagittal T1 FS images confirm the enhancing nature of the lesions and demonstrate their extension along the expected course of the distal lumboscral plexus and femoral nerve (*arrows*)

tumor, iliopsoas hematoma, iliopsoas abscess or bursitis (Fig. 9). On MRI, the intrapelvic femoral nerve can show increased signal and size and course deviation due to mass effect. Abnormalities of the nerve at the thigh are more difficult to detect. The iliopsoas muscle can demonstrate denervation signal alterations following injury of the intrapelvic femoral nerve, while the pectineus, sartorius and quadriceps muscles can be affected if injury occurs distal to the inguinal ligament. The femoral nerve is frequently involved in diabetic amyotrophy and pathological changes can also be seen in the setting of HMSN [3].

### Obturator Nerve

Injury to the obturator nerve results in weak thigh adduction and sensory loss of the medial thigh and knee. As with the femoral nerve, the most common causes are iatrogenic and they can occur in a number of settings. The nerve can be stretched following prolonged lithotomy, or retraction during THA, or it can be directly injured or transected during gynecological or genitourinary surgery (e.g., total hysterectomy and radical prostatectomy) [20] (Fig. 8). The obturator nerve can be entrapped within the obturator canal, formed by the margins of the obturator foramen and a ligamentous band called the obturator membrane, through which the obturator nerve, artery and vein pass to exit the pelvis. Enlargement of the obturator externus bursa is another recognized cause of obturator nerve compression. The obturator nerve is susceptible to injury at the level of the pubic symphysis because of its proximity to this structure and the anterior branch can be entrapped secondary to pathology of the pubic bones including fracture, osteitis pubis and adductor brevis tendinopathy. Denervation-related signal alterations can

occur within the adductor muscles, although the adductor brevis muscle can have dual innervation by both anterior and posterior branches and will be spared if only one of the branches is involved. Enlargement and increased intraneural signal of the obturator nerve can sometimes be difficult to distinguish from adjacent vessels.

### Pudendal Nerve

Pudendal nerve entrapment can result in symptoms of perineal and genital numbness and fecal and urinary incontinence, which are characteristically exacerbated by the sitting position [20]. This occurs within the pudendal or Alcock's canal, a space within the obturator fascia lining the lateral wall of the ischiorectal fossa that transmits the pudendal vessels and nerves, resulting in a clinical entity known as Alcock canal syndrome. This has a propensity to occur in cyclists as a result of chronic compression by the saddle (cyclist's syndrome), or in occupations requiring prolonged sitting. The pudendal nerve may also be stretched during childbirth, although this rarely results in permanent neurological deficit or pain. Sacral or ischiorectal space tumors, such as chordoma and rectal carcinoma, can involve the pudendal nerve, and sacrococcygeal teratoma is a tumor that has a particular predilection to involve the pudendal nerve. MRI helps to delineate perineural scarring or space occupying lesions at the site of entrapment.

### Intrapelvic Sciatic Nerve

The well-known clinical syndrome of 'sciatica' is more commonly caused by lumbar disc pathology. Patients typically present with sharp shooting pain radiating from

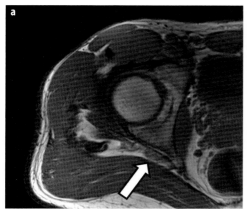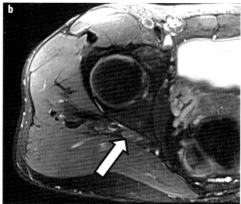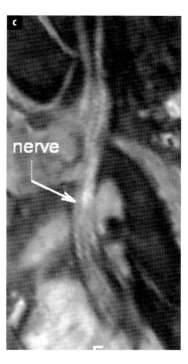

**Fig. 10 a-c.** A 27-year-old man with symptoms compatible with sciatic neuropathy following drug overdose and prolonged unwitnessed coma in supine position. Axial proton density (**a**) and FSE T2 fat-saturated (**b**) images demonstrate focal enlargement and intraneural T2 hyperintensity in the infrapiriformis sciatic nerve (*arrows*). **c** Maximal intensity projection three-dimensional PSIF (pre-excitation refocused steady-state sequence) images show focal increased signal just below the inferior border of the piriformis muscle and superior border of the superior gemellus indicative of sciatic nerve entrapment probably caused by piriformis syndrome

the buttock along the back of the thigh, in the distribution of the sciatic nerve. Patients may present with foot drop, mimicking common peroneal neuropathy. The sciatic nerve is commonly entrapped around the hip and within the sciatic notch. It can also be compressed by the piriformis muscle, resulting in 'piriformis syndrome' (Fig. 10). The peroneal component is more commonly affected than the tibial component, as it is more superficially located with less supporting connective tissue, and is fixed at two separate points. The sciatic nerve can be stretched during THA, or compressed by postoperative fluid collection or hematoma. Paralabral cysts can decompress posteriorly resulting in sciatic nerve compression. Hamstring injury may affect the adjacent nerve. Perineural cysts and neurogenic tumors are also relatively commonly in this location. Injury to the sciatic nerve can result in denervation edema-like pattern in the distal lower limb including the muscles of the knee, leg and foot. The hamstring muscles are less commonly affected due to the high take off of the branch that supplies the proximal thigh.

### Iliohypogastric Nerve

Iatrogenic disruption or damage of the iliohypogastric nerve following surgery is the most common cause of injury and usually results in pain and dysesthesia radiating to the hypogastric area. This can be seen following transverse abdominal wall incisions or suture placement, iliac bone harvesting and inguinal hernia repair [21]. Muscle tears related to sports injuries and abdominal wall expansion during pregnancy are other potential

causes. The nerve is not always visualized during MR neurography, and local anesthetic injection near the anterosuperior iliac spine can be helpful to confirm the diagnosis [21].

### Ilioinguinal Nerve

The ilioinguinal nerve is also most commonly injured during surgery, following transverse abdominal incision or suture placement, iliac graft harvesting, inguinal lymph node dissection, femoral vascular intervention or orchiectomy [22]. Muscle tears related to sports injuries and abdominal wall expansion during pregnancy are other potential causes. Patients present with pain and dysesthesia radiating from the site of injury to the inguinal area, labia majora or scrotum. The nerve is not always visualized during MR neurography, and local anesthetic injection can be helpful to confirm the diagnosis.

### Genitofemoral Nerve

The genitofemoral nerve is most commonly injured during surgery, particularly during hernia repair or gynecological procedure, but also related to abdominal incision and suture placement and lymph node biopsy or dissection. Previous appendicitis or psoas abscess can also damage the nerve. Retroperitoneal hematoma and pregnancy can also result in compression of the nerve. The clinical presentation is of pain radiating from the surgical site below the inguinal ligament to the anterior thigh, labia majora or scrotum. The nerve may not reliably be

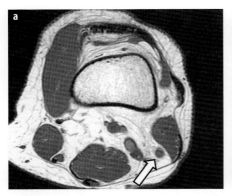
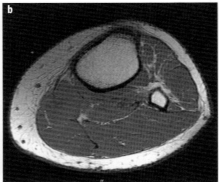
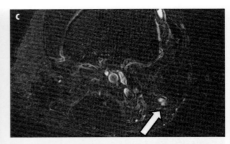
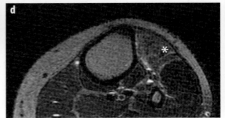

**Fig. 11 a-d.** Female patient presenting with left foot drop after varicectomy. **a, b** Axial T1 image demonstrates scar tissue encasing the common peroneal nerve (*arrow*) and fatty infiltration of the anterior tibial muscle. **c, d** Axial T2 fat-saturated neurographic images show marked intraneural T2 hyperintensity compatible with neuritis (*arrow*) and diffuse denervation edema-like changes of the anterior tibialis muscle (*)

visualized during MR neurography, with its portion traveling within the inguinal canal and along the spermatic cord more readily demonstrated. Local anesthetic injection can be helpful to confirm the diagnosis.

## Knee

### Proximal Tibial Neuropathy

Tibial neuropathy may occur within the popliteal fossa as the nerve passes over the popliteus muscles and under the tendinous arch of the soleus muscle. The tibial nerve supplies all posterior leg compartment muscles and the intrinsic plantar musculature. The following are causes of proximal tibial neuropathy: (1) popliteal fossa hematoma, (2) nerve tumors, (3) postoperative scar, and (4) Baker's cyst (Fig. 11). Clinical manifestations include weakness of the plantar and invertor musculature, as well as sensory losss in the heel and occasionally along the sural nerve distribution. MR findings include compression of the tibial nerve in the popliteal fossa, and denervation changes in the gastrocnemius and popliteus muscles [23]. Space occupying lesions in the popliteal fossa can be seen on MRI (e.g., hematoma, nerve tumors, bone tumors and Baker's cyst). Differential diagnosis includes sacral plexopathy.

### Common Peroneal Neuropathy

The common peroneal nerve branches off from the sciatic nerve at the level of the upper popliteal fossa. Its most proximal division is the lateral cutaneous nerve of the calf. The common peroneal nerve can be found posteromedial to the biceps femoris muscle in the distal popliteal fossa. At the level of the fibular neck, it gives off three terminal branches: the recurrent articular nerve, the su-

perficial peroneal nerve and the deep peroneal nerve. The superficial nerve supplies the lateral compartment muscles (peroneus longus and brevis) and the deep nerve supplies the anterior compartment muscles (anterior tibialis, extensor hallucis longus, extensor digitorum longus and brevis and peroneus tertius).

The following are causes of common peroneal neuropathy: (1) extrinsic compression due to prolonged immobilization (surgery, coma, overdose); (2) extrinsic compression due to space occupying lesions (osteochondromas, tumors, ganglion/synovial cysts, varicosities); (3) traumatic injury following fibular head fracture, knee dislocation or knee surgery (Fig. 11); and (5) post-traumatic compartment syndrome [24, 25].

Clinical manifestations include dysesthesias in the proximal third of the lateral leg as well as foot drop and a slapping gait. The symptoms are typically worsened during plantar flexion and/or inversion of the foot. MR findings include intraneural T2 hyperintensity at the level of the knee joint, space occupying lesions and denervation signs involving both the anterior and the lateral compartment muscles (Fig. 11). The differential diagnosis includes compartment syndrome, tibial stress fracture and shin deep medial tibial syndrome (shin splints).

## Ankle/Foot

### Anterior Tarsal Tunnel Syndrome

Anterior tarsal tunnel syndrome is caused by compression of the deep peroneal nerve as it travels deep to the superior and inferior extensor retinacula or at the level of the talonavicular joint as it travels deep to the extensor hallucis longus tendon. Distally, the deep peroneal nerve may also be entrapped at the level of the first and second tarsometatarsal joints as it travels in a tight tunnel

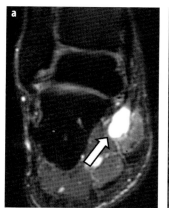 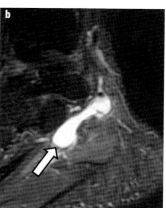 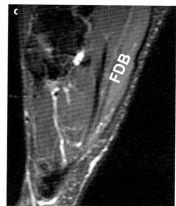 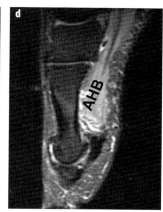

**Fig. 12 a-d.** Tarsal tunnel syndrome: medial plantar nerve compression. **a, b** Coronal and sagittal T2 fat-saturated images demonstrate a bilobed ganglion occupying the tarsal tunnel (*arrow*). Note edema-like denervation signal in the quadratus plantae muscle. **c, d** Sagittal T2 fat-saturated images show denervation edema-like changes of the flexor digitorum brevis (*FDB*) and abductor hallucis brevis (*AHB*) muscles

beneath the extensor hallucis brevis muscle. The following are causes of anterior tarsal tunnel syndrome: (1) stretching of the nerve secondary to ankle instability, (2) direct trauma to the dorsum of the foot, (3) hypertrophic extensor hallucis brevis muscle, (4) os intermetatarsum in the proximal first intermetatarsal space, (5) dorsal degenerative spurs at the talonavicular joint, and (6) tight-fitting shoes [23-25].

Clinical manifestations include dysesthesias along the dorsomedial aspect of the foot and weakness of the extensor digitorum brevis muscle. MR findings include denervation atrophy and edema of the anterior compartment muscles including the anterior tibial, extensor hallucis longus, extensor digitorum longus and peroneus tertius (Fig. 12). The differential diagnosis includes L5 neuropathy and common peroneal neuropathy.

## Superficial Peroneal Neuropathy

The superficial peroneal nerve descends down the leg within a fascial plane between the peroneus longus and extensor digitorum longus muscles. The nerve exits through the deep fascia of the lateral leg compartment about 12.5 cm above the tip of the lateral malleolus. The following are causes of superficial peroneal neuropathy: (1) overstretching during inversion and plantar flexion ankle injuries, (2) thickening of the lateral leg deep fascia, and (3) lateral compartment muscle hernia/fascial defect.

Clinical manifestations include tingling and paresthesias along the lateral aspect of the lower leg and dorsum of the foot with sparing of the first web space. Pain is typically exacerbated by activity. On physical examination, point tenderness may be elicited 10-12 cm above the lateral malleolus where the nerve exits the deep fascia. MR findings include fascial defect or fascial thickening, with or without peroneal muscle hernia. Axial imaging in plantarflexion and dorsiflexion of the foot is recommended [25].

## Tarsal Tunnel Syndrome

The tarsal tunnel is a fibro-osseous space that extends from the posteromedial aspect of the ankle to the plantar aspect of the foot. The tunnel is divided into two compartments: (1) proximal, at the level of the tibiotalar joint; and (2) distal, at the level of the subtalar joint. The tarsal tunnel contains the posterior tibial nerve and its branches. The posterior tibial nerve provides motor function to the plantar muscles of the foot and sensation to the plantar aspect of the foot and toes. The following are causes of tarsal tunnel syndrome: (1) compression of the posterior tibial nerve secondary to osseous spurs, fracture fragments or tarsal coalition; (2) space occupying lesions such as ganglia, nerve tumors, tenosynovitis, accessory or hypertrophic muscles, fibrous septations and varicosities (Fig. 12); (3) congenital foot deformitites; and (4) systemic diseases (diabetes, peripheral vascular disease) [26, 27].

Clinical manifestations include paresthesias along plantar aspect of the foot and toes, Tinel sign and muscle weakness of the plantar muscles of the foot. MR findings include increased size and signal of the tibial nerve and its branches (infrequent), denervation edema of the plantar muscles of the foot, space occupying lesions and enhancement of the tarsal tunnel on postgadolinium images. The differential diagnosis includes sacral plexopathy.

## Baxter's Neuropathy

Baxter's neuropathy is secondary to compression of the inferior calcaneal nerve. The inferior calcaneal nerve is the first branch of the lateral plantar nerve arising within the tarsal tunnel. The lateral plantar nerve is a terminal branch of the posterior tibial nerve. It supplies most of the muscles of the foot, including the abductor digiti minimi, quadratus plantae, flexor digiti minimi brevis, adductor hallucis, the interossei mucles, and the second-fourth lumbricals. It also carries sensation from the lateral sole of the forefoot and midfoot and from the fifth toe and the lateral half of the fourth toe. The terminal branches of the inferior calcaneal nerve innervate the periosteum of the medial calcaneal tuberosity, one to the abductor digiti minimi, and one to the flexor digitorum brevis muscle. The following are causes of Baxter's neuropathy: (1) entrapment by a hypertrophied abductor hallucis muscle particularly in runners, (2) compression by inferior calcaneal enthesophyte/thickened plantar fascia as the nerve courses anterior to the medial calcaneal tuberosity, and (3) stretching secondary to a hypermobile pronated foot.

Clinical manifestations include heel pain, numbness along the lateral third of the sole of the foot and weakness of the abductor digiti minimi. MR findings include denervation edema or fatty atrophy of the abductor digiti minimi muscle [28]. Abductor hallucis muscle hypertrophy and plantar fasciitis may found as potential source of inferior calcaneal nerve entrapment.

## Jogger's Foot

Jogger's foot is defined as entrapment of the medial plantar nerve in a narrow space between the abductor hallucis muscle and anatomic crossover between the flexor digitorum longus and the flexor hallucis longus tendons (Henry's knot). The medial plantar nerve is a terminal branch of the posterior tibial nerve arising within the tarsal tunnel. It supplies the flexor digitorum brevis, abductos hallucis, flexor hallucis and the first lumbrical muscles. It also carries sensation from the medial two thirds of the plantar surface of the foot including the plantar sides of the first to third toes, and the medial half of the fourth toe. The following are causes of jogger's foot: (1) heel valgus and excessive pronation while running, and (2) high medial arch [29].

Clinical manifestations include dysesthesias in the heel, medial arch and plantar aspect of the first and second toes, Tinel sign behind the navicular tuberosity and secondary hallux rigidus. MR findings include muscle denervation edema or atrophy of the abductor hallucis, flexor digitorum brevis, flexor hallucis brevis and first lumbrical. Space occupying masses can be found in the fat plane interposed between the abductor hallucis and the flexor digitorum brevis muscles.

## Morton's Neuroma

Morton's neuroma is a disorder caused by chronic entrapment of the interdigital nerve under the intermetatarsal ligament. Morton's neuroma is more often found at the second and third intermetatarsal spaces. The entrapped nerve undergoes chronic compression, endoneural edema, epineural/endoneural vascular hyalinization and perineural fibrosis evolving into a mass-like enlargement. The following are causes or mimickers of Morton's neuroma: (1) excessive pronation and dorsiflexion of the metatarsal bones, such as in wearing high-heeled shoes; (2) plantar plate injury; (3) Freiberg's infraction; (4) intermetatarsal ganglion; and (5) arthritis/synovitis of the second metatarsophalangeal joint (second ray syndrome) [30].

Clinical manifestations include intermetatarsal pain and numbness exacerbated by walking/standing and relieved by rest and shoe removal. On physical examination, a palpable mass is often accompanied by a characteristic click (Mulder's sign). MR findings include a teardrop-shaped soft tissue mass emanating from the intermetatarsal space extending plantarly (Fig. 13). The mass typically demonstrates low signal intensity on T1 weighted images and T2 weighted images with variable hyperintensity on fluid-sensitive sequences. Post-contrast enhancement is often noted.

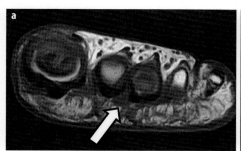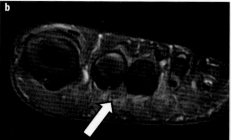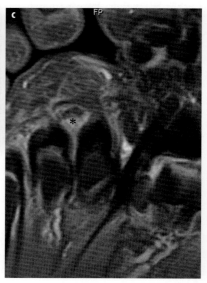

**Fig. 13 a-c.** Morton's neuroma. Coronal proton density (**a**), coronal T2 fat-saturated (FS) (**b**) and axial T2 FS (**c**) images depict an intermediate signal intensity teardrop-shaped soft tissue mass (*arrow*) located in the intermetatarsal space extending into the plantar fat pad. Note mild homogeneous bright signal on fluid-sensitive sequences compatible with hyperemia/granulation tissue (*)

## Conclusion

There are multiple potential etiologies for neurogenic pain and denervation syndromes in the pelvis and lower extremity. Clinical localization of symptoms, as well as knowledge of the neural anatomy, is of critical importance in the search for an underlying etiology. Recent advances in imaging with appropriate utilization and interpretation of dedicated MR neurography may demonstrate pathological changes within the peripheral nerves as well as elucidate the underlying pathology or cause. Muscle denervation changes are a very useful secondary sign of pelvic and lower extremity neuropathy, particularly in the absence of a detectable compressive etiology. MR neurography imaging is subject to certain pitfalls, of which the radiologist should be cognizant when interpreting these examinations. It is crucial that these examinations are not reported in isolation and that a diagnosis of neuropathy is made only on the basis of relevant imaging findings in the appropriate clinical setting.

## References

1. Filler A, Maravilla K, Tsuruda (2004) MR neurography and muscle MR imaging for image diagnosis of disorders affecting the peripheral nerves and musculature. J Neurology Clinics 22: 643–682
2. Petchprapa C, Rosenberg Z, Sconfienza LM et al (2010) MR Imaging of entrapment neuropathies of the lower extremity Part 1. The pelvis and hip. RadioGraphics 30:983-1000
3. Chhabra A, Andreisek G (2012) Magnetic Resonance Neurography. Jaypee Brothers Medical Publishers, 1st edn. New Delhi
4. Moore K, Tsuruda J, Dailey A et al (2001) The value of MR neurography for evaluating extraspinal neuropathic leg pain: a pictorial essay. American Journal of Neuroradiology 22:786-794
5. Gupta S, Nguyen HL, Morello HA et al (2004) Various approaches for CT-guided percutaneous biopsy of deep pelvic lesions: anatomic and technical considerations. Radiographics 24:175-189
6. Yukata K, Arai K, Yoshizumi Y (2005) Obturator neuropathy caused by an acetabular labral cyst: MRI Findings. AJR Am J Roentgenol 184:112-114
7. Sherman P, Matchette M, Sanders T (2003) Acetabular paralabral cyst: an uncommon cause of sciatica. Skel Radiology 32:90-94
8. Woettler K (2010) Tumors and tumor-like lesions of peripheral nerves. Seminars in Musculoskeletal Radiology 14:547-558
9. Stull MA, Moser RP Jr, Kransdorf MJ (1991) Magnetic resonance appearance of peripheral nerve sheath tumors. Skel Radiology 20:9-14
10. Sorenson E, Chen J, Daube J (2002) Obturator neuropathy: causes and outcome. Muscle and Nerve 25:605-607
11. Busis NA (1999) Femoral and obturator neuropathies. Neurolog Clinics 17:633-653
12. Cardosi R, Cox C, Hoffman M (2002) Postoperative neuropathies after major pelvic surgery. Obstet Gynecol 100:240-244
13. Navarro RA, Schmalzried TP, Amstutz HC, Dorey FJ (1995) Surgical approach and nerve palsy in total hip arthroplasty. Journal of Arthroplasty 10:1-5
14. Oldenburg M, Muller RT (1997) The frequency, prognosis and significance of nerve injuries in total hip arthroplasty. International Orthopedics 21:1-3
15. Zwolak P, Eysel P, Michael JWP (2011) Femoral and obturator nerves palsy caused by pelvic cement extrusion after hip arthroplasty. Orthopedic Reviews 3:e6
16. Kenny P, O'Brien CP, Synnott K (1999) Damage to the superior gluteal nerve after two different approaches to the hip. J Bone Joint Surg Br 81B:979-981
17. Murata Y, Takahashi K, Yamagata M (2000) The anatomy of the lateral femoral cutaneous nerve with special reference to the harvesting of iliac bone graft. J Bone Joint Surg Am 82:746-747
18. Mirovsky Y, Neuwirth M (2000) Injuries to the lateral femoral cutaneous nerve during spine surgery. Spine 25:1266-1269
19. Ahmad F, Turner SA, Torrie P (2008) Iatrogenic femoral artery pseudoaneurysms. A review of current methods of diagnosis and treatment. Clinical Radiology 63:1310-1316
20. Hough D, Wittenberg K, Pawlina W et al (2003) Chronic perineal pain caused by pudendal nerve entrapment: anatomy and CT-guided perineural injection technique. AJR Am J Roentgenol 181:561-567
21. Whiteside JL, Barber MD, Walters MD (2003) Anatomy of ilioinguinal and iliohypogastric nerves in relation to trocar placement and low transverse incisions. American Journal of Obstetrics and Gynaecology 189:1574-1578
22. Madura JA, Madura JA 2nd, Copper CM et al (2005) Inguinal neurectomy for inguinal nerve entrapment: an experience with 100 patients. Am J Surg 189:283-287
23. Hochman MG, Zilberfarb JL (2004) Nerves in a pinch: imaging of nerve compression syndromes. Radiol Clin North Am 42:221-245
24. Kim S, Choi JY, Huh YM et al (2007) Role of magnetic resonance imaging in entrapment and compressive neuropathy-what, where, and how to see the peripheral nerves on the musculoskeletal magnetic resonance image: part 1. Overview and lower extremity. Eur Radiol 17:139-149
25. Lacour-Petic MC, Lozeron P, Ducreux D (2003) MRI of peripheral nerve lesions of the lower limbs. Neuroradiology 45:166-170
26. Lau JT, Daniels TR (1999) Tarsal tunnel syndrome: a review of the literature. Foot Ankle Int 20:201-209
27. Masciocchi C, Catalucci A, Barile A (1998) Ankle impingement syndromes. Eur J Radiol 27:S70-73
28. Recht M, Grooff P, Ilaslan H et al (2007) Selective atrophy of the abductor digiti quinti: an MRI study. AJR Am J Roentgenol 189:123-127
29. Schon LC, Baxter DE (1990) Neuropathies of the foot and ankle in athletes. Clin Sports Med 9: 489-509
30. Delfaut E, Demondion X, Bieganski A et al (2003) Imaging of foot and ankle nerve entrapment syndromes: from well demonstrated to unfamiliar sites. Radiographics 23:613-623

# Specific Aspects of Sports-Related Injuries of the Pediatric Musculoskeletal System

Peter J. Strouse[1], Karen Rosendahl[2]

[1] Section of Pediatric Radiology, C. S. Mott Children's Hospital, University of Michigan Health System, Ann Arbor, MI, USA
[2] Department of Pediatric Radiology, Haukeland University Hospital, Bergen, Norway

## Introduction

Children in the western countries are increasingly involved in sporting activity, both team and solo sports. Participation is increasingly focused on a single sport or even a specific role in a specific sport. Children are thus increasingly at risk of sports-related injury. Repetitive focused activity predisposes some children to stress and repetitive trauma type injuries.

The incidence and distribution of sport-related injuries vary based on sport affiliation, participation level, gender and player position. In the UK, up to 80% of children aged between 5 and 15 years take part in organized sport, 11% of whom are involved in intensive training [1]. Approximately one child in ten will sustain a recreational injury in a given year. In general, boys are more prone to sports injuries than girls, and also sustain more severe injuries, possibly because they are more aggressive [1]. Sports involving contact and jumping have the highest injury levels, with American football in particular accounting for the majority of injuries followed by wrestling, basketball, soccer and baseball. Ski and snowboard accidents are commonly seen in regions were the activities are available.

Most high-performance pediatric athletes become involved in sport in the latter half of the first decade of life. During this time period, sports-related injuries typically consist of contusions, sprains and extremity fractures, typically plastic or Salter type fractures. Ligament and muscle injuries are rare. Injuries of the spine and head are rare.

In the first half of the second decade, things change. Children grow. Sports become more competitive and physical. Prepubertal children have open epiphyseal and apophyseal physes. The physes usually constitute the weakest link in the anatomic chain. Stressors that cause ligamentous injury in adults usually cause physeal injury in the immature athlete. The physes are also prone to stress type injury due to repetitive activity [2]. In addition to the physes, the general composition of bone is not mature. Some nonphyseal osseous injuries are relatively specific to children. In addition to long bone physeal injuries, adolescents may suffer injury to physes of the apophyses. Apophyses are growth centers that do not contribute to longitudinal growth. They are sites of muscle tendon origin or insertion.

Prior to physeal fusion, ligamentous injury is uncommon, but can occur. With physeal fusion at adolescence, injury to ligamentous structures becomes more common and injury patterns are similar to those seen in young adults.

In addition to stress injuries of physes, and more commonly, children may be subject to develop stress fracture or stress injury at various locations due to repetitive activities. Away from the growth plate, such stress injuries are similar in presentation and radiologic appearance to such injuries occurring in adults.

Some children are predisposed to stress injury or develop symptoms because of the presence of underlying congenital anomalies or variants predisposing to pathology. Nontraumatic processes such as bone tumors (i.e., osteoid osteoma, osteosarcoma) or infection may mimic traumatic injury. Traumatic injuries may act as a nidus for infection. Myositis ossificans is a not infrequent post-traumatic process in children and may mimic a soft tissue or juxtacortical neoplasm.

In this essay and presentation, we will focus on the imaging of injuries that are unique to the pediatric population. Pathologies that occur in children, but are more common in adults, will be mentioned, but not covered in detail.

## Shoulder

In the latter half of the second decade, injury to the shoulder becomes quite common, particularly with participation in contact sports such as American football and hockey [3]. Shoulder dislocations are frequent. Imaging findings in shoulder dislocation and instability in adolescents

J. Hodler et al. (eds.), *Musculoskeletal Diseases 2013-2016,*
DOI: 10.1007/978-88-470-5292-5_25 © Springer-Verlag Italia 2013

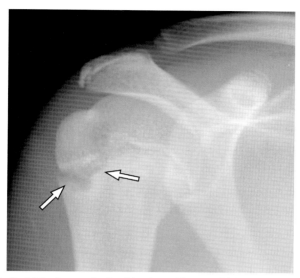

**Fig. 1.** Little leaguer's shoulder in a 15-year-old boy. Irregularity and widening of the lateral aspect of the proximal humeral physis is noted, with extrusion of cartilage into the adjacent metaphysis (*arrows*)

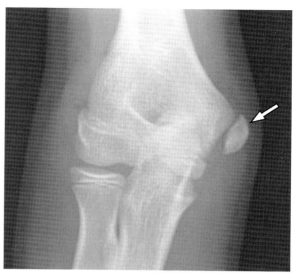

**Fig. 2.** Acute medial epicondylar apophysis avulsion (*arrow*) in a 14-year-old boy. The patient experienced acute pain while pitching a baseball

are similar to those seen in adults. Clavicle fractures are common. Acromioclavicular separation injuries are relatively uncommon in adolescents.

Injury from repetitive throwing becomes more common in later adolescence, most commonly being seen in baseball pitchers and other throwing athletes. Rotator cuff and labral injuries are uncommon but may occur. A unique injury to skeletally immature throwers is "Little Leaguer's shoulder." Little Leaguer's shoulder is stress injury of the physis of the proximal humerus caused by repetitive throwing. On radiographs, the physis of the proximal humerus is wide and slightly irregular (Fig. 1). On magnetic resonance imaging (MRI), the growth plate appears widened with irregular margins and adjacent bone marrow edema [4]. Findings may mimic other processes such as leukemia; however, the clinical history will suggest the proper diagnosis and findings are confined to one location. Symptoms and radiologic abnormalities abate with prolonged cessation of activity.

## Elbow

Younger children may suffer an array of elbow fractures, with supracondylar and lateral condylar fractures being the most common patterns. Elbow dislocations are uncommon. With an elbow dislocation in a skeletally immature patient, the location of the medial epicondylar ossification center should be carefully assessed. It is usually avulsed during the dislocation and frequently becomes trapped within the elbow joint with reduction.

The other common mechanism for medial epicondylar avulsion is a throwing injury. Medial epicondyle avulsion in the throwing juvenile athlete is classic "Little Leaguer's

elbow," as described by Brogdon in 1960 [5]. Classically, injury presents with acute symptoms during a throw with a "pop" and acute pain and point tenderness over the medial epicondyle. Radiographs show displacement of the medial epicondyle (Fig. 2). For experienced readers, comparison radiographs are not necessary. Although displacement less than 3 mm may be treated conservatively, most avulsed medial epicondylar apophyses are reduced and pinned.

Pitching limits are imposed in American youth baseball to prevent injury. Juvenile throwers are also prone to other injuries, including capitellar osteochondritis dissecans, stress injury of the medial epicondylar physis, flexor tendinopathy and ulnar collateral ligament injury [6]. The latter two injuries become more common with skeletal maturity. Stress injury of the medial epicondylar physis is often called "medial epicondylitis" or "Little Leaguer's elbow"; however, as discussed, Little Leaguer's elbow was originally described as an acute avulsion injury [6]. With stress injury of the medial epicondylar physis, the physis will appear wide and irregular. Adjacent edema may be seen within bone marrow and soft tissues on MRI.

Capitellar osteochondral injury occurs due to valgus stress [6]. The capitellum is a less common site of osteochondral injury and osteochondritis dissecans than the knee or ankle. The radiographic appearance is similar. An irregular lenticular defect is seen in the osseous capitellum. Arthrography or MRI may show a defect in the overlying cartilage. Unstable fragments may become loose bodies.

Throwing adolescents may also develop stress injury of the physis of the olecranon, likely related to the stress of triceps muscle contraction during the throwing motion [6, 7].

## Wrist and Hands

Wrist injuries in skeletally immature athletes are very common; however, most are plastic fractures (i.e., buckle fractures) of the distal radial metaphysis or Salter type fractures involving the physis. Stress injury of the distal radial physes is very common in gymnasts ("gymnast wrist"). Presentation is frequently with unilateral symptoms; however, the abnormality is usually bilateral. Similar to other physeal stress injuries, the growth plates of the distal radius are wide and irregular with adjacent metaphyseal sclerosis (Fig. 3) [8]. Adjacent bone marrow edema is seen on MRI [9]. Symptoms and radiological findings abate with prolonged cessation of activity. Continued activity may lead to premature physeal fusion, relative radial shortening with ulnar positive variance, and predisposition to carpal impingement. Age restrictions on participation in Olympic gymnastics are aimed at preventing wrist injury.

Carpal injuries are rare in children due to the lack of complete ossification "providing a cushion" and some normal ligamentous laxity. Beginning around the time of puberty, scaphoid injuries become increasingly common. Imaging of scaphoid injuries is analogous to that in adults. As in adults, the proximal pole of the scaphoid is predisposed to avascular necrosis. Injuries to other carpal bones are rare in the pediatric age group. Repetitive injury to the hook of the hamate may occur with racquet or other sports producing repetitive contact to hypothenar region; however, such injury is relatively rare in children. Injury of the carpal ligaments is uncommon in children.

Due to the presence of growth plates and the composition of the bones, active children are subject to different patterns of metacarpal and phalangeal injury of the

hand than adults. Equivalent injury mechanisms may produce Salter type fractures.

## Pelvis and Hips

There are six apophyseal growth centers on the pelvis and proximal femurs: iliac crest, anterior superior iliac spine (ASIS), anterior inferior iliac spine (AIIS), ischial apophyis, greater trochanter and lesser trochanter [10]. Each of these apophyses may avulse with sports injury. ASIS and ischial apophysis injuries are most common. The ASIS is the site of origin of the sartorius muscle. The AIIS is the site of origin of the rectus femorus muscle. The iliac crest is the site of origin of the external and internal abdominal oblique muscles, transverse abdominis muscle, gluteus medius muscle and the tensor fasciae latae. The hamstring muscles originate from the ischial apophysis. The gluteus medius and minimus muscles, the piriform muscle, the internal obturator muscle and the gemelli muscles insert on the greater trochanter, and the iliopsoas tendon inserts on the lesser trochanter. Avulsions of the apophyses thus occur with specific activity related to the function of the attached muscle. For instance, ASIS avulsions are common with kicking injuries, ischial apophysis avulsions with hurdling, and iliac crest avulsions occur with wrestling or sudden turns while running. With acute injury, the involved apophysis is displaced (Fig. 4). Stress injuries and healing acute injuries may appear similar with widening and irregularity of the apophyseal growth plate. Adjacent bone marrow and soft tissue edema may be seen with MRI. Rarely, avulsions may occur prior to apophyseal ossification. Displaced acute avulsions may heal with

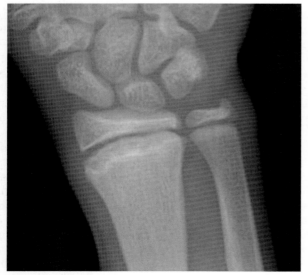

**Fig. 3.** Gymnast wrist in a 12-year-old girl. The distal radial physis is widened with irregularity of its metaphyseal margin. Symmetric abnormality was noted on the contralateral side

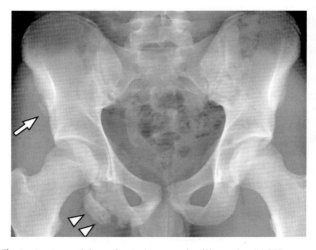

**Fig. 4.** Acute avulsion of anterior superior iliac spine (ASIS, *arrow*) and chronic avulsion of ischial tuberosity (*arrowheads*) in a 16-year-old boy soccer player. The patient presented with acute pain after a kick due to the ASIS avulsion. Due to displacement of the ischial apophysis and continued activity there is exuberant callous formation

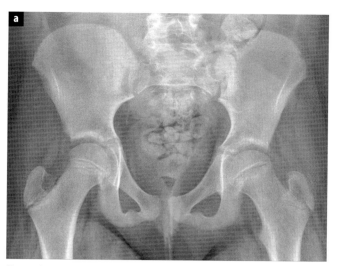 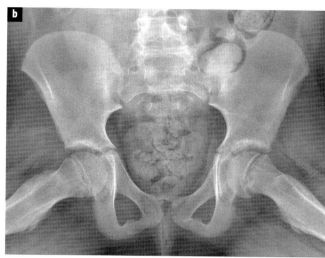

**Fig. 5 a, b.** Slipped capital femoral epiphysis in an 11-year-old girl. **a** Anteroposterior image shows widening and irregularity of the left proximal femoral growth plate. A line extended up from the lateral margin of the left femoral neck (Klien's line) intersects less femoral head than a similar line on the right. The right hip is normal. **b** Posteromedial displacement of the left femoral head relative to the left femoral neck and growth plate widening are better seen on the abduction view

exuberant callous and may be mistaken for an osseous neoplasm (Fig. 4).

Slipped capital femoral epiphysis (SCFE) occurs in children approaching the time of puberty until the growth plates are fused. Although injury may occur with sports activity, the classic body habitus of affected children is not that of the active adolescent athlete. Patients tend to be overweight and delayed in sexual maturation. SCFE may present acutely, as a chronic process or as an acute injury superimposed on a chronic slip ("acute on chronic"). If a child is unable to bear weight on the extremity, the SCFE is termed "unstable", and if able to bear weight, the SCFE is termed "stable" [11]. Early slips may be very subtle on radiography. Identification is enhanced by obtaining abduction (frog leg lateral) views and comparison to the contralateral side (Fig. 5). About 20% of patients have bilateral SCFE, but usually not symmetric at presentation. Symmetric presentation in a young child suggests an underlying condition such as an endocrinopathy.

Radiographic signs of SCFE include malalignment of the femoral head and neck, sclerosis or buttressing of the femoral neck, and loss of height of the femoral head due to rotation. ASIS avulsion may produce similar symptoms to SCFE and should be assessed for, particularly if SCFE is not evident on radiographs.

Femoral acetabular impingement can be diagnosed in adolescence [12, 13]. Cam-type deformity may be associated with vigorous participation in certain sports activities [13]. Maldevelopment of the femoral head/neck junction may also predispose. A relatively high proportion (6%) of adolescents have radiological findings suggestive of having had a mild silent slipped epiphysis (Lehmann et al. unpublished results, investigating a population based cohort of 2,072 healthy adolescents). Others suggest that an inherited anomalous development of the femoral head/neck junction with insufficient wasting predisposes [12]. Patients present with pain with extremes of flexion and locking or decreased range of motion suggestive of associated labral tears.

## Knee

Prior to physeal fusion, the physes of the knee are weaker than the ligaments. Physeal fractures of the distal femur and proximal tibia are moderately common [14]. The composition of bone is also not mature. Although not a ligamentous injury, avulsion of the tibial spine occurs with increased frequency in the skeletally immature with the same mechanism as leads to anterior cruciate ligament (ACL) injury in older patients (Fig. 6). With such injury, the ACL is usually intact but may occasionally be injured. Accompanying injuries of the collateral ligaments and menisci are not infrequent. In a young patient, the presence of a large traumatic knee joint effusion should prompt search for a tibial spine avulsion fracture, particularly if a fat/fluid level is seen.

Prior to skeletal maturity, injuries of the cruciate ligaments, collateral ligaments and menisci are uncommon. A torn lateral meniscus in a younger patient is often due to an underlying discoid meniscus (Fig. 7) [15]. It may be difficult to discern the meniscus as discoid due to the tear and displacement of fragments. With skeletal maturity, injury of cruciate ligaments, collateral ligaments and menisci become quite common. Bucket handle tears of the menisci with displaced fragments seem to be relatively common in adolescents [16].

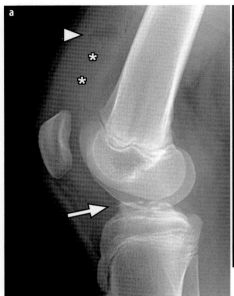

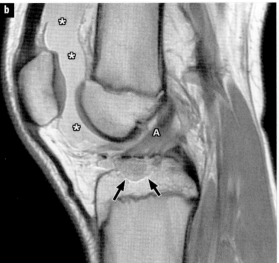

**Fig. 6 a, b.** Tibial spine avulsion in a 13-year-old girl sustained while downhill ski racing. **a** Lateral radiograph of the knee shows a large joint effusion (*asterisks*) with a fat/fluid level (*arrowhead*). Irregularity of the tibial spine suggests a fracture (*arrow*). **b** Sagittal proton density magnetic resonance image shows the tibial spine avulsion fracture (*arrows*). The anterior cruciate ligament (*A*) is attached to the fragment. A large joint effusion (*asterisks*) is noted

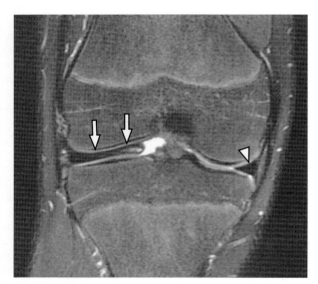

**Fig. 7.** Discoid lateral meniscus in a 15-year-old boy baseball player. Coronal proton density with fat saturation magnetic resonance image shows an enlarged lateral meniscus (*arrows*). Ill-defined increased signal is noted within the meniscus due to degeneration. The *arrowhead* shows the normal medial meniscus

Adolescents are also prone to injuries involving the extensor mechanism [17]. Transient lateral patellar dislocation is very common. Genu valgus, a shallow trochlea of the distal femoral epiphysis and patella alta predispose; notably patella alta may be accompanied by chronic low-grade knee pain due to patellofemoral stress syndrome. The injury is more common in girls. The patella usually reduces promptly and often the patient is unaware that the patella dislocated. Osteochondral injury may occur on the medial patellar facet or anterolateral aspect of the lateral femoral condyle due to impaction. Small osteochondral

fractures or fragments are occasionally seen on radiography. In addition, on MRI, bone marrow edema is seen at this site with disruption of the medial retinaculum and medial patellofemoral ligament. Stress type injury may occur at the inferior pole of the patella (Sinding-Larsen-Johansson disease, or Jumper's knee) or tibial apophysis (Osgood-Schlatter disease). The latter is a clinical diagnosis. Marked irregularity of the tibial apophysis is common and usually normal. MRI may demonstrate edema in the soft tissues and apophysis and occasionally a retropatellar tendon bursa. Acute avulsions of the tibial apophysis are rare. Avulsions of the patellar tendon may occur at the lower pole of the patella ("patellar sleeve fracture") or rarely at the upper pole.

Osteochondral lesion (osteochondritis dissecans, OCD) of the femoral condyles is a common lesion in teenage athletes. The most common location is at the lateral aspect of the medial femoral condyle anteriorly. A lenticular area of lucency is seen within the articular surface. MRI is helpful in determining the integrity of the overlying cartilage. In addition to cartilage defects, fluid undermining the lesion and cysts is indicative of instability; however, assessment of stability is less accurate in younger adolescents than adults [18]. OCD must be differentiated from normal developmental irregularity of the posterior aspect of the femoral condyles [19]. This occurs at a younger age, is devoid of symptoms, and has intact overlying cartilage without associated bone marrow edema. Juvenile OCD may represent a stress injury of the epiphyseal physis and may thus be etiologically distinct from the adult form of OCD [20].

Bipartite patella is a normal variant; however, symptoms may occur due to stress at the synchondrosis between the superolateral ossification center and the rest of the patella. Adjacent bone marrow edema is seen on MRI.

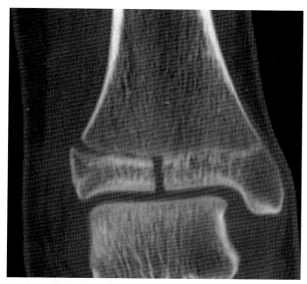

**Fig. 8.** Juvenile Tillaux fracture in a 14-year-old boy. The fracture courses transverse through the lateral aspect of the distal tibial physis and sagittal through the distal tibial epiphysis. Slight separation of the fracture fragments is seen at the articular surface

## Ankle and Foot

The juvenile Tillaux and triplane fractures are "transitional fractures" seen in patients approaching skeletal maturity. The physeal portion of the fracture courses through the unfused portion of the growth plate and therefore is characteristically anterolateral. The juvenile Tillaux fracture is a Salter III fracture of the distal tibia (Fig. 8). The anterior talofibular ligament attaches to the epiphyseal fragment. The triplane fracture has epiphyseal, physeal and metaphyseal fracture components. The epiphyseal fracture line is typically in the sagittal plane and the metaphyseal fracture line is typically in the coronal plane (since not the same fracture plane, this is *not* a Salter IV fracture). Computed tomography (CT) is commonly used to confirm the presence of a fracture and delineate the fracture anatomy for operative planning [21]. A gap of 2 mm or greater at the articular surface is considered an indication for operative fixation to reduce the risk of premature degenerative disease due to articular incongruity.

Ligamentous injuries at the ankle become increasingly common with skeletal maturity. Imaging is similar to adult patients. Lisfranc injuries are very uncommon in children but may occur. Such injuries are aggressively sought on imaging and aggressively treated to avoid permanent instability. On MRI, disruption of the Lisfranc ligament is seen between the medial cuneiform and the base of the second metatarsal. Associated tarsal or metatarsal fractures or joint disruption may be seen. Tendon injuries at the ankle are uncommon in children.

Tarsal coalition typically presents early in the second decade of life as the bones near completion of ossification and the foot becomes sturdier [22]. Patients often present with pain induced by athletic activity. Increased stress at the site of coalition produces symptoms. Talocalcaneal and calcaneonavicular coalitions far outnumber other sites and are roughly equal in incidence. Calcaneonavicular coalitions are readily diagnosed by radiography. While talocalcaneal coalitions are usually suggested on radiographs, CT or MRI is used for confirmation and delineation [22]. In addition to showing the osseous or fibrous coalition, MRI will show edema on either side of the coalition. Untreated tarsal coalition does predispose patients to talar OCD and tendinopathy.

Accessory navicular bones (type II) may produce symptoms due to stress on the synchondrosis with the navicular bone proper or due to osseous prominence [23]. Posterior ankle impingement is a common finding in athletes and dancers with repetitive extremes of plantar flexion (i.e., en pointe ballet dancers) [23]. A prominent os trigonum may predispose. MRI will demonstrate edema with soft tissues and the adjacent bones.

Avulsion fractures of the tuberosity at the base of the fifth metacarpal are common in adolescents [24]. True Jones fractures of the fifth metatarsal are infrequent. Jones fractures occur approximately 1.5 cm proximal to the tuberosity [24].

## Stress Fracture

Athletically active adolescents are prone to stress fractures due to repetitive activity [25]. Distance runners are most affected although injuries may occur with other sports and activities such as marching band. Common sites of stress fracture include the tibia, the femur, the calcaneus, and the second or third metatarsals [25]. Stress fractures of the upper extremities or pelvis are uncommon in children. Stress fractures of the first rib may occur due to prolonged carrying of heavy school backpacks. Stress fractures are characterized by sclerosis, cortical thickening and smooth, benign appearing periosteal new bone. With progression, an ill-defined fracture line may be seen. With further activity, this may rarely progress to a complete fracture. Patients not infrequently present with symptoms prior to development of radiographic findings. Initial radiographs are therefore negative. The patient may thus continue the inciting activity. MRI is thus obtained, frequently with a delay from the initial presentation and initial radiographs. It is therefore frequently helpful to repeat the radiographs for correlation with the MRI.

## Myositis Ossificans

While muscle contusions are probably common in child athletes, frank muscle tears are rare. Myositis ossificans is a poorly understood response to muscle injury, not infrequent in children. While it is post-traumatic, often a

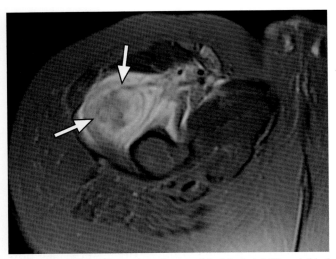

**Fig. 9.** Myositis ossificans in a 9-year-old girl. Axial T2-weighted with fat saturation magnetic resonance image shows a high signal mass (*arrows*) in the deep anterior upper thigh musculature. Abundant perilesional edema is noted

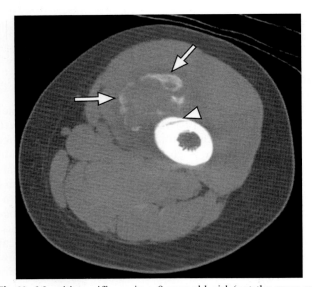

**Fig. 10.** Myositis ossificans in a 9-year-old girl (not the same patient as in Fig. 9). Axial computed tomography image shows peripheral ossification within the mass (*arrows*). Non-aggressive periosteal new bone is present on the underlying femur (*arrowhead*)

specific inciting traumatic episode is not recognized. Patients present with pain and swelling. Early radiographs are negative or show only soft tissue swelling. Imaging, therefore, often proceeds to MRI if the correct diagnosis is not suspected. On MRI, myositis ossificans may appear as a hyperintense, hyperenhancing mass with abundant adjacent edema (Fig. 9) [26]. This may mimic an aggressive neoplasm. Proper diagnosis may be suggested by location within muscle and a history of a traumatic injury. Ideally, plain radiographs or limited CT is performed and

shows characteristic peripheral ossification within the mass (Fig. 10) [27]. Differential considerations also include juxtacortical (parosteal) osteosarcoma.

## Spine

Repetitive stresses to the growing thoracolumbar spine can cause acute and overuse injuries that are unique to the pediatric age group. Plain radiographs and CT are critical for detecting vertebral fracture, and MRI is an essential adjunct for evaluating muscular, ligamentous and spinal cord injury [28].

Acute spinal injuries are rare, but responsible for up to one-quarter of all acute cervical spine injuries in children, the typical high-risk sports being American football, diving, skiing, gymnastics and trampolining [29, 30]. Although all levels can be affected, most spinal injuries below the age of 12 years involve the atlanto-axial or atlanto-occipital joints. Note that up to 2 mm "pseudo"spondylolysis at levels C2-3 and C3-4 can be seen in healthy children. Sporting injuries to the cervical spine most often occur in adolescent boys, and are isolated injuries associated with a relatively low injury severity score (ISS). In around 75% of these injuries, no radiographic abnormality can be detected (spinal cord injury without radiographic abnormality, SCIWORA), but MRI shows a high incidence of cord abnormality such as edema and/or hemorrhage (gradient echo sequences are helpful to differentiate between these two entities). Supervised flexion and extension radiographs are useful to assess stability in this situation.

Intervertebral disk herniation is rare in prepubertal children, but increasingly seen in adolescents who participate in competitive sports, with L4/L5 and L5/S1 being the most commonly affected levels. It is often associated with fracture of the ring apophyses. The role of continuous bony microtrauma is not clear. Radiographs are usually normal. On MRI, there is focal protrusion of the disc with displacement of the longitudinal ligament, reflecting focal rupture of the annulus fibrosus. Herniation of the nucleus pulposus through the vertebral end-plate into the adjacent vertebrae is termed a Schmorl node (Fig. 11). These are relatively common in the lower thoracic and upper lumbar spine of adolescents, and may be associated with pain – and with Scheuermann disease. The nucleus may also herniate between the vertebral body and the ring apophysis, termed anterior transosseous escape. This is seen particularly in adolescents and may result in failure of fusion of the ring apophysis (limbus vertebrae).

Scheuermann disease of the lumbar or thoracolumbar spine is defined as kyphosis, with at least three adjacent wedge-shaped vertebrae (more than 5 degrees). It is most frequently seen in adolescent athletes, particularly gymnasts, rowers and weightlifters. The true natural history has not been clearly established, but excessive physical stress at the time of end-plate maturation is believed to play a role. Radiologically, there are wedge-shaped vertebrae,

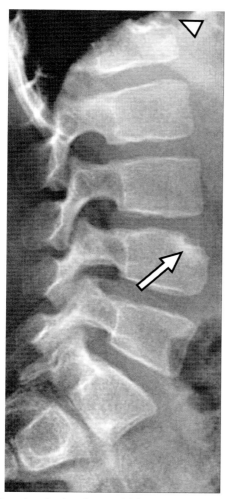

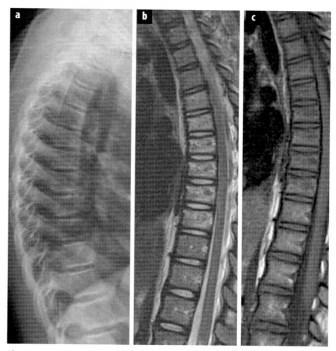

**Fig. 12 a-c.** Early Scheuermann disease in a 10-year-old male gymnast, presenting with back pain and increased thoracic kyphosis. **a** Lateral radiograph shows anterior wedging and irregular endplates of thoracic vertebrae T4 to T9. Sagittal T2-weighted (**b**) and T1-weighted (**c**) magnetic resonance images show additional marrow edema adjacent to the vertebral endplates. The findings are suggestive of Scheuermann disease, early stage

**Fig. 11.** Schmorl nodes in a 7-year-old female skier, presenting with lower back pain. Lateral radiograph showing a defect (*arrow*) in the upper end plate of the fourth lumbar vertebrae, anteriorly, and reduced disk height at level L3/L4. Similar findings are seen at T12 (*arrowhead*)

often associated with markedly irregular end-plates, Schmorl nodes and disc space narrowing (Fig. 12).

Spondylolysis is an osseous defect of the pars interarticularis between the superior and inferior facets of the vertebral body, while listhesis is the slippage of the superior vertebra on the inferior (Fig. 13). Both can be related to hyperextension and axial loading during childhood, and is thought to be a stress fatigue fracture, although occasionally it is an acute injury. Its frequency increases with age through childhood, especially between 5 and 7 years, to reach 6% in adults. Typically, the child presents with lower back pain and focal tenderness. The condition is related to gymnastics, dancing, football, weightlifting and running. Approximately 70% of spondylolistheses occur at the L5-S1 level, and only rarely occur above L3. They are usually bilateral, but occasionally they are unilateral, in which case compensatory hypertrophy of the contralateral pedicle may be seen, as increased density, on plain radiographs. If plain

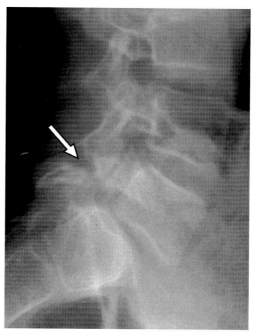

**Fig. 13.** Spondylolysis and spondylolisthesis in a 12-year-old male football player, presenting with low back pain. Lateral radiograph shows a linear defect in the pars interarticularis (*arrow*) consistent with spondylolysis at L5, with grade I anterior spondylolisthesis of L5 on S1. When a pars defect is identified radiographically, further imaging usually is not needed

radiographs are negative or inconclusive, further imaging may be warranted. A tailored CT or MRI, using "reversed angle" axial images (approximately 45 degrees caudal angulation), clearly shows the defect in the posterior arch and also delineates any foraminal encroachment by bone fragments. Magnetic resonance findings can guide treatment (i.e., distinguish between an acute or healing lesion and an inactive lesion representing a fibrous union requiring surgical fixation).

## Conclusion

Children and adolescents are increasingly involved in sports. Youth sports are increasingly competitive. Pediatric sports injury is common. Patterns of injury are different than in adults, mainly due to the presence of open physes. Knowledge of characteristic pediatric injuries and injury patterns aids in diagnosis.

## References

1. Shanmugam C, Maffulli N (2008) Sports injuries in children. Br Med Bull 86:33-57
2. Laor T, Wall EJ, Vu LP (2006) Physeal widening in the knee due to stress injury in child athletes. AJR Am J Roentgenol 186:1260-1264
3. Kocher MS, Waters PM, Micheli LJ (2000) Upper extremity injuries in the paediatric athlete. Sports Med 30:117-135
4. Obembe OO, Gaskin CM, Taffoni MJ, Anderson MW (2007) Little Leaguer's shoulder (proximal humeral epiphysiolysis): MRI findings in four boys. Pediatr Radiol 37:885-889
5. Brogdon BG, Crow NE (1960) Little leaguer's elbow. Am J Roentgenol Radium Ther Nucl Med 83:671-675
6. Klingele KE, Kocher MS (2002) Little league elbow: valgus overload injury in the paediatric athlete. Sports Med 32:1005-1015
7. Rettig AC, Wurth TR, Mieling P (2006) Nonunion of olecranon stress fractures in adolescent baseball pitchers: a case series of 5 athletes. Am J Sports Med 34:653-656
8. Chang CY, Shih C, Penn IW et al (1995) Wrist injuries in adolescent gymnasts of a Chinese opera school: radiographic survey. Radiology 195:861-864
9. Shih C, Chang CY, Penn IW et al (1995) Chronically stressed wrists in adolescent gymnasts: MR imaging appearance. Radiology 195:855-859
10. Fernbach SK, Wilkinson RH (1981) Avulsion injuries of the pelvis and proximal femur. AJR Am J Roentgenol 137:581-584
11. Loder RT, Richards BS, Shapiro PS et al (1993) Acute slipped capital femoral epiphysis: the importance of physeal stability. J Bone Joint Surg Am 75:1134-1140
12. Wenger DR, Kishan S, Pring ME (2006) Impingement and childhood hip disease. J Pediatr Orthop B 15:233-243
13. Siebenrock KA, Ferner F, Noble PC et al (2011) The cam-type deformity of the proximal femur arises in childhood in response to vigorous sporting activity. Clin Orthop Relat Res 469:3229-3240
14. Close BJ, Strouse PJ (2000) MR of physeal fractures of the adolescent knee. Pediatr Radiol 30:756-762
15. Kelly BT, Green DW (2002) Discoid lateral meniscus in children. Curr Opin Pediatr 14:54-61
16. Dunoski B, Zbojniewicz AM, Laor T (2012) MRI of displaced meniscal fragments. Pediatr Radiol 42:104-112
17. Dwek JR, Chung CB (2008) The patellar extensor apparatus of the knee. Pediatr Radiol 38:925-935
18. Kijowski R, Blankenbaker DG, Shinki K et al (2008) Juvenile versus adult osteochondritis dissecans of the knee: appropriate MR imaging criteria for instability. Radiology 248:571-578
19. Gebarski K, Hernandez RJ (2005) Stage-I osteochondritis dissecans versus normal variants of ossification in the knee in children. Pediatr Radiol 35:880-886
20. Laor T, Zbojniewicz AM, Eismann EA, Wall EJ (2012) Juvenile osteochondritis dissecans: is it a growth disturbance of the secondary physis of the epiphysis? AJR Am J Roentgenol 199:1121-1128
21. Brown SD, Kasser JR, Zurakowski D, Jaramillo D (2004) Analysis of 51 tibial triplane fractures using CT with multiplanar reconstruction. AJR Am J Roentgenol 183:1489-1495
22. Newman JS, Newberg AH (2000) Congenital tarsal coalition: multimodality evaluation with emphasis on CT and MR imaging. Radiographics 20:321-332
23. Miller TT (2002) Painful accessory bones of the foot. Semin Musculoskelet Radiol 6:153-161
24. Lawrence SJ, Botte MJ (1993) Jones' fractures and related fractures of the proximal fifth metatarsal. Foot Ankle 14:358-365
25. Jaimes C, Jimenez M, Shabshin N et al (2012) Taking the stress out of evaluating stress injuries in children. Radiographics 32:537-555
26. Kransdorf MJ, Meis JM, Jelinek JS (1991) Myositis ossificans: MR appearance with radiologic-pathologic correlation. AJR Am J Roentgenol 157:1243-1248
27. Amendola MA, Glazer GM, Agha FP et al (1983) Myositis ossificans circumscripta: computed tomographic diagnosis. Radiology 149:775-779
28. Maxfield BA (2010) Sports-related injury of the pediatric spine. Radiol Clin North Am 48:1237-1248
29. Brown RL, Brunn MA, Garcia VF (2001) Cervical spine injuries in children: a review of 103 patients treated consecutively at a level 1 pediatric trauma center. J Pediatr Surg 36:1107-1114
30. Kokoska ER, Keller MS, Rallo MC et al (2001) Characteristics of pediatric cervical spine injuries. J Pediatr Surg, 36:100-105

# Nontraumatic Musculoskeletal Abnormalities in Pediatrics

Philippe Petit[1], Simon Robben[2]

[1] Department of Pediatric Radiology, Hôpital Timone-Enfant, Marseille, France
[2] Department of Radiology, Maastricht University Medical Centre, Maastricht, The Netherlands

## Introduction

Children differ from adults with respect to anatomical, physiological and psychological response to disease. Moreover, children can have a variety of congenital and hereditary disorders. Therefore radiologists who deal with children require specific knowledge and specific skills.

Pathology with a low incidence, e.g., bone tumor, needs specific attention: imaging should be guided by considerations of common sense, limiting the risks (irradiation, sedation, unnecessary biopsy) and choosing the most efficient combination of examinations for each individual child.

In recent years, technical innovations have been added to our armamentarium, including contrast enhanced ultrasonography, whole-body magnetic resonance (MR) imaging, diffusion weighted MR sequences, and positron emission tomography-computed tomography (PET-CT). These new techniques continuously modify our strategies and our ability to detect, identify or predict the behavior of specific pathologies.

This abstract will focus on the most striking radiological features of neoplastic and inflammatory pediatric musculoskeletal disease. Other pathological processes (metabolic, endocrine, vascular, traumatic and congenital) will be discussed briefly.

## Pediatric Neoplastic Disease

### Bone Tumors

High-quality X-rays are still the first method of exploration for bone tumors, and often the only one necessary. Computed tomography (CT) has a limited role to play in pediatric patients and must be used when a real benefit is expected (i.e., diagnosis and/or treatment of osteoid osteoma).

MR imaging is the modality of choice to define the tumoral extension within the bone and in the soft tissues. For this purpose, a comprehensive knowledge of the issues of MR examination is mandatory. Ewing sarcoma and osteosarcoma are the two most frequent long bone tumors of the adolescent. They need to be explored with a dedicated MR protocol used prior to biopsy and at the end of chemotherapy. Some teams add a mid-course MR follow-up. The goals of these studies are to adequately assess the surgical osseous and extraosseous margins of resection and the answer to chemotherapy. An incomplete exploration will have a significant impact on patient survival. The important points of the protocol are:

- Q body coil covering the opposite site of the tumor to look for skip metastasis [short TI inversion recovery (STIR) or T1 in sagittal and coronal planes] [1] (Fig. 1)
- Surface coil centered on the tumor to look especially for a possible transphyseal extension. Coronal T1, axial T2, three-dimensional T1 fat-saturation gadolinium weighted sequences (Fig. 1) need to be done at the very least.

Diffusion weighted MR sequences may have an interesting role to play in early differentiation of poor and good responders to chemotherapy in osteosarcomas. Initial results that were obtained on a small series need to be confirmed before it can be used in current practice [2] (Fig. 1). 18F-fluorodeoxyglucose (18F-FDG) PET has also been used to assess the response to neoadjuvant chemotherapy in this indication. A strong correlation between a decrease in FDG uptake and tumor necrosis has been demonstrated. However, there is still no standardized uptake value threshold available that could definitely separate good responders from poor responders. The FDG-PET response is obtained too late in the treatment course to modify a potentially unsuccessful treatment [3-5].

Whole body MR (WBMR) is gaining acceptance in pediatric radiology. Despite the length of acquisition (at least 20-30 min) and the need for sedation in the youngest patients, a high spatial resolution associated with an absence of radiation are obvious advantages of MR, compared with bone scan scintigraphy and PET-CT. WBMR has been demonstrated to be more accurate than

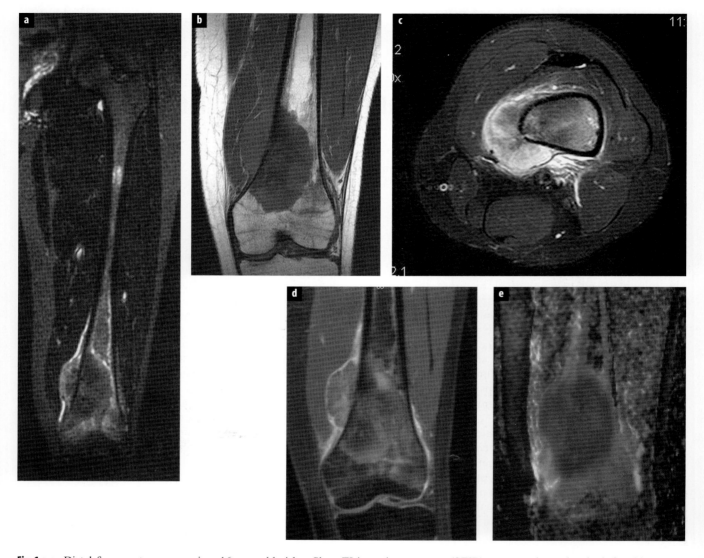

**Fig. 1 a-e.** Distal femur osteosarcoma in a 16-year-old girl. **a** Short TI inversion recovery (STIR) sequence is used to look for skip metastases. The Q body coils must be placed in order to get sufficient signal at the opposite side of the lesion. A surface coil placed on the tumor is then used to allow accurate local assessment of tumoral extension. **b** Coronal T1-weighted image. **c** Axial T2 fat-saturation image. **d** Coronal reconstruction of three-dimensional gadolinium T1 fat-saturation sequence. **e** Coronal ADC map (b0-b900) done at mid course of chemotherapy: signal measurement of the whole tumor would allow following the tumoral response

Tc scintigraphy [6, 7]. However, comparative pediatric studies between WBMR and PET-CT are scarce in the literature [6]. They have mostly concentrated on tumoral diseases (Ewing sarcoma, osteosarcoma, lymphoma, histiocytosis). Different MR sequences have been tested (T2 fat saturation, STIR, T1, diffusion) alone and in combination, and compared with PET-CT the results have been considered satisfactory [8, 9]. The addition of diffusion weighted sequences to STIR WBMR sequences has enhanced observation of the lesion and improved diagnostic accuracy for lymphomas [10]. Despite the potential application of WBMR in the investigation of metastases (Fig. 2), the major drawback is the length of exploration time (45 min).

## Soft Tissue Tumors

Regarding this topic, the eternal question that is particularly relevant is: 'how can we obviate to miss a malignant soft tissue tumor without to ask any time for a biopsy. Most of these lesions are benign (pseudotumors, vascular tumor and vascular malformations, fibrohistocytic tumors). The age of the patient, site of the lesion, clinical history and especially chronicity of the lesion are cornerstones of diagnosis. Some predisposing diseases should also be investigated (neurofibromatosis, Li Fraumeni syndrome, etc.) [11].

Malignant tumors are rare, accounting for around 1% of all soft tissue tumors in pediatrics. Rhabdomyosarcoma

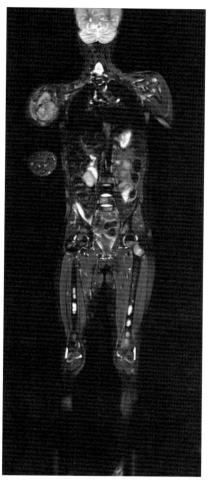

**Fig. 2.** Whole body magnetic resonance imaging of a 13-year-old girl with Ewing sarcoma of the right humerus. Fusion images of short TI inversion recovery (STIR) and diffusion weighted sequences reveal numerous bone metastases (for color reproduction see p 307)

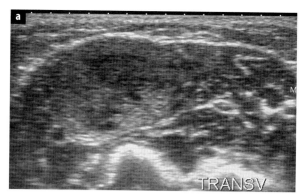

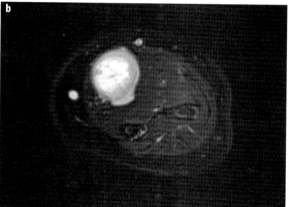

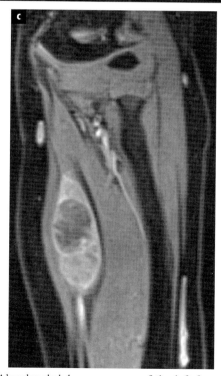

**Fig. 3 a-c.** Alveolar rhabdomyosarcoma of the left forearm in a 2-year-old girl. **a** On ultrasound, the intramuscular mass can be misdiagnosed for a recent thrombosed venous malformation. **b** Axial T2 fat-saturation weighted image reveals a frank mixed hypersignal without fresh hemorrhage. **c** T1 gadolinium coronal fat-saturation weighted image shows an enhancing intramuscular lesion with excentric necrotic area

accounts for 50% of all soft tissue sarcomas. The most frequently occurring non-rhabdomyosarcoma malignant tumors are tumors of the peripheral primitive neuroectodermal/Ewing (pPNET/Ew) sarcoma family (19%), malignant peripheral nerve sheath tumors (6.5%), infantile fibrosarcomas (6%) and synovial sarcomas (5%) [12].

The following clinical criteria indicate strong suspicion of malignancy: size greater than 5 cm, increase in size, pain and deep location of the lesion [11].

The first radiological approach is ultrasound (US) Doppler. X-rays and MR imaging are second-line investigation techniques. CT should not be carried out if there is suspicion of a soft tissue tumor, except if myositis ossificans is suspected.

Rhabdomyosarcoma (Fig. 3) can occur at any age, and the principal differential diagnosis is the intramuscular venous malformation (VM). Therefore it is important that the radiologist can clearly separate these two entities, and in order to do this US must be used to look for some specific features. The presence of fluid-fluid level in the lesion is not sufficient to provide a diagnosis of VM. On the other hand, the presence of some poor arterial flow (<15 cm/s) does not exclude a diagnosis of VM. It is then essential to look for a round-shaped phlebolith, with or without posterior shadowing. Rhabdomyosarcoma is principally composed of tissues of different echogenicity, usually with a rich arterial flow. One must take into account that even with the high sensitivity of Doppler, absence of Doppler flow does not mean that the lesion is not vascularized. However, this finding indicates a possible benign nature of the lesion. Contrast US is of interest in this setting, and particularly to separate rhabdomyosarcoma from VM [13]. However, this technique has not received Food and Drug Administration (FDA) approval for use in pediatric practice. The actual strategy used to differentiate rhabdomyosarcoma from VM is explained in the abstract of the workshop "Vascular malformations of the pediatric musculoskeletal system", in the Kangaroo course.

When the lesion has not been definitely recognized clinically, or by US and X-ray imaging, then MR exploration is mandatory [14]. Once again, this examination must be done prior to biopsy or surgery in order to accurately delineate the limits of the tumor, and sometimes to allow recognition of the lesion. We recommend to always use at least a Spin Echo (SE) T2 sequence without fat saturation to allow correct assessment of the pure fluid into the lesion. With a T2 fat-saturation sequence, necrotic malignant lesions and myxoid lesions may have a pseudocystic appearance. Gadolinium injection is always indicated, except when a VM or a lymphatic malformation has been definitely recognized on US Doppler. Criteria in favour of malignancy are: size (more than 5 cm), absence of low signal intensity on T2, signal heterogeneity on T1, peripheral and centripetal contrast enhancement, contiguous invasion of bone and/or neurovascular structures However, none of these MR criteria are 100% specific [11].

MR diffusion has not proved to be capable to either separate benign from malignant processes, or evaluate post-therapeutic changes accurately [15].

All soft tissue masses that are of uncertain origin must be subjected to a multidisciplinary approach in order to decide the type of biopsy (fine-needle aspiration, core biopsy, surgical open biopsy) necessary, and the destination of the samples (histopathology, immunohistochemistry and/or cytogenetic laboratories).

## Pediatric Inflammatory Disease (Infectious)

### Osteomyelitis

Osteomyelitis [16] is defined as an infection of the bone marrow; the most common causal organism is *Staphylococcus aureus*. Less frequently, *Streptococcus* spp., *Escherichia coli* and *Pseudomonas aeruginosa* are cultured from blood or aspirates [17]. The incidence of *Haemophilus influenzae* osteomyelitis has decreased dramatically since

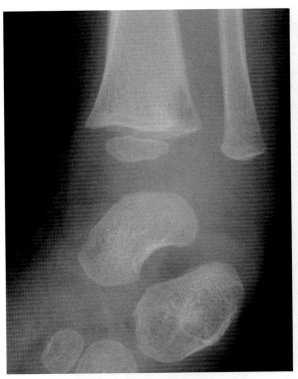

**Fig. 4** A one and a half year old girl who refuses to bear weight on her left foot, and shows fever. The lucent lesion represents metaphyseal osteomyelitis. The epiphysis was not affected

the introduction of *Haemophilus influenzae* type b (Hib) vaccination. The manifestation of osteomyelitis in children is age-dependent. In infants, diaphysial vessels penetrate the growth plate to reach the epiphysis, facilitating epiphysial and joint infections in this age group.

In older children, the growth plate constitutes a barrier for the diaphyseal vessels. Vessels at the metaphysis terminate in slow-flow venous sinusoidal lakes, predisposing the metaphysis as the initiation point for acute hematogenous osteomyelitis (Fig. 4).

The increased pressure within the medullary cavity causes the infection to spread via the Haversian and Volkmann's canals into the subperiostal space. Because the periosteum is less firmly attached to the cortex in infants and children than in adults, elevation will be more pronounced in childhood osteomyelitis. In contrast, sequestration is rare in neonatal osteomyelitis [17].

Conventional radiography is usually the initial modality used to demonstrate deep soft tissue swelling in early disease. However, bone destruction and periosteal reaction become obvious but only 7-10 days after the onset of disease. Conventional radiography is a screening method that can often suggest a diagnosis, exclude other pathology, and be correlated with other imaging findings.

Ultrasonography (US) can detect cortical defects and abscesses in the course of the disease (Fig. 5). Detection of subperiosteal abscesses is especially important because US-guided aspiration or surgical drainage has to be

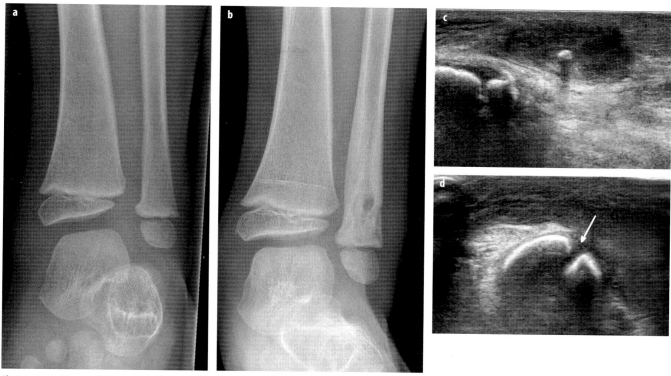

**Fig. 5 a-d.** A 5-year-old boy with intermittent swelling of the left ankle after a minor trauma 1 year ago. **a** Radiograph at the time of trauma shows no abnormalities. **b** Radiograph 1 year later demonstrates soft tissue swelling, cortical thickening and a cortical defect. Growth line in tibia probably represents the initial event. **c, d** Ultrasonography shows a sequestrum floating in a soft tissue abscess that communicates with the bone marrow through a small cortical defect (*arrow*). Chronic osteomyelitis. Cultures were positive for *Staphylococcus aureus*

considered in these patients, whereas those with osteomyelitis without abscesses can be treated with antibiotics only. CT demonstrates osseous abnormalities earlier in the course of the disease than conventional radiographs; however, this is at the expense of a higher dose of radiation. It is superior to MR imaging for visualizing bone destruction, gas in the bone and bone sequestration.

MR is, as with CT, not a screening method, but an invaluable method of demonstrating the intra- and extraosseous extent of osteomyelitis. Predictors of early osteomyelitis are ill-defined low T1 and high T2 signal intensity, poorly defined soft tissue planes, lack of cortical thickening and poor interface between normal and abnormal marrow. In chronic osteomyelitis, there is good differentiation between diseased marrow and soft tissue abnormalities [18].

The use of gadolinium increases confidence in the diagnosis and the detection of small abscesses [19, 20].

## (Spondylo)discitis

Spondylitis, spondylodiscitis and discitis in children are perhaps different manifestations of the same disease: a low-grade infection affecting the vertebral body and intervertebral disc [21]. Many organisms cause spondylodiscitis; even low-grade viral infection has been postulated in patients with no positive cultures (50%) [22]. The

clinical symptoms may be subtle, varying from limping, the inability to stand or sit upright, to frank back pain. The first radiological sign is intervertebral disc space narrowing with indistinct endplates on either side, and this eventually leads to destruction of the endplates. The best imaging technique is MR imaging, which demonstrates signal intensity abnormalities in the intervertebral disc and adjacent vertebral bodies.

## Septic Arthritis

The hip joint is the most frequent location of septic arthritis in childhood; the knee, shoulder and elbow are also common sites [17]. Early diagnosis is mandatory to prevent cartilage destruction, joint deformity, growth disturbance and eventually premature arthrosis. Most commonly, it is caused by hematogeneous seeding or, less frequently, by extension into the joint space from osteomyelitis. Etiologic organisms are *S. aureus* (most common), group A streptococci and *Streptococcus pneumoniae*. In neonates, group B streptococci and *E. coli* are important causes, whereas *Neisseria gonorrhoeae* can be a cause in adolescents [17]. The incidence of *H. influenzae* has declined since large vaccination programs were introduced. The presenting sympoms are fever, non-weight bearing, erythrocyte sedimentation rate >40, and peripheral white blood cell count of >12,000. If all these symptoms are present, the likelihood of septic arthritis is 99% [23]. Unfortunately, many children do not show such an obvious clinical picture and imaging techniques are important tools to give additional information about the suspected joint.

Conventional radiographs can be normal or they can demonstrate joint space widening with adjacent soft tissue swelling. However, sensitivity and specificity for septic arthritis is low.

US is very sensitive for the detection of joint effusion, especially in the pediatric population, and small amounts, up to 1 mL, can be detected. However, the specificity of the diagnosis is poor. The absence of joint effusion virtually excludes septic arthritis [24]. Neither the size nor the echogenicity of the effusion can distinguish an infectious from a noninfectious effusion [25, 26].

CT is less sensitive for the detection of joint effusion, but may identify areas of adjacent osteomyelitis. MR is very sensitive for the detection of synovial disease [27]. Initially, MR imaging reveals distention of the joint capsule by nonspecific T2 high intensity fluid. In later stages, the joint effusion tends to have a more intermediate signal intensity and seems to be heterogeneous. Moreover, MR can demonstrate cartilage destruction and adjacent cellulitis [28]. Combined with gadolinium injection and fat suppression techniques, sensitivity of 100% and specificity of 77% can be accomplished with MR [29].

## Soft Tissue Infections

### Cellulitis, Soft Tissue Abscesses and Necrotizing Fasciitis

Cellulitis, soft tissue abscesses and necrotizing fasciitis are infections of the skin and subcutaneous tissues, with a predilection for the extremities in children [30]. *S. aureus* and *Streptococcus pyogenes* account for the majority of the infections. Patients present with soft tissue swelling, erythema and fever.

Conventional radiographs often show nonspecific soft tissue swelling. The US appearance resembles edema of the subcutaneous fat, showing swelling, increased echogenicity of the subcutaneous fat with decreased acoustic transmission, blurring of tissue planes, progressing to hypoechoic strands between hyperechoic fatty lobules. This appearance is nonspecific and cannot be distinguished from noninfectious causes of soft tissue edema [31]. Increased vascularity at color or power Doppler US can suggest an infectious cause [32].

CT and MR findings of cellulitis include skin thickening, abnormal density/signal intensity of the subcutaneous fat and normal deep fascial and muscle compartments [17].

Depending on the type of infection and the immune system of the patient, cellulitis can progress to a soft tissue abscess. The majority of cases are caused by *S. aureus*. Superficial abscesses begin as cellulitis and subsequently liquefy to form a localized pus collection. Conventional radiographs can show nonspecific soft tissue swelling and occasionally gas in the soft tissues.

The US appearance of abscesses is highly variable: abscesses can present with or without mass effect and the liquefied contents can be anechoic, hypoechoic, hyperechoic and even isoechoic to surrounding tissues. The margins can be relatively sharp, blend in with the surrounding cellulitis, or be outlined by an echogenic rim [33]. To confirm the liquid nature of a nonanechoic mass, the presence of "ultrasonographic fluctuation" should be investigated [34]. Also, color Doppler US can be used to confirm the avascular nature of the mass [32].

The imaging findings are shown to better advantage with MR; the T1 low and T2 high signal intensity of the fluid shows good contrast with the enhancing rim. The presence of an enhancing rim on post-gadolinium-administration images has a high sensitivity and specificity for the diagnosis of a soft tissue abscess. The abscess fluid itself does not enhance. Diffusion weighted imaging can add specficity to contrast-enhanced T1-weighted images [35].

Necrotizing fasciitis is a rare, rapidly progressive and often fatal infection of the subcutaneous tissues, fascia and surrounding soft tissue structures. Early diagnosis is mandatory because the disease may have a fatal course if adequate therapy (extensive surgical debridement and antibiotics) is not commenced promptly. Causative organisms are *S. aureus* and group A streptococci.

The sonographic features of necrotizing fasciitis are: (a) fascial thickening and accumulation of fluid, (b) cloudy fluid or loculated abscess in the fascial plane, (c) subcutaneous soft tissue swelling, and (d) eventually gas in soft tissues [32]

To a certain extent, MR images of necrotizing fasciitis resemble those of infectious cellulitis; however, there is also involvement of the deep fascia and intramuscular spaces [36].

### Pyomyositis

Pyomyositis is suppurative bacterial infection in striated muscle [25, 30, 37, 38]. It is rare because striated muscle is relatively resistant to bacterial infection, and it is encountered most frequently in tropical regions. All striated muscles of the skeleton can be involved, but there is a predilection for muscles in the thigh and pelvis. Contributing factors are trauma, diabetes mellitus, chronic steroid use, connective tissue disorders, varicella infection and immunosuppression. Children are affected in one third of cases, both in tropical and nontropical regions. The most frequent causative organism is *S. aureus*. Pyomyositis can be difficult to diagnose because the infection is initially confined to the muscular compartment causing myalgia, general malaise and fever. It is often difficult for the child to locate the pain, particularly when pyomyositis involves hips or pelvis. Also the unawareness of the disease, especially in nontropical setting, can cause a delay in diagnosis.

US findings depend on the stage of the disease [39]. Stage 1 (phlegmonous) shows localized muscle edema, and distortion of the filamentous planes with ill-defined

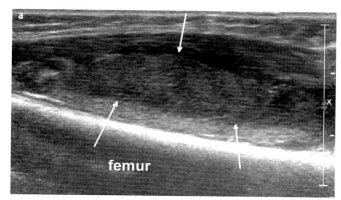

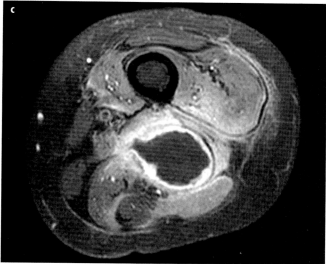

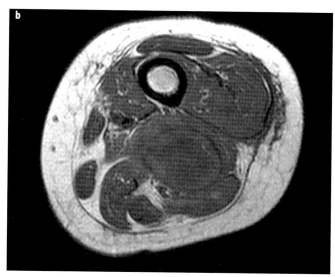

**Fig. 6 a-c.** Pyomyositis in an 11-year-old boy during chemotherapy for acute lymphatic leukemia. **a** Ultrasonography shows intramuscular liquefaction with increased echogenicity (*arrows*). **b** T1-weighted transverse image of the thigh shows intramuscular hypointense fluid collection. The bone marrow is not involved. **c** T1-gadolinium fat sat shows thick enhancing rim

areas of decreased echogenicity. Stage 2 (suppurative) shows liquefaction corresponding with abscess formation. The echogenicity of the pus may be increased, decreased or equal to surrounding tissues (Fig. 6). Doppler US and gentle compression with the transducer to visualize motion of particles can be useful in equivocal cases (see sections on osteomyelitis and soft tissue abscesses). The presence of gas within an inflamed muscle is very suggestive of abscess formation caused by anaerobic organisms.

MR imaging can identify abscesses and co-existing areas of osteomyelitis and septic arthritis. In stage 1, a heterogeneous T2 signal intensity is present in the enlarged muscle. In stage 2, abscess formation is seen as a focus of T2 high signal intensity and T1 low signal intensity. Gadolinium demonstrates peripheral rim enhancement (Fig. 6).

## Pediatric Inflammatory Disease (Noninfectious)

### Juvenile Idiopathic Arthritis

Juvenile idiopathic arthritis (JIA) [40] encompasses all forms of arthritis that begin before the age of 16 years, persist for more than 6 weeks, and are of unknown etiol-

ogy and pathophysiology. Traditionally, conventional radiographs were used to demonstrate overgrowth, cartilage loss and erosions. Pediatric scoring systems have increased the value of conventional radiographs. US and MR imaging have further improved the diagnostis of JIA by demonstrating bone marrow edema (MR), synovitis and erosions (MR and US). Recent examinations have focused on differentiating pathologic bone and cartilage abnormalities from normal developmental variants.

For further reading, see the abstract of the workshop "Imaging of Juvenile Idiopathic Arthritis" in the Kangaroo course.

### Chronic Recurrent Multifocal Osteomyelitis

Chronic recurrent multifocal osteomyelitis (CRMO) [41, 42] is believed to be the pediatric variant of SAPHO syndrome, which is a combination of synovitis, acne, pustulosis, hyperostosis and osteitis. CRMO is considered to be rare, but it may be underdiagnosed because of the absence of specific clinical symptoms, laboratory test results, or radiological findings. The etiology is unknown. It affects children and adolescents. The presenting symptom is inflammatory pain, and fever is not a common finding. Virtually all patients have increased erythrocyte sedimentation rate (ESR) and C-reactive protein (CRP), and there is a mild increase of white blood cell count in some patients. Radiological examination demonstrates focal lysis and reactive hyperostosis with periosteal reaction. MR imaging shows nonspecific bone marrow signal intensity changes (T1 hypointense and T2 hyperintense), but it is useful to demonstrate the extent of the disease. Isotope bone scans show a mean number of foci of five per patient. The lower limbs are most frequently affected, followed by the pelvis, spine and anterior chest wall (including claviculae).

It is a self-limiting disease but flares occur at variable intervals and the disease can remain active into adulthood.

## Other Pathological Processes

### Pediatric Vascular Diseases

Avascular necrosis is frequently seen in childhood. Perthes disease is well known, but any epiphysis, carpal or tarsal bone may be affected. Conventional radiography is the initial modality for imaging, and often no additional imaging is necessary. The role of US is limited to the detection of joint effusion and cartilage thickening [43]. MR imaging is more sensitive for avascular necrosis than other imaging techniques because it demonstrates bone marrow abnormalities and is used for equivocal cases or to determine the extent of the necrosis [44].

For further reading, see the abstract of the workshop "Vascular malformations of the pediatric musculoskeletal system" in the Kangaroo course.

### Pediatric Trauma

See abstract of the workshops "Specific aspects of sport-related injuries of the pediatric musculoskeletal system" and "Nonaccidental trauma and its imitators" in the Kangaroo course.

### Pediatric Endocrine and Metabolic Diseases

Endocrine and metabolic diseases [45, 46] in children can cause osseous abnormalities of the skeletal system. Vitamin D deficiency causes rickets with its typical metaphyseal abnormalities. The bones in vitamin C deficiency show white metaphyseal lines, diffuse osteopenia and large subperiosteal hemorrhages.

Hypothyroidism and hypogonadism cause retardation of skeletal maturation. Hyperparathyroidism results in diffuse osteopenia, marked subperiosteal bone resorption and renal stones.

### Congenital and Hereditary Diseases

The huge spectrum of hereditary diseases [46] includes (among others) osteochondrodysplasias, storage disease and other inborn errors of metabolism. These are beyond the scope of this abstract.

## Conclusion

Diagnosis of musculoskeletal disease in children is difficult and challenging because of the great variety of diseases and typical presentation of these diseases in children. Moreover, one should realize that there are many differences between the pediatric and adult musculoskeletal system. Knowledge of these differences will prevent any unnecessary delay in diagnosing pediatric musculoskeletal disease. Imaging studies play an important role in diagnosis.

## References

1. Brisse H, Ollivier L, Edeline V et al (2004) Imaging of malignant tumours of the long bones in children: monitoring response to neoadjuvant chemotherapy and preoperative assessment. Pediatr Radiol 34:595-605
2. Baunin C, Schmidt G, Baumstarck K et al (2012) Value of diffusion-weighted images in differentiating mid-course responders to chemotherapy for osteosarcoma compared to the histological response: preliminary results. Skeletal Radiol 41:1141-1149
3. Cheon GJ, Kim MS, Lee JA et al (2009) Prediction model of chemotherapy response in osteosarcoma by 18F-FDG PET and MRI. J Nucl Med 50:1435-1440
4. Costelloe CM, Macapinlac HA, Madewell JE et al (2009) 18F-FDG PET/CT as an indicator of progression-free and overall survival in osteosarcoma. J Nucl Med 50:340-347
5. Hawkins DS, Conrad EU, Butrynski JE et al (2009) [F-18]-fluorodeoxy-D-glucose-positron emission tomography response is associated with outcome for extremity osteosarcoma in children and young adults. Cancer 115:3519-3525
6. Ley S, Ley-Zaporozhan J, Schenk JP (2009) Whole-body MRI in the pediatric patient. Eur J Radiol 70:442-451
7. Mentzel HJ, Kentouche K, Sauner D et al (2004) Comparison of whole-body STIR-MRI and 99mTc-methylene-diphosphonate scintigraphy in children with suspected multifocal bone lesions. Eur Radiol 14:2297-2302
8. Krohmer S, Sorge I, Krausse A et al (2010) Whole-body MRI for primary evaluation of malignant disease in children. Eur J Radiol 74:256-261
9. Punwani S, Taylor SA, Bainbridge A et al (2010) Pediatric and adolescent lymphoma: comparison of whole-body STIR half-Fourier RARE MR imaging with an enhanced PET/CT reference for initial staging. Radiology 255:182-190
10. Gu J, Chan T, Zhang J et al (2011) Whole-body diffusion-weighted imaging: the added value to whole-body MRI at initial diagnosis of lymphoma. AJR Am J Roentgenol 197:W384-391
11. Brisse HJ, Orbach D, Klijanienko J (2010) Soft tissue tumours: imaging strategy. Pediatr Radiol 40:1019-1928
12. Carli M, Ceccetto G, Sotti G (2004) Soft tissue sarcomas. In: Pinkerton C, Plowman P, Pieters R (Eds) Pediatric oncology. Hodder Arnold, London
13. Loizides A, Peer S, Plaikner M et al (2012) Perfusion pattern of musculoskeletal masses using contrast-enhanced ultrasound: a helpful tool for characterisation? Eur Radiol 22:1803-1811
14. Laor T (2004) MR imaging of soft tissue tumors and tumor-like lesions. Pediatr Radiol 34:24-37
15. Khoo MM, Tyler PA, Saifuddin A et al (2011) Diffusion-weighted imaging (DWI) in musculoskeletal MRI: a critical review. Skeletal Radiol 40:665-681

16. van Schuppen J, van Doorn MM, van Rijn RR (2012) Childhood osteomyelitis: imaging characteristics. Insights Imaging 3:519-533
17. Kothari NA, Pelchovitz DJ, Meyer JS (2001) Imaging of musculoskeletal infections. Radiol Clin North Am 39:653-671
18. Oudjhane K, Azouz EM (2001) Imaging of osteomyelitis in children. Radiol Clin North Am 39:251-266
19. Averill LW, Hernandez A, Gonzalez L et al (2009) Diagnosis of osteomyelitis in children: utility of fat-suppressed contrast-enhanced MRI. AJR Am J Roentgenol 192:1232-1238
20. Kan JH, Young RS, Yu C et al (2010) Clinical impact of gadolinium in the MRI diagnosis of musculoskeletal infection in children. Pediatr Radiol 40:1197-1205
21. Swischuk E (1997) Infections of the spine and spinal cord. In: Imaging of the newborn, infant, and young child. Williams & Wilkins, Baltimore
22. Blickman JG, van Die CE, de Rooy JW (2004) Current imaging concepts in pediatric osteomyelitis. Eur Radiol 14 (Suppl 4):L55-64
23. Kocher MS, Zurakowski D, Kasser JR (1999) Differentiating between septic arthritis and transient synovitis of the hip in children: an evidence-based clinical prediction algorithm. J Bone Joint Surg Am 81:1662-1670
24. Zawin JK, Hoffer FA, Rand FF et al (1993) Joint effusion in children with an irritable hip: US diagnosis and aspiration. Radiology 187:459-463
25. Robben SG (2004) Ultrasonography of musculoskeletal infections in children. Eur Radiol 14 (Suppl 4):L65-77
26. Robben SG, Lequin MH, Diepstraten AF et al (1999) Anterior joint capsule of the normal hip and in children with transient synovitis: US study with anatomic and histologic correlation. Radiology 210:499-507
27. Kim HK, Zbojniewicz AM, Merrow AC et al (2011) MR findings of synovial disease in children and young adults: Part 2. Pediatr Radiol 41:512-524
28. Greenspan A, Tehranzadeh J (2001) Imaging of infectious arthritis. Radiol Clin North Am 39:267-276
29. Hopkins KL, Li KC, Bergman G (1995) Gadolinium-DTPA-enhanced magnetic resonance imaging of musculoskeletal infectious processes. Skeletal Radiol 24:325-330
30. Chau CL, Griffith JF (2005) Musculoskeletal infections: ultrasound appearances. Clin Radiol 60:149-159
31. Struk DW, Munk PL, Lee MJ et al (2001) Imaging of soft tissue infections. Radiol Clin North Am 39:277-303
32. Cardinal E, Bureau N, Aubin B et al (2001) Role of ultrasound in musculoskeletal infection. Radiol Clin North Am 39:191-201
33. Bureau N, RY C, Cardinal E (1999) Musculoskeletal infections: US manifestations. Radiographics 19:1585-1592
34. Loyer EM, DuBrow RA, David CL et al (1996) Imaging of superficial soft-tissue infections: sonographic findings in cases of cellulitis and abscess. AJR Am J Roentgenol 166:149-152
35. Neubauer H, Platzer I, Mueller VR et al (2012) Diffusion-weighted MRI of abscess formations in children and young adults. World J Pediatr 8:229-234
36. Kim KT, Kim YJ, Won Lee J et al (2011) Can necrotizing infectious fasciitis be differentiated from nonnecrotizing infectious fasciitis with MR imaging? Radiology 259:816-824
37. Jaramillo D (2011) Infection: musculoskeletal. Pediatr Radiol 41 (Suppl 1):S127-34
38. Trusen A, Beissert M, Schultz G et al (2003) Ultrasound and MRI features of pyomyositis in children. Eur Radiol 13:1050-1055
39. Loyer EM, Kaur H, David CL et al (1995) Importance of dynamic assessment of the soft tissues in the sonographic diagnosis of echogenic superficial abscesses. J Ultrasound Med 14:669-671
40. Magni-Manzoni S, Malattia C, Lanni S et al (2012) Advances and challenges in imaging in juvenile idiopathic arthritis. Nat Rev Rheumatol 8:329-336
41. Ferguson PJ, Sandu M (2012) Current understanding of the pathogenesis and management of chronic recurrent multifocal osteomyelitis. Curr Rheumatol Rep 14:130-141
42. Khanna G, Sato TS, Ferguson P (2009) Imaging of chronic recurrent multifocal osteomyelitis. Radiographics 29:1159-1177
43. Robben SG, Meradji M, Diepstraten AF et al (1998) US of the painful hip in childhood: diagnostic value of cartilage thickening and muscle atrophy in the detection of Perthes disease. Radiology 208:35-42
44. de Sanctis N (2011) Magnetic resonance imaging in Legg-Calve-Perthes disease: review of literature. J Pediatr Orthop 31:S163-167
45. Avni F (Ed) (2012) Imaging endocrine diseases in children. Springer-Verlag
46. Lachman RS (2007) Radiology of syndromes, metabolic disorders and skeletal dysplasias, 5th edn. Mosby, Philadelphia, PA

# NUCLEAR MEDICINE SATELLITE COURSE
## "DIAMOND"

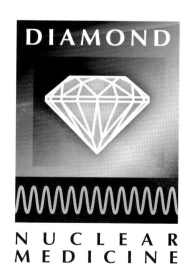

# CT Specifies Bone Lesions in SPECT/CT

Klaus Strobel

Department of Nuclear Medicine and Radiology, Cantonal Hospital Lucerne, Lucerne, Switzerland

Traditionally, planar bone scintigraphy (PS) is a very sensitive technique regarding the detection of bone lesions, but specificity is limited. In most cases PS is sufficient to exclude or detect bone metastases in tumor patients. Experienced nuclear physicians are able to differentiate degenerative from malignant lesions because of the intensity and localization of radionuclide uptake in the majority of examinations. Additional performance of single photon emission computed tomography (SPECT) increases the sensitivity of bone scintigraphy. In focal lesions that are not clear on planar or SPECT images, a supplementary SPECT/CT examination can provide a definite diagnosis in approximately 90% of lesions [1-3] (Figs. 1, 2). SPECT/CT is especially helpful in assessing lesions of the axial skeleton (Fig. 3).

The implementation of a multiple field SPECT/CT of the axial skeleton in the standard bone scan protocol pro-vides the possibility of increasing the accuracy of bone scintigraphy [4]. In addition to imaging of bone metastases, SPECT/CT offers new diagnostic possibilities in many fields of musculoskeletal imaging; particularly in the region of complex small joints, such as the wrist and the foot, SPECT/CT helps to localize and characterize lesions accurately [5]. As shown in several publications, SPECT/CT helps to specify uptake in the wrist and has a substantial impact on therapy in patients with nonspecific wrist pain and equivocal magnetic resonance imaging [6-8]. Increasingly, SPECT/CT is used to image patients with knee or hip arthroplasty, where the CT part of the study gives important additional information about prosthesis position, osteolysis and soft tissue changes [9]. Promising results have been observed for imaging of osteomyelitis of the jaw, where complementary metabolic and morphologic information is crucial for therapy planning [10, 11].

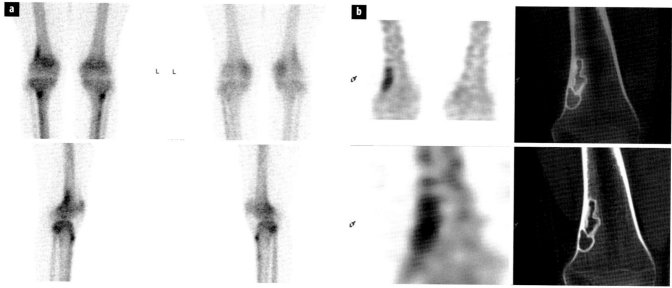

**Fig. 1 a, b.** Young patient with knee pain. **a** In addition to bilateral uptake at the tibial tuberosity, the planar scintigraphy images show an intermediate uptake at the lateral right distal femur diaphysis/epiphysis. **b** In single photon emission computed tomography (SPECT)/CT, the uptake corresponds to a lesion with the typical CT appearance of a nonossifying fibroma (for color reproduction, see p 308)

J. Hodler et al. (eds.), *Musculoskeletal Diseases 2013-2016,*
DOI: 10.1007/978-88-470-5292-5_27 © Springer-Verlag Italia 2013

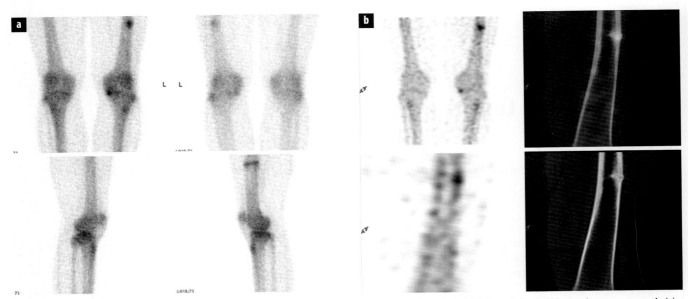

**Fig. 2 a, b.** Patient with knee pain. **a** Planar scintigraphy with uptake in the medial femorotibial joint of the left knee due to osteoarthritis, and linear uptake in the left femur diaphysis. **b** Single photon emission computed tomography (SPECT)/CT demonstrates the presence of a stress fracture (for color reproduction see p 308)

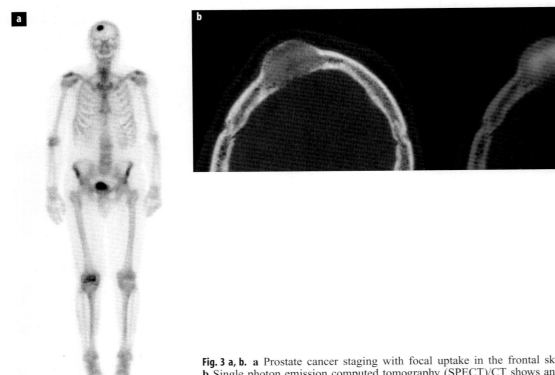

**Fig. 3 a, b.** **a** Prostate cancer staging with focal uptake in the frontal skull in planar scintigraphy. **b** Single photon emission computed tomography (SPECT)/CT shows an expansive lesion with the typical appearance of a hemangioma (for color reproduction see p 309)

SPECT/CT arthrography, where iodine contrast material is injected intra-articularly before the late phase SPECT/CT images are obtained, expands the diagnostic possibilities in multiple joints (wrist, knee, ankle), as shown in recently published case reports [12, 13] (Fig. 4).

In infection, imaging with antigranulocyte or leucocyte scintigraphy SPECT/CT accurately identifies and exactly localizes sites of infection [14, 15] (Fig. 5). Compared with planar scintigraphy, SPECT/CT provides important additional information in 36-53% of infection

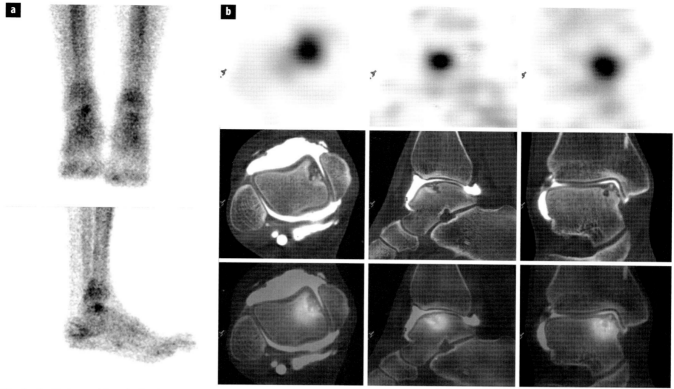

**Fig. 4 a, b.** Patient with pain in the ankle. **a** Planar scintigraphy shows focal uptake in the talus. **b** Single photon emission computed tomography (SPECT)/CT arthrography shows an osteochondral lesion in the medial talus edge with small subchondral fragments but intact cartilage surface (for color reproduction see p 309)

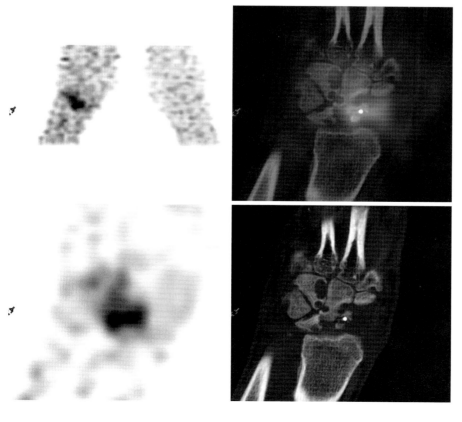

**Fig. 5.** Tc99m antigranulocyte single photon emission computed tomography (SPECT)/CT of the wrist in a patient several weeks after wrist surgery and postoperative infection. CT shows severe destruction of several carpal bones and SPECT/CT helps to localize exactly the pathologic uptake resulting from persistent infection (for color reproduction see p 310)

scans. This has been shown in diabetic foot infection, osteomyelitis and prosthetic joint infection [16-18]. Special training in CT interpretation is of course mandatory to be able to benefit from all the information given by a high-resolution CT scan as part of an intergrated SPECT/CT study.

## References

1. Even-Sapir E, Metser U, Mishani E et al (2006) The detection of bone metastases in patients with high-risk prostate cancer: 99mTc-MDP Planar bone scintigraphy, single- and multi-field-of-view SPECT, 18F-fluoride PET, and 18F-fluoride PET/CT. J Nucl Med 47:287-297

2. Strobel K, Burger C, Seifert B (2007) Characterization of focal bone lesions in the axial skeleton: performance of planar bone scintigraphy compared with SPECT and SPECT fused with CT. AJR Am J Roentgenol 188:W467-474

3. Utsunomiya D, Shiraishi S, Imuta M et al (2006) Added value of SPECT/CT fusion in assessing suspected bone metastasis: comparison with scintigraphy alone and nonfused scintigraphy and CT. Radiology 238:264-271

4. Abe K, Sasaki M, Kuwabara Y et al (2005) Comparison of 18FDG-PET with 99mTc-HMDP scintigraphy for the detection of bone metastases in patients with breast cancer. Ann Nucl Med 19:573-579

5. Pagenstert GI, Barg A, Leumann AG et al (2009) SPECT-CT imaging in degenerative joint disease of the foot and ankle. J Bone Joint Surg Br 91:1191-1196

6. Huellner MW, Burkert A, Schleich FS et al (2012) SPECT/CT versus MRI in patients with nonspecific pain of the hand and wrist - a pilot study. Eur J Nucl Med Mol Imaging 39:750-759

7. Huellner MW, Strobel K, Hug U et al (2012) SPECT/CT in diagnostics of the hand joint. Radiologe 52:621-628

8. Schleich FS, Schurch M, Huellner MW et al (2012) Diagnostic and therapeutic impact of SPECT/CT in patients with unspecific pain of the hand and wrist. EJNMMI research 2:53

9. Strobel K, Steurer-Dober I, Huellner MW et al (2012) Importance of SPECT/CT for knee and hip joint prostheses. Radiologe 52:629-635

10. Bolouri C, Merwald M, Huellner MW et al (2012) Performance of orthopantomography, planar scintigraphy, CT alone and SPECT/CT in patients with suspected osteomyelitis of the jaw. Eur J Nucl Med Mol Imaging. Epub ahead of print

11. Strobel K, Merwald M, Huellner MW et al (2012) Importance of SPECT/CT for resolving diseases of the jaw. Radiologe 52:638-645

12. Kruger T, Hug U, Hullner MW et al (2011) SPECT/CT arthrography of the wrist in ulnocarpal impaction syndrome. Eur J Nucl Med Mol Imaging 38:792

13. Strobel K, Wiesmann R, Tornquist K et al (2012) SPECT/CT arthrography of the knee. Eur J Nucl Med Mol Imaging 39:1975-1976

14. Graute V, Feist M, Lehner S et al (2010) Detection of low-grade prosthetic joint infections using 99mTc-antigranulocyte SPECT/CT: initial clinical results. Eur J Nucl Med Mol Imaging 37:1751-1759

15. Klaeser B, Spanjol M, Krause T (2012) SPECT/CT diagnostics for skeletal infections. Radiologe 52:615-620

16. Filippi L, Schillaci O (2006) SPECT/CT with a hybrid camera: a new imaging modality for the functional anatomical mapping of infections. Expert review of medical devices 3:699-703

17. Filippi L, Schillaci O (2006) Usefulness of hybrid SPECT/CT in 99mTc-HMPAO-labeled leukocyte scintigraphy for bone and joint infections. J Nucl Med 47:1908-1913

18. Filippi L, Uccioli L, Giurato L, Schillaci O (2009) Diabetic foot infection: usefulness of SPECT/CT for 99mTc-HMPAO-labeled leukocyte imaging. J Nucl Med 50:1042-1046

# FDG PET-CT Staging and Follow-up in Soft Tissue Sarcomas

Einat Even-Sapir Weizer

Department of Nuclear Medicine, Tel Aviv Sourasky Medical Center, Tel Aviv University, Tel Aviv, Israel

Sarcoma is a cancer originating from mesenchymal tissues including muscle, bone, fat and connective tissue, blood vessels and peripheral nerve. Sarcomas constitute a fifth of pediatric cancers, predominately of bone origin, while in adults sarcomas constitute only 1% of cancers and are mostly of the soft tissue type. Subtypes of soft tissue sarcomas (STS) include leiomyosarcoma, rhabdomyosarcoma, fibrosarcoma, malignant fibrous histiocytoma, liposarcoma, malignant peripheral nerve sheath tumor, malignant schwannoma, angiosarcoma, pleomorphic sarcoma, synovial sarcoma and gastrointestinal stromal tumor (GIST) [1].

Soft tissue sarcomas can occur at any site throughout the body, but almost 45% of STS are found in the extremities, especially in the lower limb, and 20% are intra-abdominal [2].

In view of the biologic heterogeneity of different subtypes of STS, there is no consensus on a single optimal imaging algorithm that should be applied in patients with STS during the course of the disease; however, data on the role of [18]F-FDG PET-CT ([18]F-fluorodeoxyglucose positron emission tomography-computed tomography) in patients with STS are being accumulated [1-9].

During the initial work-up of sarcomas, magnetic resonance imaging (MRI) is the preferable modality for description and definition of the local extent of STS [3]. Grading of STS is based on histopathological examination; yet, it is not always entirely accurate for assessment and prediction of the biological behavior and aggressiveness of the tumor. Several studies have described the use of [18]F-FDG PET-CT as complementary to biopsy in STS. Intensity of [18]F-FDG uptake measured by standard uptake value (SUVmax) of soft tissue sarcomas was found to be a tumor-grade-dependent parameter and varies among and within histologic subtypes of STS [10]. A statistically significant correlation was found between sarcoma tumor metabolism as measured by SUVmax of [18]F-FDG uptake and two major histopathologic characteristics of these tumors: mitotic count and tumor necrosis [11]. Intensity of uptake of [18]F-FDG can reliably distinguish low-grade from high-grade tumors [12, 13]. Practically, intermediate and high-grade STS are accurately identified on the basis of qualitative interpretation, almost all with SUVmax ≥2.0. The majority of low-grade STS are identified but show low-intensity uptake [3]. Baseline tumor SUVmax was found to be an independent predictor of overall survival in sarcoma patients, with high-intensity uptake being closely related to shorter overall survival [4-6, 9, 14]. Sarcomas can be very heterogeneous in composition (Fig. 1). In large masses with necrotic areas, [18]F-FDG PET-CT data can guide biopsy, decreasing the chance of sampling error by separating active tumor areas that show increased uptake and cold necrotic areas. In large low-grade tumors, [18]F-FDG-PET/CT data can identify areas with uptake of higher intensity, suggesting islands of more aggressive tumor, thus requiring a more aggressive treatment approach [1, 15]. It appears that while morphologic modalities, mainly MRI, provide good anatomic and topographic data on the primary tumor location and extent, [18]F-FDG PET-CT serves as a surrogate biomarker to determine the biological characteristics of the individual tumor.

Poor risk factors in patients with STS include high-grade tumor, large tumor size (over 5 cm in largest diameter), tumor necrosis, deep tumor location, proximal location in tumors in the lower extremity, metastatic spread, failure to achieve tumor-free margin after surgical resection, and local recurrence [1].

PET-CT, CT, bone scintigraphy and radiography are often used as complementary modalities to assess the presence of metastases. Metastatic spread of sarcomas is mainly hematogenous, although lymphatic spread may occur [2]. Lung followed by bone are the most common sites of STS metastasis. [18]F-FDG PET-CT whole body imaging is a useful modality for staging and detecting distant metastasis, with a high sensitivity and specificity and excellent negative predictive value [5]. When interpreting [18]F-FDG PET-CT images, both functional data of PET and morphological data of CT should be considered. The latter is valuable mainly for detection of lung

J. Hodler et al. (eds.), *Musculoskeletal Diseases 2013-2016*,
DOI: 10.1007/978-88-470-5292-5_28 © Springer-Verlag Italia 2013

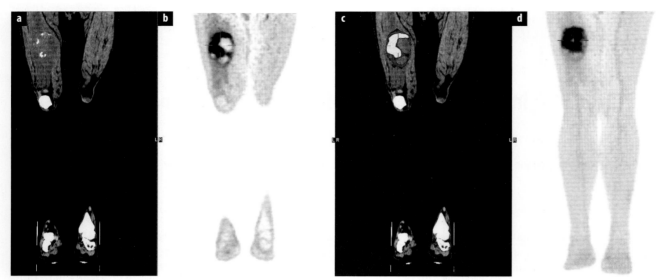

**Fig. 1 a-d.** Newly diagnosed malignant fibrous histiocytoma. From left to right, **a** computed tomography (CT), **b** positron emission tomography (PET), **c** fused PET-CT and **d** maximum intensity projection PET show the heterogeneous appearance of the mass with large areas of necrosis. These data can guide the biopsy site to areas showing increased $^{18}$F-fluorodeoxyglucose uptake (for color reproduction see p 310)

involvement, since PET may be falsely negative in the presence of small lung metastases identified by CT [5]. As for other tumors, the standard 99mTc-methylene diphosphonate (MDP) bone scan (BS) is widely used for assessment of skeletal involvement in STS, detecting bone metastases of osteoblastic type. $^{18}$F-FDG PET-CT is more accurate for detection of lytic type metastasis and early marrow involvement, for which BS is insensitive [7]. In a recent study, detection of unexpected metastasis by $^{18}$F-FDG PET-CT was reported to result in a change in treatment for 18 of 59 STS patients, mainly cancellation of surgery and referral for chemotherapy instead [5].

Patients with low-grade small STS often undergo surgery and occasionally adjuvant radiation. Surgical resection ranges from simple excision with tumor-free wide margins to complex limb salvage procedures. Patients with large intermediate-grade or high-grade large tumors are usually referred for neoadjuvant chemotherapy, with or without preoperative radiation, followed by resection and adjuvant therapy. Based on percentage of tumor necrosis in the resected tumor, a regimen of adjuvant therapy is selected so that if an adequate response is not achieved, an alternative chemotherapy regimen replaces the ineffective treatment. Chemotherapy resistance is a crucial prognostic factor. The complexity and genetic and chromosomal instability found in STS are probably the grounds for the high incidence of multidrug resistance and consequent treatment failure [16, 17].

Monitoring response to therapy is a principle role of $^{18}$F-FDG PET-CT in patients with STS particularly since the RECIST (response evaluation criteria in solid tumors) criteria for treatment response do not apply well in this cohort, as successful treatment often results in larger areas of inflammation and necrosis and no signif-

icant decrease in the tumor size [18-20]. Decrease in tumor metabolism reflected by decrease in $^{18}$F-FDG uptake has been shown to precede tumor size reduction in association with therapeutic success [1]. The novel biological anticancer drugs used in some types of sarcoma are often associated with lag in tumor shrinkage. Knowledge of the timing of performance of the PET-CT study in relation to the course and type of treatment is of great importance when interpreting the findings. When performed early after initiation of therapy, the primary clinical demand of imaging is to assess the cytostatic effect of chemotherapy in order to exclude nonresponders or modify the therapeutic protocol accordingly. Decrease or no uptake of $^{18}$F-FDG during or immediately after initiation of therapy might reflect metabolic shutdown but not necessarily death of tumor cells. As shown in a recent study on 39 STS patients, $^{18}$F-FDG PET-CT can predict survival soon after the initial cycle of neoadjuvant chemotherapy, and thus may be used as an intermediate endpoint biomarker [21].

When performed after completion of therapy, a negative $^{18}$F-FDG PET suggests no active disease even in the presence of a residual mass, as the latter can be composed of hemorrhage, edema, necrosis or scar with no active tumor tissue [8, 22]. It should be borne in mind that early after radiotherapy, inflammatory cells of granulation tissue may show increased $^{18}$F-FDG uptake with potential false-positive interpretation. Evilevitch et al. [18] investigated 42 patients with biopsy-proven high-grade STS who underwent $^{18}$F-FDG PET-CT scans before and after neoadjuvant chemotherapy. Metabolic parameters were correlated with RECIST criteria as well as histopathologic response. A decrease in $^{18}$F-FDG uptake of greater than 60% showed all histopathologic responders with sensitivity of 100% and specificity of 71%, whereas application of RECIST criteria resulted in a sensitivity of 25% and a specificity of 100%.

Approximately 10-15% of STS patients develop a local recurrence that might be difficult to identify on morphologic imaging modalities because of anatomy distorted by previous surgery and radiotherapy [2]. [18]F-FDG PET-CT was found to be valuable for detection of local recurrence despite treatment-induced altered anatomy [23].

[18]F-FDG PET/CT imaging for GIST treatment response evaluation has been incorporated into the guidelines for GIST management [24]. In responders, a rapid and almost complete shutdown of glucose metabolism, reflected by decrease or disappearance of [18]F-FDG uptake, is observed almost immediately after the start of imatinib mesylate treatment preceding a potential change in tumor size on CT in several weeks, a change that is not always present, even when treatment is successful [25]. Early metabolic response of GIST is associated with a significant longer progression-free survival [9].

In summary, [18]F-FDG PET/CT is a beneficial staging and follow-up imaging modality in this cohort. However, there is no consensus as to its introduction in the imaging algorithm nor standardization of the criteria for monitoring response to therapy. Such consensus requires a large amount of accumulated clinical data for each of the STS subtypes and long enough clinical follow-up. As PET-CT has been used for over a decade now, I believe that standardization and guidelines are soon to come.

## References

1. Eary JF, Conrad EU (2011) Imaging in sarcoma. J Nucl Med 52:1903-1913
2. Bastiaannet E, Groen H, Jager PL et al (2004) The value of FDG-PET in the detection, grading and response to therapy of soft tissue and bone sarcomas; a systematic review and meta-analysis. Cancer Treat Rev 30:83-101
3. Charest M, Hickeson M, Lisbona R et al (2009) FDG PET/CT imaging in primary osseous and soft tissue sarcomas: a retrospective review of 212 cases. Eur J Nucl Med Mol Imaging 36:1944-1951
4. Eary JF, O'Sullivan F, Powitan Y et al (2002) Sarcoma tumor FDG uptake measured by PET and patient outcome: a retrospective analysis. Eur J Nucl Med Mol Imaging 29:1149-1154
5. Fuglø HM, Jørgensen SM, Loft A et al (2012) The diagnostic and prognostic value of 18F-FDG PET/CT in the initial assessment of high-grade bone and soft tissue sarcoma. A retrospective study of 89 patients. Eur J Nucl Med Mol Imaging 39:1416-1424
6. Baum SH, Frühwald M, Rahbar K et al (2011) Contribution of PET/CT to prediction of outcome in children and young adults with rhabdomyosarcoma. J Nucl Med 52:1535-1540
7. Ricard F, Cimarelli S, Deshayes E et al (2011) Additional Benefit of F-18 FDG PET/CT in the staging and follow-up of pediatric rhabdomyosarcoma. Clin Nucl Med 36:672-677
8. Benjamin RS, Choi H, Macapinlac HA et al (2007) We should desist using RECIST, at least in GIST. J Clin Oncol 25:1760-1764
9. Stroobants S, Goeminne J, Seegers M et al (2003) 18FDG-positron emission tomography for the early prediction of response in advanced soft tissue sarcoma treated with imatinib mesylate (Glivec). Eur J Cancer 39:2012-2020
10. Benz MR, Dry SM, Eilber FC et al (2010) Correlation between glycolytic phenotype and tumor grade in soft-tissue sarcomas by 18F-FDG PET. J Nucl Med. 51:1174-1181
11. Rakheja R, Makis W, Skamene S et al (2012) Correlating metabolic activity on 18F-FDG PET/CT with histopathologic characteristics of osseous and soft-tissue sarcomas: a retrospective review of 136 patients. AJR Am J Roentgenol 198:1409-1416
12. Eary JF, Conrad EU, Bruckner JD et al (1998) Quantitative [F-18]fluorodeoxyglucose positron emission tomography in pretreatment and grading of sarcoma. Clin Cancer Res 4:1215-1220
13. Ioannidis JP, Lau J (2003) 18-FDG PET for the diagnosis and grading of soft-tissue arcoma: a meta-analysis. J Nucl Med 44:717-724
14. Schwarzbach MH, Hinz U, Dimitrakopoulou-Strauss A et al (2005) Prognostic significance of preoperative [18-F] fluorodeoxyglucose (FDG) positron emission tomography (PET) imaging in patients with resectable soft tissue sarcomas. Ann Surg 241:286-294
15. Hain SF, O'Doherty MJ, Bingham J et al. (2003) Can FDG PET be used to successfully direct preoperative biopsy of soft tissue tumours? Nucl Med Commun 24:1139-1143
16. Coley HM, Verrill MW, Gregson SE et al (2000) Incidence of P-glycoprotein overexpression and multidrug resistance (MDR) reversal in adult soft tissue sarcoma. Eur J Cancer 36:881-888
17. Komdeur R, Molenaar WM, Zwart N et al (2004) Multidrug resistance proteins in primary and metastatic soft-tissue sarcomas: down-regulation of P-glycoprotein during metastatic progression. Anticancer Res 24:291-295
18. Evilevitch V, Weber WA, Tap WD et al (2008) Reduction of glucose metabolic activity is more accurate than change in size at predicting histopathologic response to neoadjuvant therapy in high-grade soft-tissue sarcomas. Clin Cancer Res 14:715-720
19. Dimitrakopoulou-Strauss A, Strauss LG, Egerer G et al (2010) Prediction of chemotherapy outcome in patients with metastatic soft tissue sarcomas based on dynamic FDG PET (dPET) and a multiparameter analysis. Eur J Nucl Med Mol Imaging 37:1481-1489
20. Benz MR, Allen-Auerbach MS, Eilber FC et al (2008) Combined assessment of metabolic and volumetric changes for assessment of tumor response in patients with soft-tissue sarcomas. J Nucl Med 49:1579-1584
21. Herrmann K, Benz MR, Czernin J et al (2012) 18F-FDG-PET/CT Imaging as an early survival predictor in patients with primary high-grade soft tissue sarcomas undergoing neoadjuvant therapy. Clin Cancer Res 18:2024-2031
22. Schuetze SM, Rubin BP, Vernon C et al (2005) Use of positron emission tomography in localized extremity soft tissue sarcoma treated with neoadjuvant chemotherapy. Cancer 103:339-348
23. Arush MW, Israel O, Postovsky S et al (2007) Positron emission tomography/computed tomography with 18fluoro-deoxyglucose in the detection of local recurrence and distant metastases of pediatric sarcoma. Pediatr Blood Cancer 49:901-905
24. Blay JY, Bonvalot S, Casali P et al (2005) Consensus meeting for the management of gastrointestinal stromal tumors: report of the GIST Consensus Conference of 20–21 March 2004, under the auspices of ESMO. Ann Oncol 16:566-578
25. Goerres GW, Stupp R, Barghouth G et al (2005) The value of PET, CT and in-line PET/CT in patients with gastrointestinal stromal tumours: long-term outcome of treatment with imatinib mesylate. Eur J Nucl Med Mol Imaging 32:153-162

# Imaging of Metastatic Bone and Soft Tissue Lesions in Prostate Cancer with FCH PET/CT

Werner Langsteger, Mohsen Beheshti

PET-CT Center Linz, Department of Nuclear Medicine and Endocrinology, St Vincent's Hospital, Linz, Austria

The goal of current cancer care is a risk-adjusted patient-specific treatment planned to maximize cancer control while minimizing the risk of complications [1]. In prostate cancer (PCa), accurate tumor characterization and disease staging are of great importance in choosing appropriate therapeutic management from a wide array of alternatives including deferred therapy (watchful waiting), androgen ablation, radical surgery and external radiation [2, 3].

Bone is the second most common site of metastases after lymph nodes in PCa, and is related to a poor prognosis. The choice of optimal imaging modalities that best depict the bone lesions can vary depending on different patterns of bone metastases such as early bone marrow involvement, and osteoblastic, osteolytic and mixed changes and their effect on bone [4].

Positron emission tomography (PET) is increasing in popularity for staging newly diagnosed PCa and for assessing response to therapy. Many PET tracers have been tested for use in the evaluation of PCa patients and these have been based on increased glycolysis ([18F]fluorodeoxyglucose, FDG), cell membrane proliferation by radiolabeled phospholipids ([11C]choline and [18F]choline), fatty acid synthesis ([11C]acetate), amino acid transport and protein synthesis ([11C]methionine), androgen receptor expression ([18F]fluorodihydrotestosterone) and osteoblastic activity ([18F]fluoride).

[18F]fluorocholine (FCH) shows particular promise as a PCa imaging agent because of its favorable physical and pharmacokinetic properties. In this contribution, we summarize briefly the current clinical experience with FCH PET/computed tomography (CT) for PCa imaging.

## Staging

### Local Disease

In defining the extent of local disease, Kwee et al. showed that the prostate regions with the highest FCH uptake demonstrated a strong correlation with sextants with the highest volume of tumor cells, and reported receiver operating characteristics of 0.8-0.9 for FCH uptake in predicting the presence of cancer on a sextant basis in the prostate [5]. In a prospective study by our group of 130 of intermediate-risk and high-risk PCa patients, a good agreement (81%) was found between regions with maximum FCH uptake on PET/CT and sextants with maximum tumoral involvement in histopathologic examinations [3]. However, differentiation between PCa and prostatitis was not possible because intensive FCH accumulation was also seen in a few patients with prostatitis. Additionally, because of the limited resolution of PET, an assessment of capsular infiltration was not possible.

### Lymph Node Metastases

The value of FCH PET/CT in the determination of regional nodal disease has been reported by several authors. In intermediate-risk and high-risk PCa patients ($n = 16$), Beauregard et al. noted a high sensitivity of FCH PET/CT (100%) compared with FDG PET/CT (75%) and diagnostic CT (50%) for detection of distant nodal metastases [6]. FCH and FDG PET/CT had comparable sensitivity (63%) for the detection of pelvic lymph node metastases, versus 25% for diagnostic CT. In 130 PCa patients at high-risk for extracapsular disease who underwent radical prostatectomy, with 912 lymph nodes sampled, our group noted better performance of FCH PET/CT for detecting nodal involvement (Fig. 1), particularly among lymph node metastases greater than or equal to 5 mm in size (sensitivity, specificity, positive and negative predictive values of 66%, 96%, 82% and 92%, respectively) [3]. A similar study by Poulsen et al. reported sensitivity, specificity, and negative and positive predictive values of 100%, 95%, 75% and 100%, respectively, among 25 men with intermediate-risk and high-risk PCa undergoing lymphadenectomy and radical prostatectomy [7]. The latter studies focused on intermediate-risk and high-risk

J. Hodler et al. (eds.), *Musculoskeletal Diseases 2013-2016,*
DOI: 10.1007/978-88-470-5292-5_29 © Springer-Verlag Italia 2013

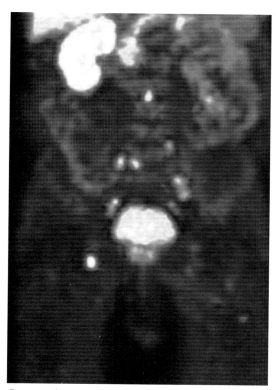

**Fig. 1.** Preoperative staging. Multiple retroperitoneal lymph node metastases in a 66-year-old patient with prostate-specific antigen 88.4 ng/mL, Gleason score 8 (for color reproduction see p 311)

PCa patients, which may account for their findings of better performance for FCH PET/CT in assessing nodal disease compared with previous studies.

## Bone Metastases

In the largest pre-operative series reported, our group found bone metastases in 13/130 patients pre-operatively; 2 of the 13 patients had bone metastases that had not been detected previously by conventional imaging (Fig. 2) [3]. The results of the study showed that FCH PET/CT would result in a therapy change for 15% of patients overall, and an upstaging change in 20% of high-risk patients. In evaluating 70 men with PCa, our group noted sensitivity, specificity and accuracy of 79%, 97% and 84%, respectively, for FCH PET/CT compared with a consensus definition of bone metastases based on conventional imaging and clinical endpoints [8]. In another prospective series of 38 patients with high-risk PCa [9], we compared the performance of FCH PET/CT with that of [18F]fluoride PET/CT (Table 1). FCH PET/CT showed significantly higher specificity than [18F]fluoride PET/CT and comparable sensitivity. However superior performance in the detection of bone marrow metastases was seen using FCH PET imaging. In those studies, discordant findings were noticed in a relatively small subset of patients with densely sclerotic lesions on CT that were negative in FCH PET and positive in [18F]fluoride PET scans (Fig. 3).

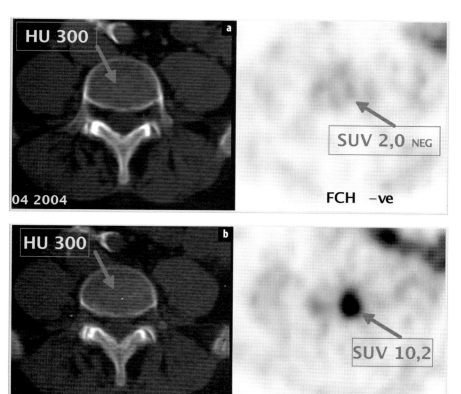

**Fig. 2 a, b.** Preoperative staging. Bone marrow metastasis in L4 in a 73year-old patient with prostate-specific antigen 8.7 ng/ml, Gleason score 8. [18F]fluorocholine (*FCH*) PET/CT negative [standardized uptake value (*SUV*) 2.0] **a**, and positive after 4 months (SUV 10.2), **b**. *HU* Hounsfield units (for color reproduction see p 311)

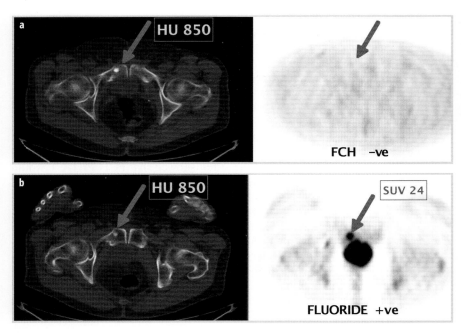

**Fig. 3 a. b.** Follow-up (prostate-specific antigen 20.5 ng/ml) 1 month after withdrawal of hormone therapy. Bone metastasis in the right os pubis [CT: sclerosis, Hounsfield units (*HU*) 850]. [$^{18}$F]fluorocholine PET/CT negative (*FCH -ve*) (**a**) and [$^{18}$F]fluoride PET/CT positive (*FLUORIDE +ve*) (**b**) [standardized uptake value (*SUV*) 24] (for color reproduction see p 312)

**Table 1.** Comparison of FCH PET/CT and [$^{18}$F]fluoride PET/CT in 38 patients (preoperative *n* = 17, postoperative *n* = 21)

| FCH PET - CT | | | |
| --- | --- | --- | --- |
| | True | False | Total |
| Positive | 97 | 1 | 98 |
| Negative | 95 | 34 | 129 |
| Estimate value | sensitivity | specifity | accuracy |
| | 74% | 99% (*P*<0,01) | 85% |

| [$^{18}$F]fluoride PET - CT | | | |
| --- | --- | --- | --- |
| | True | False | Total |
| Positive | 108 | 7 | 115 |
| Negative | 89 | 26 | 115 |
| Estimate value | sensitivity | specifity | accuracy |
| | 81% ns | 93% | 86% |

*FCH* [$^{18}$F]fluorocholine, *PET/CT* positron emission tomography /computed tomography, *ns* not significant

## Restaging

FCH PET/CT showed promising results in the detection of recurrent disease in PCa patients with increased prostate-specific antigen (PSA) after primary treatment. In a recent prospective study, we evaluated the potential of FCH PET/CT in a large population of patients (*n* = 250), correlating diagnostic accuracy with PSA levels as well as influence of androgen deprivation therapy (ADT) on FCH PET [10].

FCH PET/CT was able to correctly detect malignant lesions in 74% (185/250) of patients. In 28% of patients, only one lesion was detected (69/250). The sensitivity of the FCH PET/CT was significantly higher (*P* = 0.001) in patients with ongoing ADT [8.5%, 95% confidence interval (CI) 80-91] compared with patients not on ADT (59.5%, CI 50-69).

In addition, FCH PET/CT showed sensitivities of 77.5%, 80.7%, 85.2% and 92.8% for the trigger PSA levels of more than 0.5, 1.0, 2.0 and 4.0 ng/ml, respectively. Using a binary logistic regression analysis model, trigger PSA levels and ADT were shown to be the only significant predictors of a positive FCH PET/CT.

The results of the study demonstrated the high performance of FCH PET/CT as a noninvasive "one stop diagnostic modality" enabling us to correctly detect occult disease in 74% of patients, and to differentiate localized from systemic disease. Finally, trigger PSA levels and ADT are the two significant predictors for FCH-positive PET lesions.

## References

1. Hricak H, Choyke PL, Eberhardt SC et al (2007) Imaging prostate cancer: a multidisciplinary perspective. Radiology 243:28-53
2. Langsteger W, Heinisch M, Fogelman I (2006) The role of fluorodeoxyglucose, $^{18}$F-dihydroxyphenylalanine, $^{18}$F-choline, and $^{18}$F-fluoride in bone imaging with emphasis on prostate and breast. Seminars in Nuclear Medicine 36:73-92
3. Beheshti M, Imamovic L, Broinger G et al (2010) $^{18}$F choline PET/CT in the preoperative staging of prostate cancer in patients with intermediate or high risk of extracapsular disease: a prospective study of 130 patients. Radiology 254:925-933
4. Langsteger W, Haim S, Knauer M et al (2012) Imaging of bone metastases in prostate cancer: an update. QJ Nucl Med Mol Imaging 56:447-458
5. Kwee SA, Coel MN, Lim J, Ko JP (2005) Prostate cancer localization with $^{18}$fluorine fluorocholine positron emission tomography. J Urol 173:252-255

6. Beauregard JM, Williams SG, Degrado TR (2010) Pilot comparison of F-fluorocholine and F-fluorodeoxyglucose PET/CT with conventional imaging in prostate cancer. J Med Imaging Radiat Oncol 54:325-332

7. Poulsen MH, Bouchelouche K, Gerke O et al (2010) [$^{18}$F]-fluorocholine positron-emission/computed tomography for lymph node staging of patients with prostate cancer: preliminary results of a prospective study. BJU Int 106:639-643

8. Beheshti M, Vali R, Waldenberger P et al (2009) The use of F-18 choline PET in the assessment of bone metastases in prostate cancer: correlation with morphological changes on CT. Mol Imaging Biol 11:446-454

9. Beheshti M, Vali R, Waldenberger P et al (2008). Detection of bone metastases in patients with prostate cancer by $^{18}$F fluorocholine and $^{18}$F fluoride PET-CT: a comparative study. Eur J Nucl Med Mol Imaging 35:1766-1774

10. Beheshti M, Haim S, Zakavi R et al (2013) Impact of $^{18}$F Choline PET/CT in prostate cancer patients with biochemical recurrence – influence of androgen deprivation therapy and correlation with PSA kinetics. J Nucl Med, in press

# PET Imaging of Bone Metastases with FDG, Fluoride and Gallium-Somatostatin Analogs

Einat Even-Sapir Weizer

Department of Nuclear Medicine, Tel Aviv Sourasky Medical Center, Tel Aviv University, Tel Aviv, Israel

Imaging is aimed at identifying skeletal involvement as early as possible, to determine the extent of skeletal disease, to evaluate the presence of complications, to monitor response to therapy, and occasionally to guide biopsy. Detection of bone metastases in nuclear medicine is based on either direct visualization of tumor cells using radiotracers that accumulate in these cells, or tracers, the uptake of which reflects bone reaction secondary to the presence of malignant cells. The following summary describes the role of positron emission tomography-computed tomography (PET-CT) in assessment of bone metastases using three different PET tracers: [18]F-fluordeoxyglucose ([18]F-FDG), which directly accumulates in tumor cells of FDG-avid malignancies; [68]Ga-somatostatin, which accumulates in neuroendocrine tumors that show high expression of somatostatin receptors; and [18]F-fluoride, a bone-seeking agent that reflects secondary bone reactive changes.

The most prominent advantage of [18]F-FDG PET is its ability to detect early marrow-based spread. The normal red marrow demonstrates only low-intensity [18]FDG uptake; therefore, increased marrow uptake might suggest the presence of early malignant bone marrow deposits preceding the detection of bone metastases by bone scintigraphy (BS) and CT [1-3]. [18]F-FDG PET has been found to be superior to BS in detecting bone involvement in various malignant diseases, and also because it is highly sensitive for detection of lytic metastases, for which BS is insensitive. Thus the introduction of [18]F-FDG PET-CT in the imaging algorithms of oncologic patients often obviates the need to perform a separate BS for assessment of bone involvement [2, 4].

[18]F-FDG is considered relatively less sensitive for detection of blastic type metastases [5]. However, since in the majority of centers PET is integrated with CT, morphologic data added to the scintigraphic data allow for detection of blastic metastases on the CT images [6]. The combined functional-morphological data are also of clinical relevance in detecting complications of bone metastases. The vertebral column, for instance, is the most common skeletal region involved by metastatic spread. Tumor may invade the epidural space by direct extension from adjacent involved bone. Early diagnosis and treatment prior to the development of permanent neurological deficits is essential for a favorable outcome [7].

[18]F-FDG PET plays an important role in monitoring response of bone metastases to therapy. Sequential PET-CT studies performed in patients with breast cancer have shown that [18]F-FDG uptake reflects the immediate tumor activity of bone metastases, whereas the radiographic morphology changes vary greatly with time [8]. Disease progression is obvious on CT if new lytic lesions are identified, but is difficult to determine when sclerosis is present [9]. After successful treatment, the involved bone often becomes sclerotic, but it is not possible then to separate partial response with an ongoing active disease from the repair process by using CT. Morphological abnormality may remain permanent even when disease in the bone is no longer active. [18]F-FDG PET, on the other hand, can accurately suggest response by showing decrease in intensity of uptake regardless of the morphological appearance.

Assessing the presence of metastatic spread in patients with newly diagnosed neuroendocrine tumors (NET) is of great clinical relevance for selection of the appropriate treatment approach. If no metastases are found, the primary treatment is surgery with curative intent or debulking of the tumor mass. In cases of metastatic disease, peptide-receptor radionuclide therapy with radiolabeled somatostatin analogs may be of benefit if the tumor is showing high expression of somatostatin receptors. Imaging with labeled somatostatin at diagnosis is aimed for characterization of the somatostatin-receptor expression in the individual tumor. Planar and SPECT somatostatin receptor scintigraphy (SRS) has gained widespread acceptance as the imaging method of choice in NET patients, showing high diagnostic accuracy for detection of the primary tumor and secondary lesions. Recently, somatostatin analogs labeled with [68]Ga have been introduced for PET imaging of NET. [68]Ga is a short-lived tracer with a half-life of 68 min and is available from an inhouse

J. Hodler et al. (eds.), *Musculoskeletal Diseases 2013-2016,*
DOI: 10.1007/978-88-470-5292-5_30 © Springer-Verlag Italia 2013

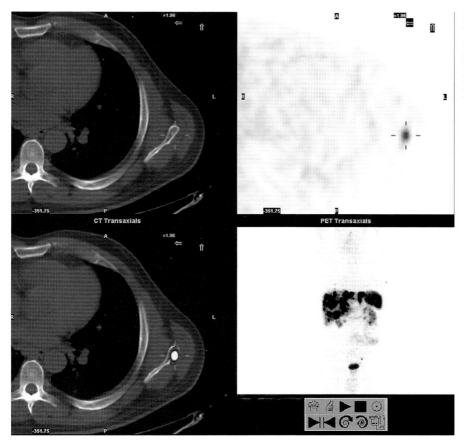

**Fig. 1.** [68]Ga- DOTANOC (DOTA-Tyr3-octreotide) positron emission tomography-computed tomography in metastatic carcinoid. Metastatic disease in the liver and bone. There is an example of an early small metastasis in the left scapule (for color reproduction see p 312)

generator of [68]Ga, with a half-life of 270.8 days, independent of an onsite cyclotron [10, 11]. The latter analogs, mostly DOTA-derivatized peptides, such as DOTA-Tyr3-octreotide (DOTATOC), show high affinity to somatostatin receptors and beneficial pharmacokinetic properties. Combined with the better resolution of PET technology, [68]Ga-somatostatin PET has been reported to show a better diagnostic accuracy for detection of bone metastases of NET compared with STS BS and CT [11, 12]. In a recent study on 89 patients with NET, SPECT STS identified only 72.5% and CT identified only 50% of the skeletal lesions identified by [68]Ga-somatostatin PET [11] (Fig. 1).

Response of bone metastases after treatment with [177]Lu-octreotate can be evaluated efficiently by SRS or [68]Ga-somatostatin PET [13]. Interestingly, in a recent study, it has been suggested that successful treatment of bone metastases can represent as lesions that increase in size on CT as a result of the repair process while showing a decrease in labeled somatostatin uptake [14].

[18]F-fluoride is a PET bone-seeking agent with uptake mechanism similar to that of the single-photon emitting tracer [99m]Tc-MDP. Fluoride ions exchange with hydroxyl groups in hydroxyapatite crystal bone to form fluoroapatite, and are deposited at the bone surface where bone turnover is greatest. Similar to [99m]Tc-MDP, accumulation of [18]F-fluoride uptake in bone metastases reflects increased regional blood flow and high bone turnover. [18]F-fluoride has better pharmacokinetic characteristics compared with those of [99m]Tc-MDP. The bone uptake of the former is twofold higher, and in contrast to [99m]Tc-MDP it does not bind to protein. The capillary permeability of [18]F-fluoride is higher and its blood clearance is faster, resulting in a better target-to-background ratio. Regional plasma clearance of [18]F-fluoride is reported to be three to ten times higher in bone metastases compared with that in normal bone [15, 16]

[18]F-fluoride PET is very sensitive for detection of osteoblastic metastases and also lytic metastases, as the latter, even when considered "pure lytic", do have minimal osteoblastic activity, which is enough for detection by [18]F-fluoride PET. It should be borne in mind that [18]F-fluoride is not tumor specific and therefore is a sensitive modality for detection of any bone abnormalities, not only malignant abnormalities.

When interpreting [18]F-fluoride PET-CT for assessment of metastatic skeletal spread, the morphologic appearance of the bone should be carefully considered on the CT data, in order to accurately separate benign and malignant sites of [18]F-fluoride uptake [17].

Several clinical reports in various malignancies have illustrated the superiority of [18]F-fluoride PET-CT over

BS for detection of bone metastases, with an excellent negative predictive value [18-21]. In patients with prostate cancer, [18]f-Fluoride PET-CT showed a greater sensitivity than [18]F-fluorocholine in the detection of bone metastasis, although the differences were not statistically significant [22]. In patients with lung cancer, it was found to be complementary to [18]F-FDG PET-CT mainly for detection of sclerotic type abnormalities [23].

There are early data suggesting that [18]F-fluoride PET can be used to assess treatment response in metastatic prostate cancer. PET was performed 6 and 12 weeks after treatment with Alpharadin® in a small pilot study of patients with prostate cancer. Measurement of serial standard uptake values allowed separation of responders and nonresponders [24].

However, use of [18]F-floride PET is not yet routine. There is a multicenter study underway in the USA to assess the use of this modality in routine use of skeletal staging in cancer, comparing [18]F-fluoride PET-CT with MDP bone scintigraphy in 500 patients with breast, prostate and non-small-cell lung cancer.

## References

1. Cook GJ, Fogelman I (2001) The role of positron emission tomography in skeletal disease. Semin Nucl Med 31:50-61
2. Even-Sapir E (2005) Imaging of malignant bone involvement by morphologic, scintigraphic, and hybrid modalities. J Nucl Med 46:1356-1367
3. Hamaoka T, Madewell JE, Podoloff DA et al (2004) Bone imaging in metastatic breast cancer. J Clin Oncol 22:2942-2953
4. Cook GJR (2010) PET and PET/CT imaging of skeletal metastases. Cancer Imaging 10:153-160
5. Cook GJR, Houston S, Rubens R et al (1998) Detection of bone metastases in breast cancer by 18FDG PET: differing metabolic activity in osteoblastic and osteolytic lesions. J Clin Oncol 16:3375-3379
6. Taira AV, Herfkens RJ, Gambhir SS et al (2007) Detection of bone metastases: assessment of integrated FDG PET/CT imaging. Radiology 243:204-211
7. Metser U, Lerman H, Blank A et al (2004) Malignant involvement of the spine: assessment by 18FFDG PET/CT. J Nucl Med 45:279-284
8. Du Y, Cullum I, Illidge TM et al (2007) Fusion of metabolic function and morphology: sequential [18F]fluorodeoxyglucose positron-emission tomography/computed tomography studies yield new insights into the natural history of bone metastases in breast cancer. J Clin Oncol 25:3440-3447
9. Katayama T, Kubota K, Machida Y et al (2012) Evaluation of sequential FDG-PET/CT for monitoring bone metastasis of breast cancer during therapy: correlation between morphological and metabolic changes with tumor markers. Ann Nucl Med 26:426-435
10. Putzer1 D, Gabriel M, Henninger B et al (2009) Neuroendocrine tumor: 68Ga-DOTATyr3- Octreotide PET in comparison to CT and bone scintigraphy. J Nucl Med 50:1214-1221
11. Gabriel M, Decristoforo C, Kendler D et al (2007) 68Ga-DOTA-Tyr3-octreotide PET in neuroendocrine tumors: comparison with somatostatin receptor scintigraphy and CT. J Nucl Med 48:508-518
12. Maecke HR, Hofmann M, Haberkorn U (2005) 68 Ga-Labeled Peptides in Tumor Imaging. J Nucl Med 46:172S-175S
13 Ezziddin S, Sabet A, Heinemann F et al (2011) Response and long-term control of bone metastases after peptide receptor radionuclide therapy with 177Lu-octreotate. J Nucl Med 52:1197-1203
14. van Vliet EI, Hermans JJ, de Ridder MA et al (2012) Tumor response assessment to treatment with [177Lu-DOTA0,Tyr3] Octreotate in patients with gastroenteropancreatic and bronchial neuroendocrine tumors: differential response of bone versus soft-tissue. JNM 53:1359-1366
15. Blake GM, Park-Holohan SJ, Cook GJR et al (2001) Quantitative studies of bone with the use of 18F-fluoride and 99mTc-methylene diphosphonate. Semin Nucl Med 31:28-49
16. Grant FD, Fahey FH, Packard AB et al (2008) Skeletal PET with 18F-fluoride: applying new technology to an old tracer. J Nucl Med 49:68-78
17. Even-Sapir E, Metser U, Flusser G et al (2004) Assessment of malignant skeletal disease: initial experience with 18F-fluoride PET/CT and comparison between 18F-fluoride PET and 18F-fluoride PET/CT. J Nucl Med 45:272-278
18. Schirrmeister H, Guhlmann A, Kotzerke J et al (1999) Early detection and accurate description of extent of metastatic bone disease in breast cancer with fluoride ion and PET. J Clin Oncol 17:2381-2389
19. Schirrmeister H, Glatting G, Hetzel J et al (2001) Evaluation of the clinical value of planar bone scans, SPECT and 18F-labeled NaF PET in newly diagnosed lung cancer. J Nucl Med 42:1800-1804
20. Even-Sapir E, Metser U, Mishani E et al (2006) The detection of bone metastases in patients with high risk prostate cancer: 99mTc MDP planar bone scintigraphy, single and multi field of view SPECT, 18F-fluoride PET and 18F-fluoride PET/CT. J Nucl Med 47:287-297
21. Bortot DC, Amorim BJ, Oki GC et al (2012) 18F-Fluoride PET/CT is highly effective for excluding bone metastases even in patients with equivocal bone scintigraphy. Eur J Nucl Med Mol Imaging 39:1730-1736
22. Beheshti M, Vali R, Waldenberger P et al (2008) Detection of bone metastases in patients with prostate cancer by 18F fluorocholine and 18F fluoride PET/CT: a comparative study. Eur J Nucl Med Mol Imaging 35:1766-1774
23. Kruger S, Buck AK, Mottaghy FM et al (2009) Detection of bone metastases in patients with lung cancer: 99mTc MDP planar bone scintigraphy, 18F-fluoride PET or 18F-FDG PET-CT. Eur J Nucl Med Mol Imaging 36:1807-1812
24. Cook G, Parker C, Chua S et al (2009) Quantitative 18F-fluoride PET to monitor response in skeletal metastases from prostate cancer treated with Alpharadin (223-Ra-chloride) Nucl Med Commun 30:374

# Single Photon Imaging, Including SPECT/CT, in Patients with Prostheses

Helmut F. Rasch[1], Michael T. Hirschmann[2]

[1] Department of Radiology and Nuclear Medicine, Kantonspital Baselland, Bruderholz, Switzerland
[2] Department of Orthopaedic Surgery and Traumatology, Kantonspital Baselland, Bruderholz, Switzerland

## Introduction

Osteoarthritis has a multifactorial genesis and represents the most frequently occurring degenerative joint disease of adult patients worldwide. The demographic change in western industrial nations has led to a rising number of patients undergoing joint arthroplasty [1-3]. As a result of younger patients receiving treatment and higher life expectancy, the incidence of revision surgery is growing. For example, the number of hip replacements in the USA increased from 220,000 to 234,000 in only 1 year (2003-2004), and the number of knee replacements from 418,000 to 478,000; this trend is ongoing [4]. The impact of these increasing patient numbers places an immense financial strain on the health system. For precise planning of therapy, and also taking into account financial costs, a comprehensive accurate diagnostic procedure is needed to optimize the therapy and treatment of these patients.

Routinely performed conventional X-rays, and also conventional computed tomography (CT) slices cannot precisely describe the position of the component in three dimensions. For example, a rotational alignment will affect the appearance of the posterior slope in cases of total knee replacement [5]. Precise identification of the position of the component is crucial because malpositioning and malorientation are two major causes of pain following total knee replacement [6, 7]; also, it has an impact on the outcome, and facilitates understanding the kinematics of modern prosthesis types [8]. In addition, the outcome after arthroplasty is related to the correct position of the component [9].

For metal artefacts, single-photon emission computed tomography/CT (SPECT/CT) is currently the only sectional image modality that provides adequate information about a prosthetic joint, considering morphological (bone structure and quality), metabolic (bone metabolism), soft tissue (presence of infection or pseudotumors) and biomechanical data (position of prosthesis component) in one examination and with adequate image quality.

## SPECT/CT: How Is It Done?

In the following sections, standard SPECT/CT procedures are described, along with hardware and practice recommendations.

The standard SPECT/CT evaluation of a joint prosthesis includes a conventional three-phase bone scintigraphy followed by combined SPECT/CT of the joint of interest. Additional short spiral scans of the adjacent joints allow reconstruction of mechanical axis and precise determination of component position. Unfortunately, this requires dedicated software packages or workstations, because these measurements cannot be performed with commercial software suites of modern scanners.

### Perfusion Study (Planar Images)

After intravenous injection of 500-700 MBq 99m-technetium-diphosphonate in a first step, perfusion images of the joint of interest are acquired to detect hyperemia. Whenever possible, simultaneous acquisition in two planar views is favored. These images are important to detect possible inflammatory processes and determine signs of algodystrophy.

### Bloodpool Study (Planar Images)

About 2 min after the primary tracer application, acquisition of the two planar views, supplemented with additional views such as lateral or medial projections, is performed. These projections visualize inflammatory changes of the joint (septic and aseptic) and the first localization of the pathology. In principle, it is possible to obtain a fast SPECT acquisition, which can be complemented with a low-dose CT scan for anatomical coregistration. Compared with SPECT-CT systems that include a full diagnostic CT component, systems that use a flat panel CT component allow imaging with a significantly higher reduction of the radiation dose without loss of image quality.

J. Hodler et al. (eds.), *Musculoskeletal Diseases 2013-2016,*
DOI: 10.1007/978-88-470-5292-5_31 © Springer-Verlag Italia 2013

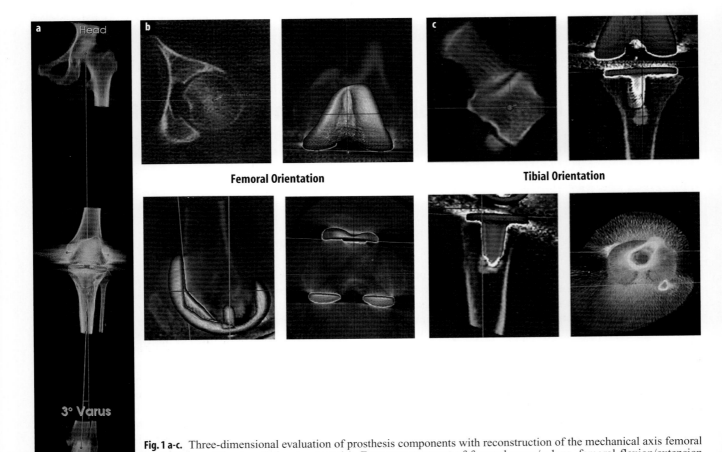

**Fig. 1 a-c.** Three-dimensional evaluation of prosthesis components with reconstruction of the mechanical axis femoral and tibial resulting in a 3 degree varus (**a**). Easy measurement of femoral varus/valgus, femoral flexion/extension and femoral rotation (**b**). The tibial component slope and the tibial rotation are defined (**c**) (for color reproduction see p 313)

## Mineral Phase (Whole Body and SPECT/CT)

Depending on the age of the patient, late-phase imaging is performed 2-4 h after injection.

Since the the SPECT data set are normalized to 100%, the whole body images give valuable information about the "real" activity or intensity of the pathological process.

There are no studies reported in the literature regarding whether additional planar views of the joint in the whole body scans are needed. In our institution, we routinely go to SPECT acquisition directly, which saves a lot of examination time and can reduce motion artefacts, especially in patients with pain.

## SPECT Aquisition

The field of view (FOV) should be centered to the joint whenever possible. In cases of revision surgery with long prosthesis components, two FOVs are sometimes needed to cover the complete prosthesis; this can be achieved by two additional SPECT aquisitions. These may also be helpful for hip prostheses so that the lumbar spine is also covered, and a differential diagnosis between prosthesis-related pain

and/or spine problems, such as activated spondylarthritis or erosive osteochondritis, can be made more easily.

The aquisition parameter should be adjusted to the scanner performance and the patient. It should be remembered that in cases of agitated patients, it is better to acquire a fast SPECT (e.g., 8-10 min) with fewer count statistics but without motion artefacts. Long acquisition times lead to motion artefacts and these scans cannot be reliably fused.

## CT Aquisition

To obtain CT scans with high-quality reconstruction in all three planes, it is necessary to use the thinnest available collimation (full diagnostic CT components usually 0.6-0.75 mm; flat panel systems down to 0.33 mm). Using advanced imaging protocols [9, 10] for three-dimensional (3D) axis reconstruction and real 3D angle measurements, acquisition of the adjacent joints is needed. These scans can be performed with thicker slices, e.g., 3 mm or hip and ankle, when analyzing component position of a partial or total knee replacement (Fig. 1). In our experience, the best image quality can be obtained with

16-slice scanners that have enough X-ray power for use in cases of bilateral prostheses, which can cause problems when using flat panel systems. The possibility of reconstructing CT data with an extended Hounsfield scale (increasing the CT windows up to 40,000 Hounsfield units) allows significantly improved bone visualization near the bone-prosthesis or cement interface. Regrettably, this feature is currently offered by only one company.

## Image Fusion

The fusion is usually performed with the vendor's software package and provides perfect matched images in most cases. In some cases, for example when technical defects of the SPECT/CT scanner occur with the CT component, it is possible to use an available dedicated CT system and fuse the images afterwards on the workstation. The modern voxel-based algorithms often produce good results; the quality of results in descending order is: hip, knee and shoulder. Because of the very complex anatomy, this method does not usually give reliable results for the foot and ankle.

## Examination Recommendations

Patient support: position your patient in a comfortable pain-free position! Because of the long examination time up to 45 min, pain can cause distinct motion artefacts, which can compromise the whole examination. In some cases, it is necessary to apply painkillers intravenously. Pain and long examination times can be disadvantageous when using special devices to standardize patient position or simulate weight-bearing images.

## Image Analysis: Look at Everything

First, analyze the scintigraphic images, including early phase images, and address the following points: the presence/absence of hyperemia; tracer distribution and spot localization; prosthesis component – one/both sides; location of hot spots to the prosthesis; bone/cement interface; intensity on the whole body scan.

Second, obtain morphological information from CT scan and address the following points: bone density; presence/absence of focal osteopenia; presence/absence of granulomas/osteolysis; component position; relation to mechanical axis; available conventional X-rays; type of prosthesis; cemented or uncemented; coating of the prosthesis, if known (e.g., hydroxyapatite). There is a strong relationship between biomechanical principles of the prosthesis model, mechanical fixation and possible uptake patterns; therefore, it is necessary talk to the orthopedic surgeon.

## Combine All Your Information

Is there a special uptake pattern? Can it be explained by malpositioning or malrotation? Also, it is important to detect stress reactions, as these can lead to a misdiagnosis of loosening.

In summary, the complex situation in many patients requires a stringent interdisciplinary approach.

## SPECT/CT in Different Regions

### Shoulder

The number of patients who receive a shoulder arthroplasty is steadily increasing [11-14]. The spectrum of devices includes resurfacing techniques, and partial prosthesis up to complex inverse prosthesis types [12, 13]. Compared with other joints, the spherical component of the head causes strong beam hardening artefacts that make it difficult to analyze the images. The orthopedic point of view focuses on the following questions:
1. Bone quality: is there osteolysis?
2. Are there signs of aseptic loosening?
3. What is the component position?
4. Are there signs of acromial impingement as possible cause of pain, which can be easily seen as zone of hypermetabolism on the acromion?
5. Bone stock glenoidal before revision surgery: is there enough bone to fix the component?
6. Are there signs of infection?
7. If there is sign of infection, carry out additional anti-granulocyte-SPECT-CT as a second examination.

The literature regarding the use of SPECT/CT in shoulder prostheses is limited to case reports [11].

Practical recommendations:
• The affected arm/shoulder should lie in a neutral position, and the other arm should be elevated above the head. This "swimmer" position reduces artefacts caused by both shoulders. The head should be turned to one side to allow the camera to scan close to the body surface.

### Hip

Hip arthroplasty is currently one of the major orthopedic arthroplasty procedures. Indications are: unexplained pain in the postoperative setting (15-20% of all patients), suspicion of loosening, suspicion of infection, and detection of other/additional causes of pain such as spine pathologies. Before analyzing the images the following questions should be answered:
1. Are the components cemented or uncemented?
2. In cases of uncemented components, what is the type of fixation: proximal or distal?
3. What type of cup fixation has been used: press-fit or screws?

It is very important to differentiate between cemented and uncemented types of prosthesis. The uncemented shafts usually show a proximal or distal fixation zone where enostal thickening of the bone associated with focal higher uptake can appear. This is equivalent to a

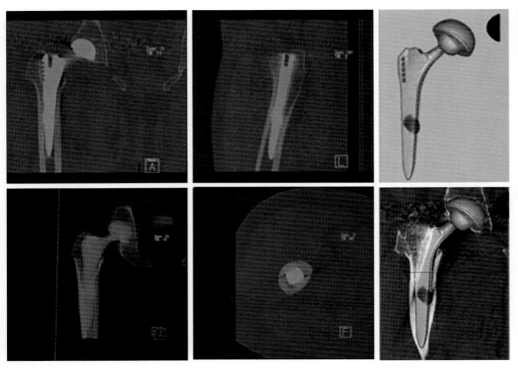

**Fig. 2.** A 54-year-old man with hip replacement on the right side 6/2008. Four years after surgery, pain is experienced under stress. SPECT-CT shows intact prosthesis components. Only slight uptake in the midshaft. Minimal varus of the shaft. Diagnosis: no loosening, slight uptake in the fixation zone and stress reaction caused by a minimal varus. The surgeon did not believe the diagnosis and the patient underwent revision. No loosening was found intraoperatively (for color reproduction see p 314)

biomechanical stress reaction and physiological bone re-modeling process, which should not be misinterpreted as aseptic loosening (Fig. 2). Usually – with the exception of the new hydroxyapatite-coated femoral shafts – a small boneless margin (smaller than 2 mm) around the shaft can be seen. Every focal widening or irregularity is suspicious of loosening. The cortical bone should be homogeneous. Distal periostal thickening distal is suspicious of micromotion of the shaft and can indicate loosening in cases of a proximal fixed prosthesis.

In cases of a cemented shaft, the cement layer should not show any sign of breaking, which is a clear sign of loosening. Osteopenic areas, especially in the trochanter, can indicate either cement problems (a thin layer that cannot distribute the pressure adequately) or component malposition, such as varus with high pressure in the trochanter minor (higher focal uptake) and less pressure in the trochanter major (less uptake). In cases of an uncemented cup, uptake can usually be seen in the cranial parts of the acetabulum, where the main force vectors are located. Any other uptake localization should lead to careful evaluation of the acetabular bone to exclude osteolysis/granulomas and pathological margins >2 mm. In cases of wide margins and large granulomas, the pathology is often seen in the CT scans only, and the scintigraphy is negative. This pathology can be missed on planar images and SPECT alone. Some cups are fixed by winding in the bone. In these cases, small focused margins and only focal missing contact between the winding and the bone is normal and is related to the operative technique. These morphological patterns do not represent

any loosening. Particularly in revision surgery, the cups are often fixed with additional screws. The analysis should consider material failure. The screws should not reach far into the pelvis as this can cause muscle problems (irritation or hematoma in the iliacus muscle) or pelvic nerve irritation. For cemented cups, the same criteria used for the shaft can be applied. Subsequently, the head should be assessed to detect signs of wearing, which is usually seen as asymmetric narrowing of the joint space. It is necessary to at least have a close look at the soft tissue (is there presence of a hematoma or pseudotumor?) and ectopic ossifications, which sometimes show an inflammatory component in the early phase or can cause mechanical problems limiting the range of motion.

Practical recommendations:
- To detect material failure such as broken screws, use the widest window that can be obtained. If possible, make additional reconstructions with an extended Hounsfield scale, otherwise dislodged broken screws can be missed.
- For evaluation of the head and exclusion of bearing problems, use radial reconstructions or a second plane through the femoral neck to see the congruency of the joint space.
- Never believe a normal whole body scan! Not every loosening shows a pathological uptake.
- Use existing conventional X-rays when available.
- Have a look to the spine: is there uptake in facet joints?
- Is there spondylosis or spinal stenosis?
- Discuss unclear findings with the orthopedic surgeon!

## Knee

The unicompartimental or total knee replacement procedure, with or without retropatellar resurfacing, is the most common arthroplasty in addition to the hip. The indications for using SPECT/CT are analogous to those for hip arthroplasty. In particular, if an initially pain-free patient develops pain symptoms month or years after arthroplasty, one should consider a diagnosis of component loosening or failure, component malpositioning or hematogenously based infection [15, 16].

As described for the hip, there is an extremely large number of different types of prosthesis and multiple different operation procedures for the knee. For a complete evaluation of a knee prosthesis, the component position plays an important role. Some data reported in the literature show a correlation between malposition and outcome after arthroplasty [5, 17]. Many mechanical situations can lead to clinical problems: abnormal varus/valgus alignment predisposes to loosening, rotational malalignment can cause anterior knee pain by patella stress, and pathological femoral extension/flexion can lead to notching or early loosening [18, 19]. For detection of loosening, the image criteria described for the hip can also be used for the knee.

Practical recommendations:

- If focal uptake does clearly not belong to the prosthesis-bone or cement-bone interface, search carefully for biomechanical problems.
- Granulomas are mostly localized at the posterior femur shield and in the posterior compartments of the tibial bone-prostheses interface. These regions should be evaluated carefully. Granulomas indicate a high risk of prosthesis loosening in the future and should be monitored at frequent short intervals.

## Foot and Ankle

In the complex anatomical region of the hindfoot, use of SPECT/CT has many advantages. The prosthesis types used in the ankle often cause large granulomas, which can best be seen along the tibial L-shaped component. The talar component is shaped like a cap, so unfortunately it is practically impossible to examine the talar bone in each compartment and under the cap. Particularly in cases of revision, the main question of whether there is any osteonecrosis under the cap cannot be answered. However, SPECT/CT can clearly visualize ectopic neo-ossification, which can cause reduced range of motion. Inlay failure and stress reaction in the adjacent joints of the hindfoot are especially found in the lower ankle. Therefore, in selected cases, SPECT/CT can be used to optimize surgical planning.

## Infection

Infection after arthroplasty is a serious complication. In particular, joint infections occur in 1-2% of the primary implants and 3-5% of revision implants [20, 21]. On conventional X-rays, infection is hard to detect and the images are mostly positive in a very late phase of the infection, which is often too late for optimal therapy. Factors associated with increased risk are skin ulcerations, steroid medication, diabetes mellitus, poor nutrition and advanced age [16]. Clinical tests to diagnose an infection include laboratory tests such as C-reactive protein, erythrocyte sedimentation rate and joint aspiration [22, 23].

A three-phase bone scintigraphy cannot distinguish between septic loosening and aseptic inflammatory situations such as allergic reaction to the metal or inlay material. A specific scintigraphic method is imaging using labelled white blood cells, or an easier method is antigranulocyte scintigraphy using antibodies to label white blood cells in vivo. The problems locating the pathology caused by low image quality have been overcome by the use of SPECT/CT. An unsolved problem is the low sensitivity in cases of low-grade infection. At present, it is not possible to clearly exclude low-grade infection with the commercially available tracers and examination techniques.

## Conclusion

SPECT/CT is, in most cases, the imaging modality of choice to evaluate joints after arthroplasty procedures. In one examination it combines metabolic, morphological and, using advanced examination settings, biomechanical data for detection of loosening, infection and component malposition or malalignment. If possible, an interdisciplinary approach with close communication between the orthopedic surgeon and nuclear medicine physician is needed to confirm the correct diagnosis.

In future, new techniques such as iterative reconstruction of the CT data to lower the radiation dose and increase image quality, or spectral imaging with its promising ability in metal artefact reduction, will offer significant improvements on the technical side of imaging. The degree to which new tracers will improve the diagnosis of infection remains to be seen.

## References

1. Räuchle M, Cemerka M, Eibenberger B, Breitenseher M (2012) Arthrosis – update. Radiologe 52:149-155
2. Singh JA (2011) Epidemiology of knee and hip arthroplasty: a systematic review. The Open Orthopaedics Journal 5:80-85
3. Bozic KJ, Kurtz SM, Lau E et al (2009) The epidemiology of revision total hip arthroplasty in the United States. J Bone Joint Surg Am 91:128-133
4. Association IHC (2006) Orthopedics Data Compendium: Use, cost and market structure for total joint replacement. August 2006
5. Holme TJ, Henckel J, Cobb J, Hart AJ (2011) Quantification of the difference between 3D CT and plain radiograph for measurement of the position of medial unicompartmental knee replacements. The Knee 18:300-305
6. Barrack RL, Schrader T, Bertot AJ et al (2001) Component rotation and anterior knee pain after total knee arthroplasty. Clinical orthopaedics and related research 392:46-55

7. Torga-Spak R, Parikh SN, Stuchin SA (2004) Anterior knee pain due to biplanar rotatory malalignment of the femoral component in total knee arthroplasty. Case report. J Knee Surg 17:113-6

8. Eckhoff DG, Bach JM, Spitzer VM et al (2005) Three-dimensional mechanics, kinematics, and morphology of the knee viewed in virtual reality. J Bone Joint Surg Am 87 Suppl 2:71-80

9. Henckel J, Richards R, Lozhkin K et al (2006) Very low-dose computed tomography for planning and outcome measurement in knee replacement. The imperial knee protocol. J Bone Joint Surg Br 88:1513-1518

10. Hirschmann MT, Schon S, Afifi FK et al (2012) Assessment of loading history of compartments in the knee using bone SPECT/CT: a study combining alignment and 99mTc-HDP tracer uptake/distribution patterns. J Orthop Res doi: 10.1002/jor.22206. [Epub ahead of print]

11. Hirschmann MT, Schmid R, Dhawan R et al (2011) Combined single photon emission computerized tomography and conventional computerized tomography: clinical value for the shoulder surgeons? I Int J Shoulder Surg 5:72-76

12. Sheridan BD, Ahearn N, Tasker A et al (2012) Shoulder arthroplasty. Part 1: Prosthesis terminology and classification. Clinical Radiology 67:709-715

13. Sheridan BD, Ahearn N, Tasker A et (2012) Shoulder arthroplasty. Part 2: Normal and abnormal radiographic findings. Clinical Radiology 67:716-721

14. Mackay DC, Hudson B, Williams JR (2001) Which primary shoulder and elbow replacement? A review of the results of prostheses available in the UK. Ann R Coll Surg Engl 83:258-265

15. Hirschmann MT, Konala P, Iranpour F et al (2011) Clinical value of SPECT/CT for evaluation of patients with painful knees after total knee arthroplasty–a new dimension of diagnostics? BMC Musculoskelet Disord 12:36

16. Dennis DA (2004) Evaluation of painful total knee arthroplasty. J Arthroplasty 19(4 Suppl 1):35-40

17. Shakespeare D, Ledger M, Kinzel V (2005) The influence of the tibial sagittal cut on component position in the Oxford knee. The Knee 12:169-176

18. Jeffcote B, Shakespeare D (2003) Varus/valgus alignment of the tibial component in total knee arthroplasty. The Knee 10:243-247

19. Ritter MA, Davis KE, Meding JB et al (2011) The effect of alignment and BMI on failure of total knee replacement. J Bone Joint Surg Am 93:1588-1596

20. Gemmel F, Van den Wyngaert H, Love C et al (2012) Prosthetic joint infections: radionuclide state-of-the-art imaging. Eur J Nucl Med Mol Imaging 39:892-909

21. Love C, Marwin SE, Palestro CJ (2009) Nuclear medicine and the infected joint replacement. Semin Nucl Med 39:66-78

22. Gollwitzer H, Diehl P, Gerdesmeyer L, Mittelmeier W (2006) Diagnostic strategies in cases of suspected periprosthetic infection of the knee. A review of the literature and current recommendations. Orthopade 35:904, 906-908, 910-916

23. Fuerst M, Fink B, Ruther W (2005) The value of preoperative knee aspiration and arthroscopic biopsy in revision total knee arthroplasty. Z Orthop Ihre Grenzgeb 143:36-41

# SPECT, CT and MR: Integration in Degenerative Musculoskeletal Diseases

Patrick Veit-Haibach

Department Medical Imaging, University Hospital Zurich, Zurich, Switzerland

## Introduction

In musculoskeletal degenerative disorders, physicians are often challenged by symptoms that are hard to locate precisely. Especially in the spine and the pelvis, as well as in the peripheral joints, the precise localization of the degeneration can be hard to detect. Additionally, symptoms can change during the course of time. After clinical examination, the imaging work-up usually starts with plain radiographs of different views (depending on the anatomical area); however, cross-sectional imaging modalities, such as magnetic resonance imaging (MRI), are frequently performed these days. The main advantage of MRI is the lack of radiation, the superb anatomical detail and, in contrast to single photon emission computed tomography (SPECT) and single photon emission computed tomography/computed tomography (SPECT/CT), the ability to show damage to cartilage, ligaments and tendons and other soft tissues. Thus, MRI is recommended by expert consensus opinion for use in several degenerative disorders as one of the primary diagnostic tools after plain radiographs. However, because MRI is able to show a large variety of lesions, it can be hard to evaluate those that are clinically relevant, especially when there is no adequate clinical history (a common problem in modern imaging) or when no dedicated musculoskeletal radiologist is available. As a consequence, some patients still lack an appropriate diagnosis after MRI, and hence they do not receive adequate therapy. Within recent years, hybrid SPECT/CT has emerged as a technique providing information on the morphological structure and metabolic activity of lesions, and providing an exact anatomical localization of pathological lesions. It has been shown in initial studies that SPECT/CT in selected indications can be a very valuable tool to provide a clinically relevant diagnosis or pinpoint the clinically relevant lesion to treat. It has also been shown that SPECT/CT can have higher inter- and intraobserver reliability than CT, bone scan or a combination of both in patients with different musculoskeletal degenerative disorders. SPECT/CT has also

shown the ability to monitor osseous metabolism after anterior cruciate ligament repair, as well as the degree of loading of the knee compartments with consecutive osteoarthritis. Additionally, also compared with MRI, SPECT/CT has been found to be helpful, for example, in hand and wrist pain as well as treatment decisions for osteochondral lesions. Finally, there are upcoming initial trials that are integrating CT-arthrography into SPECT/CT to provide a full diagnostic, hybrid method for evaluation of bony morphology and osseous metabolism, as well as soft-tissue-like cartilage surface structure and ligaments.

Here, we provide an overview on the strengths and weaknesses of SPECT/CT and MRI in degenerative disorders. We concentrate mainly on the upcoming indications of SPECT/CT, partly in comparison with MRI, since the (dis)advantages of MRI are already well known, and there are more upcoming indications in the current literature concerning the use of SPECT/CT in the diagnostic work-up.

## Clinical Indications

### Spine

A lot of literature reports have been published about the value of SPECT/CT in spine imaging and evaluation. However, one of the problems in comparing SPECT/CT and MRI directly is the lack of a robust base of comparative studies of those two modalities. The advantages of MRI are manifold: detection of bone edema as a sign of mechanical loading, visualization of the nerves and nerve roots and the cause of their compression, and spinal cysts and fatty lesions, as well as vascular malformation, to name a few. However, the evaluation of the severity of degenerative spine or facet joint lesions remains challenging, partly because of nonspecificity of symptoms, and partly because of the high number of imaging findings [1]. SPECT and SPECT/CT, on the other hand, have been

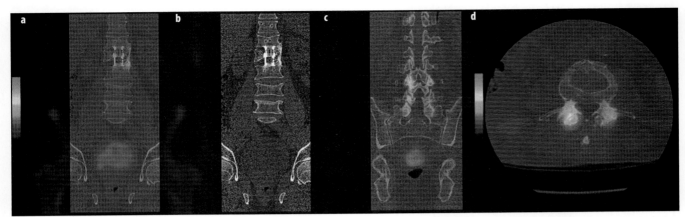

**Fig. 1 a-d.** Patient with a fracture of Th12 and consecutive cage interposition. **a** Coronal single photon emission computed tomography/computed tomography (SPECT/CT), **b** coronal CT. There is slight activity at the left lateral osseous bridge between Th12 and L1 indicating noncomplete bridging. **c** Coronal SPECT/CT, **d** axial SPECT/CT. There is additional uptake in the right facet joint of L2/3, indicating infrafusional activated arthrosis. SPECT/CT shows a higher degree of activation compared with CT, where there is no major difference morphologically concerning the degree of arthrosis (for color reproduction see p 314)

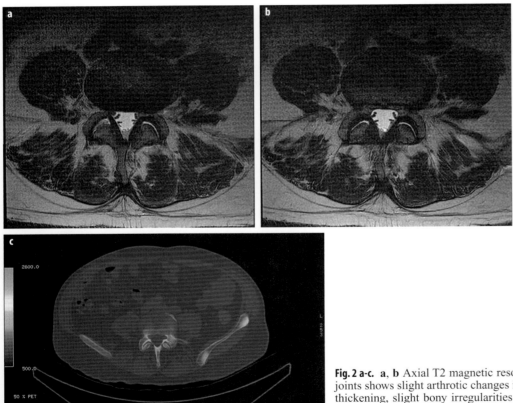

**Fig. 2 a-c. a, b** Axial T2 magnetic resonance imaging of the L4/5 facet joints shows slight arthrotic changes in both facet joints, with synovial thickening, slight bony irregularities and minimal fluid. **c** The corresponding axial single photon emission computed tomography/computed tomography (SPECT/CT) shows no activation (for color reproduction see p 315)

proven to have a role in spondylodesis, spondylosis and facet pain (Fig. 1). One study included 534 patients, of which 486 patients (91.1%) had at least one positive abnormality on SPECT scan. This included 42.8% increased uptake in the facet joint, and 29.8% in the vertebral bodies/end plates. Focal uptake in the facets in the cervical spine also increases with age [2]. MRI findings have been found to partly correlate with SPECT findings: irregular and thickened facet synovia, intra-articular fluid, synovial disturbance and intra-articular facet material have been shown to correlate with abnormalities on SPECT scan (Fig. 2). It has also been shown that the metabolic information derived from SPECT has a prognostic value concerning the prediction of response to intra-articular facet injections in the lumbar spine [3, 4]. Positive SPECT-CT images can predict clinical improvement in up to 91% of patients and can also show an alternative cause of pain in some cases, such as new fractures or multiple coexisting fractures, persisting bone remodeling in a previous cemented vertebra, and facet or discal degenerative disease [5]. SPECT/CT can not only predict outcome in infiltrative procedures, but also in surgical procedures, e.g., loosening of metallic implants (screws, cages). SPECT has been shown to be superior to CT for imaging of facet joint arthritis. Kalichman et al. reported that there is no correlation between facet joint arthritis identified by CT scan and low back pain in a community-based study population, and 62.7% of their population had facet joint arthritis on CT scan [6, 7]. SPECT/CT in these patients can differentiate between mechanical loading in the adjacent segments (e.g., in spondylodesis) and joints, continuing bone remodeling and loosening of the implants. In the latter cases, especially, CT is significantly impaired because of the presence of metallic artefacts. However, several techniques in MRI are currently being evaluated, and these should significantly improve MRI of metallic implants.

## Pelvis/Hip

There are clear differences, as well as some overlap, concerning MRI and SPECT/CT in pelvic and hip degenerations. MRI is mainly used for evaluation of the cartilage of the acetabulum and femoral head, for the evaluation of femoral acetabular impingements, as well as for the evaluation of the surrounding soft tissue structures. Enthesiopathies of the gluteal muscles attached to the greater trochanter, as well as evaluation of avascular necrosis (AVN) of the femoral head, especially in the pediatric population, are shown well by MRI. SPEC/CT can show some information about AVN, but the main indication for SPECT and SPECT/CT is degenerative osteoarthritis and prosthesis evaluation. However, there are studies indicating that SPECT/CT can also be used to assess viability of the femoral head. In a study by McMahon et al., the usefulness of SPECT/CT after Birmingham hip resurfacing was evaluated [8]. After the procedure, all study patients fell into category N (normal) (i.e., activity with the Birmingham prosthesis was 60-85% of activity shown with the normal contralateral femoral head). This was interpreted as preserved vascularity. Also in three patients with preoperative segmental AVN, scans were evaluated as category N (normal). There was no visual evidence of AVN of the femoral head during the average follow-up of 26 months. Thus, SPECT was able to show the preserved intra-osseous blood supply, probably based on the metaphyseal vessels in these arthritic hips. This important ability of SPECT/CT has also been shown in experimental studies in which stepwise artificial damage was inflicted on the structure supplying blood to the femoral

head and neck. As a result, SPECT/CT identified the group in which the femoral head turned avascular and necrotic. The decrease in perfusion after the operation and the return to normal supply levels were also monitored. Thus, SPECT/CT was able to assess the perfusion of the femoral head semiquantitatively, which might be useful in predicting the development of traumatic AVN [9]. However, there are experimentally and clinically established techniques in MRI that can show the same results as those with SPECT/CT in such patients [10]. The advantage of SPECT/CT in those patients might be that the patient has a shorter examination time (SPECT/CT can be done in 8 min). Furthermore, no research protocols are needed; the evaluation can be done within routine clinical protocols. By far the largest and most important indication is the evaluation of hip prosthesis (infection versus loosening) in patients with recurrent or ongoing pain after surgery. First, one has to determine the physiologic uptake pattern after implantation of a hip prosthesis. Generally, cemented implants can have surrounding physiological uptake up to 1 year after surgery. In uncemented implants, physiological uptake of longer than 1 year has been described as not unusual, and should not lead to an incorrect diagnosis of loosening. Early studies showed that bone scan and conventional X-ray should be evaluated in consensus, since this can increase the sensitivity in detecting prosthetic loosening (combined evaluation: sensitivity 84%, specificity 92%) [11]. When evaluating SPECT/CT in patients with suspected mechanical loosening, SPECT/CT was significantly better than planar scanning for the acetabular cup, but not for the femoral stem [12]. The advantage of current state-of-the art SPECT/CT compared with X-ray and bone scan side-by-side is of course the higher resolution, exact anatomical localization of the increased bony uptake, as well as the morphological information from CT. This additional component allows for more precise evaluation of additional causes of hip pain, e.g., periprosthetic fractures, osteolyses and heterotopic ossifications (Fig. 3). Consequently, planning of possible subsequent surgery can be determined and planned more precisely [13].

## Knee

MRI is the primary diagnostic modality in a wide range of indications in degenerative knee disorders. In particular, it shows soft tissue injuries such as meniscal tears, anterior cruciate ligament (ACL) and posterior cruciate ligament (PCL) (partial) tears, as well as cartilage thinning or erosions, with high sensitivity and accuracy. Diagnosis in most of the patients with these knee disorders is carried out primarily with MRI. However, SPECT/CT has a role in selected indications in knee disorders. Evaluation of (over)loading of knee compartments and subsequent correlation with the underlying cartilage conditions has been demonstrated in a study with 100 cases. A statistically very significant relationship was demonstrated between SPECT and the macroscopic cartilage

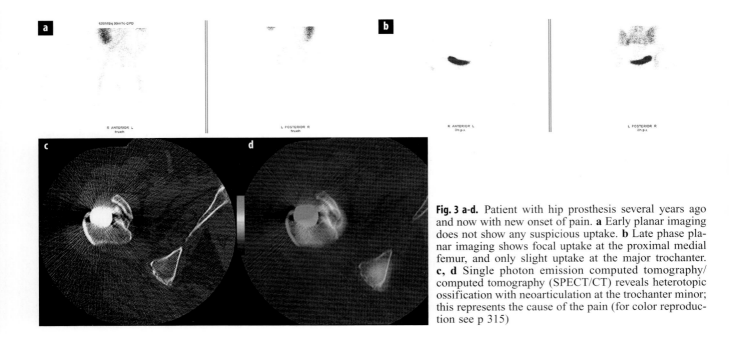

**Fig. 3 a-d.** Patient with hip prosthesis several years ago and now with new onset of pain. **a** Early planar imaging does not show any suspicious uptake. **b** Late phase planar imaging shows focal uptake at the proximal medial femur, and only slight uptake at the major trochanter. **c, d** Single photon emission computed tomography/ computed tomography (SPECT/CT) reveals heterotopic ossification with neoarticulation at the trochanter minor; this represents the cause of the pain (for color reproduction see p 315)

condition at surgery. SPECT excluded significant chondral changes (grade II-IV) with a sensitivity rate of 97%. The sensitivity of SPECT scans in detecting severe chondral lesions was 100% (medially). Overall, a SPECT bone scan provides very useful information regarding the degree of osteoarthritis in weight-bearing compartments of the knee for pre-operative planning [14]. Similar findings have been shown in several other studies that demonstrated that pre-arthroscopic or presurgical evaluation of the degree of osteoarthritis with SPECT and SPECT/CT was reliable and helpful concerning the planning of the procedure. In particular, the medial compartment can be investigated with high accuracy. Jeer et al. described significant associations between scan findings and osteoarthritis in all compartments of the knee ($P <0.05$); however, the strongest association was demonstrated in the medial compartment, while the weakest association was found in the patella-femoral compartment and lateral tibial plateau. Thus, the study found SPECT to be particularly helpful in the planning of medial tibiofemoral unicompartimental arthroplasty to confirm unicompartmental disease [15]. Correlations between the osteoarthritis and increased tracer uptake in the associated compartment were demonstrated, and correlation of the degree of osteoarthritis with the degree of tracer uptake was also established in several studies. In one study, a positive and statistically significant correlation was found between the intensity of uptake on SPECT and the severity of the arthroscopic findings in the menisci and medial femoral condyle. An $r$ value of 0.663 ($P <0.001$) was shown for the medial meniscus, an $r$ value of 0.67 ($P <0.001$) for the lateral meniscus, and an $r$ value of 0.7 ($P <0.001$) for the medial femoral condyle, indicating that the uptake

intensity positively correlated with the severity of pathology seen at arthroscopy [16]. Furthermore, the intensity of the tracer uptake correlated with the degree of malalignment, and thus SPECT/CT reflects the specific loading pattern of the knee with regard to its alignment. In the postoperative setting, SPECT/CT has also proved to be useful for a variety of indications. Interestingly, when evaluating patients after ACL repair, tracer uptake on SPECT/CT showed no correlation with instability, pivot shift or clinical laxity testing. However, the tracer uptake correlated significantly with the position and orientation of the ACL graft (e.g., a more horizontal femoral graft position showed significantly increased tracer uptake within the superior and posterior femoral regions, and a more posteriorly placed femoral insertion site showed significantly more tracer uptake within the femoral and tibial tunnel regions etc.). Thus, SPECT/CT tracer uptake intensity and distribution showed a significant correlation with the femoral and tibial tunnel position and orientation in patients with symptomatic knees after ACL reconstruction [17]. In another study that investigated the use of SPECT for displaying bone remodeling after knee arthroplasty, there was a significant correlation between 12-month SPECT uptake and preceding bone marrow density change in the medial tibia ($r = 0.5$, $P = 0.044$) [18]. At 12 months, SPECT uptake in the operated knee was notably higher compared with that of the control knee. SPECT uptake showed a statistically significant decrease from 12 months to 24 months, while SPECT uptake in the control knee remained stable. The authors concluded that increased SPECT uptake during the first 2 years after uncomplicated total knee arthroplasty is most likely to be a result of normal postoperative bone remodeling. A leveling of SPECT uptake might indicate a new balance between bone loss and regain [18]. Lastly, in another study SPECT/CT was able to change the suspected diagnosis and consequent treatment in a significant number of patients with painful knee arthroplasty. SPECT/CT imaging changed the suspected diagnosis and the proposed treatment in 19/23 (83%) knees based on, for example, identifying progression of osteoarthritis or loosening, and thus it proved to be a helpful tool in establishing the diagnosis and guiding subsequent management [19]. There has recently been a further technical development with the introduction of SPECT/CT arthrography, which overcomes the drawbacks of SPECT/CT compared with MRI by making it possible to evaluate osteochondral lesions, meniscal tears, loose bodies and tears of the cruciate ligaments [20].

## Foot/Ankle

Because of the complex anatomy, the evaluation of osseous lesions of the foot and ankle presents clinical and diagnostic challenges. Currently, as in the aforementioned indications, MRI is the imaging gold standard, especially for soft tissue lesions. Detailed, high-resolution imaging can be done on a routine basis to evaluate joint cartilage, tendons, ligaments, fascial and neuronal pathologies, impingement syndromes and stress fractures. Although bone marrow edema (a misnomer) is very nonspecific, it contributes to the diagnosis of the underlying pathology [21]. However, one of the main problems of MRI in general is its nonspecificity. In several studies and in several anatomical locations, SPECT/CT has been shown to have higher specificity as well as higher intraobserver and interobserver agreement, which is important in clinical investigations for which there is no specific musculoskeletal radiologist available. In patients with osteoarthritis of the foot and ankle, SPECT/CT has demonstrated a significantly superior intraobserver diagnostic precision for the site of active arthritis. The mean intraobserver reliability for SPECT/CT was excellent ($\kappa = 0.86$; 95% confidence interval 0.81 to 0.88) and significantly higher than that for CT and bone scanning combined. The authors concluded that SPECT/CT was a very useful imaging tool in localizing active arthritis, especially when the configuration of joints is complex [22]. Also in direct comparison with MRI, SPECT/CT proved to be partly superior in evaluation of the activity of osteochondral lesions of the talus. SPECT/CT helped preoperative planning by identifying the exact location of the active lesion, especially in multifocal disease or revision surgeries, while showing the depth of the active lesion. Patients had partly conservative treatment instead of surgery due to minimal or no activity at the evaluated lesion. In comparison, repeat MRI in this group (new onset of pain) confirmed the diagnosis of an osteochondral lesion, but did not provide further meaningful information. Also in the group of patients who did not undergo operation, while SPECT

made a diagnosis of a nonactive osteochondral lesion, MRI provided only a "morphological" diagnosis without helpful information about the activity of the lesion [23]. Other studies have confirmed the influence of SPECT/CT in comparison with MRI in these patients. In comparison with MRI alone, treatment decision making was changed in 48% of cases with SPECT/CT alone, and 52% with SPECT/CT and MRI combined. While interpretation of cartilage shows good correlation between MRI and SPECT/CT, assessment of the subchondral bone plate and subchondral bone has shown substantial differences in correlation that highlight the different information provided by these imaging techniques. Overall, compared with MRI, SPECT/CT provides additional information and influences the decision making of osteochondral lesion treatment and therefore it might be useful to perform both procedures. Lastly, SPECT/CT has been found to be useful in guidance of local infiltration in patients with foot and ankle pain. When infiltrating the area with elevated tracer uptake, a response rate of 90% could be achieved. When assessing the agreement on pain-initiating structures determined by standard clinical assessment versus SPECT/CT, a disagreement in 16 of 30 (53%) cases was found, especially in patients with pain in the midfoot. Thus, SPECT/CT had a higher predictive value of the clinical outcome than the clinical assessment. In the clinical setting, SPECT/CT might overrule the clinical assessment in cases where there is disagreement on the target lesion [24].

## Shoulder/Elbow

Currently, there is a lack of systematic data available concerning the use of SPECT/CT in the shoulder and elbow, and there are very few comparisons with MRI. Again, MRI has significant indications in shoulder imaging, e.g., evaluation of the glenoid cartilage and tendons and muscles of the rotator cuff, as well as the acromioclavicular joint, surrounding bursae and ligaments; therefore, it is considered to be the primary imaging modality and gold standard of shoulder imaging. There are only few case series that have shown, for example, that SPECT/CT can show loosening and – vice versa – exclusion of loosening of a shoulder prosthesis. However, one large study evaluated the usefulness of SPECT/CT in patients with suspected shoulder impingement. The patients who were diagnosed as having impingement syndrome, with or without rotator cuff tear, showed increased uptake on the operated side compared with the nonoperated side at several locations that were assessed. The greater tuberosity of the humerus could be used for quantitative measurement as a postoperative prognostic factor [25].

## Hand/Wrist

MRI findings for the hand and wrist are similar to those described above for the spine and the ankle. MRI has the major advantage of showing early damage to intra-

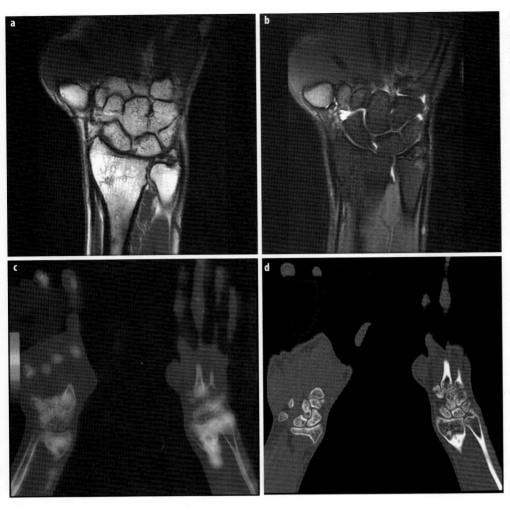

**Fig. 4 a-d.** Patient with status post-fracture of the left forearm. Osteosynthesis material has already been removed; however, the patient continues to have pain at the proximal wrist. Magnetic resonance imaging shows the consolidated forearm fracture that ends in the distal radioulnar joint (DRUJ). Additionally, there are bony irregularities in the DRUJ and the cartilage is thinned (**a** coronal T, **b** coronal proton density fat-saturated). Single photon emission computed tomography/computed tomography (SPECT/CT) shows that there is still elevated uptake in the distal forearm, representing ongoing bone remodeling. Additionally, there is uptake in the DRUJ, an indication that there is arthrosis starting to occur here also (**c** coronal SPECT/CT, **d** coronal CT) (for color reproduction see p 316)

and extra-articular soft tissue such as cartilage, ligaments and tendons, and this is often the reason for wrist pain [26]. Late consequences of soft tissue damage such as structural bone alterations and calcification of tendons and cartilage can be shown by both CT and MRI. Again, based on the variety of lesions shown by MRI, the main problem remains nonspecificity. There are now upcoming data from patients with several degenerative disorders of the hand and wrist that show that SPECT/CT can be of additional help.

In a study that compared SPECT/CT and MRI in patients with nonspecific pain (a challenging clinical condition), MRI yielded a high sensitivity (0.86), but a low specificity (0.20). In contrast, SPECT/CT yielded a high specificity (1.00) and a low sensitivity (0.71) in the detection of the leading clinical pathology. Thus, the two imaging procedures might be complementary in such patients (Fig. 4) [27]. In another study evaluating a similar patient population, SPECT/CT showed the highest accuracy as well as the highest interobserver agreement. The most accurate modality for experienced readers was SPECT/CT (77% accuracy, 90% specificity, 74% sensi-

tivity), followed by MRI (56% accuracy, 10% specificity, 65% sensitivity). The interobserver agreement of experienced readers was generally higher with SPECT/CT for lesion detection ($\kappa$ = 0.93, MRI = 0.72), localization ($\kappa$ = 0.91, MRI = 0.75) and etiology ($\kappa$ = 0.85, MRI = 0.74), while MRI yielded better results for typing of lesions ($\kappa$ = 0.75, SPECT/CT = 0.69) [28]. Significant influence on clinical decisions has also been shown in clinical practice [29]. SPECT/CT showed higher lesion detection rates compared with standard X-rays and planar bone scan. A significant impact on patient management was demonstrated in 37% of the patient population. The authors concluded that SPECT/CT might be added to the diagnostic work-up in those patients for whom standard imaging fails to detect the main pathology [29]. SPECT/CT arthrography has also been introduced recently. Such an approach combines the advantages of CT arthrography with the metabolic component of SPECT. Therefore disorders that are generally diagnosed by MRI can be detected by SPECT/CT, possibly providing additional specificity concerning the activity of the lesion [30, 31].

# References

1. Laker SR, Concannon LG (2011) Radiologic evaluation of the neck: a review of radiography, ultrasonography, computed tomography, magnetic resonance imaging, and other imaging modalities for neck pain. Phys Med Rehabil Clin N Am 22:411-428

2. Makki D, Khazim R, Zaidan AA et al (2010) Single photon emission computerized tomography (SPECT) scan-positive facet joints and other spinal structures in a hospital-wide population with spinal pain. Spine J 10:58-62

3. Dolan AL, Ryan PJ, Arden NK et al (1996) The value of SPECT scans in identifying backpain likely to benefit from facet joint injection. Br J Rheumatol 35:1269-1273

4. Pneumaticos SG, Chatziioannou SN, Hipp JA et al (2006) Low back pain: prediction of short-term outcome of facet joint injection with bone scintigraphy. Radiology 238:693-698

5. Solá M, Pérez R, Cuadras P (2011) Value of bone SPECT-CT to predict chronic pain relief after percutaneous vertebroplasty in vertebral fractures. Spine J 11:1102-1107

6. Kalichman L, Li L, Kim DH et al (2008) Facet joint osteoarthritis and low back pain in the community-based population. Spine 33:2560-2565

7. Damgaard M, Nimb L, Madsen JL (2010) The role of bone SPECT/CT in the evaluation of lumbar spinal fusion with metallic fixation devices. Clin Nucl Med 35:234-236

8. McMahon S, Young D, Ballok Z ((2006) Vascularity of the femoral head after Birmingham hip resurfacing. A technetium tc 99m bone scan/ single photon emission computed tomography study. J Arthroplasty 21:514-521

9. Shen F, Yan ZQ, Guo CA et al (2011) Prediction of traumatic avascular necrosis of the femoral head by single photon emission computerized tomography and computerized tomography: an experimental study in dogs. Chin J Traumatol 14:227-232

10. Ehlinger M, Moser T, Adam P (2011) Early prediction of femoral head avascular necrosis following neck fracture. Orthop Traumatol Surg Res 97:79-88

11. Aliabadi P, Tumeh SS, Weissman BN et al (1989). Cemented total hip prosthesis: radiographic and scintigraphic evaluation. Radiology 173:203-206

12. Chew CG, Lewis P, Middleton F et al (2010). Radionuclide arthrogram with SPECT/CT for the evaluation of mechanical loosening of hip and knee prostheses. Ann Nucl Med 24:735-743

13. Strobel K, Steurer-Dober I, Huellner MW et al (2012) Importance of SPECT/CT for knee and hip joint prostheses. Radiologe 52:629-635

14. Hart R, Konvicka M, Filan P et al (2008) SPECT scan is a reliable tool for selection of patients undergoing unicompartmental knee arthroplasty. Arch Orthop Trauma Surg 128:679-682

15. Jeer PJ, Mahr CC, Keene GC et al (2006) Single photon emission computed tomography in planning unicompartmental knee arthroplasty. A prospective study examining the association between scan findings and intraoperative assessment of osteoarthritis. Knee 13:19-25

16. Siegel Y, Golan H, Thein R (2006) 99mTc-methylene diphosphonate single photon emission tomography of the knees: intensity of uptake and its correlation with arthroscopic findings. Nucl Med Commun 27:689-693

17. Hirschmann MT, Mathis D, Rasch H et al (2012) SPECT/CT tracer uptake is influenced by tunnel orientation and position of the femoral and tibial ACL graft insertion site. Int Orthop [Epub ahead of print]

18. Soininvaara T, Nikola T, Vanninen E et al (2008) Bone mineral density and single photon emission computed tomography changes after total knee arthroplasty: a 2-year follow-up study. Clin Physiol Funct Imaging 28:101-106

19. Hirschmann MT, Konala P, Iranpour F (2011) Clinical value of SPECT/CT for evaluation of patients with painful knees after total knee arthroplasty—a new dimension of diagnostics? BMC Musculoskelet Disord 12:36

20. Strobel K, Wiesmann R, Tornquist K (2012) SPECT/CT arthrography of the knee. Eur J Nucl Med Mol Imaging 39:1975-1976

21. Nathan M, Mohan H, Vijayanathan S (2012) The role of 99mTc-diphosphonate bone SPECT/CT in the ankle and foot. Nucl Med Commun 33:799-807

22. Pagenstert GI, Barg A, Leumann AG et al (2009) SPECT-CT imaging in degenerative joint disease of the foot and ankle. J Bone Joint Surg Br 91:1191-1196

23. Meftah M, Katchis SD, Scharf SC et al (2011) SPECT/CT in the management of osteochondral lesions of the talus. Foot Ankle Int 32:233-238

24. Kretzschmar M, Wiewiorski M, Rasch H et al (2011) 99mTc-DPD-SPECT/CT predicts the outcome of imaging-guided diagnostic anaesthetic injections: a prospective cohort study. Eur J Radiol 80:e410-5

25. Park JY, Park SG, Keum JS et al (2009) The diagnosis and prognosis of impingement syndrome in the shoulder with using quantitative SPECT assessment: a prospective study of 73 patients and 24 volunteers. Clin Orthop Surg 1:194-200

26. Zanetti M, Bram J, Hodler J (1997) Triangular fibrocartilage and intercarpal ligaments of the wrist: does MR arthrography improve standard MRI? J Magn Reson Imaging 7:590-594

27. Huellner MW, Bürkert A, Schleich FS (2012) SPECT/CT versus MRI in patients with nonspecific pain of the hand and wrist – a pilot study. Eur J Nucl Med Mol Imaging 39:750-759

28. Hüllner M, Perez-Lago M, Strobel K (2012) Interobserver variability in SPECT/CT, MRI, CT, bone scan and plain radiographs in patients with unspecific wrist pain. In: Proceedings of the 25th Annual EANM Congress, October 27-31, 2012, Milan, Italy

29. Schleich FS, Schürch M, Huellner MW (2012) Diagnostic and therapeutic impact of SPECT/CT in patients with unspecific pain of the hand and wrist. EJNMMI Res 2:53

30. De Filippo M, Pogliacomi F, Bertellini A (2010) MDCT arthrography of the wrist: diagnostic accuracy and indications. Eur J Radiol 74:221-225

31. Krüger T, Hug U, Hüllner MW (2011) SPECT/CT arthrography of the wrist in ulnocarpal impaction syndrome. Eur J Nucl Med Mol Imaging 38:79

# Scintigraphy of Primary and Metastatic Tumors

Mark E. Schweitzer

Department of Medical Imaging, University of Ottawa, Ottawa, ON, Canada

## Metastatic Tumors

The most common indication for bone scintigraphy in tertiary care centers is a concern for metastatic disease. This should be done only in patients who have a high risk of metastatic disease, as false-positive examinations and little useful diagnostic yield occur in patients who are at low risk. Consequently, most patients with breast and prostate cancer should not receive a bone scan for work-up of metastatic disease.

When one is presented with an abnormal scintigram, correlation with plain film should nearly always be performed. If there is no benign explanation for the finding on conventional radiography, it is presumed to be a metastasis. If clinical quandary still exists, computed tomography (CT) can be used, in rare occasions only. Even rarer, yet, would be the need for magnetic resonance imaging (MRI) for confirmation.

In most cases, the pattern of metastatic disease would be a tip off, and most of the time the pattern on scintigraphy is characterized by multiple areas in the axial skeleton that show variable shape, variable size and variable intensity (Fig. 1).

The location should be predominantly axial, and when in long bones mostly in the proximal metaphyses. Eighty percent of patients have axial involvement, 50% in the spine, and less commonly in the cervical spine. Thirty percent have lesions in the pelvis, 20% in ribs and 15-20% in the skull. Long bone involvement is also seen in 15% of patients.

If one sees more distal metastases as well as proximal metastases, one should have a higher suspicion for an anemia causing redistribution of red marrow more distally. Distal lesions can also be seen in lung and, less commonly, breast cancer.

When presented with an image where there is a single isolated area that might be a metastatic deposit, our recommendation is to do another more sensitive examination to see if there are multiple deposits elsewhere. Only approximately 15% of these deposits are found to be

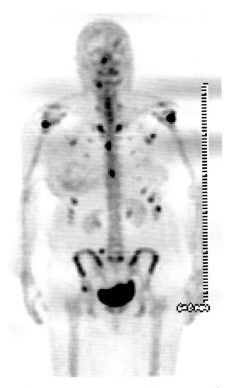

**Fig. 1.** Delayed whole body scintigram demonstrates the typical axial locations for metastatic disease

metastases. The next most sensitive test will be positron emission tomography (PET) scanning most often or, in different centers, whole body MRI. In the majority of cases these focal deposits will be multifocal when a more sensitive test is performed.

Diffuse osseous metastatic disease is termed skeletal carcinomatosis, and it is usually related to a breast or a prostate primary. On PET or skeletal scinitgraphy, a superscan is seen. The superscan is characterized by lack of renal uptake, more intense skull and metaphyseal

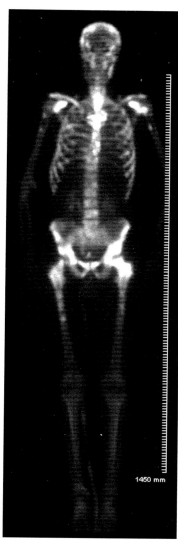

**Fig. 2.** Superscan in breast metastases with metaphyseal and skull increased uptake, and relative lack of renal and soft tissue uptake

activity, and less than usual soft tissue uptake (Fig. 2). Somewhat surprisingly, these patients can survive for a moderate amount of time.

Very rarely will metastatic deposits be cold on bone scan. Most often these are hypervascular, quite destructive lesions that yield little reactive bone formation in the natural history. The most commonly described primaries include renal cell cancer, occasional thyroid cancer and occasional colon cancer. On radiography, one will see a very lytic blown out lesion, sometimes with an accompanying soft tissue mass.

Follow-up of potentially treated metastases by scintigraphy is troublesome. It is easy when lesions are smaller or go away. However, increased activity might not represent worsening disease. On skeletal scanning, the flair phenomenon might be noted, with falsely increased activity in previously seen lesions. Usually no new locations are noted. However, very subtle lesions can heal and show the flair phenomenon and thus look like new lesions. This appearance usually reverts back to normal after about 3 months. Unfortunately, this is often too long to alter treatment, and other follow-up imaging, such as PET or MRI, is used.

## PET Scanning

PET scanning should be rarely used in the initial evaluation of metastatic disease, not because it is not accurate, but because it is usually overkill. Sometimes when a PET scan is suggested, an MRI can be done at lower cost and with higher sensitivity. In addition, PET scanning is often less useful for less biologically aggressive metastases, such as some prostate metastases and breast metastases.

However, PET scanning is useful when there are indeterminate bone scintigram findings for metastatic disease or when a whole body PET scan is done for total body staging, including both the osseous and the nonosseous portions of anatomy. The distribution is as described above for scintigraphy, and characterized by similarly variable size, variable shape and variable intensity. When a single lesion is seen on PET scanning, a focal MRI of that area should be done. If the MRI is still nonspecific, then whole body marrow imaging should be performed. There are specific false-positive lesions on PET scanning that are more common than on scinitgraphy; thus closer radiologic correlation is often needed. This can usually be done via the concomitant CT. False-positive causes of PET scanning are protean, related to its high sensitivity and include arthroses, Paget's disease, stress injuries and benign tumors.

F18 PET scanning is useful as a higher-sensitivity bone scan and gives a similar appearance for osteoblastic disease.

Most whole body bone scans performed for metastatic disease should be accompanied by transaxial single photon emission computed tomography (SPECT) imaging accompanied by CT. This enables better localization, as well as correlation with CT findings. As better quality CT scanners become increasingly available with both SPECT cameras and PET scanners, direct comparison and the knowledge required for this is becoming increasingly necessary.

## Multiple Myeloma

The more subtle the imaging findings of myeloma, the more indolent is the course of the disease. However, many patients carry a diagnosis of monogammopathy of unknown origin and these patients need to be evaluated for long periods of time. Traditionally, radiography of the skeleton performed every 6-12 months has been used to follow these patients to see if they develop osteolytic lesions. More recently, many of these patients get PET scan, whole body MRI or both.

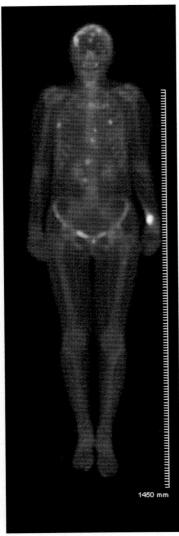

**Fig. 3.** Mutifocal uptake is seen in the spine, ribs and pelvis secondary to multiple myeloma

Traditionally on scintigraphy, one-third of myeloma is hot, one-third is cold and one-third is normal; currently, probably 50% is hot with improved scanners, by scintigraphy (Fig. 3).

The PET findings in myeloma can be relatively subtle, with limited increased standard uptake values demonstrated. When this is seen, the myeloma is relatively less virulent and corresponds to a salt and pepper pattern on MRI, with a preponderance of salt and not much pepper.

## Primary Tumors

Both primary benign and malignant osseous tumors can have abnormal scintigraphic findings. Triple phase scintigraphy should be performed in all suspected primary bone tumors, and if there is a possibility that the find-

ings are related to an atypical metastasis then delayed whole body imaging is suggested.

The primary tumors that show increased flow include aggressive osseous tumors and relatively benign but hypervascular medullary tumors such as osteoid-osteoma, chondroblastoma and osteoblastoma. The first of these will demonstrate the double donut sign on delayed imaging, where a center area of quite increased uptake is noted, surrounded by an area along the periphery of moderately increased uptake.

Fibrous dysplasia demonstrates one of the more variable scintigraphic appearances, with occasionally abnormal flow, and approximately one-third of patients showing intense on delayed uptake, similar to osteoid osteomas. Obviously, osteosarcomas and chondrosarcomas show uptake that is relatively proportional to their histologic grade.

When a patient has a malignant primary tumor, a scintigram can be done to look for skip lesions. This is really useful for osteosarcomas only, and, to a large degree, MRI has replaced this need. However many of these patients undergo whole body PET scanning, which has a secondary gain of seeing secondary skeletal lesions, but more importantly determining whether there is lung and, to a lesser degree, liver and brain spread.

In a similar fashion, soft tissue sarcomas can benefit from whole body PET scanning.

Benign tumors that demonstrate little scintigraphic uptake include giant cell tumors, unicameral bone cyst and nonossifying fibromas. In these cases, the scintigram can be used to see if a secondary fracture is present. If uptake is significantly increased a pathologic fracture is likely present.

The scintigraphic findings of most primary tumors can be extrapolated from their well-known radiographic appearances. However, several points need to be kept in mind. First, geographic precision, combined with knowledge of the age and gender of the patient, significantly lowers the differential diagnosis the most. Second, CT correlative images of the ribs, transverse processes and clavicle are the hardest to read. Third, if the CT images show no definite cause of the abnormal uptake, it is more likely to be malignant. Fourth, myeloma is often best seen on CT as multiple small holes, easiest to demonstrate at the vertebral endplates; uptake on scintigraphy will be minimal, and only subtle changes will be seen in PET in this situation. Last, window carefully when looking at the CT images and measure Houndsfield units as a window into tissue typing.

MRI correlation will be more frequently performed in the future as PET/MRI becomes more widespread.

## Suggested Reading

Brenner AI, Koshy J, Morey J et al (2012) The bone scan. Semin Nucl Med 42:11-26

Britton KE (2002) Nuclear Medicine imaging in bone metastases. Cancer Imaging 2:84-86

Buchbender C, Heusner TA, Lauenstein TC et al (2012) Oncologic PET/MRI, part 2: bone tumors, soft-tissue tumors, melanoma, and lymphoma. J Nucl Med 53:1244-1252

Ebert W, Muley T, Herb KP, Schmidt-Gayk H (2004) Comparison of bone scintigraphy with bone markers in the diagnosis of bone metastasis in lung carcinoma patients. Anticancer Res 24:3193-3201

Hahn S, Heusner T, Kümmel S et al (2011) Comparison of FDG-PET/CT and bone scintigraphy for detection of bone metastases in breast cancer. Acta Radiol 52:1009-1114

Healy CF, Murray JG, Eustace SJ et al (2011 Multiple myeloma: a review of imaging features and radiological techniques. Bone Marrow Research doi:10.1155/2011/583439

Koizumi M, Ogata E (2002) Bone metabolic markers as gauges of metastasis to bone: a review. Annals of Nuclear Medicine 16:161-168

Masriani G, Bruselli L, Kuwert T et al (2010) A review on the clinical uses of SPECT/CT. Eur J Nucl Med Mol Imaging 37:1959-1985

Narayanan V, Koshy C (2009) Metastatic bone disease – a review of literature. Austral-Asian Journal of Cancer 8:257-268

Zelinka T, Timmers HJ, Kozupa A et al (2008) Role of positron emission tomography and bone scintigraphy in the evaluation of bone involvement in metastatic pheochomocytoma and paraganglioma: specific implications for succinate dehydrogenase enzyme subunit B gene mutations. Endocr Relat Cancer 15:311-323

# PEDIATRIC RADIOLOGY SATELLITE COURSE "KANGAROO"

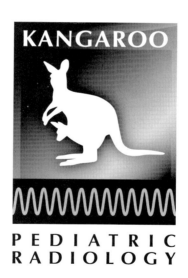

# Imaging of Juvenile Idiopathic Arthritis

Karen Rosendahl

Department of Pediatric Radiology, Haukeland University Hospital, Bergen, Norway

## Introduction

Juvenile idiopathic arthritis (JIA) is a heterogeneous condition including all forms of chronic arthritis of unknown origin, duration ≥6 weeks and with onset before 16 years of age. It is characterized by chronic synovial inflammation with potential risk of developing progressive joint destruction and serious functional disability [1-4]. It affects around 1 in 1,000 children under the age of 16 [5-8]. Typically, the child presents with a history of morning stiffness, vague pain and one or more swollen joints.

Recent research has shown that adult disease is seen in up to 75% of those having suffered JIA during childhood [9]. Moreover, the temporomandibular joint (TMJ) is involved in up to 70% of patients; in a high proportion it is overt and thus not treated specifically [10]. This may lead to pubertal growth disturbances of the TMJs, including restricted mandibular growth [9, 11, 12], with development of malocclusion and facial deformities [13]. Assessment of the TMJs, with treatment of those testing positive, has therefore become an important issue in management of children with JIA. The new understanding of JIA being more aggressive than previously believed and the introduction of new disease-modifying drugs have led to earlier and more aggressive treatment, and have fuelled the search for more accurate disease markers to better monitor therapeutic response.

## Classification

Based on clinical and laboratory findings, JIA is currently subdivided to include [14-16] (Table 1):

**Table 1.** Subgroups of juvenile idiopathic arthritis

| Subset of JIA | Frequency (%) | Age at onset | Clinical characteristics | Male/females |
|---|---|---|---|---|
| Oligo | 27-56 | Early childhood, peak 2-4 years | Four or fewer joints involved the first 6 months; lower extremity more often affected, generally good prognosis, worse prognosis if more than four joints affected after 6 months (extended oligo JIA); risk of developing iridocyclitis | F>>>M |
| Poly, RF negative | 11-28 | Early peak 2-4 years, late peak 6-12 years | Four of more joints involved the first 6 months, absence of IgM RF; heterogeneous disease with three subsets; prognosis varies with the disease subset | F>>M |
| Poly, RF positive | 2-7 | Late childhood to adolescence | Four or more joints involved the first 6 months, IgM RF positive; resembles adult rheumatoid arthritis. Involvement of small joints; progressive and diffuse joint involvement | F>>M |
| Entethesis-related arthritis | 3-11 | Late childhood to adolescence | Characterized by entesitis and arthritis. Often HLA-B27 positive; commonly hip involvement at presentation; often a mild and remitting course but may progress with sacroiliac and spinal joint involvement, resembling ankylosing spondylitis | M>>F |
| Psoriatic | 2-11 | Early peak 2-4 years, late peak 9-11 years | Arthritis and psoriatic rash or psoriasis in closefamily; controversial definition, resembles oligoarthritis, but more often with dactylitis and involvement of both small and large joints | F>M |
| Systemic | 4-17 | Throughout childhood | Arthritis and quotidian fever plus one or more of the following symptoms: characteristic rash, hepatomegaly, splenomegaly, lymphadenopathy, serositis; variable course; 5-8% develop macrophage activation syndrome | F=M |

Subgroups described in [14-16]
*F* female, *JIA* juvenile idiopathic arthritis, *M* male, *RF* rheumatoid factor

J. Hodler et al. (eds.), *Musculoskeletal Diseases 2013-2016*,
DOI: 10.1007/978-88-470-5292-5_34 © Springer-Verlag Italia 2013

- Oligoarthritis: one to four joints affected in the first 6 months of disease. This category is further divided into persistent oligoarthritis (with no more than four involved joints during the disease course) and extended oligoarthritis, involving more than four joints after the first 6 months.
- Polyarthritis: more than four joints affected within the first 6 months.
- Systemic arthritis: arthritis accompanied by systemic illness including fever.
- Psoriatic arthritis: arthritis associated with psoriasis.
- Enthesitis-related arthritis: these patients are often HLA-B27 positive.

This classification is unsatisfactory because many of the identified subgroups appear to be too inhomogeneous. Furthermore, it is difficult to distinguish, early in the disease course, between patients who are most likely to develop joint damage, and who therefore require a more aggressive treatment at an early stage, and patients who will have a mild disease course. Finally, in clinical trials, drug efficacy is judged only on clinical parameters, since measures that can allow the early identification of the progression of joint damage, and therefore of drug efficacy on disease progression, are not available in children.

## Imaging

The role of imaging is to secure the diagnosis, to assess the extent, severity and activity of the disease, and to help monitor therapeutic response and potential complications to steroid therapy and immobilization, such as compression fractures and avascular necrosis. During the past decade there has been a shift from traditional radiography towards newer techniques such as ultrasound and magnetic resonance imaging, thus without proper evaluation of their accuracy and validity.

Radiographs can show periostitis, bone erosion, cartilage loss [indirectly, through joint space narrowing (JSN)], osteoporosis and joint misalignment (Figs. 1-4), but cannot visualize synovium, joint effusion, articular cartilage, bone marrow, or ligaments and tendons directly. Plain radiographs have particularly low sensitivity for disease in early stages (Table 2) [17-24].

Joint damage evaluation has traditionally been performed by radiographic scoring methods assessing JSN and erosions; however, they are quite inaccurate, in part due to the growing skeleton [25]. Wrist disease has been associated with a more severe course of arthritis and a poorer functional outcome, and is the only joint in which suitable radiographic measures of disease progression have been reported. Much effort has been spent recently on validating existing scoring systems or devising new ones, of which a modified version of the Sharp/van der Heijde wrist score has gained most acceptance (Table 2). The original Sharp/van der Heijde score is based on the assessment of JSN in 15 different

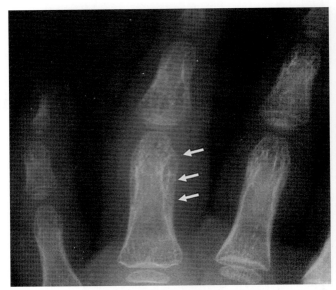

**Fig. 1.** Radiograph in 4-year-old girl with juvenile idiopathic arthritis, shows periarticular soft tissue swelling of the left fourth finger, proximal interphalangeal joint, periarticular osteoporosis and periostitis along the proximal phalanx (*arrows*)

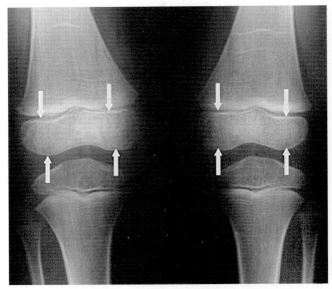

**Fig. 2.** A 5-year-old boy with active juvenile idiopathic arthritis of the right knee for 3 months. Radiograph shows accelerated growth of the knee epiphysis, as compared with the right normal side (*arrows*)

locations, and bone erosion in 16 locations for each hand/wrist, separately. JSN is scored from 0 to 4, and bone erosion from 0 to 5, and the scores are summarized to make a total score ranging from 0 to 280 [26]. Notably, carpal/metacarpal changes in younger children tend to present as bony deformation, ranging from mild squaring to severe compression, rather than definite erosions as often seen in adults (Fig. 3). This has been

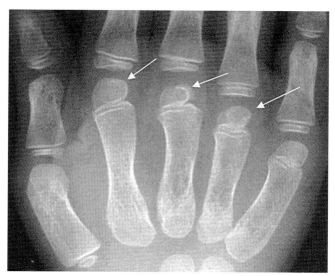

**Fig. 3.** A 4-year-old girl with juvenile idiopathic arthritis and wrist affection. Radiograph shows squaring of the metacarpal epiphysis (*arrows*)

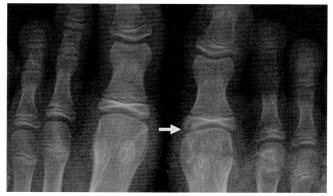

**Fig. 4.** Juvenile idiopathic arthritis in a 12-year-old boy. Radiograph shows destructive change of the metatarsophalangeal joint of the first left toe, with joint space narrowing and small erosions (*arrow*)

accounted for in Sharp/van der Heijde's scoring system in that both entities are considered pathological and scored in a similar fashion.

Rossi and colleagues noted that JSN tends to predominate over erosive change in JIA, and that erosion tends to involve locations other than those seen in adult rheumatoid arthritis [19]. For these reasons Ravelli et al. added another five locations to those described by Sharp/van der Heijde (second to fourth metacarpal bases, the capitate and the hamate), giving a total score of 330 [18]. When scoring is preceded by a meticulous standardization process, accuracy appears to be appropriate for clinical use.

Ultrasound (US) performs better than clinical examination in the diagnosis and localization of inflammatory change, such as joint effusion, bursal fluid collection and synovitis [27, 28] (Figs. 5-9). US can visualize inflammatory change relatively accurately, while assessment of chronic change is less feasible [29]. A structured assessment of synovitis and tenosynovitis, and classification of the findings, has been devised; however, the technique needs further validation [30] (Table 1). A few small uncontrolled studies have described improved sensitivity for detection of bone erosions in joints with the use of US as compared with conventional plain radiography; however, firm conclusions cannot be drawn from these studies. US may also demonstrate changes to cartilage.

Magnetic resonance imaging (MRI) can visualize both active JIA change, such as soft tissue and synovial inflammation, effusion, bone marrow edema and chronic change. Additional contrast-enhanced series can help quantify the inflammation process, and also differentiate pannus from joint effusion [20]. Furthermore MRI is the only technique for assessment of bone marrow edema [21].

The protocol should include pulse sequences for assessment of the synovium (T2-weighted and fat-saturated/gadolinium enhanced T1-weighted images) and cartilage

**Table 2.** Classification systems for active inflammatory change and chronic, structural change in juvenile idiopathic arthritis

| Classification system | Active, inflammatory change | | Chronic, structural change | |
| --- | --- | --- | --- | --- |
| | Detection of pathology | Scoring system | Detection of pathology | Scoring system |
| Clinical parameters | Joint swelling, relatively low sensitivity | Inaccurate | Joint malalignment, late finding | Inaccurate |
| Radiography | Unfeasible | | Feasible | Lack of accurate scoring systems, adapted version of the Sharp/van der Heijde wrist score |
| Ultrasound | Effusions, synovial hypertrophy, tenosynovitis, feasible | Relatively accurate | Relatively unfeasible | Inaccurate |
| MRI | Effusions, bone marrow edema, synovial, hypertrophy with hyperaemia, tenosynovitis, feasible | For wrist; devised by HeC, relatively accurate [20, 21] | Relatively unfeasible | For wrist; devised by HeC, relatively inaccurate [16, 22-24] |

*HeC* Health-a-Child multicenter study (London, Paris, Rome, Genoa) radiology group, *MRI* magnetic resonance imaging

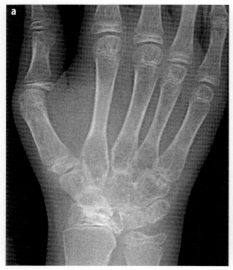
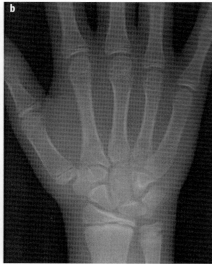

**Fig. 5 a, b.** **a** Hand radiograph in a 12-year-old girl with longstanding juvenile idiopathic arthritis (poly, rheumatoid factor positive) shows severe osteoporosis, crowding of the carpals and squaring of the metacarpal epiphysis. **b** A normal hand is shown for comparison

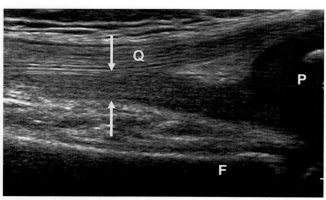

**Fig. 6.** Sagittal ultrasound view of the left knee joint in a 5-year-old girl with juvenile idiopathic arthritis shows synovial hypertrophy within the suprapatellar recess (between *arrows*) without an effusion (verified by compression technique). *F* distal femur, *P* patella, *Q* quadriceps tendon

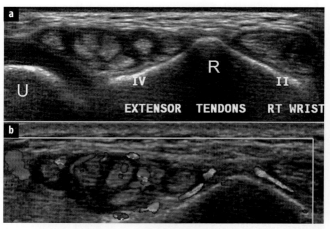

**Fig. 8 a, b.** Axial ultrasound view (standard view) of the dorsal right wrist in a 7-year-old girl with juvenile idiopathic arthritis shows tenosynovitis of the extensors (compartments 2-4) (**a**) and verified by hyperemia on color Doppler (**b**). *R* distal radius, tubercle of Lister; *U* distal ulna (for color reproduction see p 317)

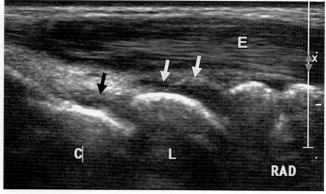

**Fig. 7.** Sagittal ultrasound view (standard view) of the dorsal wrist in a 6-year-old girl with juvenile idiopathic arthritis shows synovial hypertrophy and small effusions in the radiocarpal (*white arrows*) and midcarpal joints (*black arrow*). *C* capitate, *E* inflamed extensor tendons, *L* lunate, *RAD* distal radius (for color reproduction see p 317)

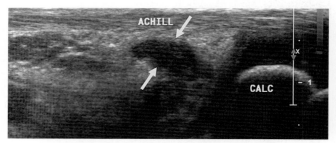

**Fig. 9.** Sagittal ultrasound view of the posterior ankle in a 9-year-old boy with enthesitis-related arthritis shows a swollen prepatellar bursa (*arrows*). *ACHILL* Achilles tendon, *CALC* calcaneus (for color reproduction see p 317)

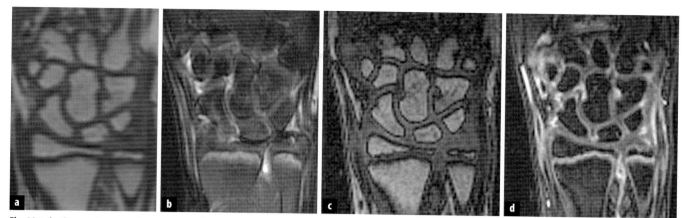

**Fig. 10 a-d.** Coronal magnetic resonance images of the wrist in a 12-year-old girl with juvenile idiopathic arthritis, including a T1-weighted image [three-dimensional (3D) spin echo] showing no erosion (**a**), a T2 fat-saturated image showing a sliver of fluid in the radioulnar joint (within normal variation) (**b**), a T1-weighted (3D spoiled gradient recalled echo sequence) before (**c**) and after (**d**) intravenous contrast administration, showing mildly increased synovial enhancement around the distal scaphoid, the trapezoid and the trapezium, consistent with focal inflammation

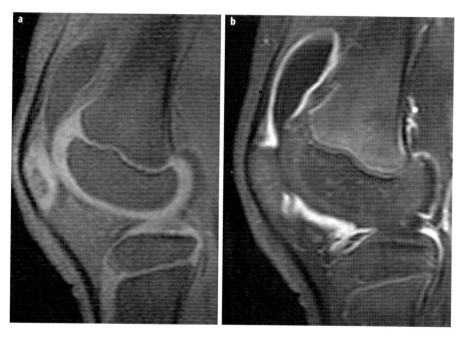

**Fig. 11 a, b.** Sagittal magnetic resonance images of the right knee in a 12-year-old boy presenting with a swollen, painful knee. **a** T1 fat-saturated image (water exited) showing a swollen, prepatellar recess. **b** Contrast-enhanced image showing vivid enhancement of a mildly thickened synovium, consistent with synovitis. The clinical picture suggested juvenile idiopathic arthritis

and bone [T1/proton density weighted and three-dimensional (3D) spoiled gradient recalled echo sequences] in different planes (Figs. 10, 11).

The value of MRI as an advanced method to evaluate disease activity and disease damage in adults with rheumatoid arthritis is under active investigation by a research consortium called Outcome Measures in Rheumatology Clinical Trials (OMERACT). However, the results drawn from OMERACT studies are not directly applicable to children, because adult rheumatoid arthritis is different from JIA and because the growing skeleton of children needs a different approach (Fig. 12). Indeed, in children ossification is incomplete and joint

space width varies with age [16, 22]. Thus, despite technical progress in the imaging of cartilage, as development of ultrashort TE sequences, driven equilibrium, Fourier transform (DEFT) imaging, and steady-state free precession (SSFP) sequences for the detection of subtle surface irregularities and tiny focal defects of the articular cartilage, diffusion weighted techniques to assess degradation of collagen fibers, delayed gadolinium-enhanced cartilage imaging (dGEMRIC) to detect changes in cartilage proteoglycan content, and T2 relaxation time mapping to detect integrity of collagen in the extracellular matrix, the potential helpfulness of these techniques is yet to be seen. The same goes for sophisticated analysis

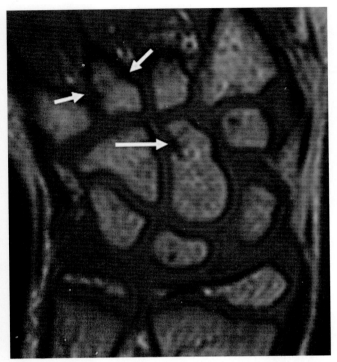

**Fig. 12.** Coronal T1-weighted image in a healthy 11-year-old boy shows bony depressions in the base of the fourth metacarpal and in the lunate (*arrows*) – within normal variation

of 3D image data to provide articular surface contour mapping, and 3D rendering as well as volumetric quantification of articular cartilage to evaluate the progression and response to treatment in patients with chronic arthritis. Progress in the assessment of synovitis, including dynamic contrast-enhanced MRI to assess the degree of inflammation, is also flawed with methodological difficulties, although voxel-by-voxel analysis of signal intensity versus time curves has proven more accurate than the region-of-interest approach in adults with rheumatoid arthritis. Other techniques for assessment of inflammation using semiautomated or automated segmentation program techniques of dynamic contrast-enhanced MRI have also been described [31, 32]. Thus, although MRI is a potential powerful imaging tool to assess joint inflammation and the progression of joint damage, standardized, validated, and feasible assessment systems are lacking.

During the years 2006 to 2010 we, as part of a large European-Union-funded multicenter study, devised a new scoring system for wrist involvement in JIA, assessing both active and chronic change, based on MRI and radiography combined. Based on a large cohort of around 350 patients aged from 5 to 15 years, we have examined feasibility and accuracy for all the different components within a scoring system, namely bone erosions, bone marrow edema, synovitis (effusion, synovial hypertrophy, increased enhancement) and tenosynovitis. In general, the accuracy, i.e., inter- and intraobserver agreement,

seems to be better for active than for chronic change (Table 2), and thorough standardization of the scoring method prior to assessment appears to be crucial. One major problem in assessing bone erosions and bone marrow change on MRI in particular was the lack of normal references (Fig. 10). Thus, during the project, such standards were created based on a population of 89 healthy children aged 5-15 years [16, 22]. Informed by these findings, we had to adjust some of the definitions used for pathological change.

In conclusion, imaging is crucial for the assessment, grading and follow-up of children with JIA. Plain radiography still plays an important role in the diagnostic work-up and in monitoring chronic change. US performs better than clinical examination in the diagnosis and localization of inflammatory change, but accurate scoring systems are lacking. US can also guide joint injections. MRI is an important tool for the detection and grading of active change, and is a promising technique for future assessment of chronic change. At present, the assessment of chronic change is flawed by the wide variation of normal bone size and shape, and the results drawn from the "adult OMERACT studies" are not directly applicable to children.

## References

1. Ruperto N, Lovell DJ, Cuttica R et al (2009) Long-term efficacy and safety of infliximab plus methotrexate for the treatment of polyarticular course juvenile rheumatoid arthritis: findings from an open-label treatment extension. Ann Rheum Dis 69:718-722
2. Ruperto N, Lovell DJ, Cuttica R et al (2007) A randomized, placebo-controlled trial of infliximab plus methotrexate for the treatment of polyarticular-course juvenile rheumatoid arthritis. Arthritis Rheum 56:3096-3106
3. Ringold S, Wallace CA (2007) Measuring clinical response and remission in juvenile idiopathic arthritis. Curr Opin Rheumatol 19:471-476
4. Oen K, Malleson PN, Cabral DA et al (2002) Disease course and outcome of juvenile rheumatoid arthritis in a multicenter cohort. J Rheumatol 29:1989-1999
5. Gabriel SE, Michaud K (2009) Epidemiological studies in incidence, prevalence, mortality, and comorbidity of the rheumatic diseases. Arthritis Res Ther 11:229
6. Kaipiainen-Seppanen O, Savolainen A (2001) Changes in the incidence of juvenile rheumatoid arthritis in Finland. Rheumatology (Oxford) 40:928-932
7. Riise OR, Handeland KS, Cvancarova M et al (2008) Incidence and characteristics of arthritis in Norwegian children: a population-based study. Pediatrics 121:e299-e306
8. Symmons DP, Jones M, Osborne J et al (1996) Pediatric rheumatology in the United Kingdom: data from the British Pediatric Rheumatology Group National Diagnostic Register. J Rheumatol 23:1975-1980
9. Arvidsson LZ, Smith HJ, Flato B, Larheim TA (2010) Temporomandibular joint findings in adults with long-standing juvenile idiopathic arthritis: CT and MR imaging assessment. Radiology 256:191-200
10. Weiss PF, Arabshahi B, Johnson A et al (2008) High prevalence of temporomandibular joint arthritis at disease onset in children with juvenile idiopathic arthritis, as detected by magnetic resonance imaging but not by ultrasound. Arthritis Rheum 58:1189-1196

11. Arvidsson LZ, Fjeld MG, Smith HJ et al (2010) Craniofacial growth disturbance is related to temporomandibular joint abnormality in patients with juvenile idiopathic arthritis, but normal facial profile was also found at the 27-year follow-up. Scand J Rheumatol 39:373-379

12. Fjeld MG, Arvidsson LZ, Stabrun AE (2009) Average craniofacial development from 6 to 35 years of age in a mixed group of patients with juvenile idiopathic arthritis. Acta Odontol Scand 67:153-160

13. Dahllof G, Martens L (2001) Children with chronic health conditions – implications for oral health. In: Koch A, Poulsen A (Eds) Pediatric dentistry. A clinical approach. Munksgaard, Copenhagen, pp 421-444

14. Petty RE, Southwood TR, Manners P et al (2004) International League of Associations for Rheumatology classification of juvenile idiopathic arthritis: second revision, Edmonton, 2001. J Rheumatol 31:390-392

15. Kahn P (2011) Juvenile idiopathic arthritis – an update on pharmacotherapy. Bull NYU Hosp Jt Dis 69:264-276

16. Müller Ording LS (2012) Establishment of Normative MRI Standards for the Paediatric Skeleton to better outline Pathology. Focused on Juvenile Idiopathic Arthritis. A dissertation for the degree of Philosophiae Doctor. University of Tromsø, Faculty of Health Sciences, Tromsø

17. Poznanski AK, Hernandez RJ, Guire KE et al (1978) Carpal length in children–a useful measurement in the diagnosis of rheumatoid arthritis and some congenital malformation syndromes. Radiology 129:661-668

18. Ravelli A, Ioseliani M, Norambuena X et al (2007) Adapted versions of the Sharp/van der Heijde score are reliable and valid for assessment of radiographic progression in juvenile idiopathic arthritis. Arthritis Rheum 56:3087-3095

19. Rossi F, Di DF, Galipo O et al (2006) Use of the Sharp and Larsen scoring methods in the assessment of radiographic progression in juvenile idiopathic arthritis. Arthritis Rheum 55:717-723

20. Damasio MB, Malattia C, Tanturri de HL et al (2012) MRI of the wrist in juvenile idiopathic arthritis: proposal of a paediatric synovitis score by a consensus of an international working group. Results of a multicentre reliability study. Pediatr Radiol 42:1047-1055

21. Tanturri de HL, Damasio MB, Barbuti D et al (2012) MRI assessment of bone marrow in children with juvenile idiopathic arthritis: intra- and inter-observer variability. Pediatr Radiol 42:714-720

22. Avenarius DM, Ording Muller LS, Eldevik P et al (2012) The paediatric wrist revisited–findings of bony depressions in healthy children on radiographs compared to MRI. Pediatr Radiol 42:791-798

23. Boavida P, Hargunani R, Owens CM, Rosendahl K (2012) Magnetic resonance imaging and radiographic assessment of carpal depressions in children with juvenile idiopathic arthritis: normal variants or erosions? J Rheumatol 39:645-650

24. Muller LS, Avenarius D, Damasio B et al (2011) The paediatric wrist revisited: redefining MR findings in healthy children. Ann Rheum Dis 70:605-610

25. Johnson K (2006) Imaging of juvenile idiopathic arthritis. Pediatr Radiol 36:743-758

26. van der Heijde D (2000) How to read radiographs according to the Sharp/van der Heijde method. J Rheumatol 27:261-263

27. Breton S, Jousse-Joulin S, Cangemi C et al (2011) Comparison of clinical and ultrasonographic evaluations for peripheral synovitis in juvenile idiopathic arthritis. Semin Arthritis Rheum 41:272-278

28. Janow GL, Panghaal V, Trinh A et al (2011) Detection of active disease in juvenile idiopathic arthritis: sensitivity and specificity of the physical examination vs ultrasound. J Rheumatol 38:2671-2674

29. Muller L, Kellenberger CJ, Cannizzaro E et al (2009) Early diagnosis of temporomandibular joint involvement in juvenile idiopathic arthritis: a pilot study comparing clinical examination and ultrasound to magnetic resonance imaging. Rheumatology (Oxford) 48:680-685

30. Malattia C, Damasio MB, Magnaguagno F et al (2008) Magnetic resonance imaging, ultrasonography, and conventional radiography in the assessment of bone erosions in juvenile idiopathic arthritis. Arthritis Rheum 59:1764-1772

31. Malattia C, Damasio MB, Basso C et al (2012) A novel automated system for MRI quantification of the inflamed synovial membrane volume in patients with juvenile idiopathic arthritis. Arthritis Care Res (Hoboken) 64:1657-1664

32. Malattia C, Damasio MB, Basso C et al (2010) Dynamic contrast-enhanced magnetic resonance imaging in the assessment of disease activity in patients with juvenile idiopathic arthritis. Rheumatology (Oxford) 49:178-185

# Nonaccidental Trauma and its Imitators

Peter J. Strouse

Section of Pediatric Radiology, C.S. Mott Children's Hospital, University of Michigan Health System, Ann Arbor, MI, USA

## Introduction

Child abuse is a worldwide problem. While some societies have higher reported incidence, children of all nations are undoubtedly affected. During the year 2009 in the USA, there were 1,770 deaths due to child abuse and approximately 125,000 children were estimated to be the victims of physical abuse [1].

Abused children present in a myriad of ways. Presenting histories are often false and misleading. Radiology often plays a key role in suggesting the diagnosis. Imaging findings may suggest an abusive injury. Initial imaging of an abused child is determined by the presentation and is aimed at identifying findings that are life threatening and that warrant immediate treatment or management to prevent further compromise. Once the patient is stabilized, and if child abuse is suspected, a skeletal survey is usually obtained to evaluate for additional findings, characterize the abnormalities and to contribute to the diagnosis of child abuse or a differential consideration.

Many processes can clinically and radiologically mimic child abuse. It is equally as important to properly exclude the diagnosis and to make the appropriate differential diagnosis as it is to suggest the diagnosis of abuse.

The chief cause of morbidity in child abuse is trauma to the central nervous system. Children can also suffer fatality due to visceral trauma. In the majority of children suffering fatal abuse injury, there is skeletal evidence of prior trauma in the form of healing fractures. Therefore, justification for radiographic skeletal surveys largely lies in finding such fractures, identifying them before a fatal incident, and aiding to facilitate proper clinical and social care of the affected child.

## Imaging Algorithms

Many of the radiographic findings of abusive trauma are subtle. Proper imaging algorithms and attention to proper technique are therefore of paramount importance. The American College of Radiology and the American Association of Pediatricians provide guidelines for the radiographic evaluation of suspected child abuse [2-4]. Box 1 lists the views obtained in a standard skeletal survey. Some recent studies have questioned the inclusion of radiographs of all areas of the body; however, although rare at some sites, abusive injuries can be seen on any one of these views and potentially on only one of these views. Whole or partial body radiographs ("babygrams") are an unacceptable substitute for a skeletal survey.

Ideally, images are reviewed by a radiologist versed in the imaging findings of child abuse and its differential diagnosis before the child leaves the imaging room. Radiographs are checked for image quality, proper positioning and labeling. The radiologist should verify that the study

---

**Box 1.** Views of a radiographic skeletal survey for suspected child abuse*

Routine:
    Skull: anteroposterior (AP) and lateral
    Lateral skull (may include C-spine)
    Lateral thoracic and lumbar spine
    Ribs: AP, right posterior oblique, left posterior oblique
    AP pelvis and lumbar spine
    AP of each femur
    AP of each tibia/fibula
    AP of each humerus
    AP of each forearm
    Posteroanterior of each hand
    AP (dorsoventral) of each foot

Optional:
    Lateral views long bones
    Coned views of joints or ribs
    Townes view of skull

*Ideally, radiographs are reviewed by a radiologist before the patient leaves the imaging suite. Poorly positioned or otherwise suboptimal images are repeated. Lateral views of long bones or coned views of a joint are obtained for positive or equivocal findings in the extremities. Coned views of the ribs may be considered for further delineation of rib findings. Townes view of the skull may be performed for better evaluation of the occipital bone and demonstration of wormian bones

---

J. Hodler et al. (eds.), *Musculoskeletal Diseases 2013-2016*,
DOI: 10.1007/978-88-470-5292-5_35 © Springer-Verlag Italia 2013

contains all the required views. Additional images can be obtained to further evaluate equivocal findings and positive findings. Most commonly, this would entail addition of lateral views of the long bones or lateral views centered at the joints. A Townes view of the skull can be obtained to better evaluate the occipital bone and to look for wormian bones, particularly if fractures are found elsewhere in the body.

In equivocal cases or in cases where there is a very high clinical suspicion for child abuse but the initial skeletal survey is negative, a follow-up skeletal survey or nuclear medicine bone scintigraphy can be helpful [5]. A follow-up skeletal survey is typically obtained 10-14 days after the initial survey and may be limited to the long bones and ribs, also including other areas of radiologic or clinical concern from the time of the initial survey. Most centers use nuclear medicine bone scans sparingly; however, they can be very sensitive for certain fractures, such as of the ribs.

Imaging obtained for evaluation of central nervous system or visceral trauma should be carefully evaluated for osseous findings. For instance, rib fractures can be evident on chest or abdominal radiographs, on the upper images of abdominal computed tomography (CT) or on CT or magnetic resonance imaging (MRI) of the spine. Head CT images should be carefully evaluated for skull fracture. While some authors have proposed whole body CT, its use is limited by radiation dose and lower spatial resolution than radiographs. Nonetheless, focused CT can be helpful in confirming rib fractures. Whole body MRI is of limited use in detecting lesions that are relatively advanced in healing [6].

Radiographic investigation is strongly indicated for all fatal cases of suspected child abuse as well as for all unexpected infant deaths [7]. A postmortem skeletal survey is performed with the same technique as in the living child. In the postmortem state, where radiation dose is no longer a concern, CT parameters can be changed to increase resolution. At this time, however, the utility of CT for postmortem evaluation is still under investigation [8].

## Specificity of Findings

Through the seminal work of Dr Paul Kleinman, and supplemented by others, the individual radiographic findings of child abuse can be characterized into high specificity, moderate specificity and low specificity (Box 2) [9, 10].

## High-Specificity Findings

### Posterior Rib Fractures

Rib fractures caused by accidental trauma are uncommon in children under 5 years of age because of the plasticity of their bones. As such, any rib fracture in a child without reliably witnessed trauma and without metabolic bone disease must be viewed with a degree of suspicion. Rib fractures can occur at any location in the rib arc. Acute transverse fractures with displacement are rare. Acute fractures are usually greenstick or buckle fractures and can be very difficult to see on radiographs, if at all. Particularly if lateral, there may be associated subpleural hematoma. Posterior rib fractures, near the spine, have the highest specificity for child abuse [9, 11]. The rib is torqued or levered over the transverse process. Posterior rib fractures become more conspicuous with callous due to healing. Frequently, fractures of the lateral rib arc are seen in conjunction with posterior rib fractures (Fig. 1).

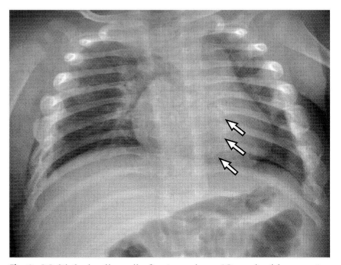

**Fig. 1.** Multiple healing rib fractures in a 10-week-old asymptomatic boy whose twin was fatally abused. The right third to ninth and left fourth to ninth ribs are expanded laterally with callous. In addition, there are subtle healing fractures of the posterior left seventh to ninth ribs (*arrows*)

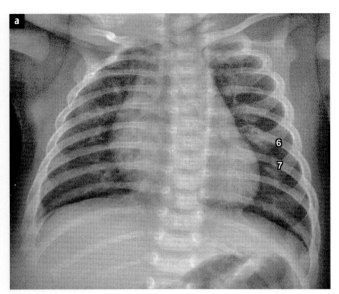

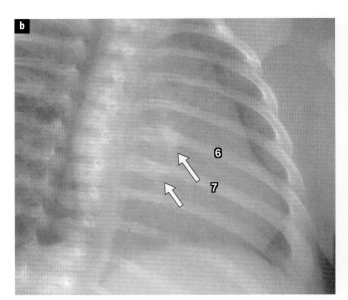

**Fig. 2 a, b.** Healing posterior rib fractures in a 6-week-old boy: **a** anteroposterior and **b** oblique views. The oblique view aids in identification of fractures of the left posterior sixth (*6*) and seventh (*7*) ribs (*arrows*)

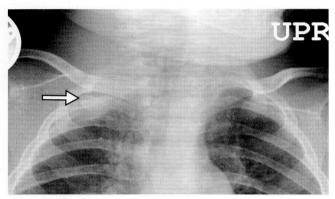

**Fig. 3.** Acute first rib fracture in a 3-month-old boy. The fracture line (*arrow*) is sharply defined with slight distraction of fragments. There is associated subpleural hematoma

These lateral rib fractures also occur with squeezing due to a compressive force on the inside arc of the rib and a distractive force on the outside arc of the rib. Oblique views aid in detection of rib fractures (Fig. 2) [12]. *Differential considerations*: rib anomalies, fractures due to metabolic disease, superimposition of sternal ossification centers, normal anterior flaring of the ribs.

## Fracture of the First Rib

Although rare in child abuse, fracture of the first rib in an infant is generally not seen as a result of other causes (Fig. 3). These fractures are likely to occur as a result of indirect forces related to shaking or rapid flexion with the scalene muscles attached to the body of the first rib and its ends fixed by the manubrium anteriorly and the spine

posteriorly [13]. *Differential considerations*: first rib anomaly, anomalous articulation of first and second ribs.

## Fractures of the Sternum, Scapula and Spinous Processes

Fractures at these sites are also rare in child abuse, but generally not seen from other causes. Specific applied forces in child abuse can predispose to these fractures. Possible mechanisms include blunt force from anterior causing sternal fracture, direct force due to the grasp of an abuser causing acromial fractures, and forced flexion due to shaking or axial impact causing spinous process fractures. *Differential considerations*: normal sternal ossification centers, acromial variants.

## Classic Metaphyseal Lesions

The term "classic metaphyseal lesion" (CML) was introduced by Kleinman to include "bucket handle fracture" and "corner fracture" type lesions of the metaphyses of long bones [9, 14]. The lesions are relatively transverse fractures through the edge of the metaphysis. Depending on the degree of displacement, the position of the limb and the angle of the X-ray beam, the acute lesion can appear as either a curvilinear fragment ("bucket handle") or as a corner fragment (Fig. 4). With healing, lesions become indistinct, there is associated sclerosis, cartilaginous ingrowth into the metaphysis can occur, and the lesion disappears [15]. Periosteal new bone formation is seen with healing only if there is associated periosteal injury. In rough decreasing order, CMLs are most common at the distal tibia and fibula, the distal femur, the proximal tibia and fibula, the distal radius and ulna, and the proximal humerus. They are uncommon at the proximal

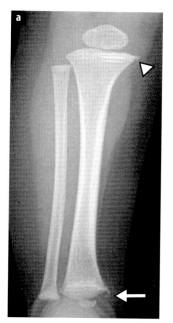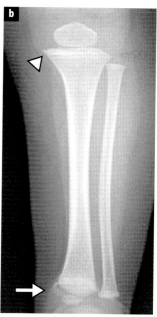

**Fig. 4 a, b.** Classic metaphyseal lesions in an 8-month-old girl. **a** Right tibia. **b** Left tibia. Bucket handle fractures are seen at each distal tibia (*arrows*). Subtle corner fractures are seen at the medial aspect of each proximal tibia (*arrowheads*)

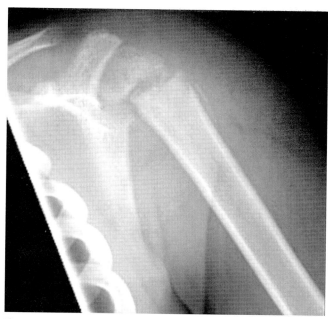

**Fig. 5.** Healing physeal fracture (Salter I) of the proximal humerus in a 35-month-old boy. The proximal humeral metaphysis is displaced lateral relative to the humeral head. The physis is widened and ill-defined. Periosteal new bone is seen at the lateral aspect of the proximal humeral metaphysis

femur and at the elbow. CMLs probably occur as a result of torsional force applied to a limb or extreme forces experienced with shaking with the extremities flailing. *Differential considerations*: normal developmental variants [16], pyhysiologic bowing, rickets, (spondylo)metaphyseal dysplasia especially types Schmid and Sutcliffe ("corner fracture type"), congenital syphilis, Menke syndrome, scurvy.

## Moderate-Specificity Findings

### Multiple Fractures and Fractures of Differing Age

While most think of multiple fractures and fractures of differing age as characteristic of abusive injury, these findings are only moderately specific. Children with metabolic bone disease and children with certain syndromes, namely osteogenesis imperfecta, are prone to fracture and can have multiple fractures and fractures of differing age. Almost uniformly, such children have a known medical history, radiography suggests an underlying bone disorder, and the fractures seen do not fall into the high-specificity patterns describe above. An otherwise well child with normal bone mineralization with multiple fractures of differing age presenting to an emergency room should promptly raise suspicion for child abuse. *Differential considerations*: metabolic bone disease including rickets, osteogenesis imperfecta, Menke syndrome, multiple episodes of accidental trauma.

### Spine Fracture

Infants can suffer spinal trauma as a result of axial or direct impact or extreme degrees of flexion. Compression fractures are most common in the lower thoracic and upper lumbar spine, but may occur throughout the spine [17]. Critical cervical spine trauma and spinal cord injury are uncommon, but may occur. *Differential considerations*: vertebral anomalies including hypoplasia, infection, neoplasm.

### Growth Plate Fractures

Fractures through the growth plate (physis) in the infant are uncommon [18]. These fractures can occur due to other causes, namely birth trauma. Physeal fractures caused by abuse are most common at the proximal humerus (Fig. 5), perhaps related to the grasp of the abuser's hands. Interestingly, these fractures seem to be more common in children aged 2-3 years. Less common sites of abusive physeal fracture occur at the proximal femur and the distal humerus. *Differential considerations*: birth trauma, infection.

### Pelvis

Fractures of the pelvis are rare in child abuse and are likely to occur as a result of blunt force trauma, including being slammed down in a sitting position. Fractures can also occur as a consequence of sexual assault. Fractures of

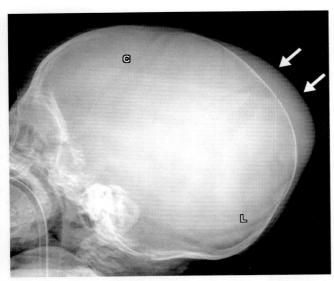

**Fig. 6.** Complex skull fracture in an 8-week-old boy who was fatally abused. Multiple fracture lines are seen within the parietal bones. Overlying soft tissue swelling is present (*arrows*). *C* coronal sutures, *L* lambdoid sutures

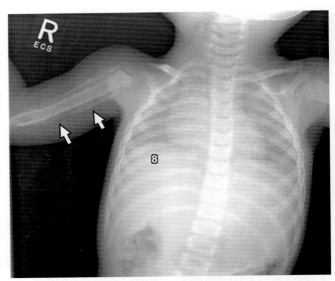

**Fig. 7.** Post-traumatic periosteal new bone in a 21-month-old girl. Exuberant periosteal new bone (*arrows*) cloaks the right humerus, extending from metaphysis to metaphysis. No underlying fracture was identified. A subtle healing fracture of the posterior right eighth rib (*8*) is noted

the pubic bones are most common [19, 20]. *Differential considerations*: normal ischiopubic synchondrosis, normal variants in pubic bone ossification.

### Digital Fractures of the Hands and Feet

Before infants begin to crawl and cruise and explore their environment, fractures of the digits of the hands and feet are distinctly uncommon. Once infants reach an age of exploration, the hands, and to a lesser extent the feet, become prone to crush injury from doors. Fractures of the phalanges, metacarpals and metatarsals are likely to occur as a result of a squeezing force. These fractures can be very subtle buckle fractures, which become more conspicuous with healing [21]. *Differential considerations*: normal contour of bones mimicking fracture.

### Complex Skull Fracture

Complex skull fractures can be bilateral, have multiple fracture lines and be depressed (Fig. 6). Such fractures do not occur with trauma in the home [22]. Complex fractures can occur as a result of falls from a substantial height or severe motor vehicle accident. *Differential considerations*: accidental trauma, normal anatomy, wormian bones.

## Low-Specificity Findings

### Periosteal New Bone

Periosteal new bone can form due to a number of reasons. Physiologic periosteal new bone is seen in healthy

infants, characteristically 1-4 months old, and typically along the diaphysis of the humerus laterally, the ulna medially, the femur laterally and the tibia medially [23, 24]. Physiologic periosteal new bone is typically bilateral and symmetric but not always, and asymmetry of positioning can render it asymmetric on radiography. Traumatic periosteal bone from abuse tends to be metaphyseal, asymmetric and can be more exuberant (Fig. 7). *Differential considerations*: physiologic periosteal new bone, Caffey's disease, prostaglandin administration, post-body wall edema, accidental trauma, infection, neoplasm.

### Long Bone Fractures

Fractures of diaphysis of the long bones are very suspicious for abuse if occurring in a nonambulatory child prior to the age of cruising [25]. Such infants typically cannot generate sufficient force or mechanism for long bone fracture. One-third to one-half of humeral and femoral diaphyseal fractures in nonambulatory infants are caused by abuse. Abusive long bone fractures can be incomplete, transverse, oblique or spiral (Fig. 8). Spiral or oblique fractures do not necessarily denote abuse and can occur from accidental injury once infants are ambulatory. Once infants gain their footing, cruise and walk, accidental long bone fractures become more common. Rarely, nonambulatory infants can suffer long bone fracture as a result of falls, being fallen on, or other rare mechanisms. In these instances, corroborative witnesses or other evidence is usually available to exclude abuse. *Differential considerations*: accidental trauma, metabolic bone disease.

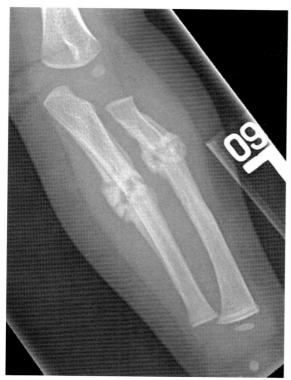

**Fig. 8.** Healing fractures of the radial and ulnar diaphyses in an 8-month-old girl (same patient as shown in Fig. 4). Abundant callous and periosteal new bone is present. This image was obtained at the time of presentation

## Clavicle Fracture

Because clavicle fractures are common as a result of birth dystocia, they are considered low specificity for abuse. Clavicle fractures from birth trauma should demonstrate callous by 10-14 days after birth [26]. The fractures are not infrequently missed at the time of neonatal evaluation. If an infant is at least 10-14 days of age and presents with a clavicle fracture without visible callous, the injury is not due to birth trauma and can be abusive in etiology [26]. Clavicle fractures caused by accidental injury are relatively uncommon in toddlers, but do occur. *Differential considerations*: birth trauma, accident trauma, congenital pseudarthrosis.

## Linear Skull Fracture

Linear skull fractures can occur as a result of traumatic birth, short falls onto a hard surface in the home or child abuse. Overlying soft tissue swelling is seen, particularly if acute. Linear skull fractures are very common in child abuse, but are not specific. Careful correlation with the clinical history and validation of the purported mechanism is necessary to exclude abuse. *Differential considerations*: birth trauma, accidental trauma, normal anatomy, accessory sutures/fissures.

## Synthesis

While each individual radiographic finding has a degree of specificity no one finding is pathognomonic for child abuse. When a child has multiple radiographic findings, the constellation of findings achieves greater specificity than the individual findings, particularly if there are multiple different high-specificity lesions. Regardless of the findings, careful correlation with a good history and physical examination are required to determine the plausibility of the findings with the purported mechanism. A low-specificity lesion becomes more suspicious if the purported mechanism is incompatible. A low-specificity lesion becomes more suspicious if presentation is delayed.

## Differential Diagnosis

Processes that can mimic child abuse on radiography are listed in Box 3. The possibility of an alternative diagnosis is considered in all cases. The most common differential diagnoses encountered are normal developmental

---

**Box 3.** Differential diagnostic considerations for the radiographic findings of child abuse

Trauma
        Accidental
        Obstetrical
        Iatrogenic
Developmental
        Normal metaphyseal developmental variants
        Variants of acromial ossification
        Accessory skull sutures and fissures
        Physiologic periosteal new bone
        Sternal ossification center (superimposition mimicking posterior rib fracture)
Metabolic bone disease
        Metabolic bone disease of prematurity
        Congenital (Menke syndrome) and acquired copper deficiency
        Rickets
        Scurvy
        I-cell disease
Iatrogenic (nontraumatic)
        Prostaglandin E1 therapy
        Vitamin A toxicity
Bone dysplasia
        Osteogenesis imperfecta
        Metaphyseal chondrodysplasia, type Schmid
        Spondylometaphyseal dysplasia, type Sutcliffe
        ("corner fracture type")
Neurogenic
        Myelomeningocele
        Congenital insensitivity to pain
Neoplastic
        Metastatic neuroblastoma
        Leukemia
Infection/inflammatory
        Osteomyelitis
        Congenital syphilis
        Caffey disease (idiopathic cortical hyperostosis)

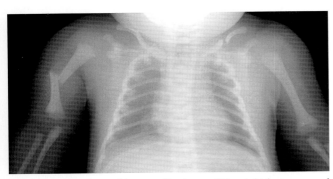

**Fig. 9.** Newborn boy with acute fractures of the right humerus and left clavicle due to obstetrical trauma. Delivery was difficult with severe dystocia

variants, physiological processes, obstetrical (Fig. 9) and iatrogenic injury, and accidental injury [27, 28]. Individually, it is rare for the other processes listed to mimic child abuse and be mistaken for child abuse due to misdiagnosis. Radiographic findings of osteopenia suggest an underlying metabolic bone disease or chronic systemic illness. Wormian bones are accessory intrasutural bones in the skull, most common in the lambdoid sutures. Significant wormian bones are 1 cm or greater in size, greater than ten in number, and arranged in a mosaic pattern [29]. Such wormian bones are rarely seen in normal children, but can be seen in some process that may mimic child abuse, namely osteogenesis imperfecta and Menke syndrome. If an alternative diagnosis is suggested, further clinical work-up, additional history or additional imaging may be diagnostic.

So-called "temporary brittle bone disease" is a hypothetical disease process that has never been proven to exist [30]. Recently, vitamin D deficiency has been put forth as a possible cause of fractures. Currently, there is no evidence that congenital or acquired vitamin D deficiency or insufficiency predisposes infants to the high-specificity findings seen in child abuse [31]. Attempts to ascribe high-specificity abusive fractures to either "temporary brittle bone disease" or vitamin D deficiency should be met with skepticism.

## Reporting

All states in the USA, and presumably most countries, have mandated reporting of suspected child abuse by law. A radiologist can be the first to suspect child abuse. Fortunately, direct reporting by the radiologist to law enforcement is rarely required as there are child protection teams that assimilate the case information and fulfill this obligation. Nonetheless, if a radiologist suspects child abuse, and no one else assumes responsibility for reporting, the radiologist is obligated to report suspected child abuse to the appropriate authority.

Imaging findings and conclusions must be expediently communicated to the referring clinician. Usually, this takes the form of direct face-to-face communication or a phone call.

Radiology reports in cases of suspected or possible child abuse must be well thought, succinct but complete, and contain proper documentation. Reports should include: (1) detailed descriptions of individual positive findings with statements of specificity, (2) an overall statement of conclusion based on the constellation of findings, (3) recommendations for additional imaging or clinical evaluation, (4) statements indicating consideration of alternative diagnoses, and (5) precise documentation of communication with the clinical service. Reports must be pristine as they are liable to become courtroom documents. Careful proofreading and editing is a must.

Radiologists will not infrequently be called upon to testify in court. Careful preparation is important, including review of the images and reports. Ideally, the case is reviewed with the legal team ahead of time so that the nature of testimony is firmly understood by both parties. It is the duty of the testifying radiologist to provide accurate testimony based on his/her own experience and what they know from the literature. Unproven hypotheses and pseudoscience have no place in the courtroom and are ultimately harmful to the wellbeing of the child.

## Conclusion

Radiography plays a major role in the diagnosis and delineation of child abuse. Nevertheless, the radiographic findings are but one part of the clinical presentation. The radiologist is obligated to provide an accurate report of the findings and resultant conclusions, to communicate it promptly, to strongly and appropriately consider alternative diagnoses, and to contribute to the work of the child protection team to properly diagnose, treat and protect the child. The contributions of a radiologist in identifying child abuse can be lifesaving.

## References

1. US Department of Health and Human Services, Administration for Children and Families, Administration on Children, Youth and Families, Children's Bureau (2010) Child Maltreatment 2009. US Government Printing Office
2. Meyer JS, Gunderman R, Coley BD et al (2011) ACR Appropriateness Criteria® on suspected physical abuse-child. J Am Coll Radiol 8:87-94
3. American College of Radiology (2011) ACR-SPR practice guideline for skeletal surveys in children. http://www.acr.org (accessed 12/4/2012)
4. Section on Radiology, American Academy of Pediatrics (2009) Diagnostic imaging of child abuse. Pediatrics 123:1430-1435
5. Kleinman PK, Nimkin K, Spevak MR et al (1996) Follow-up skeletal surveys in suspected child abuse. AJR Am J Roentgenol 167:893-896
6. Perez-Rossello JM, Connolly SA, Newton AW et al (2010) Whole-body MRI in suspected infant abuse. AJR Am J Roentgenol 195:744-750

7. The Society for Pediatric Radiology - National Association of Medical Examiners (2004) Post-mortem radiography in the evaluation of unexpected death in children less than 2 years of age whose death is suspicious for fatal abuse. Pediatr Radiol 34:675-677
8. Hong TS, Reyes JA, Moineddin R et al (2011) Value of post-mortem thoracic CT over radiography in imaging of pediatric rib fractures. Pediatr Radiol 41:736-748
9. Kleinman PK (1990) Diagnostic imaging in infant abuse. AJR Am J Roentgenol 155:703-712
10. Kleinman PK (2009) The Spectrum of non-accidental injuries (child abuse) and its imitators. In: Hodler J, Schulthess GK von, Zollikofer CL (Eds) (2009) Musculoskeletal diseases. Diagnostic imaging and interventional techniques. IDKD 2009-2012. Springer-Verlag Italia, Milano, pp 227-233
11. Kleinman PK, Marks SC, Nimkin K et al (1996) Rib fractures in 31 abused infants: postmortem radiologic-histopathologic study. Radiology 200:807-810
12. Ingram J, Connell J, Hay T et al (2000) Oblique radiographs of the chest in nonaccidental trauma. Emerg Radiol 7:42-46
13. Strouse PJ, Owings CL (1995) Fractures of the first rib in child abuse. Radiology 197:763-765
14. Kleinman PK, Marks SC, Blackbourne B (1986) The metaphyseal lesion in abused infants: a radiologic-histopathologic study. AJR Am J Roentgenol 146:895-905
15. Kleinman PK, Marks SC, Jr., Spevak MR et al (1991) Extension of growth-plate cartilage into the metaphysis: a sign of healing fracture in abused infants. AJR Am J Roentgenol 156:775-779
16. Kleinman PK, Belanger PL, Karellas A, Spevak MR (1991) Normal metaphyseal radiologic variants not to be confused with findings of infant abuse. AJR Am J Roentgenol 156:781-783
17. Kleinman PK, Marks SC (1992) Vertebral body fractures in child abuse. Radiologic-histopathologic correlates. Invest Radiol 27:715-722
18. Merten DF, Kirks DR, Ruderman RJ (1981) Occult humeral epiphyseal fracture in battered infants. Pediatr Radiol 10:151-154
19. Ablin DS, Greenspan A, Reinhart MA (1992) Pelvic injuries in child abuse. Pediatr Radiol 22:454-457
20. Perez-Rossello JM, Connolly SA, Newton AW et al (2008) Pubic ramus radiolucencies in infants: the good, the bad and the indeterminate. AJR Am J Roentgenol 190:1481-1486
21. Nimkin K, Spevak MR, Kleinman PK (1997) Fractures of the hands and feet in child abuse: imaging and pathologic features. Radiology 203:233-236
22. Meservy CJ, Towbin R, McLaurin RL et al (1987) Radiographic characteristics of skull fractures resulting from child abuse. AJR Am J Roentgenol 149:173-175
23. Shopfner CE (1966) Periosteal bone growth in normal infants. A preliminary report. Am J Roentgenol Radium Ther Nucl Med 97:154-163
24. Kwon DS, Spevak MR, Fletcher K, Kleinman PK (2002) Physiologic subperiosteal new bone formation: prevalence, distribution, and thickness in neonates and infants. AJR Am J Roentgenol 179:985-988
25. Scherl SA, Miller L, Lively N et al (2000) Accidental and nonaccidental femur fractures in children. Clin Orthop Relat Res 96-105.
26. Cumming WA (1979) Neonatal skeletal fractures. Birth trauma or child abuse? J Can Assoc Radiol 30:30-33
27. Swischuk L (2000) Not everything is child abuse. Emerg Radiol 7:218-224
28. Kleinman PK (2008) Problems in the diagnosis of metaphyseal fractures. Pediatr Radiol 38 Suppl 3:S388-394
29. Cremin B, Goodman H, Spranger J, Beighton P (1982) Wormian bones in osteogenesis imperfecta and other disorders. Skeletal Radiol 8:35-38
30. Mendelson KL (2005) Critical review of temporary brittle bone disease. Pediatr Radiol 35:1036-1040
31. Slovis TL, Chapman S (2008) Evaluating the data concerning vitamin D insufficiency/deficiency and child abuse. Pediatr Radiol 38:1221-1224

# Pediatric Musculoskeletal Diseases and their Different Manifestations in Childhood

Simon G. Robben

Department of Radiology, Maastricht University Medical Centre, Maastricht, The Netherlands

## Introduction

Children are not small adults. There are significant anatomical, physiological and psychological differences, and a large number of congenital and hereditary diseases can also be added to the list of differences.

Many of the differences have their radiological counterparts and therefore it is not surprising that radiology of children is quite different from radiology of adults. This is true for the central nervous system, digestive tract, respiratory tract and urogenital tract, and also for the musculoskeletal tract, which is the topic of this abstract.

The pediatric musculoskeletal system is characterized by the presence of growth plates, red bone marrow conversion, and high metabolism and rich vascularization. These specific features are in part the reason why pathological processes (inflammation, neoplasms, trauma, endocrine and metabolic processes) have specific radiographic characteristics in children.

## Imaging Techniques

Scintigraphy and cross-sectional imaging techniques such as ultrasonography (US), computed tomography (CT) and magnetic resonance imaging (MRI) have improved the ability to evaluate the musculoskeletal system dramatically. Selection of the optimal techniques in each individual patient is essential, and factors such as cost, radiation and need for sedation should all be considered. Conventional radiography is the initial modality to evaluate the bones because it is fast and has a low radiation dose. US is the initial modality for the evaluation of the soft tissue pathology and joint effusions because it is rapid and nonionizing. Moreover, the images are not degraded by metallic artefacts or motion artefacts (as with CT and MRI), and finally US offers the possibility of fine needle aspiration to confirm the infectious nature of a fluid collection, and histological biopsies in cases of solid tumors.

MRI and CT are not screening methods but are very useful in detailing osseous and soft tissue changes whenever conventional radiographs and US are not conclusive. CT allows a good definition of cortical and medullary bone changes. The major drawback of CT is the radiation load. MRI is superior in diagnosing soft tissue abnormalities, bone marrow changes, cartilage destruction and involvement of the growth plate. The major drawback of MRI is the need for sedation in children 6 years or less.

Scintigraphy (three-phase bone scan with Technetium 99m) has a high sensitivity for bone disease but a low specificity. Whole body MRI promises to be a good alternative.

## Children's Behavior

Neonates are easy to handle and all noninvasive imaging techniques can be used. US is the initial modality in neonates for many clinical questions. The diagnostic value of US increases when the neonate is relaxed. Always use warm echogel, and in case of emergency a pacifier with syrup should do the trick.

MRI is feasible when performed immediately after feeding. Usually, newborn infants fall into a deep sleep after a meal and this effect can be enhanced by some sleep deprivation and food deprivation prior to the meal. Intravenous access should be given several hours prior the examination. Unfortunately, this protocol fails after the age of 3-6 months. Older infants and preschool children usually need sedation for dedicated MRI examinations, although some clinical questions (control of hydrocephalus) can be answered with fast scanning techniques without the need for sedation.

CT techniques have been improved (dual source CT) and scanning times of less than 1 s are possible. Breath-holding and motion are no significant items any more and the radiation dose required is often much lower.

Once children go to school, their communication skills improve and their voice should not be neglected by only

J. Hodler et al. (eds.), *Musculoskeletal Diseases 2013-2016*,
DOI: 10.1007/978-88-470-5292-5_36 © Springer-Verlag Italia 2013

speaking with the parents. However, do not even try to negotiate with a child (e.g., the amount of barium they have to drink), you will lose.

## Growth Plates

Growth of children is facilitated by enchondral bone formation at the growth plates and membranous (appositional) growth along the shafts [1, 2]. Growth plates are cartilaginous plates separating the epiphysis from metaphysis or apophysis from metaphysis (Fig. 1) and are unique for the pediatric skeleton. Therefore, all processes that specifically affect the growth plate will be of greater clinical importance in children than in adults. In particular, premature closure (epiphysiodesis) can have disastrous effects on growth (Fig. 2). This can be caused by infection (osteomyelitis), neoplasm, trauma (Salter-Harris fractures) and ischemia (meningococcal sepsis), and it results in arrest of growth. If the epiphysiodesis is excentric, this will result in severe varus, valgus, retroflection or anteflection deformity. Epiphysiodesis can be evaluated with MRI [3].

On the other hand, overgrowth (both enchondral and membranous growth) occurs in diseases that increase blood flow to the growth plate during a prolonged period of time. This phenomenon is present in vascular malformations and juvenile idiopathic arthritis. Adults with similar diseases (rheumatoid arthritis) present with radiological features other than overgrowth.

Growth lines (synonyms: growth recovery lines, growth arrest lines, Park-Harris lines) are thin sclerotic metaphyseal lines parallel to the growth plate. Usually they represent short periods of growth arrest during which the newly formed osteoid remains longer than usual in the zone of provisional calcification. These lines are nonspecific and can be caused by trauma, systemic illness and chemotherapy. Often no cause can be found (idiopathic). Growth lines can also be formed during short periods of hypermineralization, such as in vitamin D overload or bisphosphonate therapy (in patients with osteogenesis imperfecta). Lead bands in chronic lead intoxication are, in a way, caricatures of growth lines.

Growth lines disappear during growth, and can persist into adulthood, but they will not appear during adulthood.

During childhood, growth plates progressively become smaller until they close and the epiphysis and metaphysis fuse. However, some diseases simulate a widening of the growth plate (e.g., rickets, see section below on metaphysis).

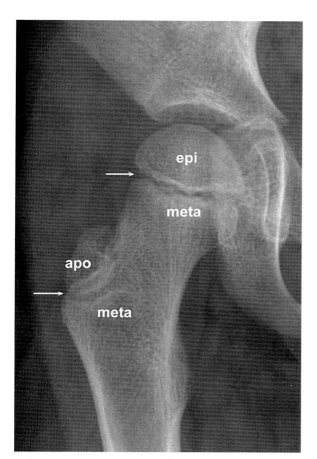

**Fig. 1.** Hip joint of a 6-year-old boy. Normal findings. *Arrows* point to growth plates. *apo* apophysis, *epi* epiphysis, *meta* metaphyis

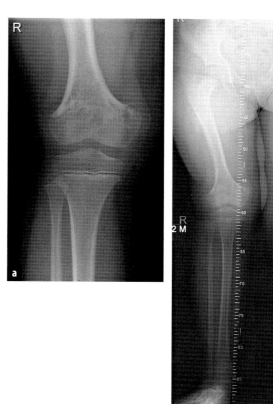

**Fig. 2 a, b.** A 7-year-old girl developed premature closure of the growth plate of the distal femur (**a**) after ostemyelitis at the age of 8 months, resulting in severe leg-length discrepancy (**b**)

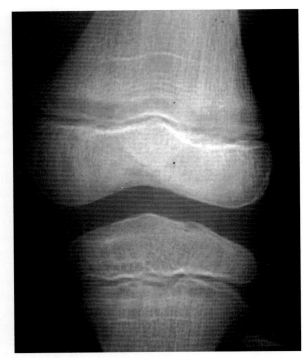

**Fig. 3.** A 5-year-old boy with a limp. Lucent metaphyseal bands at the proximal tibia and distal femur. Similar abnormalities were found at the hip. Diagnosis was acute lymphatic leukemia

## Metaphysis

Metaphyses are unique for the pediatric skeleton; after closure of the growth plate the metaphysis and epiphysis fuse and cease to exist as separate structures.

The metaphysis is characterized by high metabolism and vascularization; this is to be expected because both mineralization and enchondral bone formation take place at this location. In a sense, the metaphysis is the mirror of bone metabolism. All systemic diseases that alter bone metabolism will radiologically first become evident at the metaphysis. For instance, rickets (dietary, renal or hereditary) affects the whole skeleton but is radiologically recognized by its typical metaphyseal changes (fraying, splaying and cupping). Lead intoxication shows characteristic metaphyseal bands of increased density, whereas childhood leukemia demonstrates lucent metaphyseal bands (Fig. 3). In adults, these diseases show much less conspicuous skeletal changes and are more difficult to detect radiologically.

Because the metaphyseal vessels terminate in slow flow venous sinusoidal lakes, the metaphysis is predisposed as the starting point for acute hematogenous osteomyelitis [4]. The manifestation of osteomyelitis in children is age dependent. In infants, diaphysial vessels penetrate the growth plate to reach the epiphysis, facilitating epiphysial and joint infections in this age group [5, 6].

In older children, the growth plate constitutes a barrier for the diaphyseal vessels; in adults, the epiphysis and metaphysis each have a separate blood supply and infection from bone to joint is far less common [7].

## Epiphysis

Epiphyses are unique for the pediatric skeleton; after closure of the growth plate the epiphysis and metaphysis fuse and cease to exist as separate structures.

In contrast to the metaphysis, the epiphysis has a low metabolism and therefore little vascularization. So, from a metabolic point of view, the epiphysis is an uninteresting structure. However, there are some features that make the epiphysis radiologically interesting.

First, all epiphyses form joints, and the carpal and tarsal bones can also be considered as epiphyseal structures forming joints. Therefore diseases of epiphyseal structures can lead to severely disabling joint abnormalities. Structures that are anatomically and histologically similar but do not form joints are called apophyses (e.g., the greater trochanter; Fig. 1).

Second, these structures have a poor vascularization, not only because of their low metabolism but also because the growth plate forms an absolute barrier for blood vessels. This makes epiphyses, and carpal and tarsal bones prone to avascular necrosis. Many of these conditions have specific names, as shown in Table 1.

The radiological appearance is quite similar for all avascular epiphyses and carpal and tarsal bones: initially some widening of the joint space, followed by subchondral fractures, sclerosis and collapse, fragmentation, remineralization and finally remodeling. This process takes about 2 years and results in a somewhat flattened epiphysis with normal bone structure and normal mineralization. In adulthood, these joints are prone to early onset arthrosis.

In adults, the former epiphyses are less vulnerable because after closure of the growth plate vessels from the former metaphysis grow into the epiphysis.

Another disease that specifically affects the epiphyses (and carpal and tarsal bones) is multiple epiphyseal dysplasia, an autosomal dominant genetic skeletal dysplasia caused by mutations in the *COMP* gene and some *COL9A* genes (encoding collagen type IX). The epiphyses are small and irregular. Also, multiple epiphyseal dysplasia predisposes for early onset arthrosis.

**Table 1.** Avascular necrosis

| Site | Name |
| --- | --- |
| Femoral head epiphysis | Morbus Legg-Calve-Perthes |
| Distal lateral humerus epiphysis | Morbus Panner |
| Epiphysis MT II | Morbus Freiberg |
| Navicular of foot | Morbus Kohler |
| Lunate | Morbus Kienbock |

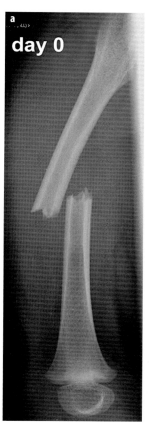
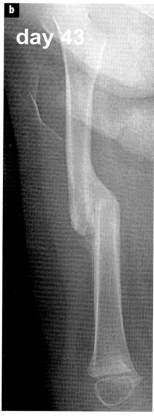
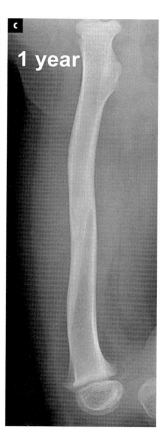

**Fig. 4 a-c. a** Midshaft femoral fracture in a 2-year-old boy. **b** Solid callus formation after 6 weeks. **c** Progressive remodeling after 1 year

## Metabolism, Bone Strucure and Vascularization

Bone metabolism and vascularization is higher in children than in adults. This results in a faster healing of fractures in children than in adults. Moreover, the process of remodeling corrects malalignment and angulation after fracture healing and can take place in 1 year (Fig. 4).

The bone of children contains a high amount of collagen and elastin, which facilitates typical childhood fractures such as greenstick fractures, torus fractures and bowing fractures.

The effects of the high metabolism on the metaphysis have been mentioned above in the section on the metaphysis.

## Bone Marrow

Bone marrow is classified as red (hematopoietic) and yellow (fatty) bone marrow depending on its composition [2, 8]. Red bone marrow contains 40% water, 40% fat and 20% protein, whereas yellow bone marrow contains 15% water, 80% fat and 5% protein. Moreover, red bone marrow has an extensive vascular network. Bone marrow is visualized with MRI. Fatty bone marrow shows high signal intensity on T1- and T2-weighted images and red bone marrow shows low intensity on T1-weighted images.

Premature and newborn children have red bone marrow, i.e., hematopoietic bone marrow. Bone marrow in children converts gradually from red bone marrow to fatty bone marrow during childhood. Conversion begins within the phalanges, and is complete by 1 year of age. Next, the diaphyses of the long bones start to convert, gradually spreading to the metaphyses. Isolated foci of residual metaphyseal red marrow in normal older children can cause confusion. These foci often have a flame-shaped configuration with their base at the growth plate and an increased T1 signal intensity relative to muscle. Another potential cause of confusion can be the speckled appearance of the childhood bone marrow of the hind- and midfoot after trauma, believed to be related to altered weight bearing. It is suggested that these T1-hypointense and T2-hyperintense speckles represent perivascular foci of red marrow [9].

In adolescence, red bone marrow is exclusively found in spine, skull and flat bones.

Epiphyses convert approximately 6 months after the appearance of the ossification center.

Many diseases affect the bone marrow: in childhood leukemia, bone marrow is gradually replaced by leukemic tissue; in sickle cell anemia, spherocytosis and thalassemia, hyperplasia of red bone marrow predominates;

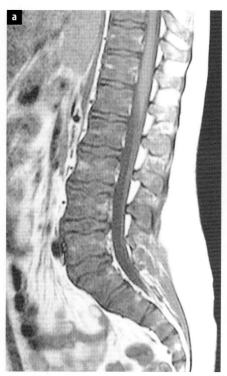
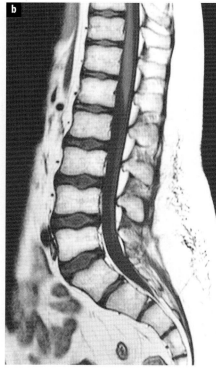

**Fig. 5 a, b.** A 14-year-old boy with acute lymphatic leukemia. **a** T1-weighted image of the lumbar spine shows absence of high fat signal intensity caused by replacement of fatty bone marrow by malignant cells. **b** After treatment, the fatty bone marrow has returned

in storage diseases, normal bone marrow is replaced by an excess of metabolites; and in aplastic anemia and after chemotherapy, myeloid tissue is depleted (Fig. 5).

The bone marrow changes in childhood leukemia cause diffuse osteopenia and, in contrast to adults, metaphyseal lucent lines on conventional radiographs (Fig. 3). These lucent lines are probably related to the high metabolism and vascularity of metaphyses.

In sickle cell anemia, the hematopoietic red bone marrow is prone to sickling and infarction because of the slow sinusoidal flow. In contrast to adults, hand-foot syndrome is a typical manifestation of sickle cell anemia in young children who still have red bone marrow in their hands and feet.

Storage diseases that manifest in childhood often show undertubulation of long bones, which is believed to be caused by the voluminous bone marrow combined with the increased bone turnover in children resulting in a re-modeling of bones to a much greater extent than in adults.

## Conclusion

Diagnosis of musculoskeletal disease in children is difficult and challenging because of the great variety of diseases and typical presentation of these diseases in children. Moreover, one should realize that there are many differences between the pediatric and adult musculoskeletal system. Knowledge of these differences will prevent any unnecessary delay in diagnosing pediatric musculoskeletal disease.

## References

1. Khanna PC, Thapa MM (2009) The growing skeleton: MR imaging appearances of developing cartilage. Magn Reson Imaging Clin N Am 17:411-21
2. Laor T, Jaramillo D (2009) MR imaging insights into skeletal maturation: what is normal? Radiology 250:28-38
3. Ecklund K, Jaramillo D (2001) Imaging of growth disturbance in children. Radiol Clin North Am 39:823-841
4. Green NE, Edwards K (1987) Bone and joint infections in children. Orthop Clin North Am 18:555-576
5. Asmar BI (1992) Osteomyelitis in the neonate. Infect Dis Clin North Am 6:117-132
6. McCarthy JJ, Dormans JP, Kozin SH, Pizzutillo PD (2005) Musculoskeletal infections in children: basic treatment principles and recent advancements. Instr Course Lect 54:515-528
7. Offiah AC (2006) Acute osteomyelitis, septic arthritis and discitis: differences between neonates and older children. Eur J Radiol 60:221-232
8. Foster KS, Chapman S, Johnson K (2004) MRI of the marrow in the paediatric skeleton. Clin Radiol 59:651-673
9. Shabshin N, Schweitzer ME, Morrison WB et al (2006) High-signal T2 changes of the bone marrow of the foot and ankle in children: red marrow or traumatic changes? Pediatr Radiol 36:670-676

# Vascular Malformations of the Musculoskeletal System

Philippe Petit[1], Michel Panuel[2]

[1] Department of Pediatric and Prenatal Radiology, Hôpital Timone Enfants, Marseille, France
[2] Department of Radiology, Hôpital Nord, Marseille, France

Vascular malformations are frequent pathologies in the pediatric age group and they can represent a real diagnostic challenge for the radiologist. In 1996, as a result of the efforts of the International Society for the Study of Vascular Anomalies, a new classification system clearly separated these developmental anomalies from the hemangiomas. The latter are benign tumors characterized by cells proliferations. Therefore, the vague term "angiomas" has now been replaced by specific entities, with adapted denomination, which present specific clinical and imaging features.

## Diagnosis Imaging Explorations

Doppler ultrasound (US) is the cornerstone of imaging exploration [1]. The use of linear high-frequency probes is essential, along with the use of low-frequency probes, in order to rule out an iceberg lesion. Absence of a Doppler signal does not mean absence of vascular flow in the lesion. In such cases, two main possibilities should always be considered: either the pulse repetition frequency is adjusted to a level that is too low to detect high speeds, or more frequently the Doppler is not sensitive enough to detect slow rates of blood flow, which can be sometimes seen in B mode.

X-rays are frequently added to US either to look for additional information in the soft tissues to help characterize the malformation [phlebolith in venous malformation (VM) (Fig. 1)], or to look for associated bony involvement. In cases of atypical US vascular lesions, the most important rule is always to consider a tumor, especially one of bony origin with soft tissue extension.

Magnetic resonance imaging (MRI) [2] has two definite roles. First, it facilitates assessment of the full extent of the malformation and accurately localizes the lesion compared with vital anatomical structures. Second, it can add useful information to that obtained from the US in order to definitely identify the malformation. Decisions

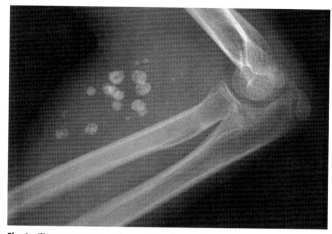

**Fig. 1.** Teenager presenting with a large intramuscular mass. X-ray demonstrates the presence of numerous phleboliths within the forearm, typical of a venous malformation

regarding the type of magnetic resonance (MR) sequences to be obtained and the need for gadolinium administration will depend on the results of the Doppler US examination. If the lesion is definitely identified by US as a VM or a lymphatic malformation (LM) there is no need for gadolinium administration.

Computed tomography is only indicated when cortical bone information is needed. This is very unusual in current practice.

Angiography is used only for exploration of arteriovenous malformation (AVM). Due to its aggressiveness, especially in pediatrics, it is almost always performed only as the first step before embolization. In some rare cases, where the feeding vessels are not sufficiently clear on MRI, angiography will be performed to accurately determine the therapeutic strategy. In this situation, the risk of an increase in activity of the lesion as a result of stimulation by the catheter should always be considered.

J. Hodler et al. (eds.), *Musculoskeletal Diseases 2013-2016,*
DOI: 10.1007/978-88-470-5292-5_37 © Springer-Verlag Italia 2013

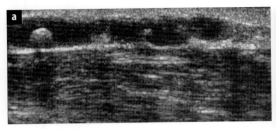
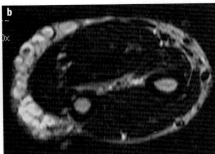

**Fig. 2 a, b.** A 7-year-old girl presenting with a venous malformation of the arm. **a** Ultrasound shows a tubular anechoic large venous structure containing a round hyperechoic structure with posterior shadowing (phlebolith). **b** T2 spin-echo sequence in the axial plane confirms the absence of deep extension of this malformation. A small phlebolith is visible as a hyposignal surrounded by the hypersignal of the stagnant fluid

## What Are the General Clinical Features?

Vascular malformations are present at birth, but might not be visible at this stage. They grow in proportion with the growth of the patient. LMs and VMs are classically discovered at a young age (neonates, babies), while AVM tends to become symptomatic later (teenagers), secondary to trauma or hormonal influence. Therefore the patient and his/her family can be unaware of LM and VM and AVM at the time of presentation. When they become known, the length of evolution, over several months or years, is very helpful in restricting the differential diagnoses, especially diagnoses of malignancy. The malformations can be isolated or they can be part of more complex syndromes (e.g., Klippel Trenaunay, Parkes Weber, Sturge Weber, Bean) [3].

## What Are the Main Types of Malformation, and How Are They Diagnosed and Treated?

### Venous Malformation

VM is the most frequent vascular malformation. It represents an embryological abnormal development of the venous system. It can be either superficial or deeply located (muscle, bone). It can be localized at all anatomical sites; the most frequent sites are the face, cervical region and limbs.

Clinically, when visible, VM appears as a blue lesion with low rate of blood flow or no detectable blood flow. Some small hard spots can be palpable, representing clots in the lesion, the phleboliths. The lesion increases in size with tourniquet or gravity and decreases in reverse positioning.

On imaging, the lesion can have several different appearances [4]. It can be a tubular-shaped structure, resembling varices running superficially or deeply, and be associated, or not, with dysplasia of the deep venous system (Fig. 2). It can be a hypoechoic mass that is superficial or intramuscular (Figs. 3, 4), focal, with no blood flow or slow rate of flow detected by Doppler US. The major differential diagnosis to consider in pediatric practice is rhabdomyosarcoma. The presence of a fluid-fluid level in the lesion is not sufficient to make a diagnosis

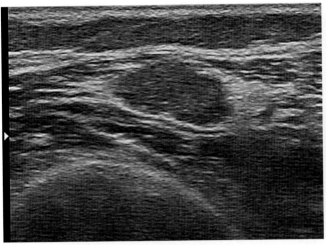

**Fig. 3.** A 16-year-old girl presenting with an acute pain of the left thigh corresponding to an acute thrombosis of a venous malformation. Ultrasound shows a hypoechoic homogeneous intramuscular mass surrounded by hyperechoic fatty tissue

of VM. On the other hand, the presence of poor arterial flow (<15 cm/s) does not exclude a diagnosis of VM. The mass, often multiloculated, can present like a bunch of grapes, with or without communication with the adjacent venous system. It is then essential to look for a round-shaped phlebolith, with or without posterior shadowing. Suspicion of VM without US confirmation can have one of two outcomes: either the patient is older than 5 years and an MRI should be performed (axial T1 and T2, axial T1 gadolinium sequences and subtraction, delayed three-dimensional T1 fat-saturated acquisitions), or he is younger than 5 years and diagnostic tests should be done:

- first, D-dimers, platelets and fibrinogen should be assayed to look for signs of local coagulopathy that favor a diagnosis of VM
- then, treatment with aspirin 75 mg/day for at least 1 week should be commenced. Patients with VM will become less symptomatic or asymptomatic and the lesion will appear compressible and less echogenic on US.

If the diagnosis remains uncertain, then a MR exploration under sedation should be carried out. If there is no

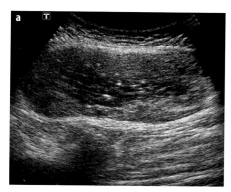
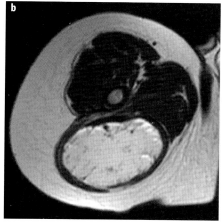
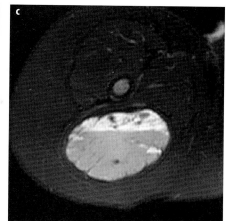
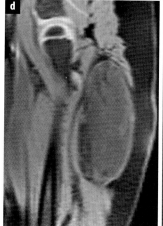
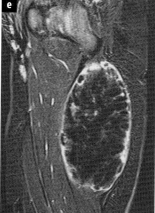
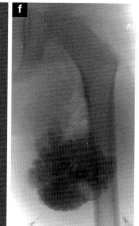

**Fig. 4 a-f.** A 2-year-old boy who presented with an asymptomatic large mass subsequently discovered an intramuscular well-limited venous malformation in the left thigh. **a** Ultrasound convex probe: well-limited heterogeneous and hypoechoic intramuscular mass containing some hyperechoic focus. **b** Magnetic resonance (MR) spin-echo (SE) T2 axial: the lesion appears almost in isosignal to fat with small hyposignal focus (phleboliths). **c** MR SE T2 fat-saturated axial image (at the same level as in **b**) reveals a fluid-fluid level. **d** MR echo gradient (EG) T1 sagittal image confirms a fluid-fluid level and absence of a hypersignal. **e** MR EG T1 sagittal image after gadolinium and subtraction on a delayed acquisition: feeding of the lesion is very poor, from peripheral to center. **f** Percutaneous embolization: injection into the malformation through butterfly needles of foam of aetoxysclerol. No venous drainage is visible

definite diagnosis after these tests, then a biopsy is mandatory. Samples must be sent for histopathology, immunohistochemistry and cytogenetic analyses.

Interventional radiology is part of the treatment armamentarium that can be used for patients with VM. Under local or general anesthesia, symptomatic or unesthetic venous malformations can be effectively treated by injection of sclerosing products, including polidocanol (liquid or foam), alcohol and sodium tetradecyl sulfate, through butterfly needles placed under US guidance (Fig. 4) [5].

## Lymphatic Malformation

LM is another frequent vascular malformation. It can be diagnosed antenatally or at birth. It consists of dilated lymphatic masses that do not have communication with the normal lymphatic system. It can be localized at all anatomical sites; the most frequent sites are the face, cervical region and limbs [6].

Clinically, the underlying skin can be normal, or present with multiple vesicles. An acute episode with hemorrhage or infection can reveal the lesion.

On US, a noncomplicated LM appears like a multiseptated cystic mass with thin walls. Micro and macro

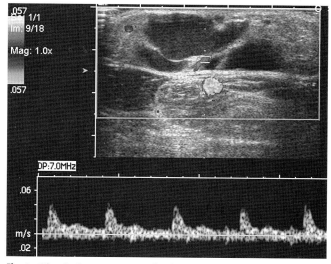

**Fig. 5.** Classical appearance of a lymphatic malformation, which appears as an anechoic multiloculated lesion with slow arterial flow in the septa (for color reproduction see p 318)

cysts can be present in the same lesion. The septa may contain small arteries with only poor rate of blood flow, or no flow may be visible within the lesion (Fig. 5). There can be difficulties in diagnosis, especially in complicated

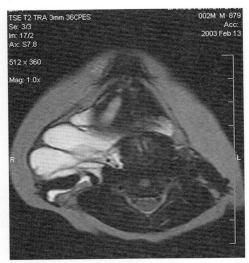

**Fig. 6.** Axial T2 section demonstrates homogeneous frank hypersignal of a lymphatic malformation of the neck

forms where the multiseptated appearance is no longer visible and a more tissular aspect is present. As with VMs, therapy with anti-inflammatory agents and antibiotics is required. US is better than MR at making a diagnosis in the complicated form of LM, because of the high power resolution of the 12-15 MHz US probes.

Regarding MRI, either the diagnosis is known with certainty before MRI, and therefore two orthogonal sequences in T2 are sufficient to assess the volume and the extent of the lesion, or the diagnosis is doubtful and then a complete MR work-up with intravenous injection of contrast media is mandatory (Fig. 6).

Percutaneous sclerotherapy is also often used for treatment [7]. Our preferred sclerosing agents include absolute alcohol, doxycycline, OK-432 and polidocanol.

## Arteriovenous Malformation

AVM is a malformation with a high rate of blood flow and abnormal communication between the arterial and venous network. This lesion has a wide spectrum of presentation. It may be quiescent or be responsible for hemorrhage and cardiac failure leading to amputation or death. Four stagings have been proposed from I (quiescent) to IV (very active). The lesion can grow and gain activity spontaneously, or after local trauma or hormonal stimulation (puberty, pregnancy) [8].

Clinically, two main signs should be looked for: warmth of the skin and a thrill.

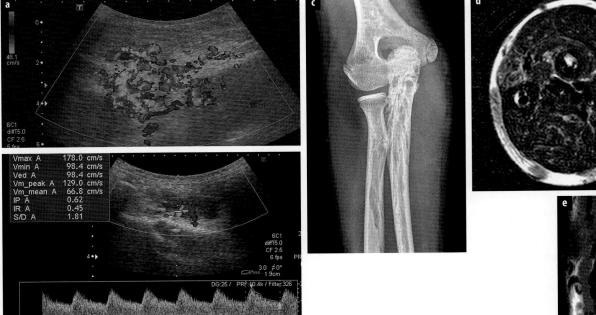

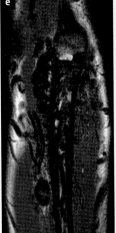

**Fig. 7 a-e.** A 12-year old girl with chronic swelling of the right elbow. Arteriovenous malformation was revealed at the time of ultrasound (US) examination. **a, b** US revealed multiple enlarged vessels, mainly arteries with high flow and low resistive index. No tissue mass was visible. **c** Anteroposterior view of the upper forearm shows sclerotic lesion of the ulna and radius indicating vascular involvement of the medullar bone. Heterogeneous water densities are also present in the subcutaneous fat. **d, e** Magnetic resonance imaging, axial T2 and coronal T1: multiple intraosseous and intramuscular flow voids are present, corresponding to high velocity flow in numerous vessels

US gives important clues for diagnosis of AVM. The lesion is not well limited, it can be located in the skin, muscle or bone, or in a combination of two or three of these tissues. It is made up of a bunch of large vessels, arteries and veins. A well-limited lesion should be considered as a tumor and needs a biopsy after MR exploration and multidisciplinary evaluation. Doppler is the key technique showing high velocity and low resistive index. However, these signs alone cannot rule out a tumor.

MR, and especially dynamic MR angiography, is well suited to demonstrate the vessels feeding the AVM, the abnormal fast venous drainage and the extent of this malformation in different tissues.

Angiography is limited to situations mentioned above.

Treatment should be considered at anytime the AVM becomes symptomatic [9]. However, a more aggressive approach is now being considered, since it has been demonstrated that all AVMs always progress over time [10]. The treatment involves endovascular embolization and surgery.

## Conclusion

Vascular malformations are frequent pathologies found in pediatric practice, from newborns to the teenagers. All radiologists will encounter these diagnoses during their career. A good knowledge of the US findings will help to accurately advise children and parents of diagnosis and treatment (Fig. 7). In complex cases and when treatment is planned, the availability of a multidisciplinary team is mandatory. If the lesion is not typical, either clinically or on imaging, then a histological test is needed.

## References

1. Dubois J, Alison M (2010) Vascular anomalies: what a radiologist needs to know. Pediatr Radiol 40:895-905
2. Moukaddam H, Pollak J, Haims AH (2009) MRI characteristics and classification of peripheral vascular malformations and tumors. Skeletal Radiol 38:535-547
3. Hyodoh H, Hori M, Akiba H et al (2005) Peripheral vascular malformations: imaging, treatment approaches, and therapeutic issues. Radiographics 25 (Suppl 1):S159-171
4. Dubois J, Soulez G, Oliva VL et al (2001) Soft-tissue venous malformations in adult patients: imaging and therapeutic issues. Radiographics 21:1519-1531
5. Goyal M, Causer PA, Armstrong D (2002) Venous vascular malformations in pediatric patients: comparison of results of alcohol sclerotherapy with proposed MR imaging classification. Radiology 223:639-644
6. Alqahtani A, Nguyen LT, Flageole H et al (1999) 25 year's experience with lymphangiomas in children. J Pediatr Surg 34:1164-1168
7. Churchill P, Otal D, Pemberton J et al (2011) Sclerotherapy for lymphatic malformations in children: a scoping review. J Pediatr Surg 46:912-922
8. Enjolras O, Logeart I, Gelbert F et al (2000) Arteriovenous malformations: a study of 200 cases. Ann Dermatol Venerol 127:17-22
9. Lee BB, Bergan JJ (2002) Advanced management of congenital vascular malformations: a multidisciplinary approach. Cardiovasc Surg 10:523-533
10. Liu AS, Mulliken JB, Zurakowski D et al (2010) Extracranial arteriovenous malformations: natural progression and recurrence after treatment. Plast Reconstr Surg 125:1185-1194

# BREAST IMAGING SATELLITE COURSE
## "PEARL"

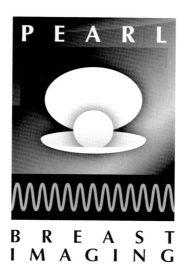

# Breast MRI BI-RADS®: Second Edition Highlights

Elizabeth A. Morris

Department of Radiology, Breast Imaging Center, Memorial Sloan-Kettering Cancer Center, New York, NY, USA

Since the first edition of the magnetic resonance imaging (MRI) section of the illustrated BI-RADS® lexicon, the field of breast MRI has grown enormously. Understandably, certain terms have been added or deleted as better terms have been identified. Additionally, concepts such as background parenchymal enhancement (BPE) have been proposed and included. A section on nonenhancing findings has been added. A section devoted to implant description and assessment is new.

## Focus

An enhancing focus is a tiny round pin-point "dot" of enhancement that is seen only on the postcontrast images. It is a round, homogeneously enhancing area with circumscribed margin. In general, foci are too small to exhibit internal enhancement characteristics. Foci can be found in women of any age and menopausal status. A focus can be benign or malignant.

In general, foci are a few millimeters in size; however, applying strict size criteria is not favored. It must be noted that cancers <5 mm can be identified in the breast on MRI. If margins and internal enhancement can be assessed, then the lesion would be considered a mass. As techniques improve, with higher resolution capabilities, fewer lesions will be described as a focus and more will be classified as a mass.

If a focus is not unique, it is likely to represent a component of the patient's background parenchymal enhancement (BPE). If it is unique and separate from the BPE, it may warrant evaluation. Margin analysis, kinetic analysis, internal enhancement and T2-weighted characteristics can be evaluated to determine whether a focus is likely to be benign or suspicious. Imaging features that favor benign etiology are circumscribed, persistent, homogeneous and very high signal intensity on bright fluid imaging. Imaging characteristics that favor malignancy are irregular, spiculated, wash out kinetics, rim or heterogeneous enhancement, and not very high in signal on bright fluid imaging.

## Mass

A mass is an area of enhancement with an epicenter and convex borders, existing as a three-dimensional (3D) structure. The committee decided not to assign a size requirement, recognizing that suspicious masses can be of all sizes. In general, as the mass size increases so does the likelihood of malignancy.

Mass descriptors for shape and margins have been adopted from the mammography BI-RADS® lexicon. In general, as with mammography, circumscribed oval or round masses are seen more with benign lesions, whereas irregular, spiculated masses are more likely to be malignant. Care should be taken with respect to morphology, as round circumscribed masses on MRI represent cancer more frequently than at mammography. There are several possible explanations for the presence of morphologically benign lesions representing cancer on MRI. First of all, MRI does not have the spatial resolution of mammography with current techniques and field strength so that margin analysis internal enhancement may suffer. Second, the cancers with benign morphology on MRI are usually small, and smaller than we might be used to detecting on mammography. As with most imaging techniques, the ability to resolve margins depends on the size of the lesion. Kinetic evaluation is important when considering these morphologically benign appearing lesions. As with other imaging techniques, the worst feature of the lesion under evaluation should be used to determine the need for biopsy.

A mass has internal enhancement that can be characterized. In general, homogeneous enhancement and nonenhancing internal septations indicate a possible benign process. While it is certainly possible to see classic appearances of certain lesions, morphologic overlap can occur between benign and malignant lesions; if there is any doubt, biopsy should be performed. The committee recognizes that when masses become large and ill-defined they might be described as regional enhancement.

Mass analysis can benefit from bright fluid sequences [i.e., T2 weighted or short-tau inversion recovery (STIR)]

J. Hodler et al. (eds.), *Musculoskeletal Diseases 2013-2016,*
DOI: 10.1007/978-88-470-5292-5_38 © Springer-Verlag Italia 2013

in addition to the postcontrast sequences obtained. In general, benign mass lesions can be increased in signal relative to fibroglandular parenchyma on bright fluid imaging, particularly cysts, lymph nodes and fibroadenomas. Cancers may or may not exhibit increased signal on bright fluid imaging. Cancer can be heterogeneously high in signal on bright fluid imaging if the tumors are necrotic, cellular or mucinous. Mucinous carcinoma and liposarcoma classically demonstrate very high signal on bright fluid sequences; however, there are usually other suspicious features, such as irregular shape or noncircumscribed margins, that warrant biopsy.

## Non-Mass Enhancement

In the first edition of the MRI section of the illustrated BI-RADS® lexicon, non-mass enhancement (NME) was used to describe BPE as well as areas that are still considered to be NME. With greater experience and understanding of BPE, some terms have been removed and the NME descriptors have been refined. NME describes enhancement in a pattern that does not have convex borders and may have intervening fat or normal fibroglandular tissue contained within the extent of the enhancement.

Clumped enhancement refers to enhancement that has the appearance of "cobble-stones" where there are small aggregates of enhancement that are variable in size and morphology. The term clumped refers to enhancement in a focal, linear or linear-branching, segmental or regional distribution. The term "clumped" on MRI is similar to the term "pleomorphic" on mammography, as it indicates enhancement in varying shapes and sizes. As ductal carcinoma in situ (DCIS) can present with this morphologic pattern, a description of clumped usually indicates a need for biopsy. The diagnosis of DCIS is usually made solely on lesion morphology, as many times the kinetic appearance does not meet minimal threshold and the time intensity curves are not typical for malignancy.

## Report Organization

### Amount of Fibroglandular Tissue

MRI is unique in that 3D volumetric data can be acquired from the image, and separation of fat and fibroglandular parenchyma is performed relatively easily. There are no data comparing mammographic density (breast composition) with MRI assessment of amount of fibroglandular tissue. Density is a term that should be applied only to mammography. The amount of fibroglandular tissue should be described as one of the following:
- Almost entirely fatty
- Scattered fibroglandular tissue
- Heterogeneous fibroglandular tissue
- Extreme fibroglandular tissue

As in the fifth edition of *BI-RADS® Mammography*, the amount of fibroglandular parenchyma is not described using percentages. Unlike mammography, where noncalcified breast lesions can be obscured by dense tissue, breast MRI is able to easily reveal an enhancing suspicious lesion independent of breast composition. Therefore, the amount of fibroglandular parenchyma does not adversely impact lesion detectability.

## Background Parenchymal Enhancement

As MRI is performed with intravenous contrast, the fibroglandular breast parenchyma can demonstrate contrast enhancement. BPE refers to the normal enhancement of the patient's fibroglandular tissue on the first postcontrast image. BPE refers to both the volume of enhancement as well as the intensity of enhancement, and an evaluation of background enhancement should take both into consideration.

The background enhancement is described as one of the following:
- Minimal
- Mild
- Moderate
- Marked

Although these categories are roughly quartiles, assigning strict percentages to indicate the degree of enhancement is likely artificial, difficult to assess without automation, and should be avoided. In general, BPE might not be evenly distributed throughout the entire breast. Due to preferential blood supply, there is the probability of greater enhancement in the upper outer quadrant of the breast and along the inferior aspect of the breast (formerly described as "sheet-like" enhancement). BPE might be more prominent in the luteal phase of the cycle if the patient is premenopausal. Therefore, for elective examinations (e.g., high-risk screening), effort should be made to schedule the patient in the second week of her cycle (days 7-14) to minimize the issue of background enhancement. Despite scheduling the patient at the optimal time of her cycle, BPE will still occur and the BPE terms should be applied. Women in whom cancer has been diagnosed and MRI is performed for staging (i.e., diagnostic) should be imaged with MRI regardless of the timing of the menstrual cycle or menstrual status.

The pattern of BPE can be variable from patient to patient, though in general the pattern of BPE for an individual is fairly constant. It is uncertain what the patterns of enhancement mean, therefore description beyond the recommended descriptors is optional. There is some evidence that BPE might indicate a level of risk for the development of breast cancer, as therapeutic measures such as anti-estrogen therapy can decrease the level of BPE. However, BPE does not appear to affect the ability to detect breast cancer.

BPE can occur regardless of the menstrual cycle or menopausal status of the patient. BPE might not be directly related to the amount of fibroglandular parenchyma present. Patients with extremely dense breasts at mammography might demonstrate little or no BPE, whereas patients with mildly dense breasts might demonstrate marked BPE. Nevertheless, most of the time, younger patients with dense breasts are more likely to demonstrate BPE.

In general, BPE is progressive over time; however, significant and fast enhancement can occur on the first post-contrast image despite fast imaging techniques. BPE on MRI is unique to a patient as is breast density at mammography. A description of background enhancement should be included in the breast MRI report.

Patterns of BPE are under investigation, as there is wide variation in the appearance from woman to woman. BPE may present as multiple foci either uniformly scattered or more focal in one area, described previously as "stippled" enhancement. Stippled enhancement is a pattern of BPE; it is usually diffuse and symmetric, however it can present as a focal finding (particularly in an area where cysts are found) suggesting focal fibrocystic disease.

### Non-Enhancing Findings

Non-enhancing findings seen on the precontrast or bright fluid images are benign. Examples include cysts, duct ectasia and some fibroadenomas and postoperative collections. Assessment of the absence of enhancement is best made on the subtraction image. Follow-up or biopsy of areas of non-enhancement is not necessary unless there are suspicious findings on another imaging modality, such as mammography or ultrasound.

## Assessment Categories

The final assessment should be based on the most suspicious finding present in each breast. A separate BI-RADS® assessment for each breast should be stated after the impression text. If the interpretation is straightforward and the same for both breasts, an overall impression that includes both breasts may be used. The overall assessment should be based on the most worrisome findings present in each breast. For example, if benign findings, such as lymph nodes or cysts, are noted along with a more suspicious finding, such as a spiculated mass, the final assessment code should be reported category 4 or 5. Similarly, if immediate additional evaluation is needed for one breast for a suspicious finding (with targeted ultrasound, for example), and there is a probably benign finding in the breast as well, the final assessment code for that breast would be category 4. If a breast with a known cancer has an additional suspicious finding warranting biopsy, then the final assessment code for that breast is category 4, not category 6.

### Category 0

Every effort should be made not to use category 0 in reading breast MRI. However, in the event that the examination is technically unacceptable (e.g., poor fat suppression, poor positioning) and would not be sufficient for interpretation, a meaningful report could not be issued and a category 0 may be issued. The MRI examination has characteristics that make it unique in comparison to mammography and ultrasound. The first and most obvious difference is the use of a contrast agent. This adds the parameter of blood flow to morphology with the associated flow metrics that may be calculated. The second is the acquisition of the exact same number and sequences whether the examination is for screening or diagnostic. As with mammography, BI-RADS® 0 should be used in the screening setting only. In interpreting breast MRI, there is enough information on the properly performed examination to decide to biopsy or recommend short-term follow-up of a specific finding. MRI, like mammography, can give a category 0 for prior MRIs before a report is issued that for auditing purposes will be replaced by the final assessment rendered in the addended report once prior examinations do become available – similar to a category 0 for technical reasons. This recommendation may change in the future when MRI screening becomes more commonplace.

A final assessment of 0 is helpful when a finding on MRI is suspicious but a benign corresponding finding on an additional study would prevent a biopsy. If a category 0 is given on MRI, then an explanatory note in the MRI report clarifying why this "suspicious" morphology is not immediately given a 4 or 5 is called for. For example, if a mass is suspicious on MRI but there is a possibility that it might represent a benign finding such as a lymph node, a targeted ultrasound that would prove that the lesion is benign would prevent a biopsy. In the case of an ultrasound recommendation following the MRI examination, the terms "MRI directed" or "MRI targeted" ultrasound are preferable to "second look" ultrasound, as it is not always certain that a "first look" ultrasound has been performed. Another example where category 0 would be useful is for a finding on MRI that is most likely fat necrosis, but the reader would like to confirm and correlate the findings to a mammogram that is not available.

When additional studies are compared or completed, a final assessment category attached to those additional studies would close out the MRI "0". When interpreting MRI it is extremely helpful to have all available imaging studies in order to give a complete report. If the additional studies can be reported in the same report, separate paragraphs indicating the pertinent findings from each imaging study can contribute to the final integrated assessment that takes into consideration the findings of all imaging studies.

### Category 1

This is a normal examination. A description of the fibroglandular tissue and background parenchymal enhancement should be included.

## Category 2

Benign findings are described in the report. Benign findings include intramammary lymph nodes, cysts, duct ectasia, postoperative collections, fat necrosis, scar, and masses, such as fibroadenomas, assessed as benign by morphology/kinetics or prior biopsy.

## Category 3

We recognize that there are few data in defining types of lesions that can be followed. There are reports that support short-term follow-up of (1) a new unique focus that is separate from the BPE but has benign morphologic and kinetic features, and (2) a mass on an initial examination with benign morphologic and kinetic features. There are data to suggest that BPE should not be followed, therefore BPE is inappropriate for follow-up. Similarly, non-mass enhancement should be characterized as either benign or malignant and given a final assessment; it should not be recommended for surveillance imaging.

## Category 4

Category 4 is used for the vast majority of findings prompting breast interventional procedures, ranging from diagnostic aspiration of complicated cysts to biopsy of fine linear and branching calcifications. According to BI-RADS® definitions expressed in terms of likelihood of malignancy, the cut points between category 3 versus category 4 assessments, and category 4 versus category 5 assessments, are 2% and 95%, respectively. Many institutions have, on an individual basis, subdivided category 4 to account for the vast range of lesions subjected to interventional procedures and corresponding broad range of likelihood of malignancy. This allows a more meaningful practice audit, is useful in research involving receiver-operating characteristic curve analysis, and is an aid for clinicians and pathologists.

Lesions that are appropriate to place in this category are: (1) suspicious non-mass enhancement such as clumped, linear, linear branching or segmental; (2) irregular, heterogeneous or rim enhancing masses; (3) foci with any suspicious morphology or kinetics. Specifically, a new focus with any suspicious feature warrants further evaluation by biopsy.

Suspicious findings on MRI warranting biopsy can be evaluated by targeted ultrasound. In general, masses are more likely to be seen on ultrasound than non-mass lesions. Biopsy of the finding should be performed with the modality that best illustrates the finding. If a correlate to the MRI finding can be reliably found on ultrasound, ultrasound biopsy might be preferable as it is usually more ubiquitous and cheaper than MR biopsy. Follow-up after both ultrasound and MRI biopsy is recommended, as missed lesions have been reported. Regarding the timing of follow-up, it has been recommended that a 6-month follow-up MRI is performed for all concordant

nonspecific benign pathology to ensure adequate sampling of the lesion. Some authors have suggested a single non-contrast T1-weighted image following ultrasound-guided biopsy for a suspicious lesion to ensure adequate and accurate sampling.

## Category 5

Category 5, highly suggestive of malignancy, was established at a time when most nonpalpable breast lesions underwent preoperative wire localization prior to surgical excision. Category 5 assessments were used for those lesions that had such characteristic features of cancer that one-stage surgical treatment might be performed immediately following frozen-section histological confirmation of malignancy. Today breast cancer diagnosis for imaging-detected lesions almost always involves percutaneous tissue sampling, so the current rationale for using category 5 assessment is to identify lesions for which any nonmalignant percutaneous tissue diagnosis is considered discordant, resulting in the recommendation for repeat (usually surgical) biopsy.

The likelihood of malignancy for category 5 assessments is ≥95%, so use of this assessment category is reserved for classic examples of malignancy. Note that there is no single MRI feature that is associated with a likelihood of malignancy of ≥95%. Just as it is found for mammography and breast ultrasound examinations, it takes a combination of suspicious MRI findings to justify a category 5 assessment.

## Category 6

This assessment category was added to the fourth edition of *BI-RADS® Mammography* for use in the special circumstance when breast imaging is performed after a tissue diagnosis of malignancy but prior to complete surgical excision. Unlike the more common situations when BI-RADS® categories 4 and 5 are used, a category 6 assessment will not usually be associated with recommendation for tissue diagnosis of the target lesion because biopsy has already established the presence of malignancy. Category 6 is the appropriate assessment, prior to complete surgical excision, for staging examinations of previously biopsied findings already shown to be malignant, after attempted complete removal of the target lesion by percutaneous core biopsy, and for the monitoring of response to neoadjuvant chemotherapy.

However, there are other scenarios in which patients with known biopsy-proven malignancy have breast imaging examinations. For example, the use of category 6 is not appropriate for breast imaging examinations performed following surgical excision of a malignancy (lumpectomy). In this clinical setting, tissue diagnosis will not be performed unless breast imaging demonstrates residual or new suspicious findings. Therefore, if a postlumpectomy examination demonstrates surgical scarring but no visible residual malignancy, the appropriate assessment is benign (BI-RADS® category 2). On the other hand, if there are, for example, residual suspicious lesions, the appropriate assessment is category 4 or 5.

There is one other potentially confusing situation involving the use of assessment category 6. This occurs when, prior to complete surgical excision of a biopsy-proven malignancy, breast imaging demonstrates one or more possibly suspicious findings other than the known cancer. Because subsequent management should first evaluate them as yet undetermined finding(s), involving additional imaging, imaging-guided tissue diagnosis or both, it must be made clear that in addition to the known malignancy there is at least one more finding requiring specific prompt action. The single overall assessment should be based on the most immediate action needed. If a finding or findings are identified for which tissue diagnosis is recommended, then a category 4 or 5 assessment should be rendered. If at additional imaging for finding(s) other than the known malignancy, it is deter-

mined that tissue diagnosis is not appropriate, then a category 6 assessment should be rendered accompanied by the recommendation that subsequent management now should be directed to the cancer. As for any examination in which there is more than one finding, the management section of the report might include a second sentence that describes the appropriate management for the finding(s) not covered by the overall assessment.

## Suggested Reading

American College of Radiology (ACR) (2013) ACR BI-RADS®, 5th edn

D'Orsi CJ, Mendelson EB, Morris EA et al (2012) Breast imaging reporting and data system: ACR BI-RADS. American College of Radiology, Reston

American College of Radiology (ACR) (2013) ACR BI-RADS® – Magnetic Resonance Imaging, 2nd edn

Morris EA, Ikeda DM, Lehman C et al (2012) Breast Imaging Reporting and Data System. American College of Radiology, Reston

# Advanced Breast Ultrasound and Interventions: An Update

Alexander Mundinger

Radiological Department and Breast Centre, Niels-Stensen-Clinics, Osnabrück, Germany

## Introduction

Ultrasound (US) technology has made progress in detecting and characterizing breast lesions, using frequencies between 7 and 18 MHz in combination with advanced tissue imaging technologies such as compound and harmonic imaging, volume scanning, modern color flow and elastography. The updated Breast Imaging Reporting and Data System (BI-RADS®) lexicon incorporates these new technological concepts and their impact on management. To date, description of a lesion should cover the new BI-RADS® US categories of vascularity and elasticity as associated findings. US constitutes the assessment method of choice for women with clinical signs and symptoms. Fundamental US enhances sensitivity for detecting cancer by 6-30% in symptomatic breast cancer patients. In risk patients with radiodense breasts, additive US to screening mammography improves the supplemental diagnostic detection rate after negative mammography by three to four per 1,000 women with dense breasts. The generally accepted role of US in population-based screening focuses on the assessment of suspicious mammographically detected lesions. US is indicated and routinely used in breast centers for preoperative staging, to monitor therapy and to keep patients under surveillance after breast conservation. US-guided core needle biopsy is the standard interventional technique for all breast lesions that correlate with findings of other imaging modalities. Sensitivity of US-guided large core needle biopsy (CNB) is 93-98%; specificity ranges from 95% to 100 %. The diagnostic accuracy of US-guided vacuum-assisted biopsy (VAB) is close to 100%. US-guided needle aspiration and CNB of the axilla should be used preoperatively to define metastatic lymph node involvement. Breast cancer screening based on automated whole breast US is an upcoming future horizon that will need sophisticated transfer of technological advancements to updated epidemiological concepts.

## Basics of Ultrasound Anatomy

Breast anatomy is the basis for understanding breast US. The breast is a modified skin gland enveloped in fibrous fascia. The undersurface of the breast lies on the deep pectoralis fascia. The superficial pectoralis fascia is located beneath the skin and nipple. The breast is composed of three major structures: skin, subcutaneous tissue and breast tissue, which contains parenchyma and stroma. The parenchyma is divided in 15-20 lobes or segments that converge at the nipple in a radial arrangement. Each lobe contains 20-40 lobules. Each lobule contains 10-100 ductules or acini. The terminal-duct lobular unit (TDLU) is the functional unit composed of a lobule and its terminal duct. Major ducts join below the nipple in a net-like pattern and widen in a portion named the lactiferous sinus before opening into the orifices of the nipple. The converging larger ducts drain the segmental ducts arising from subsegmental ducts and terminal ducts. To date, the definition of the ducts and associated TDLUs within a segment using a ductal or radial scanning examination technique complements the transversal and sagittal examination [1, 2]. Several proliferative breast diseases including ductal carcinoma in situ (DCIS) arise from the TDLUs (Fig. 1). Only DCIS cells expand throughout all ducts (Fig. 2). However, distended TDLUs due to DCIS develop rarely, while high-resolution US (HRUS) detects distended TDLUs frequently in various benign lesions. Therefore, additional information is necessary, such as a suspicious segmental distribution or the correlation to suspect imaging findings with mammography or magnetic resonance imaging (MRI). Tiny changes, as small as 2-5 mm in diameter, can be dismissed in analogy with MRI-detected foci. In contrast, such small pseudocystic changes must be assessed in the presence of concern about multifocality or duct extension of DCIS.

The echogenicity of fat is the reference for comparing other anatomical structures within breast US [1, 2]:

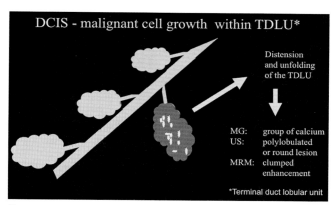

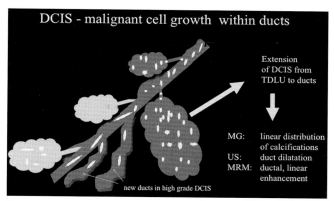

**Fig. 1.** Ductal carcinoma in situ (DCIS): malignant cell growth resulting in a distension of the terminal-duct lobular unit (TDLU). Various other benign proliferative or fibrocystic changes develop along a distinct genetic and morphological pathway and can also result in a distension of the TDLU. Associated calcifications within the TDLU develop in DCIS, fibrocystic changes, sclerosing adenosis, and other forms of adenosis. Expanded TDLUs can be depicted by mammography, ultrasound, or magnetic resonance mammography. Corresponding diagnostic criteria are listed in the text (for color reproduction see p 318)

**Fig. 2.** Ductal carcinoma in situ (DCIS): malignant extension of DCIS into the ducts and other terminal-duct lobular units (TD-LUs). New ducts can be formed in high-grade DCIS. Corresponding diagnostic criteria are given and focus on the linear extension or dilatation of ducts in all imaging modalities (for color reproduction see p 318)

- Isoechoic echogenicity is found in fat, epithelium, loose periductal and intralobular fibrous tissue and some TDLUs
- Hyperechoic echogenicity is found in skin, Cooper's ligaments, stromal fibrous tissue (interlobular) and some TDLUs
- Hypoechoic echogenicity is found in nipple, blood vessels and some TDLUs
- Anechoic echogenicity is found in dilated TDLUs (cysts), ducts and lymphatics

## Physics and Equipment

US of the breast provides physical information about the impedance of tissue interfaces that influence US transmission and reflection across the breast. The different physical base of US, X-ray mammography and MRI of the breast explains the independent and complementary diagnostic information given by each modality. The most relevant advances made in recent years are due to high-frequency US transducer equipment using frequencies between 7 and 18 MHz. Scanning with 15 MHz in comparison with 7.5 MHz results in a lateral (0.4 mm) and axial (0.2 mm) spatial resolution that is twice as high as the spatial resolution at 7.5 MHz. On the other hand, penetration depth is reduced to half. Compounding and harmonic imaging improves contrast resolution and reduces speckle artefacts. The high spatial and contrast resolution of modern breast US equipment has expanded the detection and conspicuity of subtle lesions the size of expanded TDLUs such as DCIS and microinvasive lesions. Color Doppler techniques detect and characterize blood flow within lesions, and this allows discrimination between

solid nodules and complicated cysts. Three-dimensional (3D) diagnostic imaging of the breast includes multidimensional reformations, reconstructions and tomographic US. The additional diagnostic information of 3D US focuses on demonstrating suspicious radial retractions around a tumor in the coronal plane, which is unique to this technique. Elastography reflects strain properties of lesions. Malignant nodules are generally less compressible than benign tissue. Strain, shear wave and semistatic elastography are the actual techniques to assess tissue stiffness. Elastography can downstage BI-RADS® 3 lesions independent of the applied technique. The future role of elastography continues to be evaluated. New horizons in high-end US technology encompass miniaturized and portable US systems, and automated whole breast US, and imaging fusion of US information with digital mammography, tomosynthesis, contrast enhanced dual energy mammography, MRI or positron emission tomography [3, 4].

## Indications for Breast Ultrasound

A list of updated recommendations pertaining to indications is given in Box 1 (modified according to [3]). US is the first-line imaging technique for women <40 years presenting with symptoms or clinical signs. In the presence of a suspicious lesion, US is the method of choice to guide core biopsy in order to harvest tissue. US-guided VAB is used increasingly to diagnose intraductal lesions, small architectural distortions and borderline lesions; to complete preoperative staging in patients with extensive ductal component; and for therapeutic excision. Stereotactic-guided VAB is the method of choice to sample screen-detected microcalcifications and architectural distortions not seen on US. In the dense breast, the combination of US and screening mammography improves

**Box 1.** Updated indications for high-resolution US

> Differentiation of cysts and solid tumors
> Differentiation between solid, benign and malignant lesions
> Characterization of palpable abnormalities
> Assessment of mammographic screening abnormalities
> Dense breasts showing with reduced mammographic sensitivity
> Diagnosis and follow-up of women with benign breast disease or risk lesions
> Women, during pregnancy or lactation
> Significant nipple discharge
> Under hormonal replacement therapy
> Inflamed breast and abscesses formation
> Extended screening for high-risk patients
> Second look after magnetic resonance mammography
> Guidance of interventional procedures, such as fine needle aspiration, core biopsy, diagnostic and therapeutic vacuum biopsy and preoperative tumor localization, axillary lymph node biopsy
> Preoperative staging of lesion size, skin and nipple distance for planning breast conservative surgery, mastectomy or oncoplastic reconstruction with implants, assessment of multifocality, multicentricity, intraductal extension, lymph node changes and contralateral lesions
> Preoperative staging and follow-up under neoadjuvant chemotherapy
> Surveillance after breast-conservation therapy
> Silicone implants

*US* ultrasound

cancer detection considerably compared with mammography alone, but with an increase in biopsy rate. The additional diagnostic yield of US after negative mammography is 3.2:1,000 women with dense breasts. Intraoperative surgeon-performed US focuses on accurately defining the resection segment or sector and the margin analysis of the resection specimen. MRI is useful preoperatively to assess the extent of ipsilateral disease and exclude contralateral breast cancer, particularly for women at increased risk of mammographically occult disease. Second-look US can detect up to 50% of magnetic-resonance-enhancing cancers with negative mammography [5-8].

## Examination Technique

The International Breast Ultrasound School (IBUS) and American College of Radiology (ACR) guidelines for breast US examination advise a systematic, comprehensive and reproducible examination technique, followed by documentation, description, reporting, classification and recommendation. The examination starts with proper positioning of the patient in a supine or anterior oblique position depending on the breast volume, with elevation of the ipsilateral arm. Positioning should result in a maximum flattening of the breast portion being examined. Automated tissue optimization, focal zone and field of view

settings should be optimized before scanning with the transducer perpendicular to skin. A minimum of two scan planes is recommended in whole breast US. Image analysis of a detected lesion or pseudolesion requires rotation of the transducer over the entire lesion using changing compression intensities and angulations. Radial imaging of adjacent ducts is mandatory to assess ductal extensions. BI-RADS® descriptors and further criteria of additional elastography, 3D tissue criteria, vascularization and associated lymph node morphology characterise a state-of-the-art lesions assessment by US. The o'clock position and distances to skin and nipple describe the exact localization of a lesion within the volume of the breast. Indication of palpability and imaging correlation to other modalities complete the documentation [9-12].

## Concepts of Interpretation Based on Ultrasound BI-RADS® Descriptors

The categorization of a mass finding in all modalities relates to a 3D macropathological tissue lesion. The pathology defines lesion shape, margin and texture. These features have already been described individually for the varying modalities. A uniform wording of the major diagnostic criteria for all modalities would be logical. The BI-RADS® concept took a first step in this direction and was designed primarily as a mammographic language with a clear, defined terminology. In 2003, the ACR published the Breast Imaging Atlas, which is a BI-RADS® lexicon for mammography, US and MRI. The US chapters were originally arranged under the chair of Ellen B. Mendelson [11], and the descriptors or diagnostic criteria are presented with increasing probability of malignancy. Descriptors of a mass include shape, orientation, margin, boundary, echo pattern, posterior acoustic feature and characteristics of surrounding tissue, as well as associated distinguishing findings. The combination of several descriptors predicts malignancy better than one single descriptor. However, the reader should use further explanatory elements in the guidance chapters of the atlas, such as clinical context conditions, tumor biology and epidemiological prevalence, to cover the complex field of breast lesions. Assumptions regarding the expected prevalence and individual risk for cancer in a patient drive the intuitive recommendation for or against a biopsy and influence the choice of a final BI-RADS® assessment category. In other words, the threshold for performing a biopsy is lower for a probably benign-looking lesion compared with a screening setting if advanced age, large lesion, palpability or individual high-risk situation concern the reader. BI-RADS® categories 3-5 imply a defined probability of malignancy for each category. For BI-RADS® 3, these probabilities are <2%, for BI-RADS® 4 between 3% and 94%, and for BI-RADS® 5 ≥95%. Most European US societies have adopted or modified the ACR BI-RADS® US guidelines. In addition to the 2003 US descriptors, various features have been

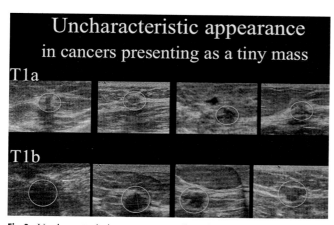

**Fig. 3.** Uncharacteristic appearance of small cancers stages T1a and T1b. All these cancers have been detected by screening mammogram and correlated to ultrasound secondarily during assessment (courtesy of Screening Centre Southwest Lower Saxony; Praxis Drewes and Partners). Several small benign lesions resemble the presentation of small cancers (for color reproduction see p 319)

---

**Box 2.** Underlying concepts of BI-RADS® US assessment categories

Categorization and management depend on the most suspicious diagnostic criterion

Benign lesions must look typically benign; no suspicious image descriptor

Malignant lesions frequently show one or more suspicious criteria

Predefined thresholds for positive predictive value or cancer risk influence the classification in categories 2-5

Overall BI-RADS® category must consider further clinical context conditions, expected prevalence and other risk factors in addition to morphological criteria of each imaging modality assessment category

Typical indicators of benignancy such as cysts, fat in a lesion (hamartoma) or benign macrocalcification (popcorn calcification with fibroadenoma) diagnosed by multimodality evaluation can downgrade overall assessment category compared with US category

Indicators of potential malignancy in other modalities can upgrade overall assessment category compared with US category

Overall assessment category should also be based on the most urgently needed procedure. This point of view ensures critical re-evaluation of final assessment category

*BI-RADS®* Breast Imaging and Reporting Data System
*US* ultrasound

---

suggested, such as elastic compressibility, movability, 3D criteria, detailed lymph node morphology and others. Further prospective multicenter studies are needed to validate the complementary diagnostic importance of such associated features as an adjunct to the basic characteristics of a lesion [12, 13]. Recently, several authors disclosed that interobserver agreement with the new BI-RADS® terminology is good, and validated the lexicon in retrospect following landmark studies in the 1990s. Only

fair agreement exists in most studies for margin evaluation. Further, a trend towards lower concordance was noted for evaluating small masses. Classification into subdivisions 4a, 4b and 4c was more or less reproducible. Despite its limitations, most authors agree that stratification predicting the likelihood of malignancy could be useful for decision making and communication with patients, and between researchers, physicians and physicians of different specialties [14-17]. The updated second edition of BI-RADS® US (2013) will re-emphasize the importance of basic features, such as mass shape, margin and orientation on one hand, and associated findings as an adjunct on the other. The amended chapters cover expanded general issues, detailed lexicon images and US descriptors, reporting system and guidance. Fig. 3 presents a training schema for beginners in the field of breast diagnostics that can be used to learn standardized BI-RADS® US reading of larger masses. This schema has no scientific proof for use in daily work-up. Box 2 highlights some underlying intrinsic and extrinsic concepts of BI-RADS® US assessment categories that must be considered in daily work.

## Concepts of Interpretation and Clinical Decision Making

The US characterization of a lesion in the daily routine follows a reproducible diagnostic algorithm and should involve fundamental US and all advanced applications of the used US system, preferably on a one-click basis.

First, the reader must define whether or not the lesion resembles a typical benign finding, such as cyst, lipoma, lymph node or previously known scar or fibroadenoma (Fig. 3). Complicated cysts with internal debris are challenging. When the debris is mobile or a fluid-debris level is seen, complicated cysts can be dismissed as benign findings, i.e. BI-RADS® US category 2 [11, 18].

Second, a typical oval-shaped, hypoechoic lesion with circumscribed margins and horizontal orientation in young women is most likely a fibroadenoma (Fig. 4). Short-term follow-up can be used. Several studies concluded that short-term follow-up of such BI-RADS® US category 3 lesions is associated with a cancer rate <2% [19-21]. Being older than 45 years, palpability or any preselection that enriched cancer cases in the collective is associated with cancer rates >2%. In a recent study, 0.8% of 4,000 women with lesions that were initially classified as probably benign proved to be malignant at follow-up. The most frequent reason for a false-negative assessment on US was failure to recognize suspicious margin characteristics (28 of 32 malignancies, 87.5%). Malignancy was more frequent in palpable (2.4%, 21 of 859) than nonpalpable lesions (0.4%, 11 of 3,141) [22]. As an isolated finding, homogeneous complicated cysts and clustered microcysts can be classified as probably benign, particularly if the lesion is new or rather small or deep, i.e., diagnostic uncertainty exists [18].

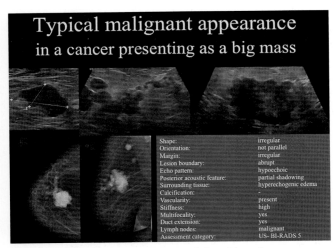

**Fig. 4.** Typical malignant appearance of ductal invasive cancer presenting as a lump in a 70-year-old patient. Mammography and ultrasound present the tumorous irregular mass, branching pattern of ductal extension, multifocal lesions, and axillary lymph node metastasis showing an expanded cortex. Description is given for the biggest mass following ultrasound Breast Imaging Reporting and Data System

### Adopted BI-RADS®-US training schema

| Margin \ Shape | Round, Oval | Lobulated | Irregular |
|---|---|---|---|
| Circumscribed | 2 (multiple) 3 (singular) | 3 (moderate) 4 (marked) | 4 |
| Indistinct Angular Microlobulated | 4 | 4 | 5 |
| Spiculated | 5 | 5 | 5 |

| Indicator of benignity |
|---|
| Typical cyst |
| Lymph node |
| Lipoma |

| Indicator of malignancy |
|---|
| Echogenic halo |
| Taller than wide |
| Strong hypoechoic |
| Shadowing |
| Ductal extension |
| Retraction pattern |
| Hypervascularity |
| Stiffness |

↓

**Upgrade or Downgrade of BI-RADS® Category**

**Fig. 5.** Adopted Breast Imaging Reporting and Data System ultrasound (BI-RADS US) training schema. BI-RADS characterization of a mass can be taught using basic descriptors and associated findings that upgrade or downgrade the overall assessment category. The teaching should support beginners in the field of breast diagnosis. This schema provides no scientific proof for use in daily workup, as it can miss cancers

Third, detailed analysis of US morphology, vascularity and elasticity of a lesion should disclose any suspicious basic descriptor or suspicious associated finding. The presence of suspicious descriptors results in a BI-RADS® US category 4 or 5 depending on the total number and character of these descriptors. A biopsy is recommended in these cases and also in benign-looking lesions that significantly increase in size during follow-up (Fig. 5) [11].

## Updated Role of Ultrasound, Including Interventions

US studies in up to 12,000 asymptomatic patients yielded tumor detection rates of only 0.3-0.4%; however, a similar size and stage was reported compared with mammographically detected clinically occult cancers. The advantage of US as an adjunct to mammography is greatest in women with palpable lesions and those at high risk, including women with dense breasts, which is a risk factor. The US signs of malignancy develop with increasing tumor size. No single diagnostic sign can pick up all cancers due to their heterogeneous appearance (Figs. 6-8). Patients with a high mammographic density (>75%) present in meta-analysis with fourfold increased risk compared with women with low radiodense breasts, and a twofold increased risk compared with women with scattered fibroglandular breasts [7]. The sensitivity of standard US for breast cancer varies from 55% to 95%. US transfers an additional diagnostic yield of 30-40% in comparison with mammography to patients with radiodense breasts in the incidence setting (Fig. 5). The updated ACR Imaging Network (ACRIN) follow-up study focuses on cancer

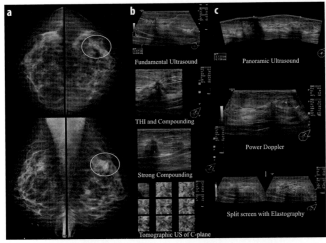

**Fig. 6 a-c.** A 48-year-old patient presenting with an architectural distortion in mammography (**a**). Corresponding mass could be missed using fundamental ultrasound (US) only. Advanced US modes (**b**, **c**) clearly show a mass with spiculations, retraction pattern in 3D US, associated flow, and moderate stiffness. Histology was ductal invasive cancer (*G1*). *THI*, tissue harmonic imaging (for color reproduction see p 319)

detection in patients with increased risk due to radiodense breasts, under surveillance after breast cancer or other conditions. Of 100 imaging-detected cancers, 23 cancers have been found only by mammography, 22 by US only, 26 by both methods, and 9 by MRI only. In national screening programs, mammography is still the method of choice for early breast cancer detection. The upcoming Austrian national screening program will add US in all women presenting with an ACR density level 3 and 4 (dense and extremely dense). To date, mammography still

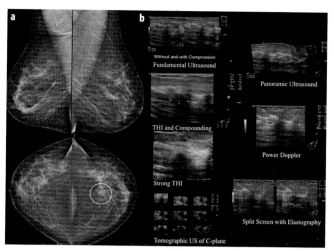

**Fig. 7 a, b.** A 47-year-old woman with mammographic mass (**a**) at 12 o'clock and corresponding ultrasound (US) (**b**) lesion presenting as an irregular hypoechoic mass, with strong shadowing, poor vascularity, and stiffness (*blue* low strain in the strain elastography image). Histology was ductal invasive cancer with low proliferation fraction. *THI,* tissue harmonic imaging (for color reproduction see p 319)

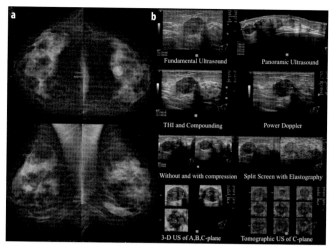

**Fig. 8 a, b.** A 51-year-old woman presenting with a recurrent mass following incomplete resection of a fibroadenoma using vacuum-assisted biopsy (VAB) 2 years earlier. Mammography shows a circumscribed round mass (**a**). Ultrasound (**b**) presents a correlative oval mass, adjacent scar with strong shadowing due to former VAB, and a second lesion. Both lesions show low vascularity and intermediate elasticity. Histology of both lesions showed fibroadenomas abundant with cells and regressive changes. *THI,* tissue harmonic imaging (for color reproduction see p 319)

provides the best compromise between advantages, disadvantages and costs [23, 24]. Breast US is indicated for further assessment of mammographic abnormalities and guiding minimally invasive biopsy. Masses in mammography and on MRI can be correlated with US confidently with increasing size, starting at a diameter of 0.5 cm [25-27]. Although advanced US is suitable for detecting subtle changes of DCIS, the detection rate of DCIS by US is low without prior knowledge of focal DCIS at mammography. Targeted US of suspected DCIS frequently finds hypoechoic lesions that represent dilated TDLUs and look similar to them, such as fibroadenoma, papilloma, ductectasia or microcystic changes. US is the method of choice when assessing and puncturing such solid-looking small masses, dilated ducts, pseudomicrocystic lesions or dense accumulations of microcalcifications that corresponded with mammographic changes. A radiogram of large-core cylinders is mandatory to correlate the US finding with index calcifications [3]. Underestimation of US-guided 14 G large core needle biopsy (LCNB) in comparison with VAB is an unsolved problem in the preoperative diagnosis of DCIS compared with the golden standard of surgical excision. Therefore, such patients rather should be directed towards VAB rather than LCNB. Underestimation rates in DCIS are reported to be between 9% and 16% for VAB, and 22% and 48% for LCNB [3, 27, 28]. For localization of nonpalpable breast cancer, intraoperative US is a reliable alternative to guide wire localization, as it achieves similar results in terms of complete tumor removal (93%), re-excision rate (11%) and excised volume [29]. Intraoperative breast US can guide segmental surgery with wide distances to the malignant lesions. High-resolution US shows a comparable diagnostic performance in preoperative staging with MRI in

invasive ductal cancer. MRI performs better in preoperative staging of lobular invasive cancer, DCIS, multifocality, multicentricity and posterior breast-wall involvement, as well as diagnosing recurrence, failing silicon prosthesis and monitoring during neoadjuvant therapy. The median additional detection yield for MRI is estimated as 16% in meta-analyses. To date, there is no evidence that preoperative MRI improves surgical care or prognosis [30-32]. The analogous statement is probably true for the role of US in preoperative staging. The presence of Doppler blood flow increases the malignancy pick-up rate, but at the expense of a significant decrease in specificity and diagnostic accuracy, and an increase in biopsy rate prognosis [33]. Contrast-enhanced US (CEUS) does not appear to be superior to conventional US as a diagnostic tool overall; however, it is a very rarely used adjunct, with no role in daily routine work. The overall true-positive rates for conventional US and CEUS have been found to be 88% and 86%, respectively. DCIS, medullary carcinoma, and intraductal papillary carcinoma achieved improved true-positive rates with 94%, 100% and 100%, respectively [34]. Elastography can increase the specificity of the US examination. Two recent meta-analyses on strain elastography reported summary sensitivities of 88% and 83%, and specificities of 83% and 84% [35, 36]. Also, several studies based on shear wave elastography have shed light on the old experience that soft should be benign and stiff resembles malignancy. In BI-RADS® 4a and 3 US lesions, the certainty of benignity is increased in an elastographic very soft lesion [37]. In contrast, the presence of an elastographic very stiff malignant lesion is associated with poor prognosis measured by histologic parameters [38]. All elastographic techniques aim to characterize breast lesions that have been previously detected and categorized according to BI-RADS® by real-time US. Therefore, the role of elastography in its various applications resembles an additional characterizing tool, such as Doppler. It has no role in population-based breast cancer screening or primary detection of US lesions. In summary, elastography will enter clinical routine and, in combination with Doppler, will increase the potential of advanced US to better characterize breast lesions.

Automated breast US acquires data of the 3D breast volume that can be analyzed on a workstation subsequent to the examination. This technology has the potential to develop US to become a primary screening tool and seems to show similar potential in characterizing lesions according to BI-RADS® US, at similar or slightly reduced diagnostic accuracy [39, 40].

Sentinel lymph node (SLN) biopsy is associated with a low local recurrence and similar survival rates to axillary lymph node dissection, and is now the standard of care. All patients with invasive breast cancer should have US of the axilla to exclude obvious nodal local spread. The presence of asymmetric focal hypoechoic cortical lobulations >3 mm, or a completely hypoechoic node with US, should direct further examination to fine-needle aspiration of the index lymph node. Cortical thickness greater than 3 mm reveals an increased risk of approximately four times for the presence of an axillary lymph node metastasis, as compared with cortical thickness less than 3 mm. Further, the absence of a hilum shows the highest specificity for axillary lymph node metastasis (94.6%), but low sensitivity [41]. US-guided biopsy of axillary lymph nodes has a sensitivity that varies between 30.6% (22.5-39.6%) and 62.9% (49.7-74.8%), and a specificity of 100% (94.8-100%) [42]. When the cytological or histological finding is positive, SLN biopsy can be omitted and primary axillary lymph node dissection be performed. In negative US findings, SLN biopsy should be performed due to the substantial number of false-negative results in patients with invasive breast cancer, although preoperative axillary US alone may exclude most cases of N2 and N3 disease [43, 44].

HRUS provides additional diagnostic information compared with mammography in postoperative surveillance after breast-conserving and oncoplastic surgery. MRI would be the method of choice for surveillance with respect to its better diagnostic performance in comparison with mammography and US [45]. However, costs and availability restrict the use of MRI to high-risk patients and differentiation between scar and recurrence with a problematic diagnostic background presented by the other modalities. Most surveillance guidelines rely on mammography alone or mammography in combination with US. To detect one locoregional recurrence or second primary breast cancer preclinically, 1,349 physical examinations versus 262 mammography and/or MRI tests were performed. Follow-up provided by only one discipline might decrease the number of unnecessary follow-up visits. Breast imaging plays a major role and physical examination a minor role in the early detection of second primary breast cancers and locoregional recurrences. The ability of physical examination to detect relapses early is low and should therefore be minimized.

## Summary

Modern breast care requires definitive nonoperative diagnosis of all potential breast abnormalities in a timely and cost-effective way. US-guided CNB has become the minimal invasive biopsy method of choice for all breast lesions (sensitivity 93-98 %; specificity 95-100%). US-guided VAB is increasingly being used for diagnosing borderline lesions, for complete preoperative staging in patients with extensive ductal component, and for therapeutic excision of biopsy-proven benign lesions, such as fibroadenomas and some papillary lesions and radial scars. The diagnostic accuracy of US-guided VAB for invasive cancers is close to 100% [3, 25, 27].

## References

1. Mundinger A (2011) Ultrasound of the breast including interventions: an update. In Hodler J, von Schulthess GK, Zollikofer CH L (Eds) Diseases of the heart, chest and breast 2011-2014. Springer-Verlag Italy, Milano, pp 259-266
2. Teboul M (2010) Advantages of ductal echography (DE) over conventional breast investigation in the diagnosis of breast malignancies. Medical Ultrasonography 2:32-42
3. Weismann C, Mayr C, Egger H, Auer A (2011) Breast sonography -2D,3D,4D ultrasound or elastography? Breast Care 6: 98-103
4. Mundinger A, Wilson ARM, Weismann C et al (2010) Breast ultrasound − update. EJC Supplements 8:11-14
5. ACR (2009) Practice guideline for the performance of ultrasound-guided percutaneous breast interventional procedures. Revised 2009. http://www.acr.org/SecondaryMainMenuCategories/quality_safety/guidelines/breast/us_guided_breast.aspx
6. American College of Radiology (ACR) (2009) Practice guideline for the performance of stereotactically guided breast interventional procedures. Revised 2009. http://www.acr.org/SecondaryMainMenuCategories/quality_safety/guidelines/breast/stereotactically_guided_breast.aspx
7. McCormack VA, Dos Santos Silva I (2006) Breast density and parenchymal patterns as markers of Breast Cancer Risk: A Meta-analysis. Cancer Epidemiol Biomarkers Prev15:1159-1169
8. Heywang-Köbrunner SH, Schreer I, Heindel et al (2008) Imaging studies for the early detection of breast cancer. Dtsch Arztebl Int 105:541-547
9. Madjar H, Rickard M, Jellins J et al (1999) IBUS guidelines for the ultrasonic examination of the breast. Eur J Ultrasound 9:99-102
10. Khouri NF (2009) Breast ultrasound. In: Harris J, Morrow M, Lippman M, Osborne C (Eds) Diseases of the breast, 4th edn. Wolter Kluwer, Lippincott Williams & Wilkins, Philadelphia, PA, pp 131-151
11. American College of Radiology (ACR) (2003) ACR BI-RADS® − Ultrasound. In: ACR Breast Imaging Reporting and Data System, Breast imaging atlas. American College of Radiology, Reston VA

12. Madjar H, Ohlinger R, Mundinger A et al (2006) BI-RADS-analogue DEGUM criteria for findings in breast ultrasound - consensus of the DEGUM Committee on Breast Ultrasound. Ultraschall Med 27(4):374-379

13. Wojcinski S, Farrokh A, Weber S et al (2010) Multicenter study of ultrasound real-time tissue elastography in 779 cases for the assessment of breast lesions: improved diagnostic performance by combining the BI-RADS®-US classification system with sonoelastography. Ultraschall Med 31:484-91

14. Lazarus E, Mainiero MB, Schepps et al (2006) BI-RADS lexicon for US and mammography: interobserver variability and positive predictive value. Radiology 239:385-91

15. Lee HJ, Kim EK, Kim MJ et al (2008) Observer variability of Breast Imaging Reporting and Data System (BI-RADS) for breast ultrasound. Eur J Radiol 65:293-298

16. Santana Montesdeoca JM, Gómez Arnáiz A, Fuentes Pavón R et al (2009) Diagnostic accuracy and interobserver variability in the BI-RADS ultrasound system. Radiologia 51:477-486

17. Abdullah N, Mesurolle B, El-Khoury M et al (2009) Breast imaging reporting and data system lexicon for US: interobserver agreement for assessment of breast masses. Radiology 25:2665-2672

18. Berg WA, Sechtin AG, Marques H et al (2010) Cystic breast masses and the ACRIN 6666 experience. Radiol Clin North Am 48:931-987

19. Gruber R, Jaromi S, Rudas M et al (2012) Histologic work-up of non-palpable breast lesions classified as probably benign at initial mammography and/or ultrasound (BI-RADS category 3). Eur J Radiol [Epub ahead of print]

20. Fu CY, Hsu HH, Yu JC et al (2010) Influence of Age on PPV of Sonographic BI-RADS Categories 3, 4, and 5. Ultraschall Med 32:8-13

21. Moon HJ, Kim MJ, Kwak JY et al (2010) Probably benign breast lesions on ultrasonography: a retrospective review of ultrasonographic features and clinical factors affecting the BI-RADS categorization. Acta Radiol 51:375-382

22. Moon HJ, Kim MJ, Kwak JY et al (2010) Malignant lesions initially categorized as probably benign breast lesions: retrospective review of ultrasonographic, clinical and pathologic characteristics. Ultrasound Med Biol 36:551-559

23. Berg WA, Zhang Z, Lehrer D et al; ACRIN 6666 Investigators (2012) Detection of breast cancer with addition of annual screening ultrasound or a single screening MRI to mammography in women with elevated breast cancer risk. JAMA 07:1394-404

24 El Saghir NS, Anderson BO (2012) Breast cancer early detection and resources: where in the world do we start? The Breast 21:423-425

25. Mundinger A (2006) Staging the breast and axilla. EJC Supplements 4:35-37

26. Lehman CD, DeMartini W, Anderson BO et al (2009) Indications for breast MRI in the patient with newly diagnosed breast cancer. J Natl Compr Canc Netw 7:193-201

27. Cho N, Moon WK, Cha JH et al (2009) Ultrasound-guided vacuum-assisted biopsy of microcalcifications detected at screening mammography. Acta Radiol 50:602-609

28. Suh YJ, Kim MJ, Kim EK et al (2012) Comparison of the underestimation rate in cases with ductal carcinoma in situ at ultrasound-guided core biopsy: 14-gauge automated core-needle biopsy vs. 8- or 11-gauge vacuum-assisted biopsy. Br J Radiol 85:e349-56

29. Barentsz MW, van Dalen T, Gobardhan PD et al (2012) Intraoperative ultrasound guidance for excision of non-palpable invasive breast cancer: a hospital-based series and an overview of the literature. Breast Cancer Res Treat 135:209-219

30. Houssami N, Hayes DF (2009) Review of preoperative magnetic resonance imaging (MRI) in breast cancer: should MRI be performed on all women with newly diagnosed, early stage breast cancer? CA Cancer J Clin 59:290-302

31. Turnbull L, Brown S, Harvey I et al (2010) Comparative effectiveness of MRI in breast cancer (COMICE) trial: a randomised controlled trial. Lancet 375:563-571

32. Peters NH, van Esser S, van den Bosch MA et al (2011) Preoperative MRI and surgical management in patients with non-palpable breast cancer: the MONET - randomised controlled trial. Eur J Cancer 47:879-886

33. Tozaki M, Fukuma E (2011) Does power Doppler ultrasonography improve the BI-RADS category assessment and diagnostic accuracy of solid breast lesions? Acta Radiol 52:706-710

34. Wang X, Xu P, Wang Y, Grant EG (2011) Contrast-enhanced ultrasonographic findings of different histopathologic types of breast cancer. Acta Radiol 52:248-255

35. Sadigh G, Carlos RC, Neal CH, Dwamena BA (2012) Ultrasonographic differentiation of malignant from benign breast lesions: a meta-analytic comparison of elasticity and BIRADS scoring. Breast Cancer Res Treat 133:23-35

36. Gong X, Xu Q, Xu Z et al (2011) Real-time elastography for the differentiation of benign and malignant breast lesions: a meta-analysis. Breast Cancer Res Treat 130:11-18

37. Berg WA, Cosgrove DO, Doré CJ et al for the BE1 Investigators (2012) Shear-wave elastography improves the specificity of breast US: the multinational study of 939 masses. Radiology 262:435-449

38. Evans A, Whelehan P, Thomson K (2012) Invasive breast cancer: relationship between shear-wave elastographic findings and histologic prognostic factors. Radiology 263:673-677

39. Prosch H, Halbwachs C, Strobl C et al (2011) Automated breast ultrasound vs. handheld ultrasound: BI-RADS classification, duration of the examination and patient comfort. Ultraschall Med 32:504-10

40. Giuliano V, Giuliano C (2012) Improved breast cancer detection in asymptomatic women using 3D-automated breast ultrasound in mammographically dense breasts. Clin Imaging [Epub ahead of print]

41. Choi YJ, Ko EY, Han BK et al (2009) High-resolution ultrasonographic features of axillary lymph node metastasis in patients with breast cancer. Breast 18:119-122

42. Alvarez S, Añorbe E, Alcorta P et al (2006) Role of sonography in the diagnosis of axillary lymph node metastases in breast cancer: a systematic review. AJR Am J Roentgenol 186:1342-1348

43. Choi JS, Kim MJ, Moon HJ et al (2012) False negative results of preoperative axillary ultrasound in patients with invasive breast cancer: correlations with clinicopathologic findings. Ultrasound Med Biol 38:1881-1886

44. Cody HS 3rd, Houssami N (2012) Axillary management in breast cancer: what's new for 2012? Breast 21:411-415

45. Pan L, Han Y, Sun X et al (2010) FDG-PET and other imaging modalities for the evaluation of breast cancer recurrence and metastases: a meta-analysis. J Cancer Res Clin Oncol 136:1007-1022

# Mammography: How to Interpret Asymmetries, Masses and Architectural Distortions

Christian Weismann

Diagnostic and Interventional Breast Department, Private University Institute of Radiology, PMU, General Hospital Salzburg, Salzburg, Austria

In order to correctly perceive and interpret mammogram images, assessment and categorization skills have to be taught in order for the reader to detect early breast cancer. Based on the detected finding, a clear recommendation is given by the final assessment category. The sensitivity of mammography is influenced by individual patient-dependent parameters (breast density, tumor growth pattern), the acquisition of the mammograms (technician), the technical quality of the image, and the experience of the reader.

**Table 1.** Mammography breast density assessment by ACR grading (BI-RADS®, fourth edition)

| ACR grading of mammographic breast tissue density | Glandular tissue component (%) | Description |
|---|---|---|
| I | <25 | Almost entirely fat |
| II | 25-50 | Scattered fibroglandular densities |
| III | 51-75 | Heterogeneously dense |
| IV | >75 | Extremely dense |

*ACR* American College of Radiologists, *BI-RADS®* Breast Imaging Reporting and Data System

## Perception

Kundel and colleagues [1] published a report on the holistic component of image perception in mammogram interpretation. In the most proficient observers, the recognition skill is based on a fast holistic mode. The holistic mode depends on an initial global analysis of the mammogram, which indicates the perturbation that is consistent with abnormality. A focal feature analysis follows. Then, the well-trained observer starts the search-to-find mode by scanning his/her gaze over the image in jumps (saccades). The less-well-trained observer is not able to perceive the input to the entire retina in a holistic mode and first starts with the more time-consuming search-to-find mode. The perception target is to pinpoint asymmetries, masses and architectural distortions quickly.

Perception is influenced by the mammographic breast tissue density. The American College of Radiology (ACR) classifies the mammographic density into four grades [2] (Table 1). ACR grade 1 is a perfect precondition for high mammographic sensitivity (up to 99%). The sensitivity decreases in cases of extremely dense mammographic breast tissue (ACR grade 4), to a level of about 50%. Therefore, under population-based mammography screening conditions, about 50% of breast cancers in ACR grade 4 density breasts are not perceivable. Ooms and colleagues [3] studied the interobserver variability regarding ACR tissue density grading (grades 1-4). The

overall weighted κ value showed substantial agreement between different observers, with a value of 0.77.

Perception is also influenced by the tumor growth pattern. The most frequently occurring histological types of breast cancers are invasive ductal and intraductal cancers in about 75% of patients, followed by invasive lobular cancers in 5-15%, mucous and medullary cancers in 5-7%, tubular cancers in 2-6%, and papillary cancers in about 2%. The cancer growth pattern may frequently produce an irregular-shaped mass with spiculations and microlobulations ("hedgehog type"), a more lobulated "benign looking" circumscribed mass ("potato type"), and several types of masses created by a mix of "hedgehog" and "potato". In addition, two different growth patterns can be described: the intracystic growing cancer and the diffuse growth type, a mix of two or more different growth patterns can exist in one cancer. The most challenging cancer growth pattern to perceive in mammograms is the diffuse type. This type has the tendency to produce nonmass asymmetries that are sometimes visible in only one mammographic view, or it can result in architectural distortion. Invasive lobular cancers can show a more diffuse growth pattern, with tissue stiffening. Frequently, additional physical examination shows harder asymmetric palpable breast tissue or an asymmetric palpable mass in the mammographic region of interest.

J. Hodler et al. (eds.), *Musculoskeletal Diseases 2013-2016,*
DOI: 10.1007/978-88-470-5292-5_40 © Springer-Verlag Italia 2013

In population-based mammography screening programs, routine mammography double reading has been proven to increase the number of visible cancers and detected cancers by 5-15% compared with single reading. In addition, computer-aided detection (CAD) can be used to reduce the rate of missed cancers. In the literature, the sensitivity of CAD for masses has been reported to be in the range 67-89% [4-6]. Gilbert and colleagues performed a retrospective comparison of single reading with CAD and double reading without CAD [7]. They showed that single reading with CAD led to a significantly higher cancer detection rate than double reading alone. The single reading with CAD found 6.5% more cancers than the double reading alone. The negative finding was an increase in recall rate for single reading plus CAD (8.6%) compared with double reading (6.5%).

## Assessment

The perturbations in a mammogram can be caused by calcifications, masses, focal or global asymmetries, architectural distortions with or without contour deformity, tubular densities or dilated ducts, nipple and/or skin retraction, skin thickening, skin lesions and axillary adenopathy. The ACR and the Breast Imaging Reporting and Data System (BI-RADS®) [2] have standardized the assessment of lesions found by mammography, ultrasound and magnetic resonance imaging (MRI) in the BI-RADS® lexicon. In the next chapter, the mammographic BI-RADS® assessment terminology of masses, architectural distortion and

**Table 2.** Mammography assessment of mass and architectural distortion using BI-RADS® descriptors (fourth edition terminology)

| BI-RADS® descriptor | | |
| --- | --- | --- |
| Mass | Shape | Round |
| | | Oval |
| | | Lobular |
| | | Irregular |
| | Margins | Circumscribed |
| | | Indistinct or ill defined |
| | | Microlobulated |
| | | Spiculated |
| | Density | High |
| | | Equal |
| | | Low |
| | | Fat containing |
| Architectural distortion | | Normal breast architecture disturbed |
| Special cases | | Intramammary lymph node |
| | | Tubular density or dilated duct |
| | | Global asymmetry |
| | | Focal asymmetry |
| Associated findings | | Skin retraction |
| | | Nipple retraction |
| | | Skin thickening |
| | | Trabecular thickening |
| | | Skin lesion |
| | | Axillary adenopathy |

*BI-RADS® Breast Imaging Reporting and Data System*

asymmetries will be highlighted. Table 2 presents the BI-RADS® descriptors and BI-RADS® terminology (valid fourth edition terminology) concerning mass and architectural distortion. At the meeting of the Radiological Society of North America (RSNA) 2012, Sickles presented the changes that are expected in the fifth edition of the BI-RADS® lexicon, which is planned for publication in 2013. These expected changes concerning the BI-RADS® desciptor "asimmetry" are implemented.

## Masses

According to the BI-RADS® Breast Imaging lexicon, a mass is defined as a three-dimensional (3D) structure with convex outward borders. Typically, a mass can be visualized on two orthogonal views. A mass with round or oval shape combined with a circumscribed margin and low or equal density (compared with breast parenchyma) has a high probability of being benign. A high-density mass with irregular shape and spiculated margin is suspicious for breast cancer. To call a margin "circumscribed", more than 75% of the mass has to be free from superpositions. Lazarus and colleagues studied the interobserver variability of different mammographic masses related BI-RADS® descriptors [8]. A moderate agreement was obtained for mass shape ($\kappa=0.48$) and mass margin ($\kappa=0.48$), and a slight agreement for mass density ($\kappa=0.18$). Concerning the fact, that a mass is perceived by the readers, a high $\kappa$-value of 0.84 resulted. Masses with indistinct margins can start initially as asymmetries.

Micro- and macrocalcifications can be associated with a mass. Pleomorphic microcalcifications in combination with a malignant invasive cancer mass indicate the presence of an extensive intraductal component (EIC) [9, 10]. This information is important for surgery because a wider cancer excision is necessary for this type of mass than for an EIC-negative mass.

## Asymmetries

Asymmetries are summarized in the BI-RADS® lexicon under "special cases". The BI-RADS® lexicon describes the term "asymmetry" as a planar structure that lacks convex outward borders, usually contains interspersed fat, and lacks the conspicuity of a 3D mass. Sickles presented the changes in the BI-RADS® asymmetry descriptor in the fifth edition of the BI-RADS® lexicon, dividing the descriptor asimmetry into four sections: asymmetry, global asymmetry, focal asymmetry and developing asymmetry. The definition of the new section asymmetry means: (1) a potential mass seen in only one projection, (2) three-dimensionality not confirmed, (3) it might represent superimposition of normal structures (summation artefact).

In the 4th edition of the BI-RADS® lexicon, global asymmetry involves a large portion of the breast, at least a quadrant. According to Sickles, it usually represents a normal variant, but may be significant when it corresponds to a palpable abnormality. In the German consensus meeting of course directors in 2009 [11], 92% voted for the evaluation of a global parenchymal asymmetry by history, clinical investigation and, if available, by comparing with previous mammograms. A focal asymmetry differs from global asymmetry in the size of the area involved; it is a space-occupying lesion seen in two different projections with concave-outward contours and usually interspersed with fat.

A focal asymmetry is more suspicious of being malignant than a global asymmetry, especially if the focal asymmetry is combined with tissue distortion [12]. It is mandatory to compare the mammogram with previous mammograms. A developing asymmetry requires additional work-up (except scar after surgery, proven trauma or proven infection at this area). If the following spot compression view does not prove that the focal asymmetry is a summation product of anatomical structures, a further evaluation with ultrasound and/or MRI is the required (BI-RADS®, fourth edition). More diffuse growing cancers, e.g., invasive lobular carcinoma, may have a tendency to appear as a focal asymmetry in one mammographic view only.

### Architectural Distortion

The normal architecture is disturbed without a visible mass. This can be caused by spiculations distorting the parenchyma radially from the point of origin. Focal retraction and deformities destroy the normal architecture. A combination of architectural distortion with masses, asymmetries and calcifications can be found. Scars after surgery lead to architectural distortion; this is considered to be harmless and does not require further work-up.

### Assessment Categories

Table 3 shows the BI-RADS® assessment categories for mammograms. It should be emphasized that category 3 is reserved for almost certain benign findings. A category 3

finding has a less than 2% probability of malignancy [2]. Follow-up after a short interval, usually 6 months, is recommended to confirm the benign underlying pathology. The three subsets of BI-RADS® 4 (4A, 4B and 4C) give a better correlation between morphological findings and expected histopathology. In a BI-RADS® 4A case, a benign histology is expected. In BI-RADS® 4B, both results, benign and malignant, can fit the expectation. In BI-RADS® 4C, the probability that the tumor is malignant is higher than the probability that it is benign. In this situation, a repeat biopsy should be considered. In the fifth edition of the BI-RADS® lexicon, the likelihood of malignancy in BI-RADS® 4A is 10%, for BI-RADS® 4B it is 50%, and for category 4C it is less than 95%. BI-RADS® 5 has a 95% and higher probability of malignancy.

In the German consensus meeting of course directors in 2009 [11], 100% of the directors voted for BI-RADS® 4 categorization in cases of architectural distortion (except a postoperative scar). Imaging does not allow differentiation between, for example, a radial scar and a tubular cancer.

A round mass with circumscribed margin of less than 75% and equal density to parenchyma should be categorized BI-RADS® 4 [11]. A single palpable mass with circumscribed margin without microcalcifications should be classed as BI-RADS® 4 [11]. A work-up of this mass is indicated.

### Early Invasive Breast Cancer

Detecting breast cancer early is an important goal for the prognosis of the patient. In the publication by Harvey and colleagues [12], they show a practical approach to finding early invasive breast cancers in mammograms. They emphasize to look for asymmetry, contour deformity (architectural distortion), lesions in the retromammary fat, and associated findings (skin and/or nipple retraction, skin thickening, trabecular thickening, skin lesion, axillary adenopathy). The mammogram should always be compared with previous mammograms. Morphological stability of a

**Table 3.** BI-RADS® mammography assessment category with description and recommendations (BI-RADS® fourth edition)

BI-RADS® categories for mammography

| Category | Assessment | Description | Recommendation |
|---|---|---|---|
| 0 | Incomplete | Further imaging evaluation necessary | Final categorization after imaging work-up |
| 1 | Negative | Nothing to comment on (normal) | Routine follow-up |
| 2 | Benign finding | No malignant features | Routine follow-up |
| 3 | Probably benign finding | Malignancy is highly unlikely | Short interval follow-up |
| 4 | Suspicious abnormality | Low to moderate probability of cancer | Biopsy should be considered |
| 4A | Suspicious abnormality | Low suspicion for malignancy | Biopsy should be considered |
| 4B | Suspicious abnormality | Intermediate suspicion of malignancy | Biopsy should be considered |
| 4C | Suspicious abnormality | Moderate concern for malignancy (but not classic) | Biopsy should be considered |
| 5 | Highly suggestive of malignancy | Almost certainly cancer | Appropriate action should be taken |
| 6 | Known cancer | Biopsy proven malignancy | Appropriate action should be taken |

*BI-RADS®* Breast Imaging Reporting and Data System

lesion is inferior to a suspicious morphology. If a suspicious mass, asymmetry or architectural distortion is found (BI-RADS® 4 or 5), an assessment is mandatory, e.g., lateral projection view, spot compression views or ultrasound. The final assessment depends on the most suspicious imaging feature; in cases where there is a feature suspicious for malignancy, a large core needle biopsy or a vacuum aspiration biopsy under stereotactic or ultrasound guidance is the usual recommendation (BI-RADS® 4 or 5).

# References

1. Kundel HL, Nodine CF, Conant EF, Weinstein SP (2007) Holistic component of image perception in mammogram interpretation. Radiology 242:396-402
2. American College of Radiology (2003) Breast imaging reporting and data system (BI-RADS), 4th edn. American College of Radiology, Reston, VA
3. Ooms EA, Zonderland HM, Eijkemans MJC et al (2007) Mammography: interobserver variability in breast density assessment. The Breast 16:568-576
4. Schulz-Wendtland R, Wenkel E, Wacker T, Hermann KP (2009) Quo vadis? Trends in der digitalen Mammografie (Quo vadis? Trends in digital mammography). Geburtsh Frauenheilk 69:108-117
5. Funovics M, Schamp S, Helbich TH et al (2001) Evaluation eines computerassistierten Diagnosesystems in der Erkennung des Mammakarzinoms (Evaluation of a computer assisted diagnosis system to detect breast cancer). Fortschr Röntgenstr 173:218-223
6. Malich A, Marx C, Facius M et al (2001) Tumour detection rate of a new commercially available computer-aided detection system. EJR 11:2454-2459
7. Gilbert FL, Astley SM, McGee MA et al (2006) Single reading with computer aided detection and double reading of screening mammograms in the United Kingdom national breast screening program. Radiology 241:47-53
8. Lazarus E, Mainiero MB, Schepps B et al (2006) BI-RADS Lexicon for US and mammography: interobserver variability and positive predictive value. Radiology 239:385-391
9. Healey EA, Osteen RT, Schnitt SJ et al (1989) Can the clinical and mammographic findings at presentation predict the presence of an extensive intraductal component in early stage breast cancer? Int J Radiation Oncology Biol Phys 17:1217-1221
10. Holland R, Connolly JL, Gelman R et al (1990) The presence of an extensive intraductal component following a limited excision correlates with prominent residual disease in the remainder of the breast. J Clin Oncol 8:113-118
11. Müller-Schimpfle MP, Heindel W, Kettritz U et al (2010) Konsensustreffen der Kursleiter in der Mammadiagnostik am 9.5.2009 in Frankfurt am Main - Thema: Herdbefunde (Consensus meeting of course directors in Breast imaging, 9 May 2009 in Frankfurt am Main – topic: masses). Fortschr Röntgenstr 182:671-675
12. Harvey JA, Nicholson BT, Cohen MA (2008) Finding early invasive breast cancers. Radiology 248:61-76

# Microcalcifications of the Breast: An Approach to Radiologic Classification

Markus Müller-Schimpfle[1], Robin Wilson[2]

[1] Department of Radiology, Neuroradiology and Nuclear Medicine, Frankfurt/Main-Hoechst Hospital, Frankfurt/Main, Germany
[2] Department of Clinical Radiology, The Royal Marsden Hospital, London, UK

Microcalcifications in the breast are common. A vast majority of microcalcifications are benign and can be clearly recognized as such without resort to biopsy [1]. A small proportion are obviously malignant, but there is a significant proportion of breast microcalcifications that cannot be accurately determined on the basis of imaging alone and require further assessment and often image-guided biopsy [1, 2]. The recognition and biopsy of suspicious microcalcifications is important, as the detection of ductal carcinoma in situ (DCIS) and small invasive cancers associated with microcalcification provides the opportunity to positively influence the outcome of these breast cancers through early treatment before the disease has spread beyond the breast [3-5]. The challenge is to detect and diagnose the microcalcifications that matter, and differentiate them from those that are benign.

Since the first description of black spots in the center of a carcinoma in 1913 by Salomon, a lot of work has been done to detect, characterize and classify microcalcifications systematically [6]. Particularly during the second half of the last century, the studies by Lanyi, Leborgne and Le Gal had a major influence on the diagnosis of microcalcifications of the breast [7-9]. However, accurate diagnosis of microcalcifications in the breast on the basis imaging alone remains difficult [10].

With the Breast Imaging Reporting And Data System (BI-RADS®), parameters have been defined that help to sort masses and microcalcifications into standardized diagnostic categories [11, 12]. However, data on the prospective classification of microcalcifications according to the BI-RADS® lexicon are rare [13-15]. Furthermore, there are no recommendations for the clinician on how to link descriptive findings listed in the BI-RADS® lexicon to the BI-RADS® assessment categories. With re-

I. Typically benign (incl. punctated)

II. Amorphous

II. Coarse heterogeneous (>0.5 mm)

III. Fine pleomorphic (<0.5 mm)

III. Fine linear, branching

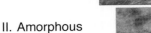

**Fig. 1.** Microcalcifications: from benign to malignant morphology. *Green frame*: microcalcifications with typically benign morphology (I); *orange frame*: microcalcifications with indeterminant morphology (II); *red frame*: microcalcifications with typically malignant morphology (III) (for color reproduction see p 320)

spect to levels of suspicion, the classification of masses seems more reliable than the classification of microcalcifications [16].

In order to accurately characterize microcalcifications in the breast, apart from the two-view standard mammograms (mediolateral oblique and craniocaudal views) additional lateral and craniocaudal compression magnification views are often useful and recommended for diagnosis.

The classification applies to a group of more than four microcalcifications (<2 mm size of a single calcification) within a volume of 1-2 cm³ [11, 12, 16, 17]. A pragmatic approach to classifying microcalcifications is suggested as follows [18, 19]:

A. Classification of the type of microcalcifications into three groups (Fig. 1):
   I. Typically benign (green in Fig. 1): vascular, popcorn-like, lucent-centered, round, rim, rod-like,

---

This is an updated version of the chapter by Müller-Schimpfle M (2012) Microcalcifications of the Breast: An Approach to Radiologic Classification. In: Hodler J, von Schulthess GK, Zollikofer ChL (eds) Diseases of the Brain, Head & Neck, Spine 2012-2015. Springer-Verlag Italia, Milano, pp. 307-310.

J. Hodler et al. (eds.), *Musculoskeletal Diseases 2013-2016,*
DOI: 10.1007/978-88-470-5292-5_41 © Springer-Verlag Italia 2013

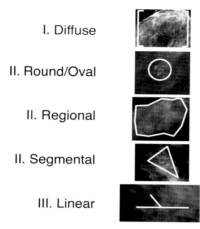

I. Diffuse

II. Round/Oval

II. Regional

II. Segmental

III. Linear

**Fig. 2.** Microcalcifications: from benign to malignant distribution. *Green frame*: microcalcifications with benign distribution (I); *orange frame*: microcalcifications with indeterminant distribution (II); *red frame*: microcalcifications with typically malignant distribution (III) (for color reproduction see p 320)

| Distribution | Morphology | | |
| --- | --- | --- | --- |
| | Typically benign | Indifferent | Typically malignant |
| Disseminated | 2 | 3 | 4B |
| Round/oval | 3 | 4A | 4C |
| Regional | 4A | 4B | 4C |
| Segmental | 4A | 4C | 4C |
| Linear/branching | 4B | 4C | 5 |

MODIFICATORS
- Number    - Additional findings    - Location    - Follow up    - Risk

**Fig. 3.** The Microcalcification matrix serves as a guide for classifying grouped microcalcifications according to morphology and distribution, additionally considering modification aspects (modificators) [13, 14] (for color reproduction see p 320)

curvilinear, suture calcifications; "typically benign" according to [6, 7].

II. Indeterminate (orange): amorphous or coarse heterogeneous; "intermediate concern, suspicious calcifications" according to [11, 12].

III. Typically malignant (red): fine pleomorphic according to [12], fine linear or fine-linear branching [12], casting according to [11], combinations of granular types with casting types (earlier also called polymorphous: fine linear plus granular, or fine linear plus branching, or branching and granular); "higher probability of malignancy" according to [11, 12].

B. Classification of the distribution of microcalcifications into five groups (Fig. 2):

I. Diffuse (equal distribution over the whole breast parenchyma).

II. Round or oval (as in blunt duct adenosis), "clustered", if not otherwise specified, typically within a volume of 1 cm³.

III. Regional (typically with a volume of >1 cm³), not conceivably related to the ductal system.

IV. Segmental, related to the segment of the ductal system.

V. Linear (ductal distribution, typically oriented towards the nipple), branching (linear distribution with additional side branches).

These "distribution modifiers" are evaluated as suggested in the BI-RADS® lexicon. The BI-RADS® lexicon itself neither defines nor quantifies the varying influence of the distribution modifiers on the assessment categories. Some distribution modifiers (regional versus segmental) have not been shown to be of different statistical significance in the literature [20, 21]. Using data found in current literature, the distribution modifiers are attributed to varying probability levels of malignancy

[7, 8, 10, 20-22]. Thereby, we have developed the standardized scheme we use for classification of microcalcifications according to the BI-RADS® morphology and distribution parameters [19]. This matrix system is demonstrated in Fig. 3.

## BI-RADS® and Indications for Biopsy

While some microcalcifications will be visible on ultrasound, the vast majority of those that require biopsy need to be sampled under stereotactic X-ray guidance using either upright add-on or prone table biopsy systems. It is important to ensure accurate sampling of the microcalcifications and the adjacent breast tissue, and for this reason vacuum-assisted core biopsy (VAB) is the preferred method. Indications for biopsy of calcifications vary but the BI-RADS® system does facilitate some consistency:

- BI-RADS® 2 (typically benign); biopsy is not usually indicated.
- BI-RADS® 3 (probably benign finding); two different approaches are common: the first involves short interval follow-up (e.g., 6-month intervals for the first two examinations, 12 months for the subsequent two examinations, with a total follow-up time of 3 years). Additional risk factors that should prompt biopsy rather than follow-up are: a strong family history of breast cancer; a personal history of invasive breast cancer, DCIS, lobular neoplasia or atypical ductal/lobular hyperplasia.
- BI-RADS® 4 and 5 (suspicious abnormality (Figs. 4-6) and highly suspicious findings (Fig. 7). VAB is performed to confirm the diagnosis of cancer, to reduce the rate of underdiagnosis (biopsy: DCIS; operation: invasive cancer; this has potential implications for

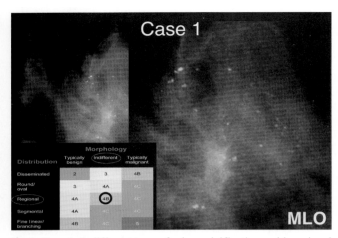

**Fig. 4.** Case 1: Indifferent type of microcalcifications with regional distribution (BI-RADS, 4B). Histology: fibrocystic changes, sclerosing adenosis, usual ductal hyperplasia. *MLO*, mediolateral oblique view (for color reproduction see p 320)

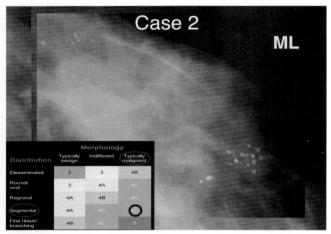

**Fig. 5.** Case 2: Typically malignant type of microcalcifications with segmental distribution (BI-RADS, 4C). Histology: invasive ductal cancer. *ML*, mediolateral view (for color reproduction see p 321)

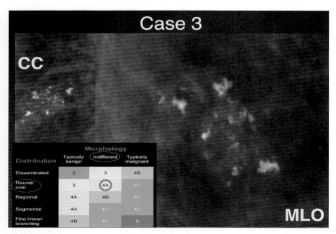

**Fig. 6.** Case 3: Indifferent (including coarse heterogeneous) type of microcalcifications with round/oval distribution (BI-RADS, 4A). Histology: fibroadenoma, fibrocystic changes. *CC*, craniocaudal view; *MLO*, mediolateral oblique view (for color reproduction see p 321)

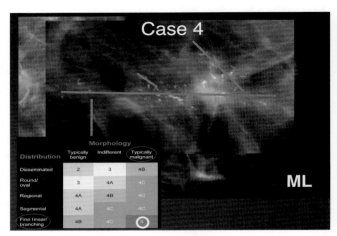

**Fig. 7.** Case 4: Typically malignant type of microcalcifications with linear and branching distribution (BI-RADS, 5). Histology: ductal carcinoma in situ (high grade). *ML*, mediolateral view (for color reproduction see p 321)

lymph node biopsy) and to define the extent and type of disease to inform the surgical options (breast conservation therapy, mastectomy) with biopsy at the two most distant regions of the lesion, if applicable.

There are a number of different vacuum biopsy systems available that are suitable for sampling tissue containing calcifications and most are compatible with either prone biopsy or add-on upright systems [23]. The technique for stereotactic breast biopsy is well described elsewhere (15, 24, 25). Lignocaine with adrenaline is the preferred local anesthetic as it reduces hematoma formation and provides longer-lasting anesthesia, particularly as multiple large cores of tissue are usually required for accurate diagnosis. It is imperative that the core samples are subjected to X-ray examination to confirm that sufficient and representative microcalcifications have been retrieved. In case of complete removal of the microcalcifications, one can either insert a marker at the end of the VAB procedure or wait for the histology report and then insert a marker (e.g., Cook coil) into the biopsy hole by ultrasound guidance. Markers that are visible on both ultrasound and mammography are preferred, as they facilitate localization if surgery is then required under ultrasound guidance.

The move from film/screen analog mammography to full field digital mammography has seen an increase in the rate of recall at screening because of the detection of indeterminate microcalcifications. In recent years it has also been recognized that failure to identify or recall isolated small clusters of microcalcifications results in missed diagnosis of DCIS and the missed opportunity to detect breast cancer when it is curable [26]. An aggressive approach to calcifications results in the diagnosis of very small invasive carcinomas, most often of higher histological grade, that would otherwise have been diagnosed much later and often after metastasis has occurred. However, it is also important not to carry out unnecessary biopsy of clearly benign disease.

## Summary

The standardization in description and classification of lesions achievable by adopting the BI-RADS® lexicon is very useful in helping target biopsy to those microcalcifications that carry a significant risk of representing significant disease. However, there is considerable intraobserver variability in the application of the descriptors and considerable experience is required to use this type of characterization system [21, 22]. Even the systematic approach of the current 4th edition of the BI-RADS® lexicon, which includes descriptors of different types of microcalcifications, lacks a translation of these microcalcification types into the BI-RADS® assessment categories. In a study addressing this topic, Berg et al. discussed that they continued to see variability in the use of the term punctate (according to the 3rd edition of the BIRADS lexicon) and suggested, that "a cluster of round punctate calcifications may be probably benign, but similar calcifications in a segmental or linear distribution would be at least suspicious" [22]. The use of regular personal comparative audit of all biopsies of calcifications will lead to rapid improvement in specificity, but it is unusual to achieve a greater than 25% positive predictive value for malignancy for calcification without significantly reducing overall sensitivity.

The combined assessment of morphology and distribution of microcalcifications is suggested in the BI-RADS® lexicon, but no rules for such an assessment are defined. The systematic work-up of calcifications suggested in this chapter tries to narrow the gap between the microcalcification description on the one hand, and the BI-RADS® categorization on the other (see Table 1).

In conclusion, microcalcifications are a very important marker of breast disease and differentiation of benign from malignant causes is fundamental to proper management and detection of early breast cancer. The BI-RADS® lexicon allows for more consistent description of breast microcalcifications and facilitates the allocation of diagnostic categories that lead to more standardized biopsy recommendations. Nevertheless, how to link the descriptive findings to the assessment categories still seems to be a difficult diagnostic task in the evaluation of microcalcifications, and is presumably more difficult than for masses. The classification of microcalcifications proposed in this chapter helps to standardize the clinical approach to calcifications and balance the need for high sensitivity while maintaining acceptable specificity in diagnosis.

## References

1. Evans AJ, Pinder SE, Wilson ARM, Ellis IO (2002) Breast calcifications. Greenwich Medical Media
2. Wilson ARM, Evans AJ (2000) Surgery - Practical problems: diagnosis of microcalcifications demonstrated on mammography. In: Corson JD, Williamson RCN (Eds) Surgery. Mosby, London
3. Evans AJ, Pinder SE, Ellis IO, Wilson ARM (2001) Screen detected Ductal Carcinoma in Situ (DCIS): Over-diagnosis or an obligate precursor of invasive disease? Journal of Medical Screening 8:149-151
4. Evans AJ, Pinder SE, Wilson ARM et al (1997) The detection of ductal carcinoma in situ at mammographic screening enables the diagnosis of small, grade 3 invasive tumours. British Journal of Cancer 75:542-544
5. Evans AJ, Pinder S, Ellis IO et al (1994) Screening-detected and symptomatic ductal carcinoma in situ: mammographic features with pathologic correlation. Radiology 191:237-240
6. Salomon A (1913) Beiträge zu Pathologie der Mammacarcinome. Arch Klin Chir 101:573-668
7. Lanyi M (1986) Diagnostik und Differentialdiagnostik der Mamma-Verkalkungen. Springer, Berlin Heidelberg New York
8. Leborgne R (1951) Diagnosis of tumors of the breast by simple roentgenography: calcifications in carcinomas. AJR Am J Roentgenol 65:1-11
9. Le Gal M, Durand JC, Laurent M, Pellier D (1976) Management following mammography revealing grouped microcalcifications without palpable tumor. Nouv Presse Med 5:1623-1627
10. de Lafontan B, Daures JP, Salicru B et al (1994) Isolated clustered microcalcifications: Diagnostic value of mammography – Series of 400 cases with surgical verification. Radiology 190:479-483
11. American College of Radiology (ACR) (1998) Illustrated Breast Imaging Reporting And Data System (BI-RADSTM), 3rd edn. American College of Radiology, Reston , pp 53-181
12. American College of Radiology (ACR) (2003) ACR BI-RADS® – Mammography, 4th edn. In: ACR Breast Imaging Reporting And Data System, Breast Imaging Atlas. American College of Radiology, Reston, pp 61-259
13. Sickles EA (1991) Periodic mammographic follow-up of probably benign lesions: results in 3,184 consecutive cases. Radiology 179:463-468
14. Orel SG, Kay N, Reynolds C, Sullivan DC (1999) BI-RADS categorization as a predictor of malignancy. Radiology 211:845-850
15. Siegmann KC, Wersebe A, Fischmann A et al (2003) Stereotactic vacuum-assisted breast biopsy--success, histologic accuracy, patient acceptance and optimizing the BI-RADSTM-correlated indication. Rofo 175:99-104
16. Hall FM, Storella JM, Silverstone DZ, Wyshak G (1998) Non palpable breast lesions: recommendations for biopsy based on suspicion of carcinoma at mammography. Radiology 167:353-358
17. Kopans DB (1989) Breast imaging. JB Lippincott, Philadelphia, pp 118-122
18. Müller-Schimpfle M, Wersebe A, Xydeas T et al (2005) Microcalcifications of the breast: how does radiologic classification correlate with histology? Acta Radiol 46:774-781
19. Müller-Schimpfle M (2008) Consensus meeting of course experts in breast diagnosis 5 May 2007 in Frankfurt am Main--topic: microcalcinosis. Rofo 180:66-68
20. Fondrinier E, Lorimier G, Guerin-Boblet V et al (2002) Breast microcalcifications: Multivariate analysis of radiologic and clinical factors for carcinoma. World J Surg 26:290-296
21. Liberman L, Abramson AF, Squires FB et al (1998) The Breast Imaging Reporting and Data System: positive predictive value of mammographic features and final assesment categories. AJR Am J Roentgenol 171:35-40
22. Berg WA, Campassi C, Langenberg P, Sexton M (2000) Breast imaging reporting and data system: inter- and intraobserver variability in feature analysis and final assessment. AJR Am J Roentgenol 174:1769-1777

23. Wilson ARM, Kavia S (2009) Comparison of large-core vacuum-assisted breast biopsy excision systems. In: Renzo Brun del Re (Ed) Minimally invasive breast biopsies, recent results in cancer. Research 173. Springer Verlag, Berlin

24. O'Flynn EAM, Wilson ARM, Michell MJ (2010) Breast biopsy: state of the art. Clinical Radiology 65:259-270

25. Wilson ARM, Evan AJ (2006) Percutaneous breast biopsy. In: Bocker W (Ed) Preneoplasia of the breast – a conceptual approach to proliferative breast disease. Elsevier, Munich

26. Evans AJ, Wilson ARM, Burrell HC et al (1999) Mammographic features of Ductal Carcinoma in situ (DCIS) present on previous mammography. Clinical Radiology 54:644-646

# APPENDIX: FULL COLOR FIGURES

*This section reproduces in colors those figures that for technical reasons are found in a black and white version in the various chapters.*

## Imaging of the Hand and Wrist

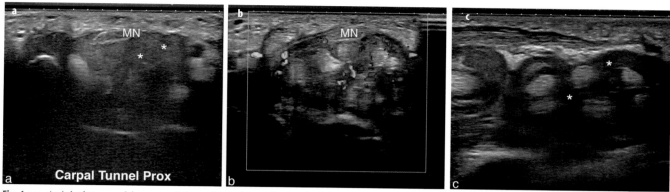

**Fig. 4 a-c.** Axial ultrasound images of the volar wrist at the level of the carpal tunnel (**a**, **b**) and palm of the hand (**c**) demonstrate a diffuse soft tissue mass (*asterisks*, **a**) around the superficial and deep flexor tendons extending distally in the palm of the hand (**c**). Part of the hypoechogenicity is based on anisotrophy (**b**); however, a definite soft tissue mass is present, with hyperemia secondary to an infection. Clinically, carpal tunnel syndrome was evident. *MN* median nerve

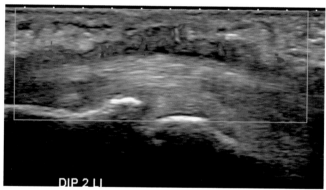

**Fig. 5.** Flexor tendon tenosynovitis. Longitudinal ultrasound image of the index finger at the level of the distal interphalangeal joint. Synovial thickening with hypervascularization is apparent

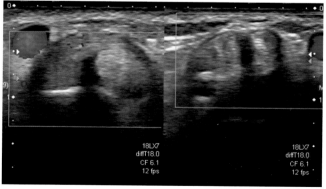

**Fig. 6.** De Quervain's tenosynovitis. Axial ultrasound images of the wrists demonstrate the first extensor compartments, with a normal image (*right*) for comparison. The radial artery is visualized with color Doppler, adjacent to the abductor pollicis longus and extensor pollicis brevis tendons. The image on the *left* demonstrates tendon thickening surrounded by hypoechoic synovium with subtle hypervascularization

## Pelvis and Groin

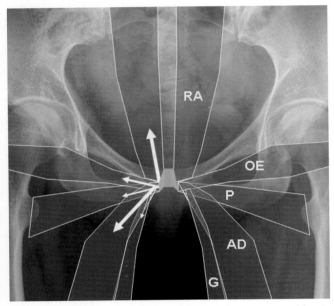

**Fig. 7.** Diagram showing anatomy of the muscle groups attaching to the pubis. *RA* rectus abdominis, *OE* obturator externus, *P* pectineus, *AD* adductors, *G* gracilis. *Arrows* show force vectors upon the pubis resulting from muscle action

## Ultrasonography: Sports Injuries

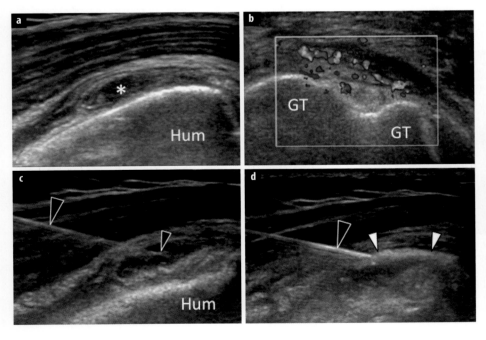

**Fig. 1 a-d.** Subacromial bursitis. Coronal oblique (**a**) and axial (**b**) sonograms show the subacromial synovial bursa presenting a thick hypervascularized wall and some fluid content (*asterisk*). **c** MSUS-guided intrabursal injection. Note the needle (*black arrowheads*) correctly positioned under the real-time guidance of ultrasound. The tip of the needle (*small black arrowhead*) lies inside the bursa. **d** After injection of a small amount of steroid-lidocaine, note the drug (*white arrowheads*) filling the bursa. No injection into the surrounding tissues is noted. *Hum* humerus, *GT* greater tuberosity of the humeral head

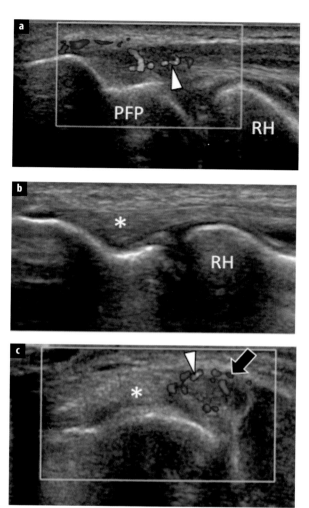

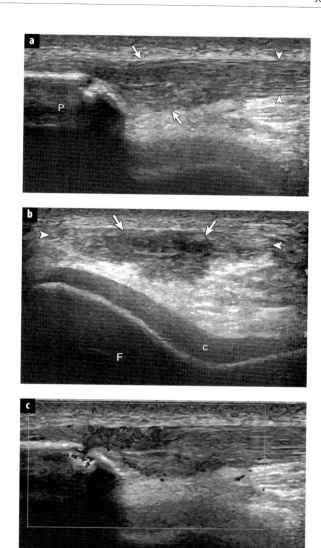

**Fig. 6 a-c.** Tendinopathy of the common extensor tendon at the elbow. All sonograms were obtained over the common extensor tendon. **a** Coronal color Doppler sonogram obtained over the anterior part of extensor. **b** Coronal sonogram obtained over the posterior part of the tendon. **c** Axial color Doppler sonogram. Note swelling, irregular hypoechoic appearance and hypervascular changes (*arrowheads*) limited to the anterior part (*arrow*) of the common extensor tendon. The posterior part (*asterisk*) of the tendon is normal. *RH* radial head, *PFP* posterior fat pad of the elbow joint

**Fig. 8 a-c.** Patellar tendon tendinosis (Jumper's knee). Ultrasound images of the long axis (**a**) and short axis (**b**) to the patellar tendon (*arrowheads*) show hypoechoic tendinosis (*arrows*) and bone irregularity of the patella (*P*). **c** Note hyperemia from neovascularity on the color Doppler image. *F* femur, *c* articular cartilage

# Cartilage: How Do We Image It? From Basic to Advanced MRI Protocols

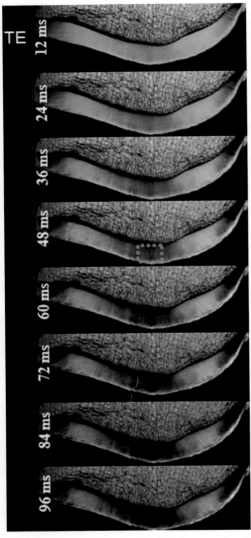

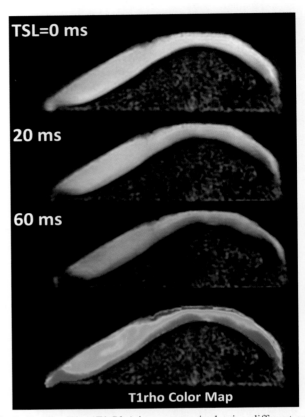

**Fig. 2.** Patellar T1ρ (*T1-Rho*) images acquired using different spin lock times (*TSL*) and corresponding T1ρ map

**Fig. 1.** Multi-echo T2 images at the level of the osteochondral junction (patellar specimen). Post-processing of the following images allows generation of corresponding T2 maps

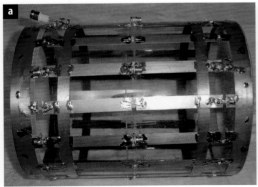

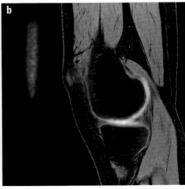

**Fig. 3 a, b.** **a** Dedicated dual tuned 23 Na$^+$/$^1$H magnetic resonance imaging (MRI) coil. **b** 3T Na$^+$ MRI sagittal image of the knee, directly measuring cartilage glycosaminoglycan content. (Courtesy of Professor Garry Gold, Stanford University USA)

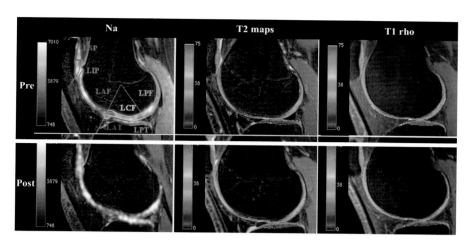

**Fig. 4.** Na$^+$, T2 and T1-rho knee cartilage maps from the Stanford basketball study. Post-season degenerative changes of the patellofemoral joint cartilage are demonstrated, in keeping with higher rates of injury at this level in jumping athletes. (Courtesy of Professor Garry Gold, Stanford University, USA)

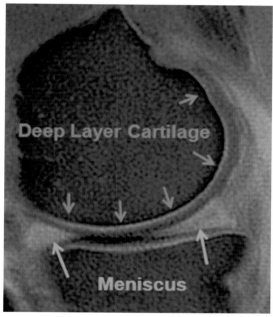

**Fig. 5.** Ultra-short echo time sagittal image of the knee. High signal is observed within the articular cartilage and meniscus (*arrows*). Note the elegant depiction of the deep articular cartilage layer (*small arrows*) along with the osteochondral junction area

## Neuropathies of the Upper Extremity

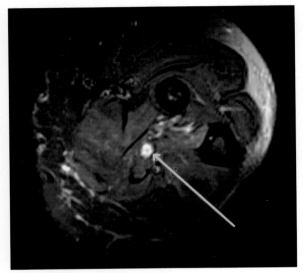

**Fig. 2.** Abnormal signal intensity of the enlarged median nerve (*arrow*) in the forearm of a 54-year-old man with nerve ischemia. Note the loss of fasculations (Courtesy of Prof. A. Chhabra)

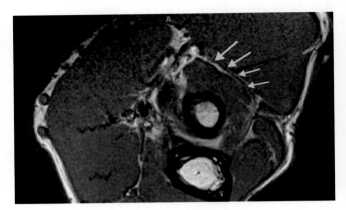

**Fig. 3.** A 32-year-old man with posterior interosseous nerve syndrome. The nerve is entrapped at the Arcade of Frohse (*arrows*) (Courtesy of Prof. A. Chhabra)

## Entrapment Neuropathies of the Lower Extremity

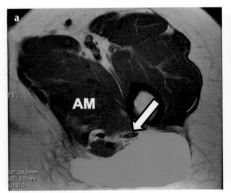
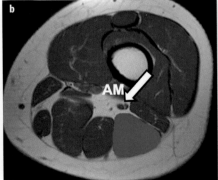
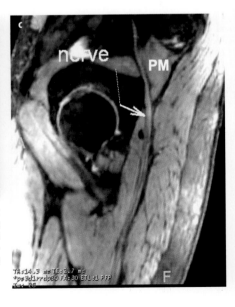

**Fig. 2 a-c.** Normal sciatic nerve. Axial T1 magnetic resonance images, just below the lesser trochanter (**a**) and at the proximal thigh (**b**), demonstrate the sciatic nerve (*arrow*) descending in the thigh between the adductor magnus (*AM*), gluteus maximus (*green*) and biceps femoris long head (*blue*) muscles. **c** Sagittal maximal intensity projection three-dimensional PSIF (pre-excitation refocused steady-state sequence) image depicts the sciatic nerve (*arrow*) exiting the pelvis at the level of the greater sciatic notch beneath the piriformis muscle (*PM*)

# Nontraumatic Musculoskeletal Abnormalities in Pediatrics

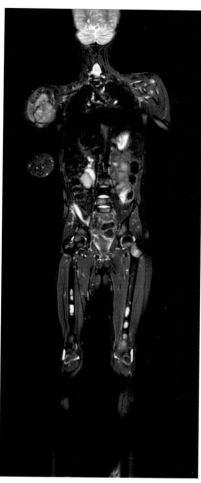

**Fig. 2.** Whole body magnetic resonance imaging of a 13-year-old girl with Ewing sarcoma of the right humerus. Fusion images of short TI inversion recovery (STIR) and diffusion weighted sequences reveal numerous bone metastases

# CT Specifies Bone Lesions in SPECT/CT

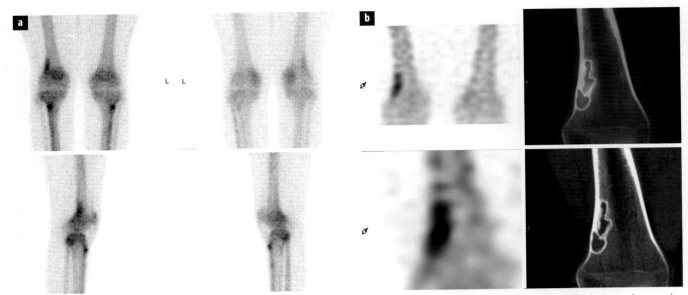

**Fig. 1 a, b.** Young patient with knee pain. **a** In addition to bilateral uptake at the tibial tuberosity, the planar scintigraphy images show an intermediate uptake at the lateral right distal femur diaphysis/epiphysis. **b** In single photon emission computed tomography (SPECT)/CT, the uptake corresponds to a lesion with the typical CT appearance of a nonossifying fibroma

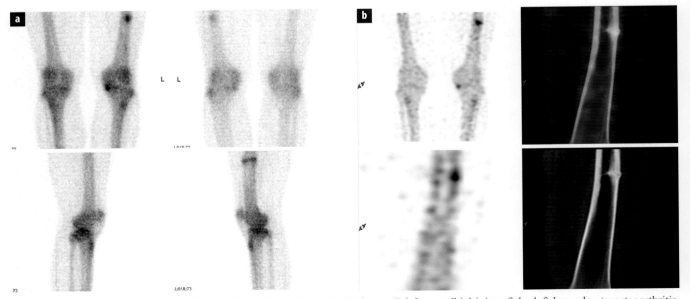

**Fig. 2 a, b.** Patient with knee pain. **a** Planar scintigraphy with uptake in the medial femorotibial joint of the left knee due to osteoarthritis, and linear uptake in the left femur diaphysis. **b** Single photon emission computed tomography (SPECT)/CT demonstrates the presence of a stress fracture

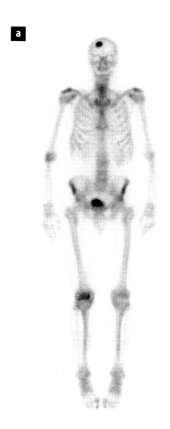

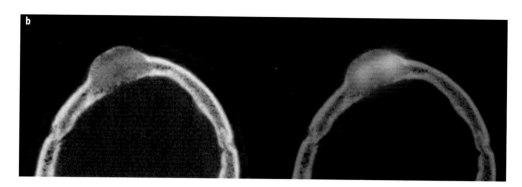

**Fig. 3 a, b. a** Prostate cancer staging with focal uptake in the frontal skull in planar scintigraphy. **b** Single photon emission computed tomography (SPECT)/CT shows an expansive lesion with the typical appearance of a hemangioma

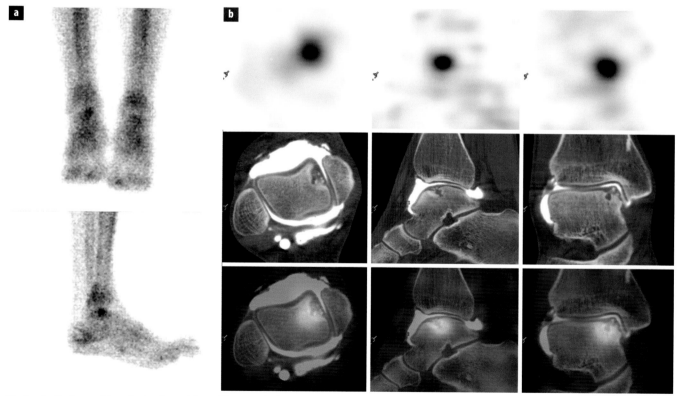

**Fig. 4 a, b.** Patient with pain in the ankle. **a** Planar scintigraphy shows focal uptake in the talus. **b** Single photon emission computed tomography (SPECT)/CT arthrography shows an osteochondral lesion in the medial talus edge with small subchondral fragments but intact cartilage surface

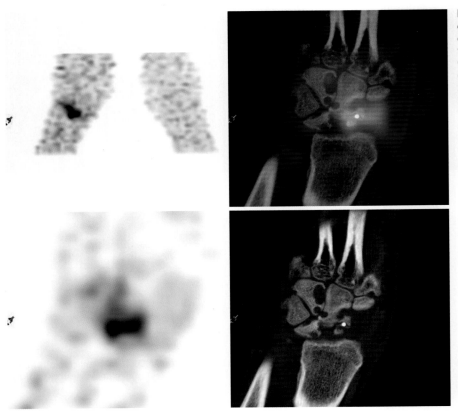

**Fig. 5.** Tc99m antigranulocyte single photon emission computed tomography (SPECT)/CT of the wrist in a patient several weeks after wrist surgery and postoperative infection. CT shows severe destruction of several carpal bones and SPECT/CT helps to localize exactly the pathologic uptake resulting from persistent infection

## FDG PET-CT Staging and Follow-up in Soft Tissue Sarcomas

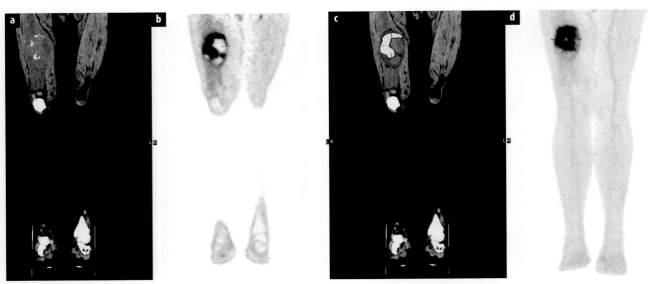

**Fig. 1 a-d.** Newly diagnosed malignant fibrous histiocytoma. From left to right, **a** computed tomography (CT), **b** positron emission tomography (PET), **c** fused PET-CT and **d** maximum intensity projection PET show the heterogeneous appearance of the mass with large areas of necrosis. These data can guide the biopsy site to areas showing increased $^{18}$F-fluorodeoxyglucose uptake

# Imaging of Metastatic Bone and Soft Tissue Lesions in Prostate Cancer with FCH PET/CT

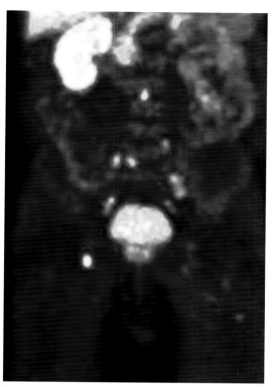

**Fig. 1.** Preoperative staging. Multiple retroperitoneal lymph node metastases in a 66-year-old patient with prostate-specific antigen 88.4 ng/mL, Gleason score 8

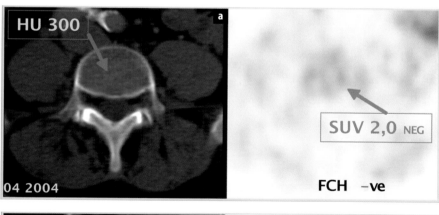

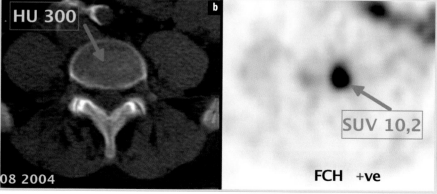

**Fig. 2 a, b.** Preoperative staging. Bone marrow metastasis in L4 in a 73year-old patient with prostate-specific antigen 8.7 ng/ml, Gleason score 8. [$^{18}$F]fluorocholine (*FCH*) PET/CT negative [standardized uptake value (*SUV*) 2.0] **a**, and positive after 4 months (SUV 10.2), **b**. *HU* Hounsfield units

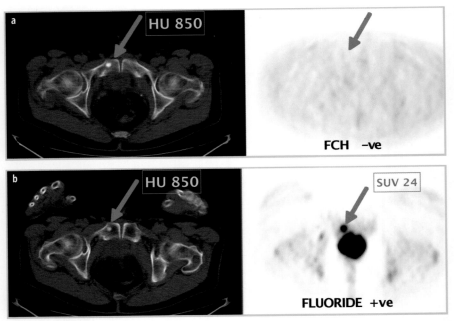

**Fig. 3 a. b.** Follow-up (prostate-specific antigen 20.5 ng/ml) 1 month after withdrawal of hormone therapy. Bone metastasis in the right os pubis [CT: sclerosis, Hounsfield units (*HU*) 850]. [$^{18}$F]fluorocholine PET/CT negative (*FCH -ve*) (**a**) and [$^{18}$F]fluoride PET/CT positive (*FLUORIDE +ve*) (**b**) [standardized uptake value (*SUV*) 24]

# PET Imaging of Bone Metastases with FDG, Fluoride and Gallium-Somatostatin Analogs

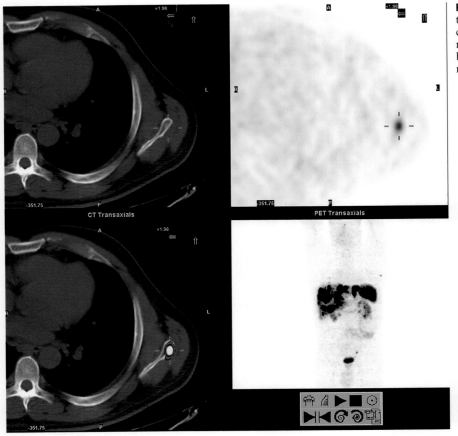

**Fig. 1.** $^{68}$Ga- DOTANOC (DOTA-Tyr3-octreotide) positron emission tomography-computed tomography in metastatic carcinoid. Metastatic disease in the liver and bone. There is an example of an early small metastasis in the left scapule

# Single Photon Imaging, Including SPECT/CT, in Patients with Prostheses

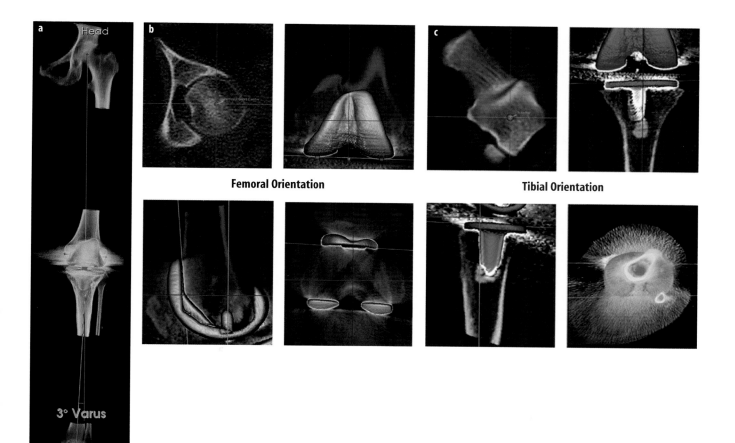

**Fig. 1 a-c.** Three-dimensional evaluation of prosthesis components with reconstruction of the mechanical axis femoral and tibial resulting in a 3 degree varus (**a**). Easy measurement of femoral varus/valgus, femoral flexion/extension and femoral rotation (**b**). The tibial component slope and the tibial rotation are defined (**c**)

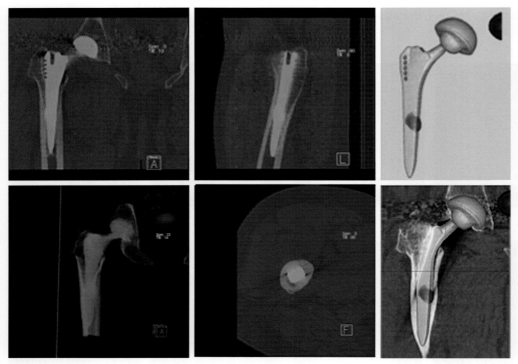

**Fig. 2.** A 54-year-old man with hip replacement on the right side 6/2008. Four years after surgery, pain is experienced under stress. SPECT-CT shows intact prosthesis components. Only slight uptake in the midshaft. Minimal varus of the shaft. Diagnosis: no loosening, slight uptake in the fixation zone and stress reaction caused by a minimal varus. The surgeon did not believe the diagnosis and the patient underwent revision. No loosening was found intraoperatively

## SPECT, CT and MR: Integration in Degenerative Musculoskeletal Diseases

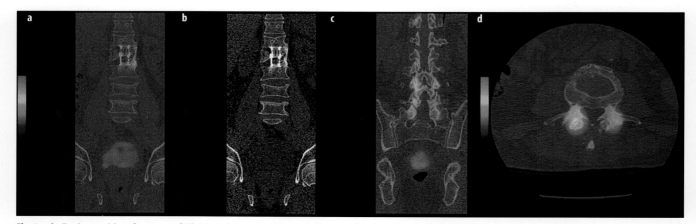

**Fig. 1 a-d.** Patient with a fracture of Th12 and consecutive cage interposition. **a** Coronal single photon emission computed tomography/computed tomography (SPECT/CT), **b** coronal CT. There is slight activity at the left lateral osseous bridge between Th12 and L1 indicating noncomplete bridging. **c** Coronal SPECT/CT, **d** axial SPECT/CT. There is additional uptake in the right facet joint of L2/3, indicating infrafusional activated arthrosis. SPECT/CT shows a higher degree of activation compared with CT, where there is no major difference morphologically concerning the degree of arthrosis

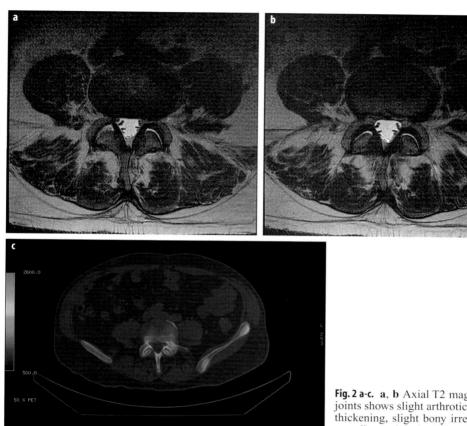

**Fig. 2 a-c. a, b** Axial T2 magnetic resonance imaging of the L4/5 facet joints shows slight arthrotic changes in both facet joints, with synovial thickening, slight bony irregularities and minimal fluid. **c** The corresponding axial single photon emission computed tomography/computed tomography (SPECT/CT) shows no activation

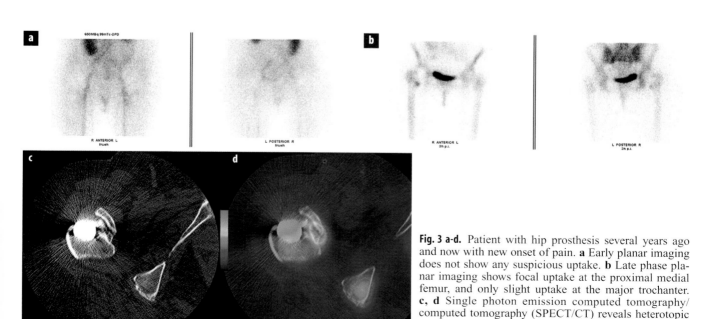

**Fig. 3 a-d.** Patient with hip prosthesis several years ago and now with new onset of pain. **a** Early planar imaging does not show any suspicious uptake. **b** Late phase planar imaging shows focal uptake at the proximal medial femur, and only slight uptake at the major trochanter. **c, d** Single photon emission computed tomography/computed tomography (SPECT/CT) reveals heterotopic ossification with neoarticulation at the trochanter minor; this represents the cause of the pain

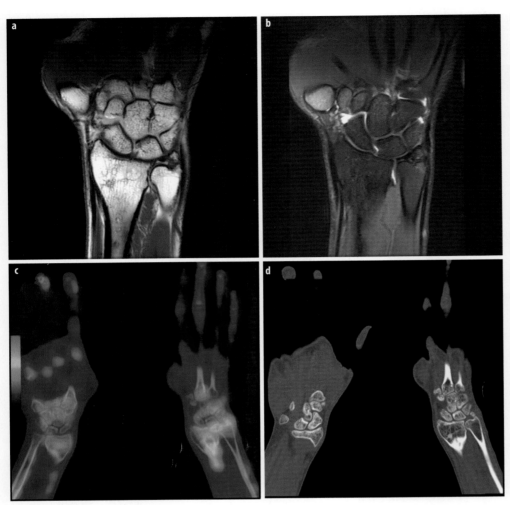

**Fig. 4 a-d.** Patient with status post-fracture of the left forearm. Osteosynthesis material has already been removed; however, the patient continues to have pain at the proximal wrist. Magnetic resonance imaging shows the consolidated forearm fracture that ends in the distal radioulnar joint (DRUJ). Additionally, there are bony irregularities in the DRUJ and the cartilage is thinned (**a** coronal T, **b** coronal proton density fat-saturated). Single photon emission computed tomography/computed tomography (SPECT/CT) shows that there is still elevated uptake in the distal forearm, representing ongoing bone remodeling. Additionally, there is uptake in the DRUJ, an indication that there is arthrosis starting to occur here also (**c** coronal SPECT/CT, **d** coronal CT)

# Imaging of Juvenile Idiopathic Arthritis

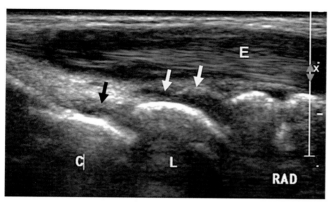

**Fig. 7.** Sagittal ultrasound view (standard view) of the dorsal wrist in a 6-year-old girl with juvenile idiopathic arthritis shows synovial hypertrophy and small effusions in the radiocarpal (*white arrows*) and midcarpal joints (*black arrow*). *C* capitate, *E* inflamed extensor tendons, *L* lunate, *RAD* distal radius

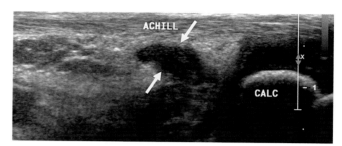

**Fig. 9.** Sagittal ultrasound view of the posterior ankle in a 9-year-old boy with enthesitis-related arthritis shows a swollen prepatellar bursa (*arrows*). *ACHILL* Achilles tendon, *CALC* calcaneus

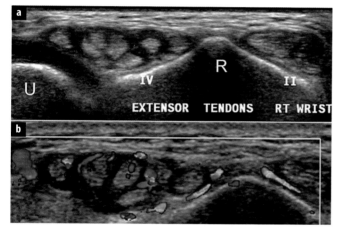

**Fig. 8 a, b.** Axial ultrasound view (standard view) of the dorsal right wrist in a 7-year-old girl with juvenile idiopathic arthritis shows tenosynovitis of the extensors (compartments 2-4) (**a**) and verified by hyperemia on color Doppler (**b**). *R* distal radius, tubercle of Lister; *U* distal ulna

## Vascular Malformations of the Musculoskeletal System

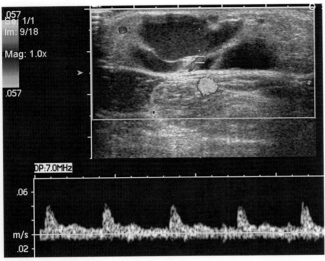

**Fig. 5.** Classical appearance of a lymphatic malformation, which appears as an anechoic multiloculated lesion with slow arterial flow in the septa

## Advanced Breast Ultrasound and Interventions: An Update

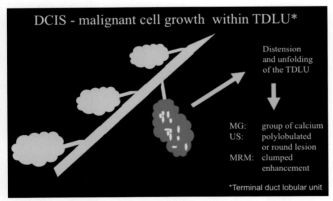

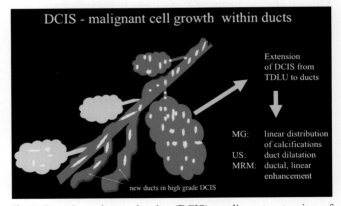

**Fig. 1.** Ductal carcinoma in situ (DCIS): malignant cell growth resulting in a distension of the terminal-duct lobular unit (TDLU). Various other benign proliferative or fibrocystic changes develop along a distinct genetic and morphological pathway and can also result in a distension of the TDLU. Associated calcifications within the TDLU develop in DCIS, fibrocystic changes, sclerosing adenosis, and other forms of adenosis. Expanded TDLUs can be depicted by mammography, ultrasound, or magnetic resonance mammography. Corresponding diagnostic criteria are listed in the text

**Fig. 2.** Ductal carcinoma in situ (DCIS): malignant extension of DCIS into the ducts and other terminal-duct lobular units (TD-LUs). New ducts can be formed in high-grade DCIS. Corresponding diagnostic criteria are given and focus on the linear extension or dilatation of ducts in all imaging modalities

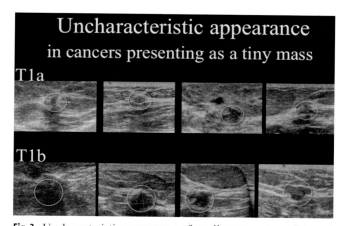

**Fig. 3.** Uncharacteristic appearance of small cancers stages T1a and T1b. All these cancers have been detected by screening mammogram and correlated to ultrasound secondarily during assessment (courtesy of Screening Centre Southwest Lower Saxony; Praxis Drewes and Partners). Several small benign lesions resemble the presentation of small cancers

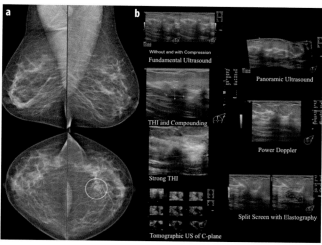

**Fig. 7 a, b.** A 47-year-old woman with mammographic mass (**a**) at 12 o'clock and corresponding ultrasound (US) (**b**) lesion presenting as an irregular hypoechoic mass, with strong shadowing, poor vascularity, and stiffness (*blue* low strain in the strain elastography image). Histology was ductal invasive cancer with low proliferation fraction. *THI,* tissue harmonic imaging

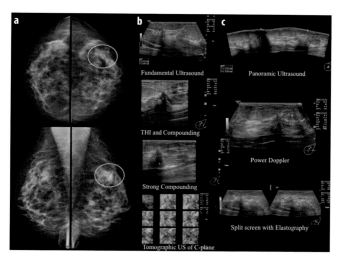

**Fig. 6 a-c.** A 48-year-old patient presenting with an architectural distortion in mammography (**a**). Corresponding mass could be missed using fundamental ultrasound (US) only. Advanced US modes (**b, c**) clearly show a mass with spiculations, retraction pattern in 3D US, associated flow, and moderate stiffness. Histology was ductal invasive cancer (*G1*). *THI,* tissue harmonic imaging

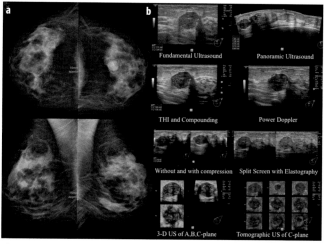

**Fig. 8 a, b.** A 51-year-old woman presenting with a recurrent mass following incomplete resection of a fibroadenoma using vacuum-assisted biopsy (VAB) 2 years earlier. Mammography shows a circumscribed round mass (**a**). Ultrasound (**b**) presents a correlative oval mass, adjacent scar with strong shadowing due to former VAB, and a second lesion. Both lesions show low vascularity and intermediate elasticity. Histology of both lesions showed fibroadenomas abundant with cells and regressive changes. *THI,* tissue harmonic imaging

# Microcalcifications of the Breast: An Approach to Radiologic Classification

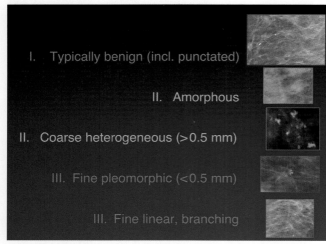

**Fig. 1.** Microcalcifications: from benign to malignant morphology. *Green frame*: microcalcifications with typically benign morphology (I); *orange frame*: microcalcifications with indeterminant morphology (II); *red frame*: microcalcifications with typically malignant morphology (III)

**Fig. 3.** The Microcalcification matrix serves as a guide for classifying grouped microcalcifications according to morphology and distribution, additionally considering modification aspects (modificators) [13, 14]

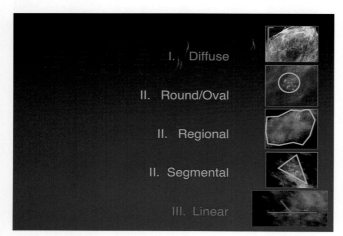

**Fig. 2.** Microcalcifications: from benign to malignant distribution. *Green frame*: microcalcifications with benign distribution (I); *orange frame*: microcalcifications with indeterminant distribution (II); *red frame*: microcalcifications with typically malignant distribution (III)

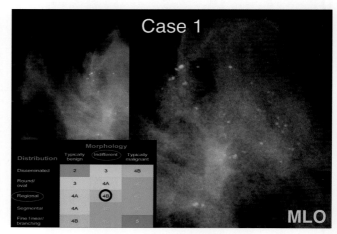

**Fig. 4.** Case 1: Indifferent type of microcalcifications with regional distribution (BI-RADS, 4B). Histology: fibrocystic changes, sclerosing adenosis, usual ductal hyperplasia. *MLO*, mediolateral oblique view

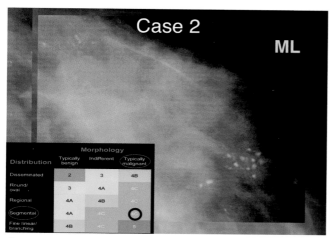

**Fig. 5.** Case 2: Typically malignant type of microcalcifications with segmental distribution (BI-RADS, 4C). Histology: invasive ductal cancer. *ML*, mediolateral view

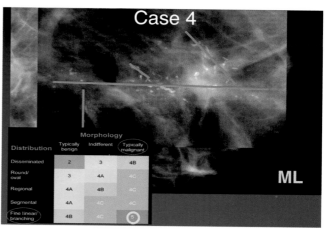

**Fig. 7.** Case 4: Typically malignant type of microcalcifications with linear and branching distribution (BI-RADS, 5). Histology: ductal carcinoma in situ (high grade). *ML*, mediolateral view

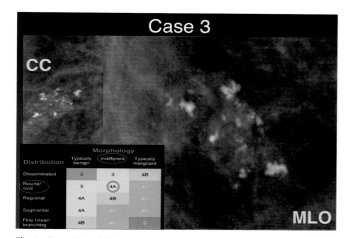

**Fig. 6.** Case 3: Indifferent (including coarse heterogeneous) type of microcalcifications with round/oval distribution (BI-RADS, 4A). Histology: fibroadenoma, fibrocystic changes. *CC*, craniocaudal view; *MLO*, mediolateral oblique view